Diseases of the Brain, Head & Neck, Spine

Diagnostic Imaging and Interventional Techniques

AF671754

J. Hodler • G.K. von Schulthess • Ch.L. Zollikofer (Eds)

DISEASES OF THE BRAIN, HEAD & NECK, SPINE

DIAGNOSTIC IMAGING AND INTERVENTIONAL TECHNIQUES

40th International Diagnostic Course in Davos (IDKD)
Davos, March 30-April 4, 2008

including the
Nuclear Medicine Satellite Course "Diamond"
Davos, March 28-30, 2008

Pediatric Satellite Course "Kangaroo"
Davos, March 29-30, 2008

presented by the Foundation for the
Advancement of Education in Medical Radiology, Zurich

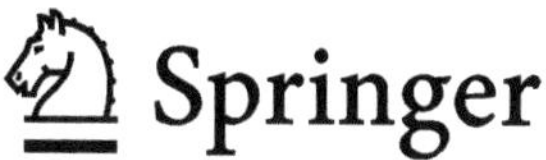

J. HODLER
Radiology, Orthopedic University
Hospital Balgrist,
Zurich, Switzerland

G. K. VON SCHULTHESS
Nuclear Medicine,
University Hospital,
Zurich, Switzerland

CH. L. ZOLLIKOFER
Kilchberg/Zurich, Switzerland

Library of Congress Control Number: 2008922062

Springer is a part of Springer Science+Business Media

springer.com

© Springer-Verlag Italia 2008

ISBN: 978-88-470-0839-7 Springer Milan Berlin Heidelberg New York
e-ISBN: 978-88-470-0840-3

This work is subject to copyright. All rights are reserved, whether the whole or part of the material is concerned, specifically the rights of translation, reprinting, re-use of illustrations, recitation, broadcasting, reproduction on microfilms or in other ways, and storage in data banks. Duplication of this publication or parts thereof is only permitted under the provisions of the Italian Copyright Law in its current version, and permission for use must always be obtained from Springer. Violations are liable for prosecution under the Italian Copyright Law.

The use of general descriptive names, registered names, trademarks, etc., in this publication does not imply, even in the absence of a specific statement, that such names are exempt from the relevant protective laws and regulations and therefore free for general use.

Product liability: The publisher cannot guarantee the accuracy of any information about dosage and application contained in this book. In every individual case the user must check such information by consulting the relevant literature.

Cover design: Simona Colombo, Milan, Italy
Typesetting: C & G di Cerri e Galassi, Cremona, Italy
Printing and binding: Grafiche Porpora, Segrate (MI), Italy

Printed in Italy

Springer-Verlag Italia S.r.l., Via Decembrio 28, 20137 Milan

Preface

The International Diagnostic Course in Davos (IDKD) offers a unique learning experience for imaging specialists in training as well as for experienced radiologists and clinicians wishing to be updated on the current state of the art and the latest developments in the fields of imaging and image-guided interventions.

This annual course deals with neuroimaging of the brain, head, neck, and spine. During the last few years, there have been considerable advances in this subject, driven by clinical as well as technological developments. The authors, internationally renowned experts in their field, have contributed chapters that are disease-oriented and cover all relevant imaging modalities, including magnetic resonance imaging, computed tomography, and positron emission tomography, as well as image-guided interventions. As a result, this book offers a comprehensive review of the state-of-the art in neuroimaging. It is particularly relevant for general radiologists, radiology residents, neurologists, neurosurgeons, and other clinicians wishing to update their knowledge in this discipline.

The Syllabus is designed to be an "*aide-mémoire*" for the course participants so that they can fully concentrate on the lectures and participate in the discussions without the need of taking notes.

Additional information can be found on the IDKD website: www.idkd.org

J. Hodler
G.K. von Schulthess
Ch.L. Zollikofer

Table of Contents

Workshops

Nuclear Medicine Satellite Course "Diamond"

Pediatric Satellite Course "Kangaroo"

List of Contributors

Abu Eid M., 141
Bagley L.J., 83
Ball W.S., 259
Baud C., 272
Becker M., 159
Bonneville J.-F., 123
Borghesi A., 176
Brant-Zawadzki M., 112
Bronen R.A., 83
Brouwer P.A., 74
Buck A., 213
Byrne J., 33
Casselman J.W., 134
Castillo M., 49
Couture A., 272
Curtin H.D., 167
Essig M., 58
Farina D., 176
Fiehler J., 27
Flanders A.E., 191
Gassner I., 265
Goffin K., 219
Herholz K., 215
Hesselink J.R., 77
Jensen M.E., 12
Knopp E.A., 3
Koeller K.K., 38
Kucharczyk W., 123
Kuwert T., 240
Loevner L.A., 172
Lövblad K.-O., 226
Manelfe C., 195
Maroldi R., 176
Meier C.A., 243
Mikulis D., 92
Modic M.T., 186
Montanera W., 3
Parizel P.M., 65
Phillips C.D., 65
Pramanik B.K., 130
Ramos Taboada L., 141
Ravanelli M., 176
Riehm S., 141
Ross J.S., 200
Saguintaah M., 272
Sarrazin J.-L., 195
Schuknecht B., 149
Smoker W., 149
Strobel K., 251
Sundgren P.C., 191
Symons S., 186
Tatsch K., 234
Thurnher M.M., 27
van Buchem M.A., 45
Van Laere K., 219
Van Paesschen W., 219
Veillon F., 141
Veyrac C., 272
Wetzel S., 92
Wiesmann M., 36
Willinsky R., 21
Wilms G., 103
Young Poussaint T., 114, 277
Yousem D.M., 130

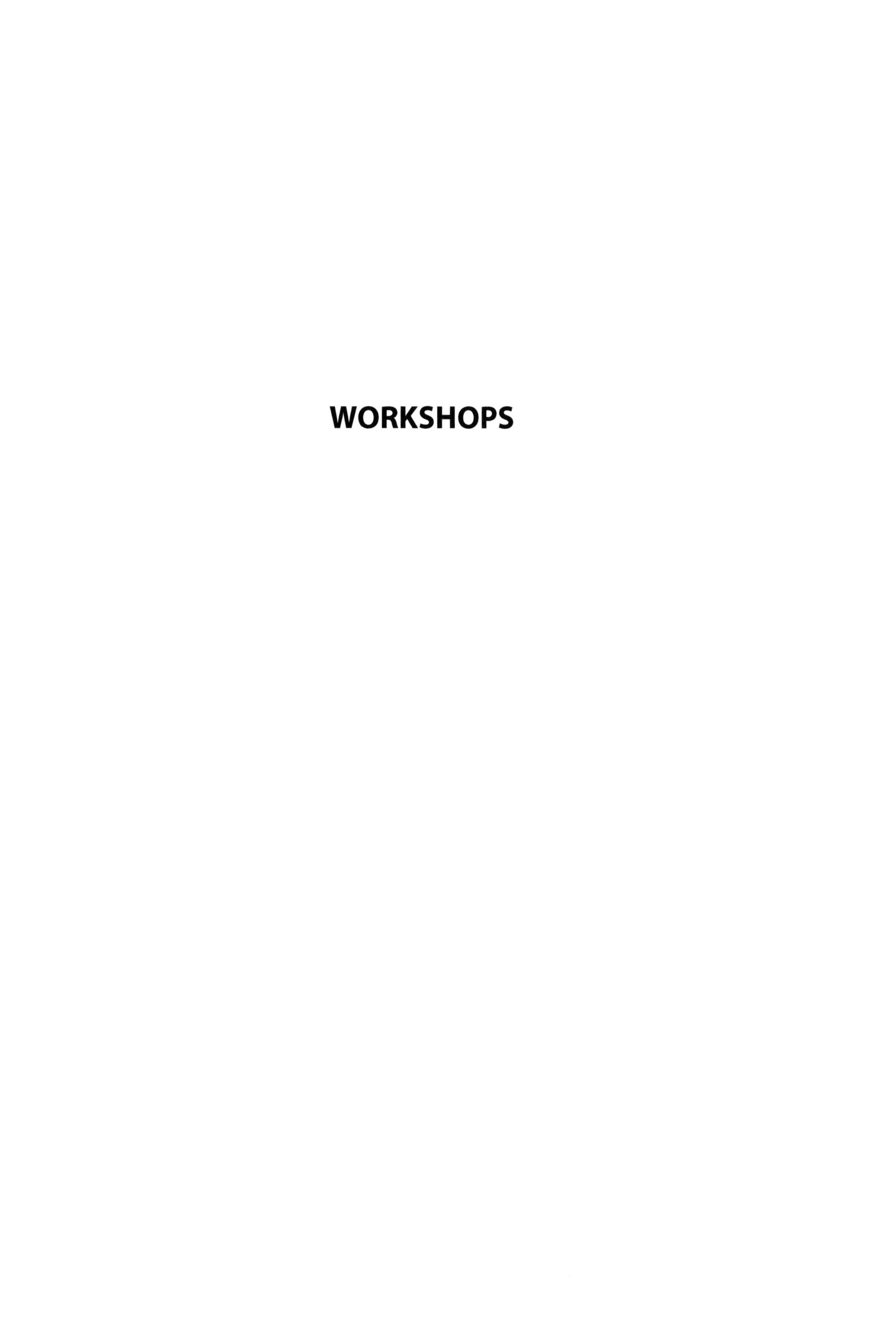

WORKSHOPS

Brain Tumors

Edmond A. Knopp[1], Walter Montanera[2]

[1] Magnetic Resonance Imaging Department, New York University School of Medicine, New York, NY, USA
[2] Department of Medical Imaging, St. Michael's Hospital, University of Toronto, Toronto, ON, Canada

Introduction

The designation "brain tumor" is commonly applied to a wide variety of intracranial mass lesions, each distinct in their location, biology, treatment, and prognosis. Since many of these lesions do not arise from brain parenchyma, the more appropriate term would be "intracranial tumors". Since the category encompasses both neoplasms and non-neoplastic mass lesions, the word "tumor" is used in its broadest sense, indicating a space-occupying mass.

Epidemiological data suggest that the annual incidence of intracranial tumors is 11-19 per 100,000 persons. Metastases to the brain from a systemic primary cancer outside the central nervous system are even more common. Intracranial tumors can cause focal or generalized neurological symptoms. Headache, nausea, vomiting, and, occasionally, cranial nerve palsy (6th nerve) may result from increased intracranial pressure. Focal symptoms and signs (e.g., paresis, visual deficit, and aphasia) usually reflect the intracranial location of the tumor and the affected area of the brain. The frequency and duration of symptoms and signs will also vary with the type of tumor. Rapidly growing tumors may cause symptoms earlier, with less overall tumor bulk than a more slowly growing tumor.

Headache occurs in about half of patients with brain tumors and is typically worse in the morning and improves after erect posture. Seizures are common (15-95%) and may be focal or generalized. Focal symptoms such as hemiparesis or dysphasia are usually subacute in onset and progressive.

The only unequivocal risk factor for intracranial tumors is past cranial radiation and has been linked to both glial and meningeal neoplasms. Primary central nervous system lymphoma has tripled in incidence over the past two decades, largely due to the increased incidence in patients with acquired immunodeficiency syndrome. However, the incidence of lymphoma is also rising in the immunocompetent population although no known environmental or behavioral factor has been identified.

Imaging Features of Intracranial Tumors

The prognosis and treatment of intracranial tumors are highly dependent on tumor histology. Predicting histology from pre-operative imaging procedures depends largely on establishing the correct location of the origin of the mass. Specifically, the radiologist must first establish whether the mass arises from within the brain parenchyma (intra-axial), or outside the brain parenchyma (extra-axial), whereby symptoms are usually due to brain compression. Radiologically identifiable anatomical clues that a tumor is extra-axial in location include the following:

a. Widening of ipsilateral subarachnoid space
b. CSF cleft between mass and brain parenchyma
c. Deviation of pial vessels between mass and brain tissue
d. Buckling of white matter
e. Bony changes (e.g., hyperostosis in meningioma)

Once established as intra-axial or extra-axial, the specific location of the mass becomes equally important in imaging analysis since certain histological types of intracranial tumor tend to occur with higher frequency in specific locations. Thus, accurate compartmentalization of the mass will limit the differential diagnosis to a relevant few types of tumors (Table 1) and help direct further imaging evaluation and treatment.

Beyond the location of the mass, it is important to note other imaging features in the magnetic resonance (MR) and computed tomography (CT) analysis of intracranial tumors in order to further increase the likelihood of arriving at an accurate diagnosis and to accurately evaluate the effect of the mass on the adjacent brain tissue. Histological features such as calcium or fat can be easily seen on cross-sectional imaging. The density of the mass on CT or the signal intensity on T2-weighted MR imaging can offer a clue to cell composition and relative water content (e.g., nucleus:cytoplasm ratio). Compressive effects on adjacent brain tissue, extent of vasogenic edema accompanying the mass, and complicating hydrocephalus are easily and non-invasively assessed. Certain tumors have a higher likelihood of presenting with hemorrhage, which can be readily diagnosed on CT or MR. Furthermore, these conventional imaging tools can be used to predict the vascularity

Table 1. Regional classification of common intracranial tumors

Intraventricular	Ependymoma Subependymoma Choroid plexus papilloma Central neurocytoma Colloid cyst Giant cell astrocytoma
Pineal region	Pineocytoma Germ cell tumor Pnet Tectal glioma Meningioma Dermoid Arachnoid cyst
Sella/suprasellar	Pituitary adenoma Craniopharyngioma Meningioma Rathke's cyst Chiasmatic glioma Dermoid/epidermoid Germ cell tumor
Cavernous sinus	Meningioma Schwannoma Pituitary adenoma Metastasis
Cerebellopontine angle	Schwannoma Meningioma Epidermoid Arachnoid cyst Paraganglioma Metastases
Skull base	Chordoma Chondrosarcoma Paraganglioma Metastasis/myeloma Sino-nasal carcinoma Esthesioneuroblasoma Lymphoma/ leukemia
Foramen magnum	Meningioma Schwannoma Brainstem glioma Ependymoma

of intracranial tumors that do not present with hemorrhage. Intravenous contrast agents add further to the conventional imaging analysis of intracranial tumors by increasing conspicuity and demonstrating enhancement characteristics that help increase specificity.

Advanced Imaging Techniques in Intracranial Tumors

With the advent of faster imaging techniques, MR imaging can now depict various aspects of brain function in addition to brain anatomy.

Brain Diffusion

Diffusion imaging uses echo planar sequences. What is being imaged is the macromolecular motion of water within the extracellular space. In the normal brain, this space is defined by the boundaries of axonal pathways. The axon bundles will restrict the patterns of motion of water. This restriction occurs in a variety of directions in normal brain. In abnormal brain, these patterns are perturbed. Diffusion imaging relies on these perturbations. The most significant limitation is due to motion. Since motion is being imaged, the sequences have to be inherently motion-sensitive. Echo planar methods limit the amount of extrinsic motion but they do not completely eliminate it.

The principle application for diffusion imaging is in the identification of hyperacute infarct. This determination can be made well in advance of T2 changes (minutes rather than hours). With infarct as the example, the principles used are as follows.

At the onset of ischemia, there is breakdown of cell-membrane Na-K ATPase pumps. This results in an influx of Na into the cell. Water then follows, resulting in cell swelling. All of this occurs within minutes of cessation of blood flow. At this time the cells are still viable; however, the extracellular space is compressed secondary to the swollen cells. The water in this compressed extracellular space is restricted in its ability to move. It is this restriction that the diffusion sequence detects. One can therefore see how diffusion imaging can detect hyperacute infarct.

The major problem with the interpretation of these images lies in the anisotropic patterns of motion; therefore imaging has to be done in three orthogonal planes in order to achieve anisotropy. Once this is achieved, the method is inherently reproducible and easy to interpret.

A second application of diffusion techniques is in the differentiation of edema (vasogenic) from gliotic change. This has implications in tumor imaging and subsequent follow-up. Infiltrative brain parenchyma, while having a diffusion abnormality, will not give as significant a signal change on a diffusion-weighted (DW) imaging as vasogenic edema. If more advanced diffusion techniques are used, such as diffusion tensor imaging and tractography, more subtle infiltrative changes are visible based upon the distortions in normal brain anisotropy. As glial neoplasms infiltrate along axonal pathways they will cause an inherent change in the fractional anisotropy along with the visible changes seen on tractography. In addition, tractography (alone and in conjunction with functional MR imaging) is becoming extremely valuable in the presurgical work-up and in planning for tumor resection. This visualization of white matter pathways and their relationship to the neoplasm allows neurosurgeons to better plan and discuss surgical options with their patients.

Diffusion techniques readily enable solid lesions to be differentiated from true cystic lesions. This in certain instances can aid in preoperative surgical planning.

Brain Perfusion

Perfusion imaging of the brain is a means to define the cerebral (capillary) blood volume by imaging following the administration of a bolus of contrast. This is different from conventional spin echo (SE) post-contrast imaging. In SE imaging, one is looking at the breakdown of the blood-brain barrier (in a similar fashion to CT). Perfusion imaging is carried out during the first pass of contrast through the capillary bed and is finished before a significant amount of contrast crosses a disturbed blood-brain barrier.

The echo planar sequences routinely employed rely on the susceptibility changes in the image due to the presence of gadolinium. These changes are manifest as a drop in signal intensity proportional to the "volume" of capillaries present. This method can be used in two major areas of imaging.

The first is tumor imaging. In this instance, perfusion "maps" enable one to determine the volume of the capillaries in the lesion in question as well as "normal" brain. This is useful in the differentiation of areas of higher grade within neoplasms and has implications in choosing the sites for biopsy. Tumor boundaries might also be better characterized. Perfusion methods also allow one to differentiate therapeutic necrosis (secondary to radiation as well as high-dose chemotherapy). In these instances, the contrast-enhancing mass, while not having an intact blood-brain barrier, does not have any increase in capillary volume; in fact this is significantly reduced (if not absent). This manifests itself perfusion techniques as a "cold" region.

The second (and more widely used) application is in the determination of hyperacute infarct. This is mentioned here only for the sake of completeness. With infarct, there is diminution of blood flow and an overall decrease in the affected capillary blood volume. These changes will occur prior to any significant T2 abnormality. In this regard, the perfusion map will show the infarct as a "cold spot".

There are however, limitations in perfusion scanning. The primary limitation reflects the need to administer gadolinium. In order to achieve a high intravascular level of gadolinium in a short finite period of time, the contrast must be administered in a rapid bolus and in flush fashion. Standard rates of administration are on the order of 5 ml/s. This rate is difficult to standardize with a hand injection. The use of a power injector simplifies this but adds significantly to the cost. A large-bore IV is needed (20 g). The second major limitation has to due with the necessity to post-process the data. Perfusion maps based upon statistical significance need to be calculated.

Previous work suggests that within a given tumor various grades of malignancy can co-exist. It has also been shown that tumor grade is related to the integrity of the blood-brain barrier and to the density and character of the tumor neovascularity . Although the integrity of the blood-brain barrier has been studied with CT and MR imaging, this characteristic alone has not been sufficient to predict tumor grade. With the advent of MR imaging methods that measure relative cerebral blood flow (perfusion), it should be possible to explore the degree of neovascularity. Aronen et al. used MR perfusion techniques to obtain a cerebral blood volume map of gliomas and demonstrated that there is a correlation between the degree of perfusion (maximal cerebral blood volume) and tumor mitotic activity and vascularity. In their studies, however, one sample was randomly obtained from each tumor either via biopsy or resection and it was not possible to directly correlate tumor pathology with radiographic features. In contrast, our methodology of stereotactic serial biopsy assures precise sampling of the lesion and allows for targeting based upon imaging features.

Clinical MR Spectroscopy

Clinical Perspective

Proton spectroscopy (MRS) extends the diagnostic utility of the MR brain examination beyond the typical structural images of anatomy and provides another functional dimension based on biochemical information. In a noninvasive manner, MRS yields valuable functional information that adds diagnostic value to the traditional MRI exam.

The functional nature of the spectroscopy examination augments other functional MR techniques such as diffusion, perfusion and BOLD MR imaging studies. Together, these new diagnostic techniques are expanding the role of diagnostic MR in the brain.

Technical Perspective

- Single-voxel spectroscopy (1D) interrogation of brain metabolites in a single location selected by the operator. Typical times are 2-8 min depending on voxel dimensions.
- Chemical-shift imaging spectroscopy (2D-multivoxel) extends the spectroscopic technique to multi-voxel arrays covering a large volume of interest in a single measurement. This technique permits the localization of chemical changes relating to various disease states. An important note is that the spectral data can be examined as single spectra, spectral maps, or as metabolite images. Typical times are 6-12 min.
- 3D CSI (true 3D or multislice 2D) is similar to CSI but with volumetric coverage.

SVS Pulse Sequences

STEAM (Stimulated Echo Acquisition Mode)

- 90°-90"-90"-echo
- "Gradient echo" with low signal-to-noise ratio (SNR)

Advantages:
- Short TE allows detection of metabolites with short T2 relaxation times (glutamate/glutamine, myo-Inositol, lipids)
- More effective water suppression

Disadvantages:
- Lower SNR
- Extremely sensitive to motion

PRESS (Point Resolved Spectroscopy)

- 90°-180°-180°-echo
- "Spin echo" with high SNR

Advantages
- Higher SNR

Disadvantages
- Long TE (135)
- Longer acquisition times
- May "miss" metabolites with short TE

Common Biochemicals Detected by Proton Magnetic Resonance Spectroscopy in Brain

N-acetylaspartate (NAA): -CH3 moiety of N-acetylaspartate: marker for active neuronal tissue.

Lactate (Lac): -CH3 moiety of lactate: marker for low tissue oxygen and anaerobic glycolysis.

Creatine (Cr): -CH2 and -CH3 moieties of creatine and creatine phosphate, important bioenergetics compounds in all living cells.

Choline (Cho): -N (CH3)3 moiety of all choline compounds, including choline, acetylcholine, phosphatidyl choline and others; important cell-membrane components.

Lipid: -CH2 and -CH3 moieties of adipose tissue storage fats (triglycerides). The fatty acyl groups in phospholipid membrane bilayer appear as broad components in the baseline.

Myo-Inositol (MI): -CH moieties of Inositol isomers.

Glutamine (Glu) and glutamate (Gln): -CH2 moieties of glutamate, glutamine.

Glucose (Glc): -CH moieties of glucose.

N-acetylaspartate (NAA)

- Marker for neuronal viability and density
- Manufactured in neurons and transported along axons.
- Highest metabolic peak
- Frequency shift of 2.0 ppm
- Increased in Canavan's disease
- Decreased in physiologic (low at birth) and aging, neoplasia, hypoxia, ischemia, infarct, epilepsy, infection/inflammation, neurodegenerative processes.

Creatine (Cr)

- Generally used as an internal standard/reference.
- Signal amplitude remains constant in most situations
- Creatine-creatine kinase-phosphocreatine is central to ADP/ATP energy pathway.
- Second highest peak, assigned 3.03 ppm
- Increased in the setting of trauma and aging
- Decreased with metastases

Choline (Cho)

- Involved in synthesis of phospholipids and membrane compounds
- Indicator of cellular turnover
- Third highest peak, assigned 3.2 ppm
- Increased in a wide variety of conditions: physiologic, recovery from insult, gliosis, neoplasia, demyelination and inflammation/infection
- Decreased in dementia, stroke and asymptomatic liver disease

Glutamine and Glutamate

- Astrocyte markers. Glutamate is an excitatory neurotransmitter, but in excess concentration is neurotoxic
- Disruption of Gln/Glu regulation has been implicated in the initiation of a cascade leading to neuronal damage/death
- Both increased in ischemia, recovery from ischemia, and liver disease
- Decreased primarily in Alzheimer disease

Lactate (Lac)

- Seen in processes involving cellular necrosis; normally not found in the brain
- Observed in pathologic processes characterized by increased anaerobic metabolism
- Doublet configuration, assigned 1.32 ppm

Lipids

- Elevated in pathologic processes such as infection, inflammation, tumor necrosis, and stroke
- Lipids within brain are associated with myelin, sphyngomyelins, phospholipids, and lecithins
- Extracerebral lipids can contaminate volume of interest!

Myo-Inositol

- Almost exclusively found in astrocytes; major role is as an osmolyte
- Chemically resembles glucose and has a variable amplitude, assigned 3.56 ppm
- increased in Alzheimer disease, neonates vs. adults, hyperosmolar state
- Decreased in hepatic encephalopathy and hyponatremia

Basic Patterns in MRS

CSF

- Cerebral metabolites are virtually absent from CSF
- Lactate and glucose are present in normal CSF
- If included in volume of interest (VOI), reduction in SNR of cerebral metabolites

Hypoxic-Ischemic Cascade

- Loss of NAA
- Appearance of lactate

- Increased Glx
- Excess Lipid frequently found
- Ultimately, loss of creatine

Abscess

- Metabolites not usually detected
- Acetate 1.92 ppm
- Leucine, Isoleucine, valine
- Succinate, pyruvate
- Lactate/lipids

HIV Toxoplasmosis

- Increased lactate/lipids 1.3/0.9
- Decreased mI
- Decreased NAA, Cr, Cho
- Diagnostic accuracy approximately 100%

HIV CNS Lymphoma

- Increased choline
- Increased lactate, lipids
- Decreased mI, NAA, Cr
- Diagnostic accuracy 75%

Progressive Multifocal Leukoencephalopathy

- Increased mI, Cho
- Decreased Cr, NAA
- Lower levels of lactate, lipids
- Diagnostic accuracy 83%

Cerebral Neoplasms (Generalizations)

- Low/absent NAA
- Low Cr
- Elevated Cho
- Elevated Lipid
- ± Lactate

Neuropathology

Histology (Norfray et al., 1999)

- Grading Chol/Cr ratios
- Low-grade/hamartomas: <1.5
- Intermediate gliomas: 1.5-2.0
- High-grade gliomas: >2.0

Chol/NAA ratios

- Normal 0.75
- Low Grade Glioma 1.86
- Ependymoma 1.8
- PNET 7.5
- Choroid Plexus Ca 8.4
- High Grade Glioma 16.6

Radiation Necrosis

- Low in all metabolites, lactate, lipids
- As opposed to recurrent tumor
- Increased choline
- Correlation with PET

Primary vs. Secondary Neoplasms

In primary glial tumors, peri-tumoral MRS demonstrates elevated choline. In secondary tumor/metastases, choline is not elevated in peritumoral tissue. This correlates with the MR perfusion findings showing increased regional cerebral blood volume (rCBV) in the peritumoral region of primary neoplasms but not of secondary ones. The basis in this difference is the presence of infiltrative tumor cells in the first instance and the presence of edema in the second.

Intracranial Tumors and Age of Presentation

Central nervous system tumors rank second in incidence only to lymphoreticular neoplasms during childhood. Approximately 15-20% of all intracranial tumors occur in children below 15 years of age. Most intracranial tumors in children represent primary lesions, with cerebral metastases being rare. The histological spectrum of intracranial tumors and their location in children vary considerably compared to in adults (Table 2). A higher proportion of childhood intracranial tumors occur in the posterior fossa, accounting for the majority of intracranial tumors in the 2- to 10-years age group. Any analysis of intracranial tumors must include consideration of patient age, in recognition of the most frequent histologies that occur in various age groups.

Table 2. Common primary intra-axial brain tumors

Pediatric	Supratentorial	Pleomorphic xanthoastrocytoma (PXA) Primitive neuroectodermal tumor (PNET) Dysembryoplastic neuroectodermal tumor (DNET) Ganglioglioma
	Infratentorial	Juvenile pilocytic astrocytoma Primitive neuroectodermal tumor (pnet) Brainstem astrocytoma
Adult	Supratentorial	Fibrillary astrocytoma Anaplastic astrocytoma Glioblastoma multiforme Oligodendroglioma
	Infratentorial	Hemangioblastoma

Common Intra-axial Tumors

Astrocytoma

These are the most common primary intra-axial mass in the adult population. While there are various grading schemes in use throughout the world, the basic premise is the same. These tumors range from low-grade lesions to highly aggressive malignant neoplasms. The differences reflect the degree of cellularity along with the presence of mitotic activity, vascular hyperplasia, and necrosis. These lesions grow by a pattern of infiltration during which they secrete a wide variety of substances that promote the survival of the tumor cells. Hence, these tumors are capable of recruiting their own blood supply. As they dedifferentiate, they will enhance. According to the WHO 4 tier classification scheme, grade I tumors are termed pilocytic; grade II tumors include fibrillary astrocytoma; grade III tumors are anaplastic, with vascular hyperplasia and mitosis; and grade IV tumors are glioblastoma multiforme, exhibiting necrosis in addition to fulfilling the criteria of grade III tumors. Grade IV tumors are considered so aggressive that they "out-grow" their own blood supply.

Oligodendroglioma

As the name implies, these tumors take origin from the oligodendroglia. They are significantly less common than astrocytomas, comprising < 10% of primary intra-axial tumors. Typically, they are seen to contain CT visible calcification in upwards of 80% of cases. They tend to be located subcortically. As is the case with astrocytomas oligodendrogliomas also vary from low-grade to high-grade. However, these tumors tend to have a better prognosis, being somewhat more chemosensitive than their pure astrocytic counterparts. They also exist in a mixed form, in which there are varied proportions of oligodendroglial cells and astrocytes. An increased degree of the oligodendroglial component corresponds to a better prognosis.

Ganglioglioma

These tumors comprise a mixed cell population, taking origin from glial and neuronal cell lines. These are the most common of "mixed tumors. Ganglioma tend to be low-grade and have a good prognosis. However, in some cases they can be somewhat more aggressive and dedifferentiate into higher-grade lesions. Typically, the patient presents with a seizure and is found to have a lesion in a cortical location. Most commonly these tumors are located in the temporal lobes. In addition, there is thinning of the overlying bony calvarium, an indicator of the longstanding nature of these lesions.

Hemangioblastoma

In adults, these lesions are the most common primary infratentorial tumors. They are low grade, essentially benign neoplasms. Incomplete resection, however, can lead to recurrence. Typically, hemangioblastoma presents as a cystic mass with a solid mural nodule that is highly vascular. The cyst wall does not enhance. The tumor's appearance is similar to that of juvenile pilocytic astrocytoma. The principal differentiating feature is age. Hemangioblastomas tend to present in young middleaged males (30-40 years) and can be multiple, in which case they are typically associated with von Hippel Lindau syndrome.

Primitive Neuroectodermal Tumor

These tumors were previously referred to medulloblastomas but were eventually renamed because of their primitive nature along with their neuroectodermal cell origin. While they are the most common posterior fossa neoplasms in children, there is a second peak of incidence in adults. Classically they occur in relation to the cerebellum but also to the supratentorial brain. PNETs represent a spectrum of disease with a varied degree of aggressiveness. The atypical teratoid rhabdoid tumor is the most aggressive form.

Juvenile Pilocytic Astrocytoma

These tumors are more commonly referred to as pilocytic astrocytoma. They are distinct from the more infiltrative low-grade astrocytomas, including histopathologically. JPAs are non-aggressive tumors in which gross surgical resection should be curative. Their imaging features are a combination of low- and high-grade lesions; they are well circumscribed yet enhance. The advanced imaging characteristics of JPAs (perfusion and spectroscopy) tend to mimic those of higher-grade lesions. Thus, it is paramount that, in such cases (and, in fact, in all cases) advanced MR data be interpreted along with the conventional images. Obviously, patient history helps as well.

Metastases

By far and away, these are the most common supratentorial (infratentorial as well) neoplasms in adults, comprising upwards of 40% of such tumors. About half of these lesions are reported to be solitary; however, with the use of higher doses of gadolinium (as well as higher field strength) this number is decreasing. In decreasing order with respect to numbers, metastases tend to arise from the lung, breast (in women), melanoma, kidney, and from primaries of the gastrointestinal tract. Metastases tend to be located at the gray-white junction with a fair amount of vasogenic edema (recognized by the sparing of the arcuate fibers along with edema's frond-like appearance). Increased T1 signal can mean either melanin or blood product. Mucinous adenocarcinoma metastases will tend to have low signal on both T2 and FLAIR imaging. Calcification can occur typically in lung or breast metastases.

Common Extra-axial Tumors

Meningioma

Meningioma is the most common extra-axial neoplasm of adults. Its incidence is highest in middle-aged females. Meningiomas are thought to originate from arachnoid cap cells and their distribution parallels that of the cap cells, which are most abundant in arachnoid granulations. The parasagittal and convex dura, sphenoid ridge, parasellar and cerebellopontine angle are common locations. Varying histological types and varying composition lead to variability in the imaging features. Meningiomas are usually hyperdense relative to brain on CT. Calcification can be detected in roughly 20% of these tumors and a bony reaction in the adjacent skull is relatively common. If present, it usually consists of hyperostosis (due to stimulation of a bony reaction with or without tumor invasion) and, less frequently, bone destruction. Enhancement on CT or MR imaging is usually relatively homogenous, with occasional cystic components, areas of necrosis, or calcium within. Meningiomas have a propensity for invasion of dural venous sinuses and encasement of carotid arteries when originating in the cavernous sinus. In the latter, meningioma can also cause caliber narrowing of the vessel. Edema in the brain region adjacent to meningioma is variable and more frequent in larger lesions.

Schwannoma

The tem "neurogenic tumor" refers primarily to schwannoma and, much less commonly, to neurofibroma. Schwannomas originate from Schwann cells, whose myelin processes surround axons of cranial nerves. They are most frequently found at the transition zone between oligodendroglial and Schwann cell coverings of the axons. Schwannomas originate much more frequently from sensory than from motor nerves. They account for 6-8% of primary intracranial neoplasms, are more frequent in adulthood (peaking in the 5th and 6th decade), and are slightly more common in females. Presenting symptoms will depend upon the nerve affected. As these tumors are well-delineated and encapsulated, they affect the cranial nerve of origin and adjacent brain by compression rather than by invasion. The vestibular division of the eighth cranial nerve is the most frequent origin (internal auditory canal and cerebellopontine angle), followed by the 5th and 7th cranial nerves. On CT, schwannomas are isodense or slightly hypodense relative to brain. Calcification and hemorrhage are very rare. MR imaging usually demonstrates an iso- to hypointense extra-axial mass on T1-weighted sequences, becoming hyperintense on T2-weighted sequences. Schwannomas usually enhance intensely on both CT and MR imaging. Smaller tumors often enhance homogenously, whereas heterogeneity is more common in larger tumors due to intralesional necrosis or cyst formation. Arachnoid cysts can also be seen in association with the surface of these lesions. In most cases, cerebellopontine-angle tumors form acute angles with the porous acousticus and the tumor extends into the internal auditory canal, often with canal expansion. This distinguishes Schwannomas from meningiomas, which are also common in this location. Schwannomas may affect bony foramina by slowly expanding and remodeling the foramen.

Cysts and Tumor-Like Intracranial Masses

Several intracranial mass lesions are not true neoplasms but are traditionally included among "brain tumors" because they represent space-occupying intracranial lesions. Dermoids and epidermoids are included in this group. Each represents a non-neoplastic "inclusion cyst" presumably arising from ectodermal cell rests during embryogenesis. Epidermoids consist of an ectoderm-derived epithelial lining (without ectodermal appendages). As the cyst wall desquamates, this material collects within the cyst. The cyst slowly expands and insinuates within cisternal spaces and fissures. Epidermoids are most frequently found off the midline and in the cerebellopontine angle, less frequently around the sella. They may show CT and MR imaging characteristics similar to CSF, and typically do not enhance following contrast administration. Use of DW imaging can reliably distinguish these lesions from arachnoid cysts. Dermoids are similar inclusions cysts, but their lining may also contain ectodermal-derived appendages (hair, teeth, sweat glands, etc). They are more typically found near the midline and may be associated with a dermal sinus. Secretions and their breakdown products often result in contents that are oily and contain lipid metabolites, giving rise to imaging features similar to fat. CT usually shows a low-density extra-axial mass, often with peripheral calcification. The above-mentioned ectodermal appendages can contribute to heterogeneity. Although the cyst wall may show some enhancement, the center of the mass should not enhance with contrast material. Dermoids may occasionally rupture intracranially and release their oily contents into the subarachnoid space. The clinical presentation may simulate acute subarachnoid hemorrhage and imaging will demonstrate dispersal of the oily contents into the subarachnoid space. Other non-neoplastic extra-axial lesions include arachnoid cyst (CSF-filled cavity within the arachnoid membrane); colloid cyst (anterior III ventricle at the foramen of Monroe); neuroepithelial cyst (most likely intraventricular and of choroidal origin); and neurenteric cyst (cyst wall composed of gut/respiratory epithelium, remnant of neurenteric canal during embryogenesis).

Paraganglioma

Cranial paragangliomas may arise at the jugular foramen (glomus jugulare) or in the middle ear cavity (glomus tympanicum). These tumors derive from glomus bodies (neural crest derivatives) and patients often present with pulsatile tinnitus. Glomus jugulare tumors originate in the adventitia of the jugular foramen and will occlude the jugular vein with growth. At the time of diagnosis, there is usually infiltration of tumor into the bony margins of the jugular foramen, with a pattern of permeative bone destruction. CT and MR show an enhancing soft-tissue mass centered on the jugular foramen (jugulare) or inferior portion of the middle ear cavity (tympanicum). A soft-tissue component may grow intracranially toward the cerebellopontine angle. In these highly vascular tumors, there is direct visualization of prominent vessels within the mass, as evidenced by MRI "flow voids" or a "salt and pepper" appearance.

Craniopharyngioma

Thought to arise from metaplasia of squamous epithelial remnants of Rathke's pouch, these tumors are usually centered in the suprasellar cistern. They may extend into the sella, retroclival region, or up into the third ventricle. Although most common in children, craniopharyngiomas may occur at any age. In addition to their characteristic location, the tumors often exhibit cyst formation, calcification, and solid enhancing components.

Chordoma

Chordomas arise from remnants of the notochord andy are most common in the sacrum. Cranial chordomas occur almost exclusively in the clivus. They are locally aggressive tumors that destroy bone and may grow into the nasopharynx, parasellar region. or prepontine cistern. MR and CT demonstrate an enhancing soft-tissue mass centered on the clivus and exhibiting bone destruction as well as areas of calcification. They are almost always hyperintense on T2-weighted MR sequences and may exhibit internal "septations".

Tumor Follow-Up

Follow-up of patients with intracranial neoplasms tends to be dictated by the clinical situation and generally falls into two groups: medical and surgical.

We scan patients undergoing surgical resection within 24 h of surgery using routine imaging. In this time-frame, the post-operative changes affecting the blood-brain barrier are not manifest and any enhancement seen is thought to represent residual enhancing tumor. It is imperative that a non-contrast T1 image is obtained, as a fair amount of hyperintense blood product may be present. First conventional follow-up is carried out 6 weeks later. Scanning within this interval can be fraught will difficulty due to the exuberant contrast enhancement present. It should be noted that if the lesion was non-enhancing preoperatively it will not enhance in the month following surgery. Further follow-up will be dictated by the clinical therapeutic protocol with which the patient is being treated. Pure surgical lesions (with gross total resection) tend to be followed at 6 weeks, 3 months × 2, then 6 months × 2, and yearly.

In patients undergoing further medical therapy, the precise timing of follow-up depends upon the treatment protocol. Typically, in those patients actively receiving chemotherapy follow-up is between 4 and 6 weeks, with courses of chemotherapy in between. In this instance, follow-up should include at least one advanced method (perfusion or spectroscopy) since the therapeutic effect can mimic disease progression and needs to be differentiated from it. The same holds true for radiation. When patients are no longer actively receiving aggressive treatment, follow-up occurs in 3-month intervals.

In all instances the presence of any imaging changes with mass effect should prompt further investigation with advanced methods. It is also important to understand the patterns of tumor spread when looking at follow-up images. Primary lesions, being highly infiltrative, will spread along paths of less resistance, i.e., along axonal bundles, and, more importantly, in a subependymal fashion. If a lesion is adjacent to the ventricular system, care must be taken to assess the subependymal surfaces for subtle linear FLAIR abnormalities tracking around the ventricular system, which may eventually enhance as well. It cannot be assumed that it's just "white matter disease".

When a suspicious finding is made there are two options: if tumor recurrence is diagnosed with certainty, then this finding must be acted upon. If however, a diagnosis of recurrence cannot be made with 100% confidence, then closer follow-up in 4-6 weeks is warranted.

Suggested Reading

Al-Okaili RN, Krejza J, Wang S et al (2006) Advanced MR imaging techniques in the diagnosis of intraaxial brain tumors in adults. Radiographics. 26 Suppl 1:S173-S189

Atlas SW, Lavi E, Fisher PG (2002) Intraaxial brain tumors. In: Atlas SW (ed) Magnetic resonance imaging of the brain and spine. Lippincott Williams & Wilkins, Philadelphia, pp 565-693

Atlas SW, Lavi E, Golberg HI (2002) Extraaxial brain tumors. In: Atlas SW (ed) Magnetic resonance imaging of the brain and spine. Lippincott Williams & Wilkins, Philadelphia, pp 695-772

Bode MK, Ruohonen J, Nieminen MT et al (2006) Potential of diffusion imaging in brain tumors: a review. Acta Radiol 47(6):585-594

Castillo M, Mukherji SK (2000) Diffusion-weighted imaging in the evaluation of intracranial lesions. Semin Ultrasound CT MR 21:405-416

Cha S, Knopp EA, Johnson G et al (2000) Dynamic, contrast-enhanced T2*-weighted MR imaging of recurrent malignant gliomas treated with thalidomide and carboplatin. AJNR Am J Neuroradiol 21:881-890

Cha S, Knopp EA, Johnson G et al (2002) Intracranial mass lesions: dynamic contrast-enhanced susceptibility-weighted echo-planar perfusion MR imaging. Radiology 223:11-29

Chenevert TL, Meyer CR, Moffat BA et al (2002) Diffusion MRI: a new strategy for assessment of cancer therapeutic efficacy. Mol Imaging 1:336-343

DeAngelis LM (2001) Brain tumors. N Engl J Med 344:114-123
Ding B, Ling HW, Chen KM et al (2006) Comparison of cerebral blood volume and permeability in preoperative grading of intracranial glioma using CT perfusion imaging. Neuroradiology 48(10):773-81
Earnest F 4th, Kelly PJ, Scheithauer BW et al (1988) Cerebral astrocytomas: histopathologic correlation of MR and CT contrast enhancement with stereotactic biopsy. Radiology 166:823-827
Ellika SK, Jain R, Patel SC et al (2007) Role of perfusion CT in glioma grading and comparison with conventional MR imaging features. AJNR Am J Neuroradiol 28(10):1981-1987
Fine HA (1995) Novel biologic therapies for malignant gliomas. Antiangiogenesis, immunotherapy, and gene therapy. Neurol Clin 13:827-846
Fitzpatrick M, Tartaglino LM, Hollander MD et al (1999) Imaging of sellar and parasellar pathology. Radiol Clin North Am 37:101-121
Grossman RI, Yousem DM (2003) Neoplasms of the Brain. In:Thrall JH ed. Neuroradiology: the requisites. Mosby-Elsevier, Philadelphia, pp 97-172
Hollingworth W, Medina LS, Lenkinski RE et al (2006) A systematic literature review of magnetic resonance spectroscopy for the characterization of brain tumors. AJNR Am J Neuroradiol 27(7):1404-1411
Kleinman G, Zagzag D, Miller D (1994) Diagnostic use of immunohistochemistry in neuropathology. Neurosurg Clin N Am 5:97-126
Knopp EA, Cha S, Johnson G et al (1999) Dynamic contrast-enhanced T2*-weighted MR imaging of glial neoplasms. Radiology 211:791-798
Koeller KK, Smirniotopoulos JG, Jones RV (1997) Primary central nervous system lymphoma: radiologic-pathologic correlation. Radiographics 17:1497-1526
Lassman AB, DeAngelis LM (2003) Brain metastases. Neurol Clin 21:1-23
Law M, Cha S, Knopp EA et al (2002) High-grade gliomas and solitary metastases: differentiation using perfusion MR imaging and proton spectroscopic MR imaging. Radiology 222:715-721
Law M, Yang S, Wang H et al (2003) Glioma grading: sensitivity, specificity, and predictive values of perfusion MR imaging and proton MR spectroscopic imaging compared with conventional MR imaging. AJNR Am J Neuroradiol 24(10):1989-1998
Le Bihan D, Douek P, Argyropoulou M et al (1993) Diffusion and perfusion magnetic resonance imaging in brain tumors. Top Magn Reson Imaging 5:25-31
Louis DN, Ohgaki H, Wiestler OD (eds) (2007) WHO classification of tumours of the central nervous system, 4th edn. IARC, Lyon
Luh GY, Bird CR (1999) Imaging of brain tumors in the pediatric population. Neuroimaging Clin N Am 9:691-716
Maiuri F, Iaconetta G, de Divitiis O et al (1999) Intracranial meningiomas: correlations between MR imaging and histology. Eur J Radiol 31:69-75
Nelson SJ, McKnight TR, Henry RG (2002) Characterization of untreated gliomas by magnetic resonance spectroscopic imaging. Neuroimaging Clin N Am 12:599-613
Norfray JF, Darling C, Byrd S et al (1999) Short TE proton MRS and neurofibromatosis type 1 intracranial lesions. J Comput Assist Tomogr 23(6):994-1003
Poussaint TY (2001) Magnetic resonance imaging of pediatric brain tumors: state of the art. Top Magn Reson Imaging 12:411-433
Provenzale JM, Mukundan S, Barboriak DP (2006) Diffusion-weighted and perfusion MR imaging for brain tumor characterization and assessment of treatment response. Radiology 239(3):632-649
Schiffer D (1991) Pathology of brain tumors and its clinicobiological correlates. Dev Oncol 66:3-9
Schiffer D (2000) Glioma malignancy and its biological and histological correlates. J Neurosurg Sci 34:163-165
Sheporaitis LA, Osborn AG, Smirniotopoulos JG et al (1992) Intracranial meningioma. AJNR Am J Neuroradiol 13:29-37
Sibtain NA, Howe FA, Saunders DE (2007) The clinical value of proton magnetic resonance spectroscopy in adult brain tumours. Clin Radiol 62(2):109-119
Young RJ, Knopp EA (2006) Brain MRI: tumor evaluation. J Magn Reson Imaging 24(4):709-724
Zamani AA (2000) Cerebellopontine angle tumors: role of magnetic resonance imaging. Top Magn Reson Imaging 11:98-107

Evaluation of the Cerebral Vessels: Endovascular Therapy

Mary E. Jensen

Department of Radiology, University of Virginia Health Systems, Charlottesville, VA, USA

This article focuses on the major clinical findings, therapeutic options, and endovascular treatments available for some of the more common vascular diseases involving the intracranial circulation. The imaging modalities used in the diagnosis of the major vascular anomalies affecting the cerebral vasculature are discussed elsewhere in this volume.

Cerebral Aneurysms

Rupture of a cerebral aneurysm is the most common cause of non-traumatic subarachnoid hemorrhage (SAH), affecting 1 in 10,000 persons each year and creating significant morbidity and mortality. Ruptured aneurysms account for 3% of all strokes, but more than 5% of stroke deaths are due to aneurysmal hemorrhage. More than 50% of the patients suffering from aneurysmal SAH will die within the first 30 days of rupture. Over the past 50 years, the benefit of surgical clipping of ruptured aneurysms relative to the risk has been well-demonstrated clinically. Accurate diagnosis with catheter angiography (and now non-invasive imaging), introduction of the operating microscope, the timing of aneurysm surgery, and therapies designed to combat vasospasm have markedly reduced poor outcomes. Even so, relatively few individuals who experience an episode of SAH escape totally unscathed.

In 1990, the first patient with a ruptured aneurysm was treated endovascularly using the Guglielmi Detachable Coil (GDC) System (Boston Scientific, Fremont, CA). Following initial clinical experiences at select sites, a 3-year, multi-center clinical trial was completed. In 1995, the device received FDA approval for use in patients with ruptured aneurysms who were not surgical candidates. The device gained popularity in clinical use, particularly in patients with deep aneurysms, severe co-morbidities, or poor clinical grades. Over the years, second-generation coils with "biologically active" or hydrogel-based coatings were developed with the intent of improving the efficacy and durability of endovascular treatment. Adjunct devices to aid in the closure of wide-necked aneurysms through balloon- and/or stent-assisted coiling were also developed and marketed (Fig. 1).

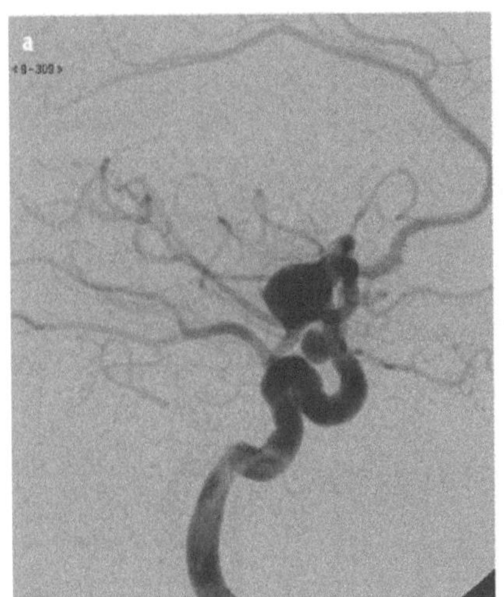

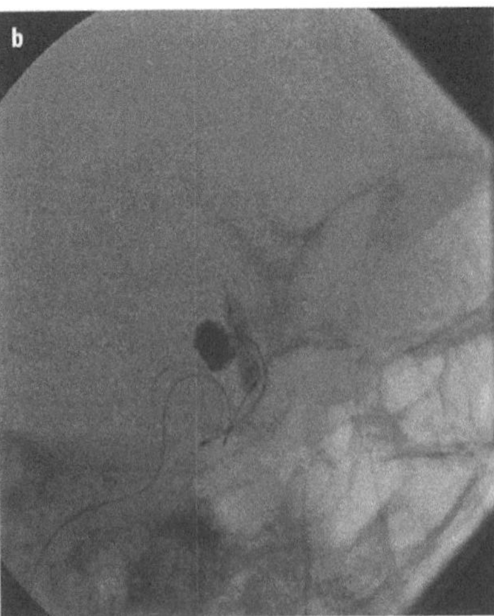

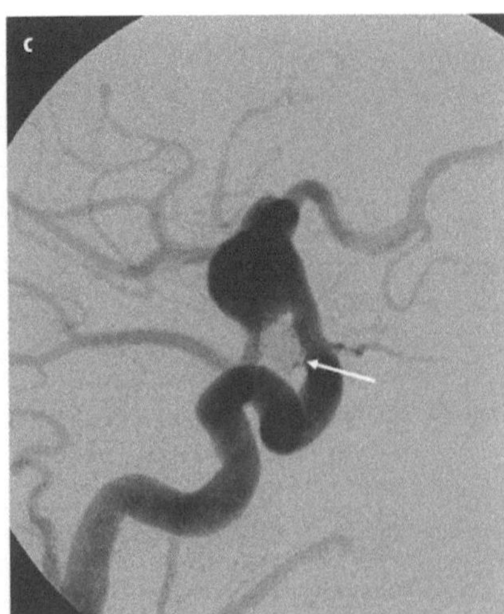

Fig. 1 a-c. This 65-year-old female presented with subarachnoid hemorrhage and was found to have a wide-necked paraclinoid aneurysm and a fusiform aneurysm of the distal left supraclinoid carotid artery (**a**). After a successful temporary balloon occlusion test, the paraclinoid aneurysm was endovascularly coiled using a balloon remodeling technique (**b**). After coiling (**c**), only minimal filling of the aneurysm at the proximal neck (*arrow*) is noted

Despite all the technological advances and clinical data demonstrating the safety and efficacy of endovascular closure of ruptured aneurysms, randomized trial data comparing aneurysm clipping to coiling were lacking until 2002. That year saw the publication of the results of the International Subarachnoid Aneurysm Trial (ISAT). This multi-center, prospective, randomized trial compared endovascular coil treatment with surgical clipping in terms of the safety and efficacy of these procedures and is the most comprehensive study to date. Enrollment began in 1994 and was prematurely halted in April 2003 by the steering committee when it was determined that the primary endpoint (25% fewer dead or dependent patients in the endovascular group, with a modified Rankin score of 3-6, at 1 year) had been reached. The study enrolled 2,143 patients at 43 centers. The majority of these patients (88%) was in good neurologic condition and had aneurysms <11 mm (92% of patients). The primary criterion for enrollment was a patient with SAH due to a ruptured aneurysm, and agreement between the neurosurgeon and endovascular therapist that the aneurysm could be treated by either method.

ISAT showed that patients treated endovascularly had substantially better outcomes than patients in the surgical group. The study demonstrated a relative risk reduction of 22.6% (95% CI 8.8-34.2) and an absolute risk reduction of 6.9% in death or disability with endovascular coiling over surgical clipping at 1 year. The survival advantage in the endovascular group was maintained at 1 year, and up to 7 years, with an absolute risk reduction of 7.4%. The rate of seizures was also substantially lower in the endovascular group. Surgical clipping outperformed endovascular coiling only with respect to retreatment rates, with the likelihood for retreatment 6.9 times higher in the endovascular group.

Several criticisms were directed against the study, including the exclusion of a large number of eligible patients, disparity of operator experience between the interventional neuroradiologists and the neurosurgeons, differences between the timing of endovascular coiling vs. surgical clipping, and the number of incompletely treated aneurysms in the endovascular group (34 vs. 18%), resulting in a higher, but not statistically significant, rebleeding rate in the endovascular population (2.4 vs. 1% in the surgical group). A more recently published article regarding long-term follow-up and retreatment of aneurysms in the ISAT cohort showed that, overall, rebleeding rates were low and not statistically different (3 of 1012 in the neurosurgery group vs. 7 of 1096 in the endovascular group) between the two cohorts. Rebleeding was more likely to occur early (within 3 months) in the neurosurgery group and was thought to be due to undetected, incompletely clipped aneurysms. The endovascular group showed a longer latency of rebleeding (12-68 months), with very late development of "de novo" aneurysms adjacent to the treated aneurysms in two patients.

Based upon the available level of evidence, it can be concluded that in patients with ruptured aneurysms treatable by either endovascular or surgical means, endovascular coil occlusion is preferred due to its demonstrated superior clinical and neurologic outcomes. Obviously, each institution will have to decide which treatment to promote based upon a variety of factors, including availability of services and operator ability.

The natural history of unruptured saccular aneurysms is less clear, making the management of these lesions more controversial. As non-imaging techniques improve, become more widely available, and are performed more frequently, incidental unruptured aneurysms are often detected. The International Study of Unruptured Intracranial Aneurysms (ISUIA) was designed to determine the natural history of unruptured aneurysms and to measure the risk associated with their treatment. Over a 7-year period, 4060 patients were evaluated: 1,692 patients with 2,686 aneurysms were not treated, 1,917 patients underwent craniotomy, and 451 were treated with coil embolization. Two major determining factors for rupture risk were aneurysm size and location. In the untreated cohort, the risk of SAH ranged from 0 to 40% based upon size and location in the anterior circulation, while the risk of SAH ranged from 2.5 to 50% using the same size criteria in the posterior circulation and posterior communicating arteries. In the treated cohorts, surgical morbidity and mortality ranged from 10.1 to12.6% while endovascular morbidity and mortality ranged from 7.1 to 9.8%. Outcome percentages varied according to patient age, aneurysm size, and location. Treated patients under 50 years of age had the lowest surgical risk (5-6% at 1 year), although increased surgical risk was noted in patients over 50, making endovascular therapy safer than surgery in this age group.

In the untreated cohort, 3% of patients had a SAH during the study period and almost all hemorrhages occurred within 5 years of diagnosis. The majority of ruptured aneurysms were >7 mm in diameter; the risk of rupture of smaller aneurysms involving the anterior circulation remained at 0.1%.

Clearly, the recommendations for a course of action in patients with unruptured aneurysms are less obvious. A number of factors should be considered before making the decision to treat or to observe. These factors include size of the aneurysm, multiplicity of aneurysms, history of prior SAH, patient age, family history of cerebral aneurysms, underlying conditions that predispose for aneurysm formation and rupture (e.g., autosomal dominant polycystic kidney disease), and concurrent pathology of other cerebrovascular disorders (e.g., arteriovenous malformations in the brain). If treatment is the recommendation, then patients should be fully informed about the risks and benefits of surgical and endovascular options. If observation is the recommendation, follow-up imaging on a 3- to 5-year basis, preferably with magnetic resonance angiography (MRA) to diminish radiation risks, should be done.

The above studies address only saccular aneurysms, which account for 90% of all aneurysms. Diagnosis and treatment of non-saccular aneurysms can be more daunting and fraught with increased risk. Non-saccular aneurysms include fusiform, dissecting, and blister/bleb aneurysms. In these lesions, the long axis of the aneurysm usually parallels the parent artery, and no discernible neck is seen. Pathologically, fragmentation of the internal elastic lamina with intramural hemorrhage and thrombus formation is noted in fusiform aneurysms, giving them a histologic appearance similar to that of atherosclerotic disease. Medial cystic necrosis with dissecting hemorrhage causing stenosis of the true lumen and formation of a dilated pseudoaneurysm covered by thin adventitia are the hallmark histologic findings of dissecting aneurysms. Blister/bleb type aneurysms typically occur on the anterior wall of the supraclinoid internal carotid artery and are not associated with branch points. Histologically, these aneurysms are focal wall defects covered only with thin fibrous tissue.

Giant saccular and non-saccular aneurysms may be approached using surgical or endovascular reconstructive or deconstructive techniques. Surgical reconstructive treatments include clipping part or all of the aneurysm lumen, with parent artery preservation, or wrapping the aneurysm dome in cotton. If parent artery preservation is not possible, the aneurysm and/or the parent artery may be occluded endovascularly following a successful temporary balloon occlusion (TBO) test. Alternatively, if the TBO test is not successful, surgical bypass may be performed followed by aneurysm occlusion. With the development of intracranial stents, reconstruction of the parent artery channel and coil embolization of the aneurysm lumen is now possible. Alternatively, overlapping stents may be placed in such a manner as to markedly diminish flow into the aneurysm lumen, resulting in progressive thrombosis of the lesion (Fig. 2). The use of high-density liquid agents (Onyx HD 500; ev3, Irvine, CA) in conjunction with balloon remodeling and/or intracranial stenting is another method currently under investigation in the treatment of giant or large wide-necked aneurysms.

As with any type of therapy, endovascular techniques carry certain risks that are proportionate to the type and complexity of the aneurysm being treated. A major risk is thrombus formation on the catheters or devices, resulting in distal embolization or adjacent vessel occlusion. Thromboembolic events can be minimized by pre-treating patients with unruptured aneurysms with anti-platelet agents and through heparinization during treatment of both ruptured and unruptured aneurysms. Other complications include aneurysm rupture, device malfunction or migration, vascular perforation or dissection, and anesthesia-related risks. Due to the possible need for emergency placement of external ventricular drainage, endovascular therapists must be able to place a drain themselves or have emergency neurosurgical back-up available.

Subarachnoid-Induced Vasospasm

The most common delayed complication of SAH is the development of cerebral vasospasm, which can be seen angiographically in 30-70% of patients with aneurysmal SAH. Clinical symptoms occur in 20-45% of patients, and vasospasm increases significant morbidity and mortality in affected patients by 20-30%. Development of vasospasm can occur any time after SAH, but is most common after 4-14 days with a peak of 7-10 days. Oxyhemoglobin stimulates the release of endothelin, a potent vasoconstrictor, and inhibits the endogenous vasodilator nitric oxide. Development of vasospasm is usually associated with the

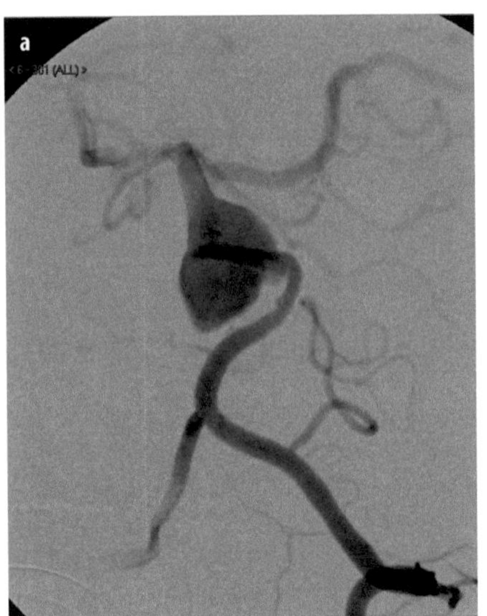

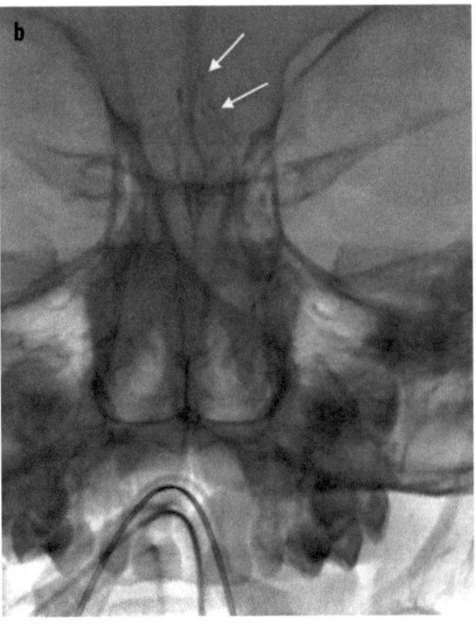

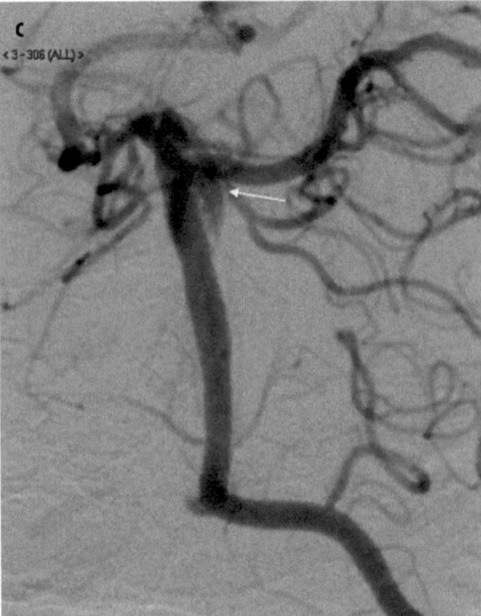

Fig. 2 a-c. This 2-year-old boy presented with developmental delay and incoordination. An AP oblique angiogram of the left vertebral artery (**a**) shows a fusiform basilar artery aneurysm involving the mid and distal basilar artery. The aneurysm was treated with three telescoped Enterprise stents (Cordis Neurovascular, Miami Lake, FL) (**b**) traversing the aneurysmal segment from the left posterior cerebral artery to the distal left vertebral artery. The distal tines of the first two stents are denoted by the *arrows*. Follow-up angiogram 6 months later (**c**) shows thrombosis of the aneurysm with a small, posteriorly located remnant sac (*arrow*). The basilar artery and its branches remain patent

amount of subarachnoid blood in the basal cisterns. Histologically, smooth muscle constriction and vessel wall edema, infiltration, and fibrosis result in luminal narrowing and decreased vascular compliance, leading to diminished peripheral flow, ischemia, and ultimately infarction.

Vasospasm may be detected by serial transcranial Doppler studies, but this technique identifies vasospasm with only 67% specificity compared to digital subtraction angiography (DSA). In addition, false-positives may occur in patients receiving hypertensive agents, and the reading can vary greatly depending upon operator experience and the suitability of the temporal bone window. Thus, DSA remains the gold standard for the evaluation of vasospasm, as it is accurate and allows immediate endovascular treatment by balloon angioplasty and/or intra-arterial injection of vasodilators if needed. However, DSA carries a slight risk of stroke and the patient may require anesthesia in order to perform the study safely. In addition, DSA is limited in its ability to quantify blood flow or predict ischemic risk. The use of non-invasive computed tomography angiography (CTA)/perfusion CT may help eliminate unnecessary invasive DSA. CTA has been reported to have 64% sensitivity and 96% specificity in the determination of location and severity of SAH-induced vasospasm. In a recent study by Wintermark et al., a CT survey in which CTA and perfusion CT were used, the most accurate non-invasive predictor of angiographic vasospasm was a combination of a sensitive mean transit time (MTT) threshold of 6.4 s with an abnormal CTA appearance of the corresponding artery. Perfusion CT was useful (accuracy of 94.8%) in determining which patients would benefit from endovascular treatment.

Treatment strategies for vasospasm include prophylactic and symptomatic therapies. Nimodipine, a calcium channel antagonist, is routinely given prophylactically as it has been shown to improve outcomes after SAH in controlled trials. Other medications that may benefit patients treated for vasospasm include magnesium sulfate, statins, and endothelin A receptor antagonists.

Controversy remains regarding the prophylactic use of triple-H therapy (hypervolemia, hypertension, hemodilution). However, hypervolemia and hypertension have been shown to be effective interventions for clinically evident vasospasm, and may reverse neurologic deficits related to cerebral ischemia. Hemodilution remains the most controversial component of triple-H therapy and a recent retrospective study demonstrated that patients with higher admission and mean hemoglobin levels had better outcomes after SAH.

If aggressive medical therapy fails to reverse ischemic deficits, prompt endovascular intervention is indicated. Vasospasm of larger vessels may be effectively treated with balloon angioplasty and the benefits of this procedure have been shown to be durable. Diffuse vasospasm involving smaller arterial branches may be treated with intra-arterial infusion of vasodilators, such as verapamil or nicardipine. Unfortunately, these dilatory effects tend to be short-lasting and multiple retreatments may be necessary.

Arteriovenous Malformations

Pial arteriovenous malformations (AVMs) encompass a variety of similar lesions that exhibit arteriovenous shunting but differ in size, location, morphologic features, and clinical presentation. The detection rate of pial AVMs is difficult to determine but is estimated to be 1.34 per 100,000 patient-years. Pial AVMs account for 1-2% of all strokes, 9% of SAHs, and 33% of intraparenchymal hemorrhages in young adults.

These lesions are congenital in nature and are thought to be caused by a defect or malfunction of the embryonal capillary maturation process. They are also associated with certain hereditary disorders, such as hereditary hemorrhagic telangectasia, in which 4-13% of affected patients have cerebral AVMs which are often multiple.

Although present at or shortly after birth, most AVMs do not become symptomatic until adulthood. Hemorrhage is the most common presenting symptom and is seen in approximately 50% of patients. The annual hemorrhage rate has been estimated at 2-4% and increases to 6-18% in the first year after the initial hemorrhage. Mortality from an AVM bleed is 6-18%. Other presenting symptoms include seizures (20-25%), headache (15%), and focal neurologic deficits (5%). Children under the age of 2 years may present with congestive heart failure and increasing head circumference due to hydrocephalus.

Arteriovenous malformations are more likely to occur in a supratentorial location (85%) than the posterior fossa (15%). Cortical AVMs are the most common (72%); they may be located in the gyrus or sulcus or involve both areas. Deep AVMs are seen in 27% of patients whereas purely subcortical lesions are rare.

Computed tomography is often the first radiologic study as it is very sensitive to acute hemorrhage. Hemorrhage may occur in the brain parenchyma adjacent to the AVM, with extension into the ventricles or subarachnoid space. SAH without parenchymal involvement is most likely to be due to rupture of an associated proximal aneurysm. In addition to hemorrhage, calcifications, parenchymal changes, such as focal atrophy, and isodense or hyperdense serpiginous structures corresponding to enlarged vessels may be seen on CT. CTA can be used to identify feeding arteries, draining veins, and associated aneurysms in addition to providing volumetric determination of the nidus.

Magnetic resonance imaging (MRI) is essential for the precise localization and topographic evaluation of AVMs, in addition to evaluating for the presence or absence of acute, subacute, or chronic hemorrhage. Associated parenchymal changes, such as edema, ischemia, gliosis, atrophy, or mass effect, are better visualized on MRI. MR angiography is useful for evaluating the size and vascular supply of the AVM although, as with CTA, non-invasive imaging techniques may not allow the true nidus to be differentiated from angiomatous change (described below).

The most exacting imaging evaluation of AVMs is DSA. In addition to morphologic information, flow-related data are obtained. DSA is superior to non-invasive techniques in the evaluation of anatomic factors that increase the risk of hemorrhage. Associated factors that are best determined on DSA include aneurysms located on the feeding vessels or in perinidal or intranidal locations, small nidal size (<3 cm), deep venous drainage, venous stenosis or varix, and the presence of a single draining vein. DSA is also better at detecting those anatomic factors associated with decreased hemorrhagic risk, including the presence of intranidal fistulae, feeder-artery stenosis, and the development of arterial angioectasia, also known as "angiomatous change". In arterial angioectasia, there is capillary dilatation of the collateral pial circulation in the vicinity of the AVM. It occurs adjacent to the nidus and on non-invasive imaging may be included inadvertently in nidal localization and measurement.

The angiographic protocol for AVM evaluation is rigorous. Internal carotid, external carotid, and vertebral arteries are selectively injected. The arterial feeders, nidus and draining veins are analyzed with rapid filming in multiple projections. Superselective injections of individual feeders may be required to determine discreet nidal elements, such as intranidal aneurysms and fistulae. These injections, done through a microcatheter, are usually performed as part of an embolization.

The imaging strategy is related to the clinical presentation. In patients presenting with hemorrhage, the first examination is CT. In patients who are undergoing immediate craniotomy, CTA may be added to determine the underlying cause of the bleed and to localize any lesion that may be present. Otherwise, DSA is done as the next step to obtain a definitive diagnosis and to determine the treatment strategy. If immediate treatment is not required, MRI may be performed to expand on the anatomic data provided by DSA.

For unruptured AVMs, CT is not indicated and MRI/MRA is the first imaging study obtained. Treatment decisions are often based upon AVM size, eloquence of adjacent brain, and the pattern of venous drainage. In many instances, there is sufficient information acquired from MRI/MRA for treatment planning. If not, then DSA is performed. If embolization is part of the therapeutic plan, the diagnostic angiogram and embolization are done at the same time. DSA is also performed prior to surgical intervention and for stereotactic localization of the AVM.

Pial AVMs are embolized for a variety of reasons: in preparation for surgical resection; for endovascular cure in small lesions; for palliation of large, unresectable AVMs; and as an adjunct to radiosurgery. The treatment strategy, targeted elements, and selected embolic agent all depend on the desired goal. In pre-operative embolization, often the deep feeders and fistulous connections are selected for treatment in order to eliminate the vasculature that is most likely to impede surgical resection. Embolic agents include polyvinyl alcohol particles and silk suture for nidal penetration, and microcoils for arterial occlusion. As for liquid agents, resection is easier with ethylene vinyl copolymer (Onyx) than with cyanoacrylates (n-BCA).

It has been estimated that only 10-14% of all pial AVMs are cured by embolization, and suitable lesions usually are fed by only a single pedicle. Treatment requires a permanent agent such as Onyx, cyanoacrylate, or sclerosing material (e.g., alcohol). Follow-up studies are necessary to insure that the AVM does not recanalize.

In the palliative treatment of large lesions, hemorrhagic elements such as aneurysms are often targeted in an effort to diminish the patient's hemorrhagic risk. Intranidal aneurysms are occluded by embolization of that portion of the nidus in which they reside. Aneurysms outside of the nidus may be embolized with liquid agents if they are on a feeding vessel leading directly to the nidus, or the feeder may be coil-occluded. For aneurysms located on the larger skull-base arteries, standard aneurysm coils and techniques are used. If symptoms are related to vascular steal, elimination of macrofistulae is often the goal. Liquid agents are more penetrating than particles or coils, but in high-flow situations they may pass through the fistula and obstruct the draining vein. In these cases, a microcoil is placed at the point of fistulization and acts as a template to trap the liquid agent, preventing excessive venous embolization.

The goal of pre-radiosurgical embolization is to increase the effectiveness of the radiosurgery by reducing the diameter of the nidus to <3 cm and by occluding the radioresistant elements; e.g., macrofistulae. Another goal is to reduce the risk of hemorrhage during the treatment latency period by targeting angioarchitectural abnormalities that might bleed, e.g., intranidal aneurysms. Small series from the late 1990s supported adjunctive embolization, but recanalization rates of 15% were reported with polyvinyl alcohol (PVA) and cyanoacrylate use. In addition, embolization may complicate radiosurgical targeting if the resultant shape is irregular or is divided into compartments. Lastly, embolization may be responsible for out-of-field recurrences if the embolized segment is not included in the target. In short, a reduction in the number of feeding pedicles or overall flow without occlusion of the nidus does not improve the ultimate outcome of radiosurgery. Embolization is only effective if it results in a permanent reduction of a discrete part of the nidus. For this reason, only permanent agents that completely fill the entire lumen of the targeted nidus will be effective.

Embolization of pial AVMs is a risky endeavor; several series reported permanent morbidity in the range of 4-15% and mortality of 1-4%. In addition, recent studies have shown that the AVM obliteration rate may be negatively affected by embolization, and that any benefit of diminished hemorrhagic risk during the latency period may be counterbalanced by the prevalence of complications with embolization.

Dural Arteriovenous Fistulae

Dural arteriovenous fistulae (DAVFs) are the most common type of intracranial AVF and account for 10-15% of all intracranial vascular malformations. Anatomically, shunting occurs from dural arterial feeders to dural sinuses or cortical veins with or without an intervening mesh of small vessels. Arterial feeders are primarily meningeal or periosteal, although transosseous and pial branches can be recruited. The feeding pedicles communicate with the draining sinus or cortical vein through single or multi-hole fistulae located in the dural wall. DAVFs are thought to be acquired lesions associated with sinus thrombosis and recanalization through induction of increased angiogenesis. The primary pathological factor in DAVFs is the development of venous hypertension from obstruction to normal venous outflow. Obstruction may be functional (from high venous pressures generated by the shunt), structural (from venous stenoses or thrombosis from high-flow venopathy) or a combination of both.

Patient presentation is based upon the location of the DAVF and the development of venous outflow obstruction. The most common location for a DAVF is at the transverse-sigmoid junction. Patients usually complain of tinnitus as their presenting symptom, and a bruit is often heard on auscultation over the mastoid region. The second most common location is in the cavernous sinus, where ocular symptoms such as proptosis and diplopia are most commonly reported. Other locations include the tentorial-incisural area, the convexity-superior sagittal sinus region, and the orbital-anterior cranial fossa; occasionally, other places, such as the marginal sinus, are involved.

A variety of classification systems have been described, with emphasis placed upon the presence of cortical venous drainage ("aggressive" lesions), or its absence ("benign" lesions). The decision to treat a dural AVF is based upon its classification. Aggressive lesions have a high rate of morbidity and mortality (15 and 10.4%, respectively) from either parenchymal hemorrhage or non-hemorrhagic neurological deficits caused by venous congestion, and therefore must be treated. Fistulae in the tentorial region or anterior cranial fossa are particularly dangerous as they are the lesions most likely to cause intracerebral hemorrhage.

Assessment of the venous circulation and associated veno-occlusive disease is required to properly classify a DAVF and to recommend a therapeutic course. The most accurate way to define the circulatory changes associated with these lesions is with DSA. Proper angiographic evaluation requires analysis of all potential arterial feeder sources and the venous drainage pattern. Due to extensive collateralization between different meningeal territories, arterial feeders may arise from multiple branches. Therefore, all arteries that potentially supply a certain anatomical location must be selectively injected for accurate angiographic evaluation. Whereas arterial evaluation confirms the diagnosis and localizes the lesion, it is the assessment of the venous phase that determines the treatment and the therapeutic modality to be used. All arterial feeders, the location and size of the fistulous segment, the venous drainage pattern, and the presence of venous occlusion or stenoses should be reported.

Benign DAVFs rarely become aggressive lesions and are usually just monitored, as long as the symptoms are tolerated and do not interfere with function. Mild diplopia may be corrected with eyeglass prisms, and use of a white-noise machine may help insomnia caused by tinnitus. Imaging re-evaluation using time-resolved contrast enhanced MRA may be considered, particularly if the patient's symptoms change. Benign DAVFs are considered for treatment when symptoms become severe; e.g., chemosis, ophthalmoplegia, or affect quality of life.

Spontaneous thrombosis of a DAVF is rare but has been reported. These lesions are usually "benign" in nature, and the reason for closure is unclear. Spontaneous regression of the fistulous connections and thrombosis of the venous outlets have been proposed as possible mechanisms. Treatment options include open surgery, radiosurgery, endovascular closure, and combined therapies. Surgical skeletonization of the sinus, venous disconnection, and/or packing of the affected sinus have been described but are usually reserved for cases that cannot be treated by endovascular means. For low-risk, symptomatic DAVFs requiring palliative treatment, a staged combination of radiosurgery and transarterial embolization provides excellent symptom relief and a high rate of closure. Palliative embolization must be approached carefully, as incomplete treatment of fistulae may result in a more robust recanalization of the shunt with conversion of a benign lesion into an aggressive one.

Endovascular therapy is the treatment of choice in most cases of aggressive DAVFs or severely symptomatic benign DAVFs. Closure may be achieved through transarterial occlusion of all feeding arteries or transvenous occlusion of the affected sinus.

Various embolic agents, such as particles, liquid silicone, absolute alcohol, platinum microcoils, and cyanoacrylates, have been used for transarterial embolization. PVA particles are easy to use and usually safe in sizes >150 µm, but vascular occlusion is typically proximal to the point of fistulization with eventual reopening of the shunt. The same holds true for the transarterial use of microcoils. Recanalization is less likely with liquid agents, but the complication rate increases due to the penetrating nature of these materials. The unpredictable nature of cyanoacrylate polymerization may result in deposition proximal to the fistulous connection or unintended venous embolization of the normal intracranial veins or the pulmonary circulation. Cranial nerve palsies and tissue necrosis are also more likely with cyanoacrylate or absolute alcohol embolization.

There have been several recent reports of complete closure via the transarterial route using a new material, Onyx (ev3, Irvine, CA), an ethylene vinyl copolymer dissolved in DMSO. The copolymer precipitates as the DSMO diffuses, resulting in a controlled mechanical obstruction of the feeding artery and the involved sinus (Fig. 3). The material has the added benefit of being non-

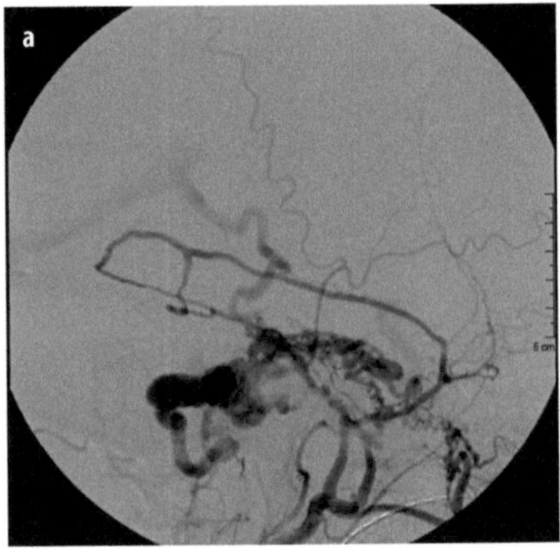

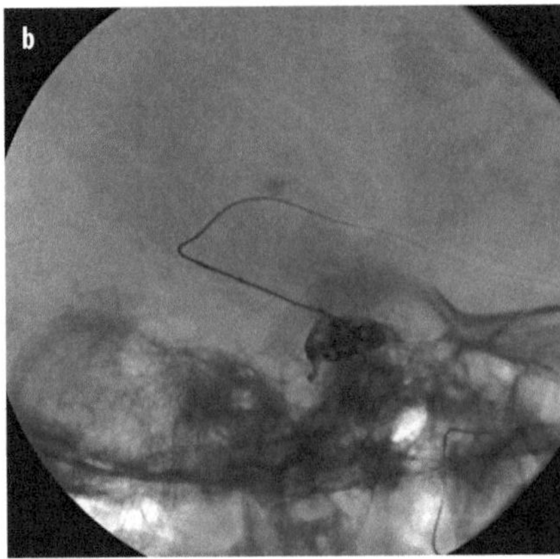

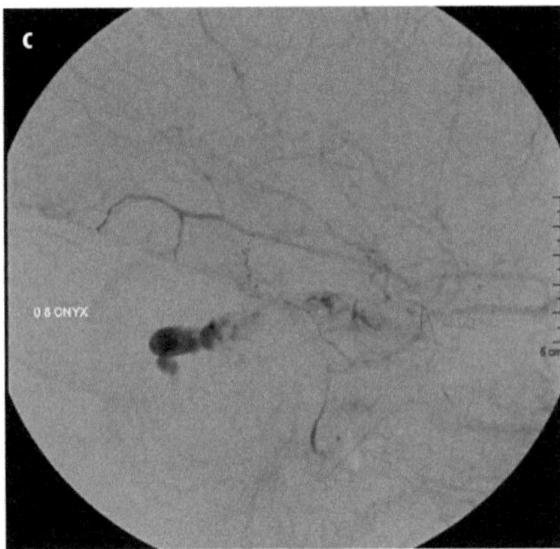

Fig. 3 a-c. A 61-year-old female complained of progressive tinnitus and imbalance. Lateral view of a right external carotid artery injection (**a**) shows a tentorial dural arteriovenous fistula fed by the posterior division and petrosal branches of the middle meningeal artery (MMA) and the pharyngeal branch and artery of the foramen rotundum of the internal maxillary artery. Venous drainage is to cortical and deep veins. The posterior division of the MMA was catheterized to the point of fistulization and injection of Onyx resulted in casting of the fistula nidus (**b**). Final lateral common carotid (**c**) angiogram shows elimination of the fistula and stasis of contrast in the venous varix

adhesive, which allows long injections times without permanent affixation of the microcatheter tip.

Transvenous embolization of the affected sinus using platinum microcoils is extremely effective in eliminating DAVFs. The entire involved segment must be occluded or the fistula will remain open. In cases of isolated shunts, the sinus is accessed via a burr-hole, direct surgical exposure, or percutaneous puncture, followed by embolization. Incomplete closure may result in the redirection of flow to cortical veins, with subsequent hemorrhage or venous congestion. In addition, navigation through the pial venous system places the patient at a small risk of SAH if vascular perforation were to occur.

Endovascular closure rates vary and are based upon the approach taken, the embolic agent used, and location of the fistula. Transvenous occlusion of carotid-cavernous dural fistulae resulted in cure rates of ≥87% in several series. Cure rates of transverse-sigmoid region fistulae are slightly lower, around 80%, using the transvenous approach but compare favorably to transarterial embolization, which typically has a cure rate of <60%. However, the transarterial success rate improves with the use of Onyx in selected lesions.

Intracranial Atherosclerotic Disease

Intracranial atherosclerotic stenoses account for 8-9% of all ischemic strokes, with 60,000 new events occurring each year. Factors that predispose patients to the development of ICAD include race, ethnicity, insulin-dependent diabetes, cigarette smoking, hypercholesterolemia, and hypertension. Many atherosclerotic stenoses are diagnosed in the setting of acute stroke. However, ICAD is often discovered either during the non-invasive imaging evaluation of patients with transient ischemic attack (TIA) symptoms or incidentally. The natural history of these lesions is dynamic, with evidence that atherosclerotic stenoses progress, regress, or remain stable over time.

A defined treatment protocol for symptomatic intracranial stenoses is difficult to determine based upon the currently available data. The Warfarin-Aspirin Symptomatic Intracranial Disease (WASID I and II) trials looked at the effectiveness of warfarin or aspirin in the prevention of stroke in patients with TIAs or minor stroke, and a major intracranial stenosis ≥50%. Although warfarin was slightly more effective than high-dose aspirin (1300 mg per day) in preventing stroke, warfarin caused more significant systemic hemorrhages than aspirin. More importantly, no statistically significant benefit was seen in either group; rather, patients continued to have a 9-12% annual risk of major stroke or death despite optimal medical management. The stroke risk was highest in patients with severe stenoses (≥70%) and in patients enrolled early (<17 days) after the initial neurologic event.

The development of microballoons and stents specifically created for the treatment of intracranial stenoses has added another treatment option for ICAD. However, the available data are restricted to case reports, small series, and the limited trials performed to obtain Humanitarian Device Exemption (HDE) approval for specific devices such as the Wingspan stent (Boston Scientific, Natick, MA). In the Wingspan trial, technical success of stent deployment reached 98%, with a 30-day and 6-month ipsilateral stroke or death rate of 4.5 and 7.5%, respectively. A second study of composite data from four institutions using the Wingspan device was published in 2007. Seventy-eight symptomatic patients with 82 stenoses >50% were treated; the technical success rate was 98.8%. Major morbidity and death were 6.1% at 30 days. However, the study has been plagued by reports of in-stent restenosis (Fig. 4) of >30% in up to 40% of patients; thus, the long-term durability of this technique is in question.

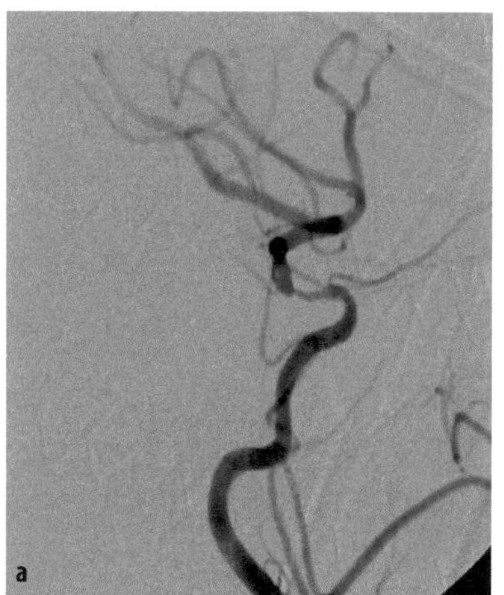

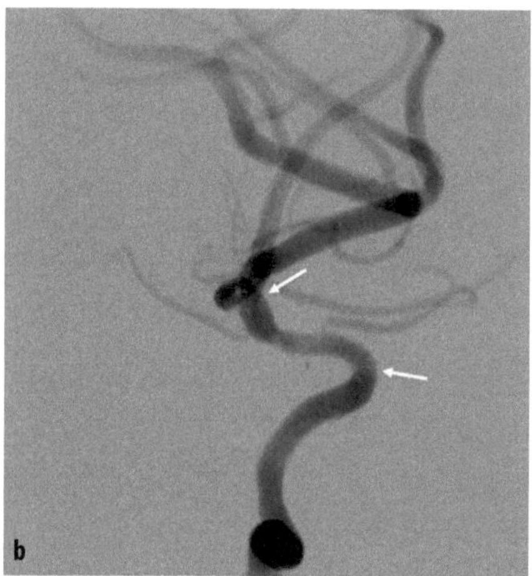

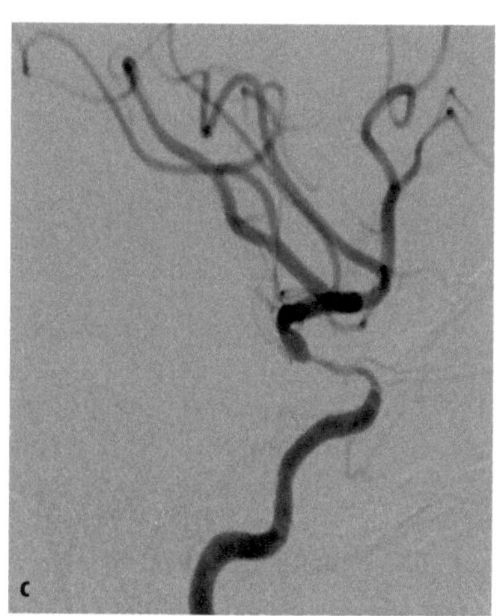

Fig. 4 a-c. This 38-year-old female was found to have progressive transient ischemic attacks involving the right hemisphere. Lateral right common carotid angiogram showed a focal stenosis of the supraclinoid carotid measuring 70% with post-stenotic dilatation (**a**). Angioplasty and placement of a Wingspan stent restored the lumen to normal size. The *arrows* mark the proximal and distal tines of the stent (**b**). Three months later, the patient's symptoms returned and repeat angiogram (**c**) showed significant in-stent stenosis involving the initially diseased portion but now extending all along the course of the stent

Treatment of Acute Ischemic Stroke: Thrombolysis and Mechanical Embolectomy

Stroke is the third leading cause of death in the USA and Europe. Over 750,000 new strokes and >200,000 deaths are reported in the USA each year. Most strokes are ischemic and stroke is the primary cause of adult disability. At present, intravenous administration of recombinant tissue plasminogen activator (r-tPA), a thrombolytic agent, is the only FDA-approved therapy for acute stroke. It must be administered within the first 3 h of symptom onset. Recanalization rates in intravenous thrombolysis depend on the vessel occluded, with decreasing rates of recanalization noted with increasing vessel size. In the Combined Lysis of Thrombus in Brain ischemia with Transcranial Ultrasound and Systemic TPA (CLOTBUST) trial, complete recanalization rates were highest in distal middle cerebral artery (MCA) occlusions (44.2%), with proximal MCA, basilar artery, and internal carotid artery (ICA) terminus ± MCA recanalization rates of 30, 33, and 18%, respectively.

Application of thrombolytic agents directly to the clot via intra-arterial infusion has been described in multiple series. However, the only intra-arterial thrombolytic agent that has been studied in a randomized, controlled manner is recombinant pro-urokinase (Prolyse in Acute Cerebral Thromboembolism Trials I and II). PROACT-II demonstrated a 15% absolute benefit in the number of patients who achieved a modified Rankin score of <2 at 90 days ($p = 0.043$). Recanalization was achieved in 66 vs. 18% of patients in the heparin only (control) group ($p<0.001$) at 2 h; the rate of symptomatic hemorrhage in the treatment group was 10 vs. 2% in the control group at 24 h. Unfortunately, the FDA has not approved pro-urokinase for the treatment of acute stroke, despite its similar functional outcomes compared to the results of the NINDS IV r-tPA trial.

Several trials combining intravenous and intra-arterial administration of thrombolytics, e.g., the Emergency Management of Stroke (EMS) and Interventional Management of Stroke (IMS-I) trials, or involving the adjunctive use of endovascular devices (IMS-II, IMS-III trials) have been completed or are on-going. The functional outcomes for treated patients were not better in the EMS or IMS-I trial than in the NINDS Stroke Study, in which patients received IV thrombolysis alone. However, in the IMS-II trial, which tested combined IV/intra-arterial (IA) r-tPA thrombolytic therapy using a novel IA ultrasound infusion system (EKOS, Bothell, WA), functional outcomes at 3 months were significantly better than those obtained in either NINDS control or IV-thrombolysis-treated patients. IMS-III is now underway to further test combined IV/IA therapy in conjunction with the EKOS device and the MERCI thrombectomy device (Concentric Medical, Mountain View, CA).

Another area of interest in acute stroke management is the potential role of perfusion-weighted imaging in the stratification of patients for aggressive therapy. The use of perfusion-weighted MRI or CT imaging to assess the response to intravenous thrombolysis and/or as a basis for intra-arterial treatment may help to improve clinical outcomes. On-going and completed acute stroke studies that use imaging as part of the protocol include MR RESCUE, ROSIE, ROSIE-CT, DEFUSE, EPITHET and trials consisting of perfusion-CT-guided IV thrombolysis at 3 and 6 h. At this time, however, there is not enough data available to make clinical treatment decisions based upon perfusion imaging findings.

In addition to intra-arterial thrombolysis, endovascular mechanical disruption and thrombus extraction have been explored. In the Mechanical Embolus Removal in Cerebral Embolism (MERCI) trial, a novel corkscrew-like device was used to capture and remove emboli from large and medium vessels within 8 h of symptom onset. In the FDA trial, the treatment group was compared to the treatment and placebo groups from the PROACT-II trial. The device was associated with rapid opening of the artery, but the efficacy in recanalization achieved with the MERCI system was similar to that achieved with IA pro-urokinase in the PROACT-II trial (45 and 66%, respectively). The device was also studied in a multi-center, prospective, single arm trial (Multi-MERCI) consisting of 123 patients suffering from moderate to severe, large-vessel ischemic strokes were treated at 15 hospitals with a combination of mechanical thrombectomy and intra-arterial thrombolysis. Recanalization was demonstrated in 54.9% (90/164) after use of the MERCI device alone. Recanalization was achieved in 68.3% (112/164) following use of the device and thrombolysis. Clinically significant procedural complications occurred in 5.5% (9/164) of patients; 90-day Modified Rankin Scale (mRS) scores ≤2 were observed in 36% of all patients. Mortality at 90-days was 34%, which may be explained by the relatively long time to treatment (median of 4.2 h) and the severity of the strokes.

While acute stroke is the subject of many on-going studies and trials, its treatment remains elusive and patient specific. The best hope for a patient in the throes of an acute stroke is immediate transportation to a primary stroke facility, where accurate diagnosis and appropriate care can be administered promptly.

Suggested Reading

Albers GW, Thijs VN, Wechsler L et al (2006) Magnetic resonance imaging profiles predict clinical response to early reperfusion: the diffusion and perfusion imaging evaluation for understanding stroke evolution (DEFUSE) study. Ann Neurol 60:508-517

Berman MF, Sciacca RR, Pile-Spellman J et al (2000) The epidemiology of brain arteriovenous malformations. Neurosurgery 47:389-396

Campi A, Ramzi N, Molyneux AJ et al (2007) Retreatment of ruptured cerebral aneurysms in patients randomized by coiling or clipping in the international subarachnoid aneurysm trial (ISAT). Stroke 38:1538-1544

Davis SM, Donnan GA, Butcher KS, Parsons M (2005) Selection of thrombolytic therapy beyond 3 h using magnetic resonance imaging. Curr Opin Neurol 18:47-52

del Zoppo GJ, Higashida RT, Furlan AJ et al (1998) PROACT: a phase II randomized trial of recombinant pro-urokinase by direct arterial delivery in acute middle cerebral artery stroke. PROACT investigators. Prolyse in acute cerebral thromboembolism. Stroke 29:4-11

Fiorella D, Levy EI, Turk AS et al (2007) US multicenter experience with the wingspan stent system for the treatment of intracranial atheromatous disease: periprocedural results. Stroke 38:881-887

Furlan A, Higashida R, Wechsler L et al (1999) Intra-arterial prourokinase for acute ischemic stroke. The PROACT II study: A randomized controlled trial. Prolyse in acute cerebral thromboembolism. JAMA 282:2003-2011

Guglielmi G, Vinuela F, Dion J, Duckwiler G (1991) Electrothrombosis of saccular aneurysms via endovascular approach. Part 2: preliminary clinical experience. J Neurosurg 75:8-14

Hartmann A, Mast H, Choi JH et al (2007) Treatment of arteriovenous malformations of the brain. Curr Neurol Neurosci Rep 7:28-34

Higashida RT, Halbach VV, Dowd CF et al (2005) Initial clinical experience with a new self-expanding nitinol stent for the treatment of intracranial cerebral aneurysms: The Cordis Enterprise stent. AJNR Am J Neuroradiol 26:1751-1756

IMS II Trial Investigators (2007) The interventional management of stroke (IMS) II study. Stroke 38:2127-2135

IMS Study Investigators (2004) Combined intravenous and intra-arterial recanalization for acute ischemic stroke: the interventional management of stroke study (IMS). Stroke 35:904-911

Ko NU, Vates GE, Smith WS (2003) Correlation of CT angiography in vasospasm secondary to aneurysmal subarachnoid hemorrhage. Neurology 60(suppl 1):A230-A231

Ledezma CJ, Hoh BL, Carter BS et al (2006) Complications of cerebral arteriovenous malformation embolization: multivariate analysis of predictive factors. Neurosurgery 58:602-611

Lewandowski CA, Frankel M, Tomsick TA et al (1999) Combined intravenous and intra-arterial rt-PA versus intra-arterial therapy of acute ischemic stroke: emergency management of stroke (EMS) bridging trial. Stroke 30:2598-2605

Marks MP, Wojak JC, Al-Ali F et al (2006) Angioplasty for symptomatic intracranial stenosis: clinical outcome. Stroke 37:1016-1020

Molyneux A, Kerr R, Stratton I et al (2002) International subarachnoid aneurysm trial (ISAT) of neurosurgical clipping versus endovascular coiling in 2,143 patients with ruptured intracranial aneurysms: a randomised trial. Lancet 360:1267-1274

Molyneux AJ, Kerr RS, Yu LM et al (2005) International subarachnoid aneurysm trial (ISAT) of neurosurgical clipping versus endovascular coiling in 2,143 patients with ruptured intracranial aneurysms: a randomised comparison of effects on survival, dependency, seizures, rebleeding, subgroups, and aneurysm occlusion. Lancet 366:809-817

Satomi J, van Dijk JM, Terbrugge KG et al (2002) Benign cranial dural arteriovenous fistulas: outcome of conservative management based on the natural history of the lesion. J Neurosurg 97(4):767-770

Smith WS, Sung G, Starkman S et al; MERCI Trial Investigators (2005) Safety and efficacy of mechanical embolectomy in acute ischemic stroke: results of the MERCI trial. Stroke 36(7):1432-1438

Stapf C, Mast H, Sciacca RR et al (2003) The New York Islands AVM Study: design, study progress, and initial results. Stroke 34:e29-e33

Stapf C, Mast H, Sciacca RR et al (2006) Predictors of hemorrhage in patients with untreated brain arteriovenous malformation. Neurology 66:1350-1355

The National Institute of Neurological Disorders and Stroke rt-PA stroke Study Group (1995) Tissue plasminogen activator for acute ischemic stroke. N Engl J Med 333:1581-1587

Turk AS, Levy EI, Albuquerque FC et al (2008) Influence of patient age and stenosis location on Wingspan in-stent restenosis. AJNR Am J Neuroradiol 29(1):23-27

van Dijik JMC, TerBrugge K, Willinsky RA, Wallace MC (2002) Clinical course of cranial dural arteriovenous fistulas with long-term persistent cortical venous reflux. Stroke 33:1233-1236

van Gijn J, Rinkel GJ (2001) Subarachnoid haemorrhage: diagnosis, causes and management. Brain 124:249-278

Wiebers DO, Whisnant JP, Huston J 3rd et al (2003) Unruptured intracranial aneurysms: natural history, clinical outcome, and risks of surgical and endovascular treatment. Lancet 362:103-110

Wintermark M, Ko NU, Smith WS et al (2006) Vasospasm after subarachnoid hemorrhage: utility of perfusion CT and CT angiography on diagnosis and management. AJNR Am J Neuroradiol 27:26-34

Wojak JC, Dunlap DC, Hargrave KR et al (2006) Intracranial angioplasty and stenting: Long-term results from a single center. AJNR Am J Neuroradiol 27:1882-1892

Evaluation of the Cerebral Vessels

Robert Willinsky

Toronto Western Hospital, University of Toronto, Toronto, ON, Canada

Introduction

In the last decade there has been a dramatic shift to non-invasive imaging of the cerebral vessels. This is justified since selective catheter angiography (digital subtraction angiography, DSA) has a risk of neurological complications despite advances in techniques and safer contrast agents. Carotid Doppler is an excellent screening tool to study the carotid bifurcation in patients with transient ischemic attacks and stroke. Transcranial Doppler is useful to detect early vasospasm in patients with subarachnoid hemorrhage. Multi-slice computed tomography (CT) angiography (CTA) and magnetic resonance angiography (MRA) have become effective methods to image the cerebral arteries and veins. DSA is now employed selectively in treatment planning after non-invasive imaging has been used for diagnosis.

CT Angiography

With the advent of multi-slice CT and improved post processing, CTA has played an increasingly important role in the evaluation of the cerebral vessels. CTA is excellent in evaluating patients with carotid stenosis. It can detect a hairline residual lumen, referred to as the "string sign", in patients with near occlusion. Typically, the string sign, which was described on DSA, has been difficult to show by MRA.

CTA is a fast and reliable method to evaluate patients with intracranial hemorrhage, especially subarachnoid hemorrhage. CTA shows most cerebral aneurysms that are detected using DSA. CTA may also reveal thrombosis or calcification in the wall of a large or giant aneurysm. Post-processing allows assessment of the aneurysm with maximum intensity projections (MIP) and surface-rendered 3D projections in multiple planes. In many cases, CTA will be sufficient to allow treatment planning. If the aneurysm is unsuitable for endovascular treatment, the patient may be treated surgically without the need for DSA. CTA is able to demonstrate vasospasm after subarachnoid hemorrhage thus avoiding DSA in patients who are initially given a trial of medical therapy.

MR Angiography

This technique plays a major role in cerebrovascular imaging. Gadolinium enhanced auto-triggered elliptic centric-ordered MRA (ATECO) has superior resolution compared to time-of-flight (TOF) MRA. This has been shown in the evaluation of carotid bifurcation, the intracranial arteries, and the intracranial veins. MRA to evaluate carotid stenosis has eliminated the need for DSA in the majority of patients. MRA of the extracranial and intracranial arteries is a standard part of the magnetic resonance imaging (MRI) evaluation of patients with stroke. Since ATECO is not dependent on the direction of flow, it yields excellent visualization of tortuous vessels and vessels with slow or turbulent flow. ATECO can determine whether there is an intracranial arterial occlusion in patients being evaluated for possible intra-arterial thrombolysis. At 3T, high-resolution imaging of the intracranial arteries with contrast has demonstrated vessel wall disease and has been helpful in differentiating atherosclerotic disease from vasculitis (Fig. 1). Wall disease is best seen on contrast-enhanced axial T1 images. T1 fluid-attenuated inversion recovery (FLAIR) is a black-blood acquisition that eliminates the signal from flowing blood, enabling specific visualization of the wall.

MRA is a good technique to screen high-risk individuals for aneurysms. Again, ATECO is superior to TOF MRA since the turbulent flow in an aneurysm may not be detected by the latter method. However, for screening purposes we prefer non-contrast TOF MRA due to its safety and ease of performance. At 3 T, non-contrast TOF MRA is similar to contrast-enhanced MRA at 1.5T. Remnants of the aneurysm neck in patients previously treated by coiling are best detected by gadolinium-enhanced MRA.

Time-resolved gadolinium-enhanced MRA is useful in the evaluation of arteriovenous fistula of the brain and spinal cord (Fig. 2). Confirmation of a fistula on the basis of the results from this non-invasive technique allows for appropriate treatment planning. Catheter angiography can be done at the same time as the endovascular treatment.

ATECO magnetic resonance venography (MRV) is the imaging modality of choice to evaluate the cerebral veins

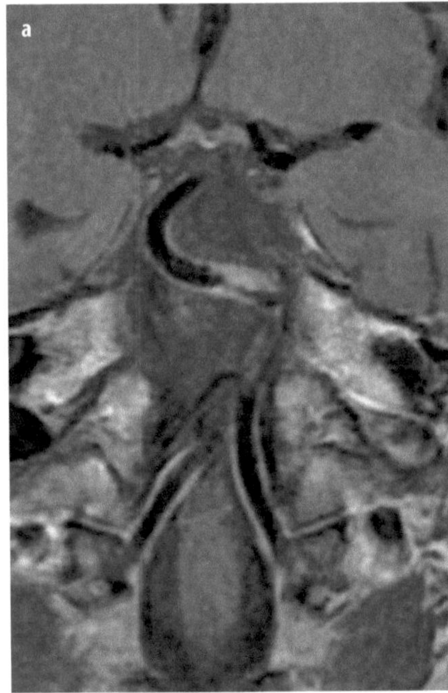

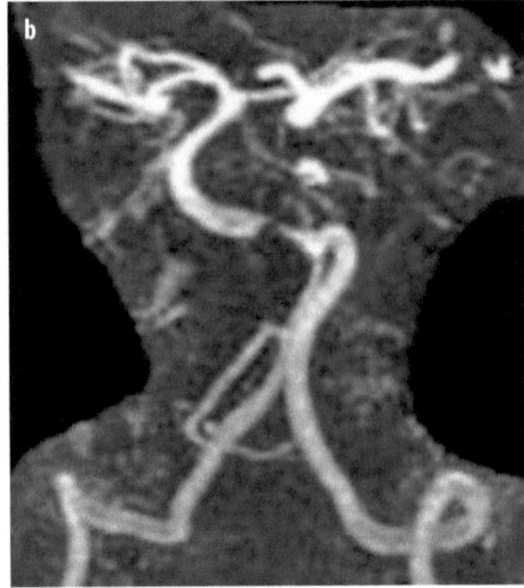

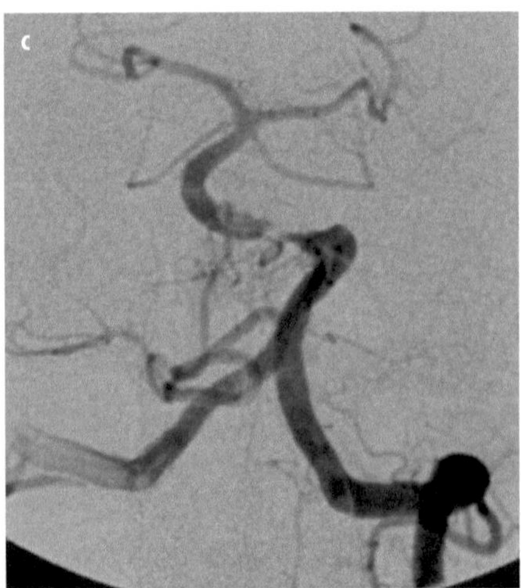

Fig. 1 a-c. Vessel wall imaging at 3T in a patient with symptomatic atherosclerosis in the basilar artery. **a** Coronal contrast-enhanced T1 FLAIR shows the enhancing atherosclerotic plaque. Corresponding contrast enhanced MRA (**b**) and catheter angiograms (**c**)

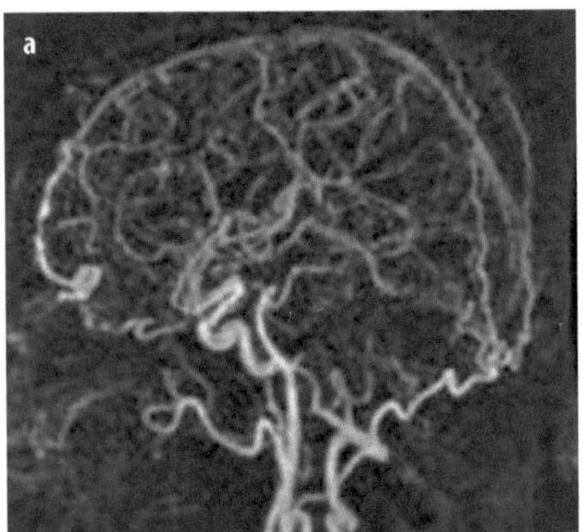

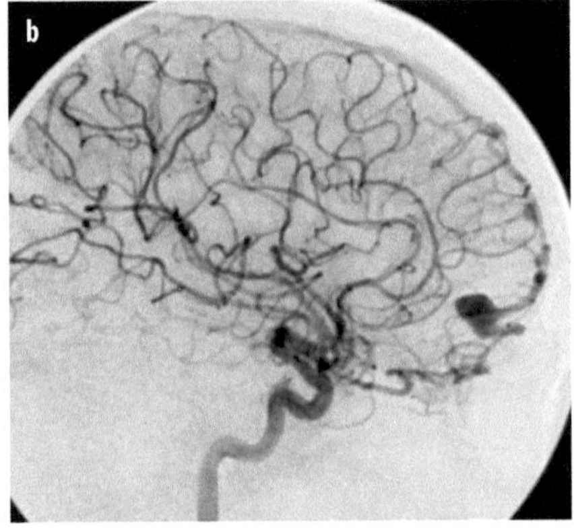

Fig. 2 a, b. Time-resolved contrast enhanced MRA ("Tricks") shows anterior cranial fossa dural arteriovenous fistula. **a** Lateral maximum intensity projection (MIP) from Tricks shows early venous filling of a dilated venous pouch above the crista galli. **b** Corresponding lateral view of the catheter angiogram in the right internal carotid artery

and venous sinuses in sinovenous thrombosis. It is far superior to TOF and phase-contrast methods. In addition, the brain parenchyma can be assessed at the same time.

Digital Subtraction Angiography

Traditionally DSA has been the "gold standard" to evaluate the cerebral vessels. This remains true for the evaluation of the cerebral arteries, circulation time, and collateral flow but is no longer true for the evaluation of the venous system. ATECO MRV is superior to DSA. Since DSA uses selective arteriograms, there is "washout" of the cerebral veins and venous sinuses from unopacified blood. In ATECO MRV, all the veins are opacified equally.

DSA allows assessment of the circulation time. This is helpful in arterial occlusive disease, arteriovenous shunts, venous occlusive disease, and the venous congestion related to dural arteriovenous fistula with cortical venous reflux. In brain micro-arteriovenous malformations (AVMs), the only clue to the presence of shunt is the finding of an early draining vein. This would be difficult to detect using CTA or ATECO MRA.

Collateral flow develops in response to occlusive disease in the arteries and veins. Collateral flow and the direction of flow are best assessed using DSA. Non-invasive imaging with CTA or MRA may detect the presence of a vessel but not the direction of flow. Assessment of collateral flow and circulation time is important in arterial stenosis and chronic venous occlusive disease. When venous collaterals enlarge and become tortuous, they may be evident on non-invasive imaging. On DSA, this pattern is referred to as "pseudophlebitic".

Rotational DSA and 3D reconstruction provide excellent detail of the morphology of a cerebral aneurysm and its adjacent vessels. Treatment decisions regarding surgery vs. coiling can often be based on the CTA. Rotational angiography is used to fine tune the endovascular approach and is helpful in better understanding complex and wide-neck aneurysms.

Cavernous Malformations

Cavernous malformations (CMs), or cavernomas, are vascular malformations of the central nervous system (CNS) composed of well-circumscribed, sinusoidal, vascular channels containing blood in various stages of thrombosis. In many patients (17-54%) the lesions are multiple and the condition is often familial (autosomal dominant). Presentation includes seizures (31%), hemorrhage (18.4%), and focal neurological deficits (15%), with the remainder being incidental findings.

Developmental venous anomalies (DVAs) are associated with CMs or may be found in isolation. DVAs represent an extreme variant of the normal venous drainage. They drain normal brain and must be preserved when CMs are excised. On MRI, DVAs appear as radiating, linear flow-voids ("caput medusa" pattern) centered on a large collecting vein. DVAs may also be found in association with telangiectasias, which are vascular malformations at the capillary level. Telangiectasias are often only well-seen on a gradient-echo sequence, have no mass effect, and diffusely enhance (Fig. 3).

MRI is the diagnostic tool of choice for detecting and identifying CMs. On non-contrast CT, they frequently appear as focal areas of increased density within the brain, often without mass effect. The characteristic MRI appearance is a well-defined, lobulated lesion with a reticulated core of heterogeneous signal intensity on T1- and T2- weighted sequences, resulting from thrombosis, fibrosis, calcification, and hemorrhage. On T2-weighted or gradient-echo images, there is a peripheral ring of hypointensity that corresponds to the deposition of hemosiderin in the surrounding brain parenchyma. CMs are angiographically occult.

In patients in whom a CM is suspected but the radiologic image is not pathognomonic, serial imaging is of value if immediate surgical intervention is not warranted. Differential diagnoses include neoplasms and hematomas. If there is a recent bleed or thrombosis in a CM, its typical features may not be evident. Perilesional and extralesional hemorrhage may be evident outside the hemosiderin ring.

Dissection of the Extracranial Cervical Arteries

Dissection of the carotid or vertebral artery can be spontaneous or traumatic. Spontaneous dissections of the carotid or vertebral artery account for 2% of all ischemic strokes, but in young and middle-aged patients they account for 10-25% of all such cases. Spontaneous dissections occur in people of all ages but there is a peak incidence in the fifth decade of life.

Dissections are more common in patients with heritable connective-tissue disorders, including Ehlers-Danlos type IV, Marfan's syndrome, polycystic kidney disease, and osteogenesis imperfecta. Angiographic changes of fibromuscular dysplasia are found in 15% of patients with spontaneous dissections of the carotid or vertebral artery. Bilateral dissections, either carotid or vertebral, are not rare.

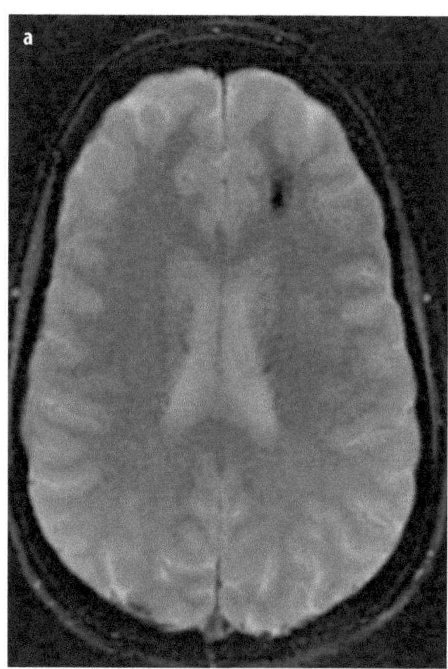

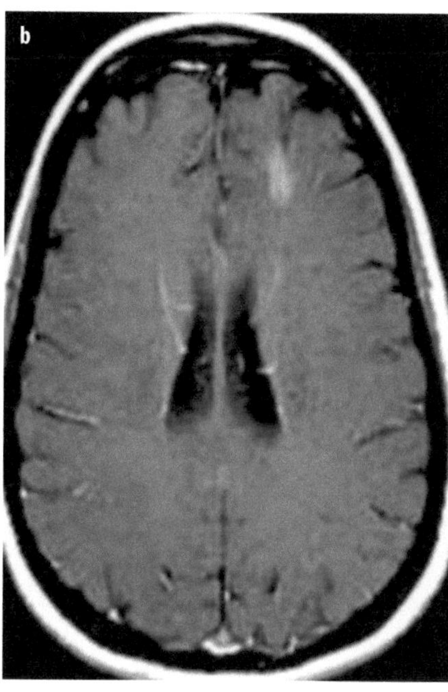

Fig. 3 a, b. Telangiectasia. Gradient-echo technique (**a**) shows a focal area of hypointensity that blushes on the post-contrast T1 study (**b**). These lesions are typically not well seen on T2 or FLAIR sequences and have no mass effect. They may have an associated developmental venous anomaly

Dissections of the carotid or vertebral artery arise from a tear of the intima. The intramural hematoma may be subintimal or subadventitial. The typical patient with carotid dissection presents with pain on one side of the face or neck, a partial Horner's syndrome (miosis, ptosis), and the delayed onset of stroke. Patients with vertebral dissection often have pain in the back of the neck, an occipital headache, and the delayed onset of posterior fossa ischemic symptoms. A lateral medullary syndrome (Wallenberg's syndrome) is commonly found.

DSA has been the traditional diagnostic test used to detect a dissection. Definitive signs of dissection are the presence of two lumens or demonstration of an intimal flap. Indirect signs are more commonly seen and include a long, irregular tapered stenosis, long tapered occlusion, or a dilatation (pseudoaneurysm) with a proximal stenosis. Carotid dissections tend to start beyond the bulb and often stop at the skull base. Vertebral dissections often occur at the C1-C2 vertebral levels and may extend into the intradural segment.

MRI is replacing DSA as the primary investigation of carotid or vertebral artery dissections. It can show the intramural hematoma, especially if fat saturation techniques are used (Fig. 4). ATECO MRA can be used to clarify the extent of the abnormality and to detect pseudoaneurysms.

Dissection of the Intracranial Arteries

Intracranial dissections are often spontaneous and may present as subarachnoid hemorrhage or stroke. The most common location is the intradural vertebral artery. Other common sites include the proximal posterior cerebral artery and the proximal posterior inferior cerebellar artery. Patients who present with hemorrhage are at high risk for re-bleeding. Non-invasive imaging may reveal an aneurysm or a long irregular stenosis. DSA often shows an irregular fusiform dilatation with a stenosis proximal to the dilatation. Assessment of collateral flow is critical since treatment often involves sacrifice of the diseased segment.

Cerebral Sinovenous Thrombosis

The clinical presentation of CVT is closely related to the location and extent of the thrombosis (cortical vs. dural sinus, superficial vs. deep). The clinical sequelae of CVT are related to the temporal evolution of the disease, the patient's venous anatomy, and the effectiveness of collateral venous pathways. The most frequent symptoms and signs of CVT are headaches, vomiting, and papilledema, the latter reflecting increased cerebral venous pressure. Patients may go on to develop seizures, decreased level of consciousness, or focal neurological deficit.

Tissue damage and stasis (trauma, surgery, and immobilization), hematologic disorders (protein C, S deficiencies; increased resistance to activated protein C), malignancies, collagen vascular disease (systemic lupus erythematosus, Behcet's syndrome), pregnancy, and some medications (oral contraceptives, hormone replacement therapy, corticosteroids) are predisposing factors for CVT.

Imaging findings of CVT can be categorized as direct, when there is visualization of a cortical or dural sinus thrombus, or indirect, when there are ischemic changes related to the venous outflow disturbance. Thrombus within the dural sinus or cortical vein can be identified as an elongated high-attenuation lesion on non-enhanced CT ("cord sign"). If the thrombus is located in the superior sagittal sinus, then a triangular filling defect ("empty delta sign") can be demonstrated on post-contrast images. The combination of MRI and contrast-enhanced MRV allows for the accurate diagnosis of CVT.

Venous infarction may be evident on CT as a diffuse low-attenuation lesion. Mass effect is common and 40% of symptomatic patients show CT evidence of hemorrhage. Bilateral, parasagittal, hypoattenuating lesions on CT are a

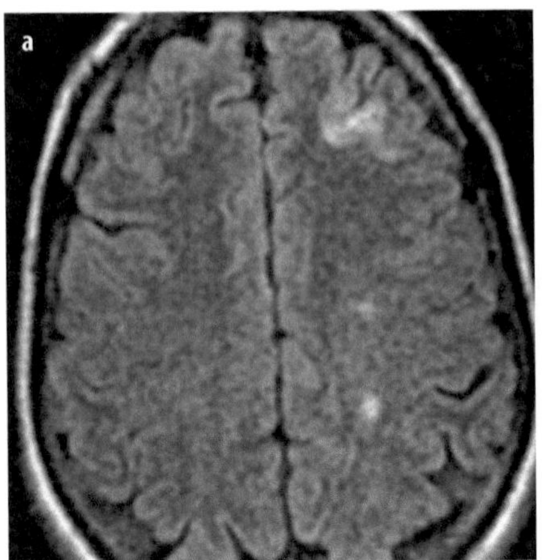

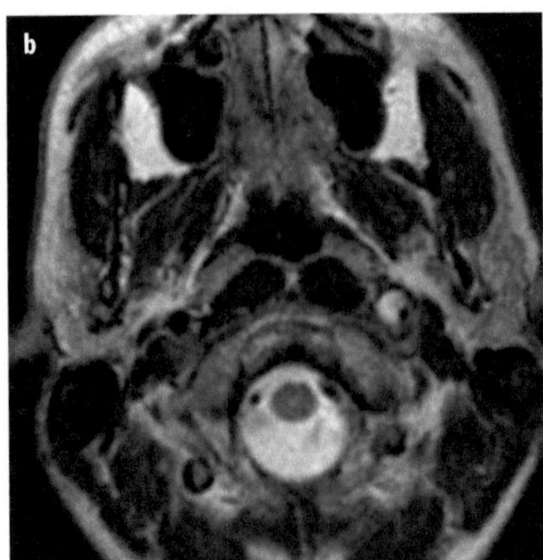

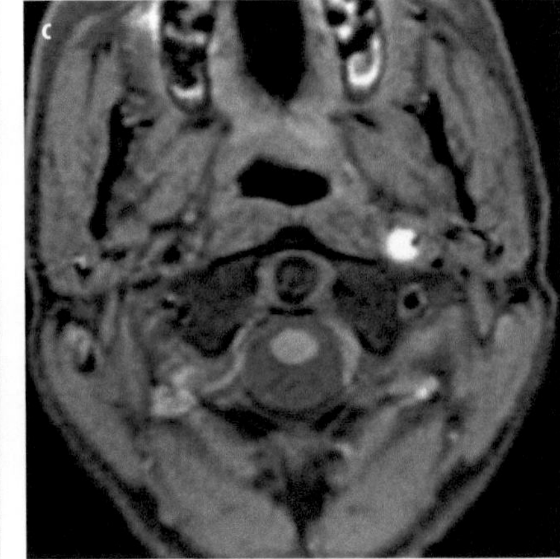

Fig. 4 a-c. Internal carotid dissection. **a** Axial FLAIR shows watershed distribution infarcts. Axial T2 (**b**) and T1 with fat saturation (**c**) show eccentric clot (methemoglobin) with a narrowed lumen (flow void) within the internal carotid artery

common feature of venous thrombosis in the superior sagittal sinus. These lesions do not conform to an arterial distribution but do involve the cortex. Isolated involvement of the temporal lobe is common and present in CVT of the transverse sinus. Bilateral thalamic hypoattenuating lesions on CT may be evident in deep venous thrombosis; on non-contrast CT, thrombus may be seen in the straight sinus.

MRI is very sensitive to the parenchymal changes that occur in CVT. Cortical and subcortical lesions with high signal intensity on FLAIR and T2-weighted imaging are highly suggestive of CVT when the lesions do not correspond to an arterial territory. Restricted diffusion in CVT may not have the same prognostic value as it does in arterial stroke and there may be reversibility of venous ischemia in CVT. These findings correlate with the important clinical improvement that may occur after an initial major neurological deficit related to CVT.

Intracranial Dural Arteriovenous Fistulas

Dural arteriovenous fistulas (DAVFs) represent 10-15% of all intracranial arteriovenous lesions. They consist of one or more true fistulas, i.e., direct arteriovenous connections without an intervening capillary bed, localized within the dura mater. DAVFs have been categorized as being benign or aggressive depending on their venous drainage and clinical symptoms. Benign DAVFs drain into the dural sinuses only, whereas aggressive DAVFs have reflux into the cortical veins. Aggressive DAVFs are associated with non-hemorrhagic neurological deficits, hemorrhage, and death, while chronic headache, pulsatile bruit, and orbital symptoms, including cranial nerve deficit due to cavernous sinus lesions (ophthalmoplegia), are indicative of benign DAVFs. Aggressive DAVFs have an annual risk of intracranial hemorrhage or non-hemorrhagic neurological deficits of 8.1 and 6.9%, respectively, adding up to a 15.0% annual event rate. Aggressive DAVFs must be treated whereas benign DAVFs may not require treatment if the symptoms are stable and well-tolerated.

The term venous congestive encephalopathy describes the conditions of those patients who present with neurological deficits caused by venous hypertension secondary to cortical venous reflux from a DAVF. This entity is analogous to the venous congestive myelopathy of the spinal cord in the presence of a spinal DAVF. On MRI T2-weighted images, hyperintensity in the parenchyma can be seen as a result of the venous hypertension and passive congestion of the brain. In the cerebral and cerebellar hemispheres, the deep white matter seems to be the most vulnerable, and after treatment these findings may be partially reversible. In the cerebellum, a peripheral diffuse enhancement pattern surrounding the central T2 hyperintensity is characteristic of DAVFs with cortical venous reflux. The combination of central T2 hyperintensity with a surplus of pial vessels is highly suggestive of a vascular malformation and mandates a time-resolved gadolinium-enhanced MRA.

Moyamoya Disease

Moyamoya disease is a primary vascular disease characterized by progressive stenosis and eventual occlusion of the supraclinoid portion of the internal carotid artery and the adjacent segments of the middle and anterior cerebral arteries. In response, an abnormal vascular network of small collateral vessels develops to bypass the area of occlusion. This disease affects children as well as adults. Adults tend to present with hemorrhage. The most frequent symptoms in children are multiple transient ischemic attack; some episodes result in a fixed deficit. Seizures are a common presentation of patients under the age of 6 years. The small collateral vessels at the base of the brain are enlarged lenticulostriate vessels. These collaterals may be evident on MRI and on DSA and represent the "puff of smoke" appearance characteristic of this disease. DSA may reveal transdural anastomoses and collateral pial vessels crossing watershed territories. Cerebral vascular reactivity studies using MRI are done to assess the vascular reserve and the need for a vascular bypass.

Central Nervous System Vasculitis

This condition is an inflammation of blood vessel walls that results in ischemia. Vasculitis affecting the CNS alone is referred to as primary angiitis of the CNS. Secondary vasculitis occurs in association with a variety of conditions, including infections, drug abuse, lymphoproliferative disease, and connective tissue diseases. Patients typically present with stroke, encephalopathy, or seizures.

MRI findings suggestive of vasculitis are multiple, bilateral lesions in the cortex and white matter. The presence of gray matter involvement should help differentiate the white matter lesions from demyelination. In approximately 20% of proven cases, DSA shows abnormalities in the cerebral arteries, including segmental narrowing, microaneurysms, and vascular beading. In vasculitis affecting the large and medium-sized cranial arteries, wall imaging with contrast may show circumferential thickening and enhancement.

Suggested Reading

Alvarez-Linera J, Benito-Leon J, Escribano J et al (2003) Prospective evaluation of carotid artery stenosis: elliptic centric contrast-enhanced MR angiography and spiral CT angiography compared with digital subtraction angiography. AJNR Am J Neuroradiol 24:1012-1019

Farb R, Scott JN, Willinsky R et al (2003) Intracranial venous system: gadolinium-enhanced three-dimensional MR venography with auto-trigerred elliptic centric-oredered sequence-initial experience. Radiology 226:203-209

Lev MH, Romero JM, Goodman DNF et al (2003) Total occlusion versus hairline residual lumen of the internal carotid arteries: accuracy of single section helical CT angiography. AJNR Am J of Neuroradiol 24:1123-1129

Meckel S, Maier M, San Millan Ruiz D et al (2007) MR angiography of dural arteriovenous fistulas: diagnosis and follow-up after treatment using a time-resolved 3D contrast-enhanced technique. AJNR Am J Neuroradiol 28:877-884

Rivera P, Willinsky R, Porter P (2003) Intracranial cavernous malformations. In: Willinsky MD (ed) Neuroimaging clinics of North America. Venous disorders of the central nervous system. WB Saunders, Philadelphia, pp 27-40

VanDijk JMC, Willinsky R (2003) Venous congestive encephalopathy related to cranial dural arteriovenous fistulas. In: Willinsky MD (ed) Neuroimaging clinics of North America. Venous disorders of the central nervous system. WB Saunders, Philadelphia, pp 55-72

Yoon DY, Lim KJ, Choi CS et al (2007) Detection and characterization of intracranial aneurysms with 16-channel multidetector row CT angiography: a prospective comparison of volume-rendered images and digital subtraction angiography. AJNR Am J Neuroradiol 28:60-67

Brain Ischemia

Majda M. Thurnher[1], Jens Fiehler[2]

[1] Department of Radiology, Medical University of Vienna, Vienna, Austria

[2] Klinik und Polikinik für Neuroradiologische Diagnostik und Intervention, Universitättsklinikum Hamburg-Eppendorf (UKE), Hamburg, Germany

A central issue in treating patients with *acute stroke* is the existence of potentially salvageable tissue. The goal of imaging is to diagnose the precise type of stroke so that appropriate management can be promptly implemented. Diagnostic imaging of acute stroke should reliably help to: (1) exclude intracranial hemorrhage; (2) differentiate between irreversibly affected brain tissue ("dead brain") and reversibly impaired tissue ("tissue at risk") that might benefit from early treatment; and (3) identify stenosis or occlusion of major extra- and intracranial arteries [1].

Computed tomography (CT) is still considered the "gold standard" for detecting cerebral hemorrhage. Its 24/7 availability is one of the major advantages of CT. Typically, 60% of infarcts will be seen 3-6 h after clinical onset, and all infarcts will be seen after 24 h. Early CT depicts hypodensity of the brain parenchyma, which reflects cytotoxic edema secondary to failure of ion pumps in response to an inadequate supply of ATP. The attenuation in HU on CT scans is directly proportional to the degree of cytotoxic edema. An increase in tissue water content of 1% will result in a 2.5% decrease in parenchymal attenuation. Early CT signs of infarct are the dense middle cerebral artery (MCA) sign; the insular ribbon sign; obscuration of the lentiform nucleus; and hypoattenuation of the brain parenchyma [2-6].

Loss of the insular ribbon on unenhanced CT scans is a very common early sign of infarction in the MCA territory. This is due to the anatomic supply of the insular cortex, which is the region most distant from the potential collateral flow from the anterior (ACA) or posterior (PCA) cerebral artery distributions [6]. Obscuration of the lentiform nucleus is another early CT sign of MCA or internal carotid artery (ICA) infarction and reflects cellular edema that arises in the basal ganglionic region [2]. Increased density in a cerebral artery represents thrombus or embolus. Hyperdensity will be seen along the course of the artery, but usually diminishes or disappears after 1-2 weeks (Fig. 1) [4].

The analysis of the early signs of stroke on CT, in a large cohort of patients within 6 h after the onset of stroke, have shown that hypodensity on CT is highly specific for irreversible ischemic brain damage if detection occurs within the first 6 h. Patients without early CT signs usually have a more favorable clinical course [7]. CT is an excellent technique not only for detecting cerebral hemorrhage, but also for identifying initially hemorrhagic infarcts.

About 15% of MCA infarction is initially hemorrhagic. Secondary hemorrhage is also not uncommon in MCA infarcts, usually after 1-3 days or after thrombolytic therapy.

The one-third rule for acute middle cerebral artery stroke (1/3 MCA rule) is usually considered before treating patients with recombinant tissue plasminogen activator (rTPA). It is a volumetric estimation of the size of the cerebral infarction of the MCA [8]. A 10-point quantitative topographic CT scan score, the Alberta Stroke Program Early CT Score (ASPECTS), has also been introduced and rated as a systematic, robust, and practical method [8].

Intracranial and neck vessels can be evaluated with CT angiography (CTA) [9]. CTA of the intracranial vessels can demonstrate the presence and the exact location of occlusions, carotid dissection, vertebralis dissection, and plaque formations. Additionally, source images from CTA have higher sensitivity than unenhanced CT (Fig. 2).

Perfusion CT is a relatively new technique that allows rapid quantitative and qualitative evaluation of cerebral perfusion. Perfusion CT (PCT) studies are obtained by monitoring the first pass of iodinated contrast agent through the cerebral vasculature. There is a linear relationship between the concentration of contrast material and attenuation [10, 11]. Contrast agent vs. time concentration curves are generated in an arterial region of interest (ROI), a venous ROI, and in each pixel. Perfusion studies have some important benefits: (1) normal or near-normal diffusion and CT data cannot preclude a large ischemic penumbra; and (2) 26% of patients require perfusion studies for the diagnosis. An interesting study comparing PCT and diffusion-weighted imaging (DWI) in the detection of acute stroke was recently presented at a meeting of the Radiological Society of North America (RSNA) [12]. The results, comparing 76 patients with stroke, showed that, compared to DWI, PCT is highly sensitive and specific for the detection of hyperacute nonlacunar strokes in the 3-h intravenous tPA window (Fig. 3) [12].

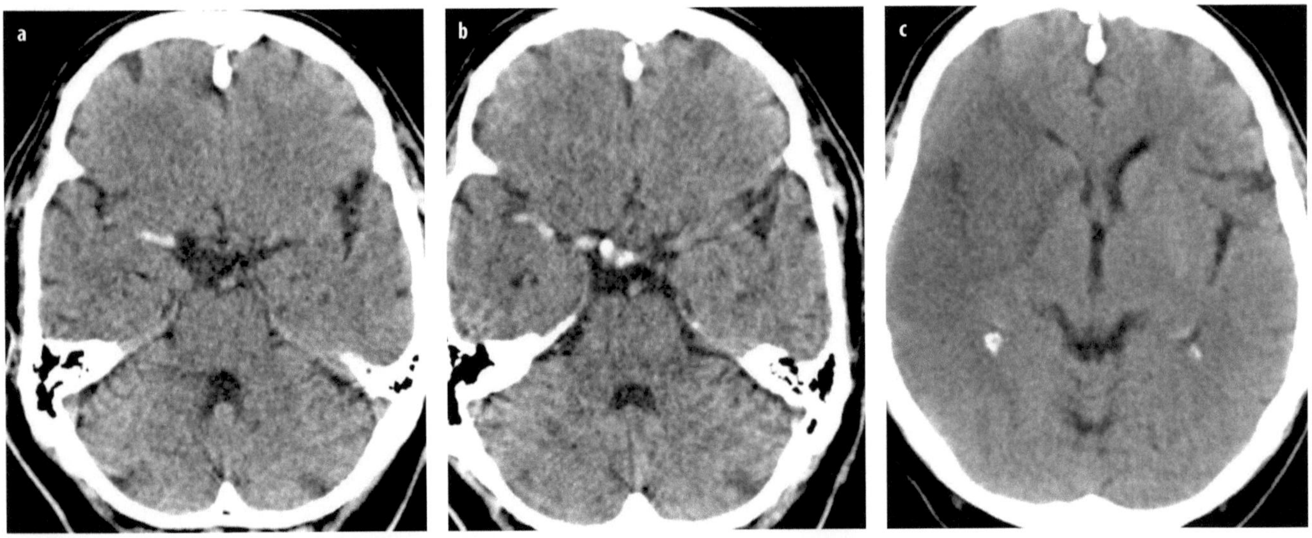

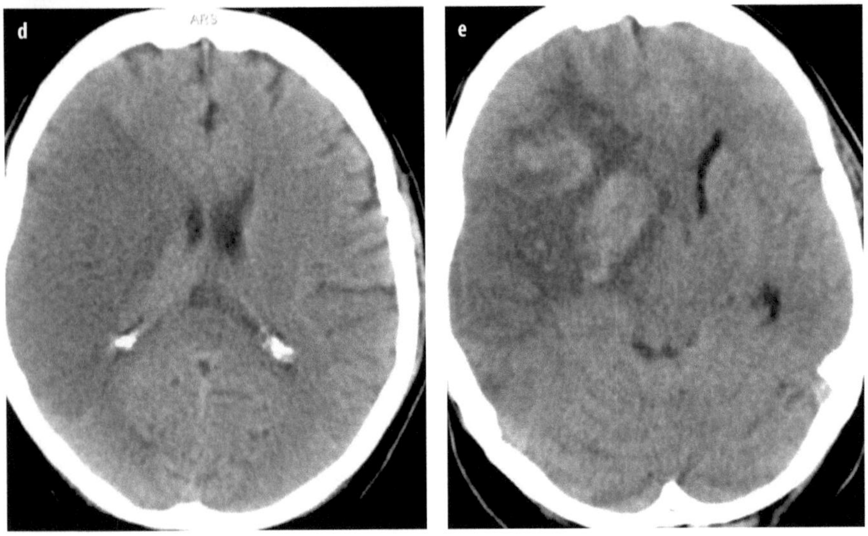

Fig. 1 a-e. Acute right MCA infarct in a 60-year-old male patient. **a**, **b** On initial unenhanced CT scan of the brain, hyperdensity along the right middle cerebral artery ("dense MCA") is noted (early CT sign of MCA infarct). **c**, **d** On follow-up CT scan 1 day later, hypodensity in the vascular territory of the right MCA is clearly depicted. **e** Hemorrhagic transformation of the MCA infarction is detected 48 h after the onset of symptoms

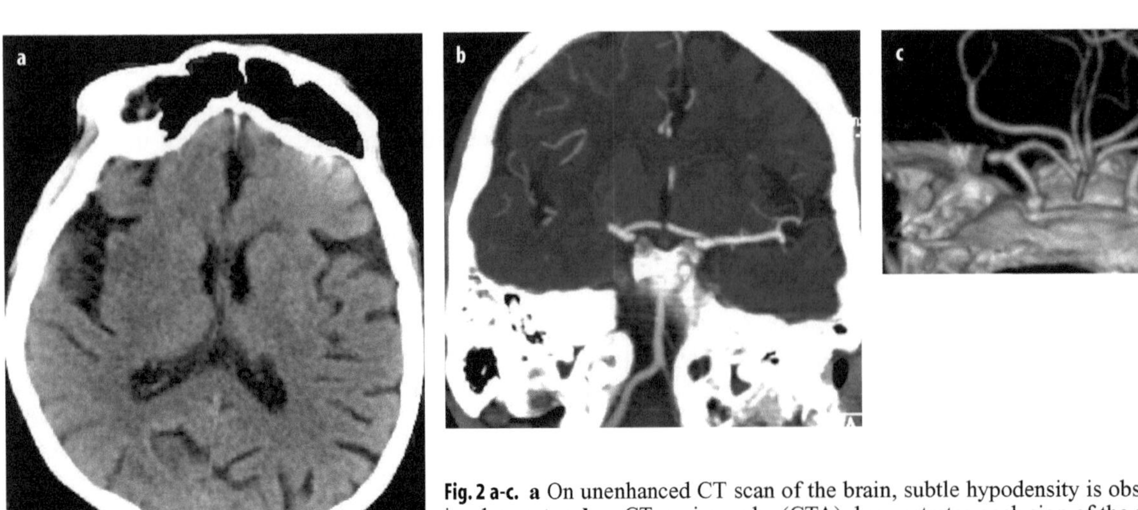

Fig. 2 a-c. **a** On unenhanced CT scan of the brain, subtle hypodensity is observed in the right insular cortex. **b**, **c** CT angiography (CTA) demonstrates occlusion of the right middle cerebral artery

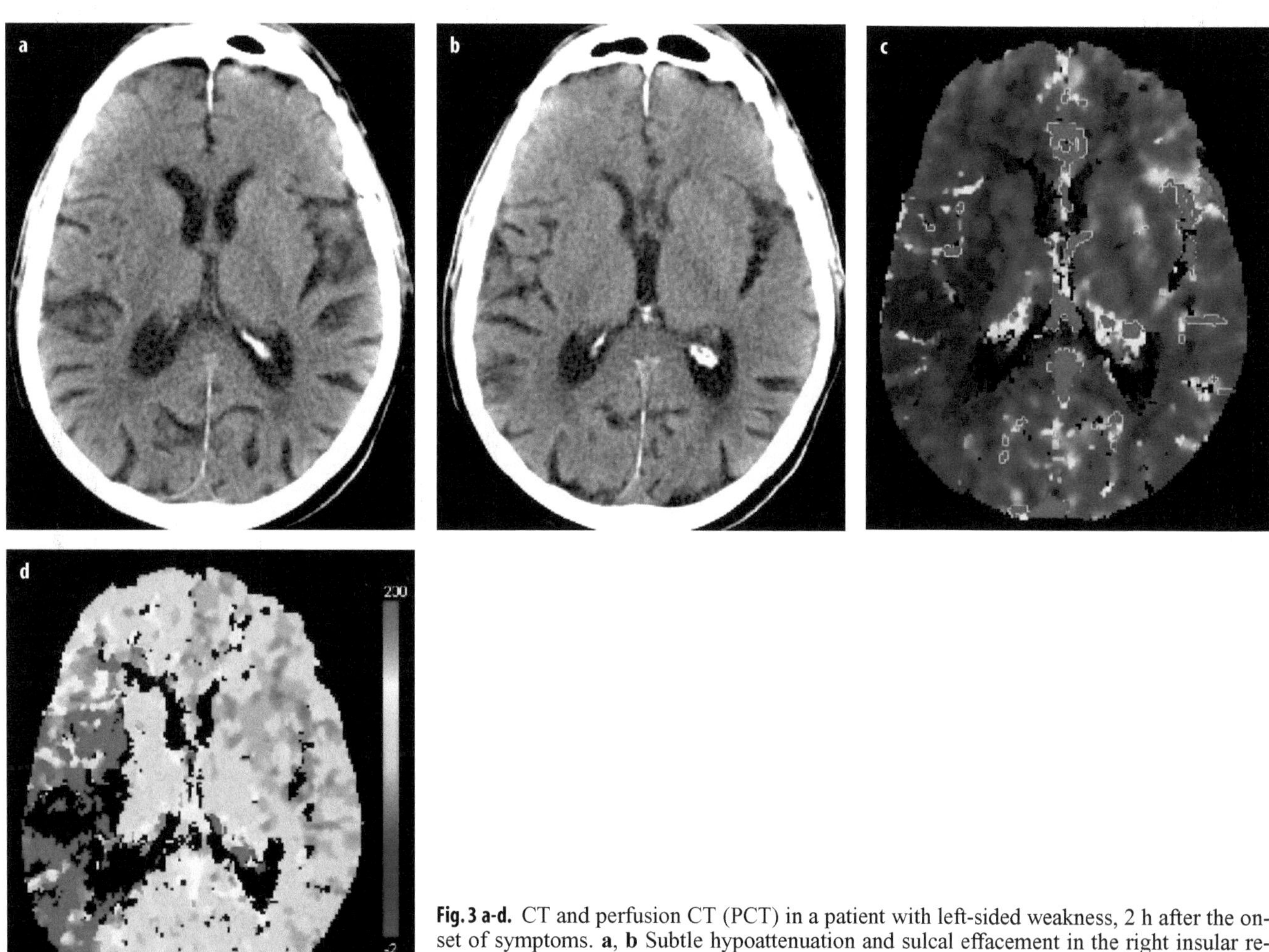

Fig. 3 a-d. CT and perfusion CT (PCT) in a patient with left-sided weakness, 2 h after the onset of symptoms. **a**, **b** Subtle hypoattenuation and sulcal effacement in the right insular region are noted on unenhanced CT of the brain. **c**, **d** Low perfusion is detected in the region of the right MCA on PCT maps (time-to-peak, cerebral blood volume). (Courtesy of Bidyut K. Pramanik, New York University, NY, USA)

Damage to the blood-brain-barrier (BBB) after ischemic stroke can be quantitatively evaluated with PCT by calculating *permeability*. Elevated permeability is associated with an increased risk for hemorrhagic transformation. One study reported the usefulness of permeability measurements in predicting hemorrhagic transformation in acute stroke [13].

On conventional magnetic resonance imaging (MRI) sequences, regions of increased signal intensity are seen on proton density (PD), T2, and fluid-attenuated inversion-recovery (FLAIR) magnetic resonance images a few hours after the onset of stroke symptoms. Approximately 80% of infarction will be detected on MRI within 24 h. However, MRI may be negative until 2-4 hours post-ictus. Increased signal intensity (SI) on PD/T2WI and FLAIR reflects changes in intracellular water, membrane dysfunction (Na/K pumps), and diminished binding of water. This suggests that the changes in SI on MRI represent irreversible injury, cell death, and infarction. Recent studies reported increased intensity in cerebral blood vessels on FLAIR images and intravascular SI loss on gradient echo images (GRE), with a sensitivity varying between 40 and 100% [14]. The increased intravascular signal intensity on FLAIR images is most likely due to a combination of factors: slow flow; flow-related enhancement; and clot SI (oxyhemoglobin) [15].

Magnetic resonance angiography (MRA) can be used to evaluate intracerebral and neck vessels. The best results have been reported when contrast-enhanced MRA (CE-MRA) is employed.

Diffusion-weighted MRI (DWI) is a technique sensitive to the restriction of Brownian motion of extracellular water due to the imbalance caused by cytotoxic edema [16, 17]. Acute ischemic lesions are characterized by a high signal on DWI and a low apparent diffusion coefficient (ADC) value due to the shift of water from the extracellular to the intracellular compartment (Fig. 4). Restricted diffusion in acute ischemic lesions is attributed to: accumulation of intracellular water; cytotoxic edema; disruption of high-energy metabolism; and loss of ion homeostasis. DWI is nearly always positive 1 h after the clinical onset of symptoms [18]. Visual assessment of diffusion images

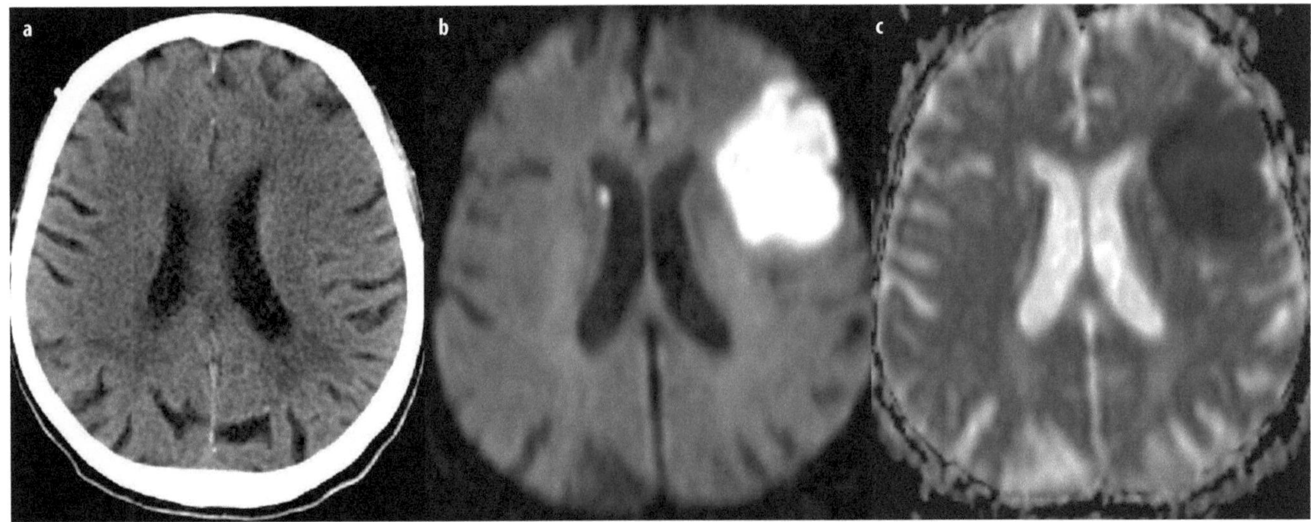

Fig. 4 a-c. Comparison of nonenhanced computed tomography (NECT) and diffusion-weighted MRI (DWI) in the detection of acute ischemia (both imaging modalities performed 3 h after onset). **a** NECT scan of the brain shows subtle hypodensity in the left frontal region. **b** Increased signal intensity is shown on DWI in the affected region. **c** Low apparent diffusion coefficient (ADC) value on the ADC map suggests restricted diffusion in acute ischemia

is uncomplicated and fast. Signal intensities on T2 increase over time. ADC gradually decreases over time, but remains significantly decreased relative to the value of the contralateral normal brain for the first 7 days [19-21].

Enhanced *perfusion MR imaging* has become one of the most important noninvasive neuroradiological MRI techniques in the last several years. Dynamic T2*-weighted gradient echoplanar imaging (EPI) sequences are used to examine cerebral perfusion of the whole brain, utilizing the T2-effect of conventional MR contrast medium. Contrast molecules behave as paramagnetic particles and induce local changes in the magnetic field [22].

The medical concept of *penumbra* was first described in 1970, based on experiments done in baboons. Following an ischemic insult, a penumbral region exists around densely ischemic, irreversibly damaged tissue. The "core" of the infarct is represented by areas of diminished blood flow and cell death; this tissue rapidly undergoes irreversible injury. However, cells in the peripheral zones are supported by collateral circulation. This peripheral region, termed the "ischemic penumbra", contains tissue that may be salvaged with prompt institution of the appropriate therapy. Reduction of cerebral blood flow from 50 ml/100g per min to 20 ml/100 g per min leads to impaired function but preserved tissue integrity (penumbra). A reduction in cerebral blood flow <20 ml/100 g per min results in oligemia. The recognition of possibly reversible and salvageable tissue around the infarct is the most important part of imaging in acute stroke [23, 24]. Penumbra is characterized by a DWI-PWI (per-

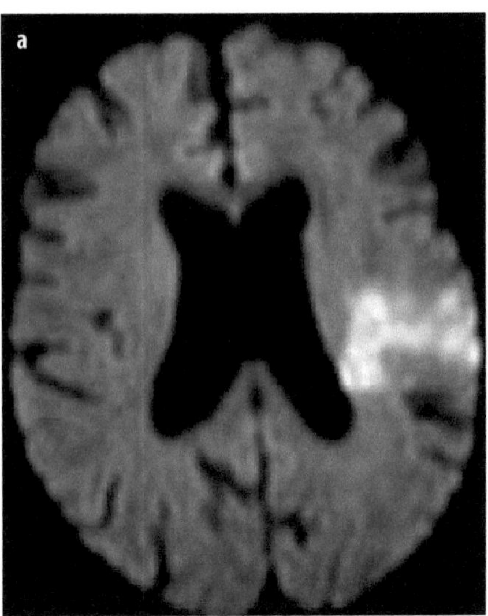

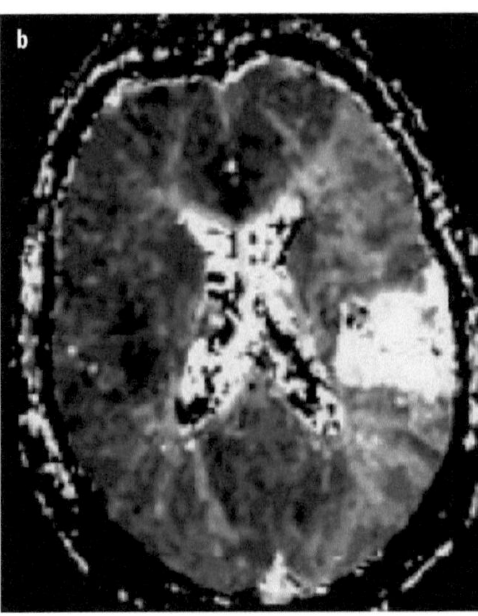

Fig. 5 a, b. Diffusion-perfusion mismatch in a patient with acute stroke. **a** High signal intensity is noted on diffusion-weighted MRI (DWI) in the left parietal region, which is indicative of restricted diffusion in the acute ischemic lesion and represents "dead tissue". **b** On perfusion MR, a much larger area of low perfusion is shown (left MCA territory)

fusion-weighted MRI) mismatch: (1) areas with abnormal signal on DWI and low perfusion progress to infarction; and (2) areas that are normal on DWI, with perfusion reduced to the penumbral level, have the ability to either recover or progress to infarction (Fig. 5) [25].

The recently use of desmoteplase in an acute ischemic stroke phase II trial illustrated three important things: (1) thrombolysis beyond 3 h is effective if an appropriate tool (i.e., stroke MRI) for patient selection is applied; (2) reperfusion on stroke MRI parallels clinical outcome, showing that stroke MRI findings may be used as a surrogate parameter for outcome; and (3) the therapeutic effect on clinical and MRI outcomes does not depend on time to treatment. Patient selection may actually be more important than time [26]. Desmoteplase is a novel plasminogen activator that selectively activates fibrin-bound plasminogen and is currently being investigated for the treatment of acute ischemic stroke within a time window of 3-9 h after symptom onset.

According to currently available knowledge, the key pathophysiological concept in stroke management is the distinction of hypoperfused tissue into three operational compartments: tissue that will inevitably die (core); tissue that will, in principle, survive (oligemia); and tissue that may either die or survive (the ischemic penumbra) [27].

Finally, what tests should be performed in acute stroke: CT, MRI, or both? DWI is clearly superior to CT in the detection of acute ischemic lesions. However, among patients with moderate to severe acute ischemic stroke, the ability of CT to detect signs of early infarction was comparable with DWI, in a recently published study [28]. Furthermore, studies have shown that DWI is not predictive of lesion growth; it cannot predict outcome nor is DWI-PWI mismatch predictive of lesion growth [29]. The results of recent studies have raised doubts about the significance of the DWI-PWI model of penumbra. Perfusion overestimates "tissue at risk", and DWI does not represent irreversible injury [30-32].

Current knowledge about imaging in stroke increases constantly. To date, findings indicate that: DWI does not only represent irreversibly injured tissue, and a DWI abnormality can include the core and the penumbra; thrombolysis beyond 3 h can still be effective; reperfusion on stroke MRI parallels clinical outcome; the therapeutic effect on clinical and MRI outcomes may not depend on time to treatment. High specificity and inter-rater reliability may make MRI mismatch scores an ideal rapid screening tool for potential thrombolysis patients [33].

References

1. Thurnher MM, Castillo M (2005) Imaging in acute stroke. Eur Radiol 15:408-415
2. Tomura N, Uemura K, Inugami A et al (1988) Early CT finding in cerebral infarction: obscuration of the lentiform nucleus. Radiology 168:463-467
3. Unger E, Littlefield J, Gado M (1988) Water content and water structure in CT and MR signal changes: possible influence in detection of early stroke. AJNR Am J Neuroradiol 9:687-691
4. Pressman BD, Tourje EJ, Thompson JR (1987) An early sign of ischemic infarction: increased density in a cerebral artery. AJNR Am J Neuroradiol 8:645-648
5. Schuierer G, Huk W (1988) The unilateral hyperdense middle cerebral artery: an early CT-sign of embolism or thrombosis. Neuroradiology 30:120-122
6. Truwit CL, Barkovich AJ, Gean-Marton A et al (1990) Loss of insular ribbon: another early CT sign of acute middle cerebral artery infarction. Radiology 176:801-806
7. Von Kummer R, Bourquain H, Bastianello S et al (2001) Early prediction of irreversible brain damage after ischemic stroke at CT. Radiology 219:95-100
8. Pexman JH, Barber PA, Hill MD et al (2001) Use of the Alberta Stroke Program Early CT Score (ASPECTS) for assessing CT scans in patients with acute stroke. AJNR Am J Neuroradiol 22(8):1534-1542
9. Tomandl BF, Klotz E, Handschu R et al (2003) Comprehensive imaging of ischemic stroke with multisection CT. Radiographics 23:565-592
10. Hoeffner EG, Case I, Jain R et al (2004) Cerebral perfusion CT: technique and clinical applications. Radiology 231:632-644
11. Miles KA (2003) Acute cerebral stroke imaging and brain perfusion with the use of high-concentration contrast media. Eur Radiol 13:M117-M120
12. Lin K, Kazmi KS, Law M et al (2006) Comparison of perfusion CT with DWI for detection of hyperacute ischemic stroke. Abstract RSNA
13. Lin K, Kazmi KS, Law M et al (2007) Measuring elevated microvascular permeability and predicting hemorrhagic transformation in acute ischemic stroke using first-pass dynamic perfusion CT imaging. AJNR Am J Neuroradiol 28:1292-1298
14. Schellinger P, Chalela JA, Kang DW et al (2005) Diagnostic and prognostic value of early MR imaging vessel signs in hyperacute stroke patients imaged < 3 hours and treated with recombinant tissue plasminogen activator. AJNR Am J Neuroradiol 26:618-624
15. Wolf RL (2001) Intraarterial signal on fluid-attenuated inversion recovery images: a measure of hemodynamic stress? AJNR Am J Neuroradiol 22:1015-1016
16. Huisman TA (2003) Diffusion-weighted imaging: basic concepts and application in cerebral stroke and head trauma. Eur Radiol 13:2283-2297
17. LeBihan D, Breton E, Lallemand D et al (1986) MR imaging of intravoxel incoherent motions: application to diffusion and perfusion in neurological disorders. Radiology 161:401-407
18. Schlaug G, Siewert B, Benfield A et al (1997) Time course of the apparent diffusion coefficient (ADC) abnormalities in human stroke. Neurology 49:113-119
19. Mullins ME, Schaefer PW, Sorensen AG et al (2002) CT and conventional and diffusion-weighted MR imaging in acute stroke: study in 691 patients at presentation to the emergency department. Radiology 224:353-360
20. Lansberg MG, Thijs VN, O'Brien MW et al (2001) Evolution of apparent diffusion coefficient, diffusion-weighted, and T2-weighted signal intensity of acute stroke. AJNR Am J Neuroradiol 22:637-644
21. Burdette J, Ricci PE, Petitti N, Elster AD (1998) Cerebral infarction: time course of signal intensity changes on diffusion-weighted MR images. AJR Am J Roentgenol 171:791-795
22. Nasel C, Azizi A, Veintimilla A et al (2000) A standardized method of generating time-to-peak perfusion maps in dynamic-susceptibility contrast-enhanced MR imaging. AJNR Am J Neuroradiol 21:1195-1198
23. Astrup J, Siesjo B, Symon L (1981) Thresholds in cerebral ischemia: the ischemic penumbra. Stroke 12:723-725
24. Markus HS (2994) Cerebral perfusion and stroke. J Neurol Neurosurg Psychiatry 75:353-361

25. Gonzales RG (2006) Imaging-guided acute ischemic stroke therapy: from "time is brain" to "physiology is brain". AJNR Am J Neuroradiol 27:728-735
26. Rowley HA (2005) Extending the time window for thrombolysis: evidence from acute stroke trials. Neuroimaging Clin N Am 15(3):575-587
27. Muir KW, Buchan A, von Kummer R et al (2006) Imaging of acute stroke. Lancet 5:755-768
28. Barber PA, Hill MD, Eliasziw M et al (2005) Imaging of the brain in acute ischemic stroke: comparison of CT and DWI. J Neurol Neurosurg Psychiatry 76(11):1528-1533
29. Mezzapesa DM, Petruzzellis M, Lucivero V et al (2006) Multimodal MR examination in acute ischemic stroke. Neuroradiology 48(4):238-246
30. Hand PJ, Wardlaw JM, Rivers CS et al (2006) MR diffusion-weighted imaging and outcome prediction after ischemic stroke. Neurology 66: 1159-1163
31. Köhrmann M, Jüttler E, Fiebach JB et al (2006) MRI versus CT-based thrombolysis treatment within and beyond the 3h time window after stroke onset: a cohort study. Lancet Neurol 5:661-667
32. Schellinger PD, Fiebach JB (2005) Perfusion-weighted imaging / diffusion-weighted imaging mismatch on MRI can now be used to select patients for recombinant tissue plasminogen activator beyond 3 hours. Controversies in stroke. Stroke 36:1098-1101
33. Butcher K, Parsons M, Allport L et al; EPITHET Investigators (2008) Rapid assessment of perfusion-diffusion mismatch. Stroke 39(1):75-81

Hemorrhagic Vascular Pathology - I

James Byrne

Department of Neuroradiology, Nuffield Department of Surgery, University of Oxford, Oxford, UK

Introduction

There are a variety of vascular pathologies that affect the brain and intracranial tissues and cause hemorrhagic *stroke*, i.e. a sudden, non-convulsive, loss of neurological function. However the term can be extended to include all types of spontaneous intracranial hemorrhage, such as subarachnoid hemorrhage, which may or may not cause a focal neurological deficit.

The causes of first-ever-in-a-lifetime stroke have been shown to be ischemic in 80%, due to intracerebral hemorrhage in 15%, subarachnoid hemorrhage in 5% and uncertain in 5% of patients reported in studies performed after CT became available. The uncertain category includes patients with possible secondary hemorrhages within areas of cerebral infarction and those without CT or autopsy diagnosis.

This brief chapter is intended to outline a logical strategy for managing the imaging of patients presenting after spontaneous intracranial hemorrhage and the diagnosis of vascular pathology. Details of the patient's acute and past medical histories may point to the cause of intracranial bleeding but in most instances it is imaging that distinguishes the victims of hemorrhagic from those with ischemic stroke. This crucial distinction triggers completely different diagnostic and therapeutic management paths.

The diagnosis of stroke is clinical and usually straight forward. Patients are referred for emergency CT brain scan and this should be performed without radiographic contrast as soon as possible. Identification of acute hemorrhage confirms the diagnosis of hemorrhagic stroke. The protocols described herein serve to identify underlying vascular pathologies. The immediate imperative is to diagnose lesions that require interventions to prevent rebleeding or progression. These lesions are most commonly vascular; in some circumstances, emergency interventions may be life-saving. It is therefore important for imaging to be appropriate and timely.

How Should the Patient with Hemorrhagic Stroke Be Investigated?

The first step is to triage patients into those likely to have an underlying structural lesion carrying a risk of rebleeding, those likely to have a "non-structural" cause that requires urgent diagnosis and treatment and those with a low incidence of an underlying lesion and therefore do not require urgent interventions. This process starts with the initial unenhanced CT brain scan and is summarised in the flow diagram below. The scheme outlined is based on determining the site and distribution of hemorrhage, i.e. whether it is within the brain (intracerebral hemorrhage) or in an extracerebral compartment (subarachnoid, intraventricular or subdural). In many instances hemorrhage may extend into more than one compartment; therefore, the scan must be analysed to identify both the origin of bleeding and the likely site of a structural vascular pathology (Fig. 1).

Causes of Spontaneous Intracranial Hemorrhage

The causes of bleeding are considered by the primary site of the hemorrhage they cause.

Intracerebral Hemorrhage

Location

Basal ganglia or thalamus:

- Atherosclerosis (commonly associated with systemic hypertension)
- Lipohyalinosis
- Arteriovenous malformation (AVM), including cavernous malformations and cryptic AVMs
- Tumor
- Isolated angiitis of the CNS
- Bleeding diathesis/hematological disorders
- Moyamoya

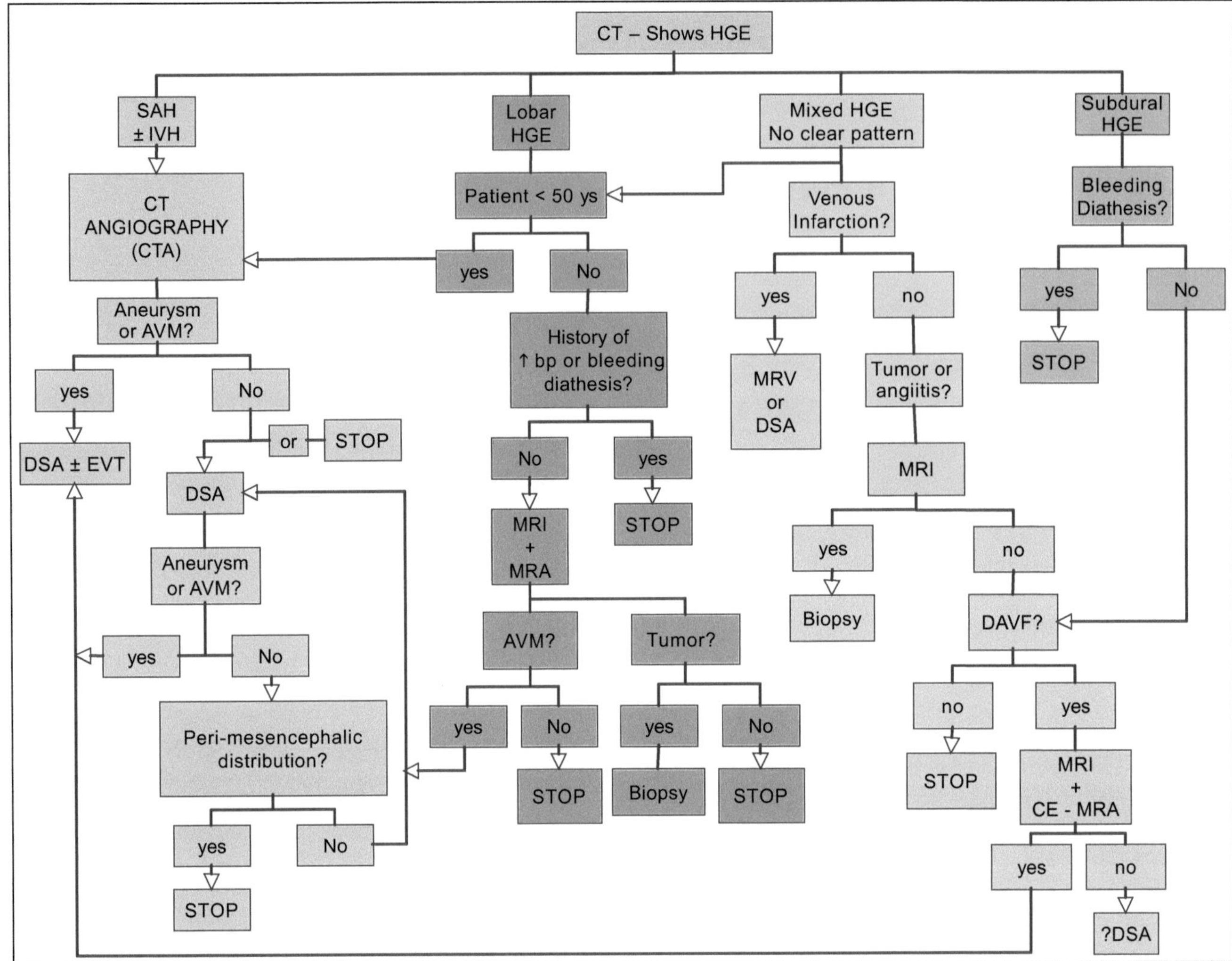

Fig. 1. Diagram of investigation after spontaneous intracranial hemorrhage. *CT*, Computed tomography; *HGE*, hemorrhage; *SAH*, subarachnoid hemorrhage; *IVH*, intraventricular hemorrhage; *AVM*, arteriovenous malformation; *MRV*, magnetic resonance venography; *DSA*, digital subtraction angiography; *EVT*, endovascular treatment; *MRI*, magnetic resonance imaging; *MRA*, magnetic resonance angiography; *DAVF*, dural arteriovenous malformation; *CE-MRA*, contrast enhanced magnetic resonance angiography

Lobar:
- Hemorrhagic transformation of ischemic stroke
- AVM, including cavernous malformations and cryptic AVMs
- Tumor
- Saccular aneurysm (distal or infectious types)
- Venous thrombosis
- Amyloid angiopathy
- Isolated angiitis of the CNS
- Substance abuse (e.g. amphetamine/cocaine)
- Bleeding diathesis/hematological disorders
- Paraneoplastic syndromes
- Hereditary hemorrhagic telangiectasia

Cerebellum and brainstem:
- Atherosclerosis and lipohyalinosis
- AVM, including cavernous malformations and cryptic AVMs
- Tumor
- Amyloid angiopathy
- Bleeding diathesis/hematological disorders

Subarachnoid Hemorrhage

Commonly:
- Saccular aneurysm
- Arterial dissection
- Angiogram-negative perimesencephalic hemorrhage

Rarely:
- Brain or spinal AVM/arteriovenous fistula
- Dural arteriovenous fistula
- Pituitary apoplexy
- Infections aneurysms
- Marfan's syndrome/pseudoxanthoma elasticum with aneurysm
- Cocaine abuse
- Sickle cell disease (children)
- Bleeding diathesis (e.g. excessive anticoagulation)

Subdural Hemorrhage

- Saccular aneurysm
- Rupture of small transpial veins
- Moyamoya
- Dural arteriovenous fistula
- Dural metastases
- Bleeding diathesis/hematological disorders

Suggested Reading

Davis S, Fisher M, Warach S (eds) (2003) Magnetic resonance imaging in stroke. Cambridge University Press, Cambridge, UK

Moritani T, Ekholm S, Westesson PL (2003) Diffusion-weighted MR imaging of the brain. Springer, Heidelberg New York

Warlow CP, Dennis MS, van Gijn J et al (eds) (1996) Stroke. A practical guide to management. Blackwell Science, Oxford

Hemorrhagic Vascular Pathology - II

Martin Wiesmann

Department of Neurosurgery, Ludwig-Maximilians-University, Munich, Germany

Introduction

Intracranial hemorrhage is a frequent indication for neuroimaging and accounts for about 10% of all strokes. Computed tomography (CT) remains the standard method to detect intracranial hemorrhage, although radiologists need also be familiar with the magnetic resonance imaging (MRI) appearance of hematomas.

The first step is to confirm or exclude the presence of a hemorrhage, identify the anatomic compartment it is located in, and approximate the age of the hemorrhage. The next step is to triage patients into those likely to have an underlying cause that requires urgent diagnosis and treatment, and those who do not require urgent interventions. To do this, neuroimaging findings need to be considered in combination with the age and medical history of the patient.

Imaging Intracranial Hemorrhage

To understand the appearance of blood clots on CT and MRI, some knowledge of the mechanism of clot formation is helpful. Initially, an intracerebral hematoma consists of intact red blood cells (RBCs) containing mainly oxygen-saturated hemoglobin (oxyhemoglobin, OxyHb). The hemoglobin is then gradually deoxygenated. At 48 h post-hemorrhage, the clot consists almost entirely of deoxyhemoglobin (DeoxyHb). The hematoma is surrounded by a rim of edema. In the early subacute phase (3-7 days) DeoxyHb is gradually converted to methemoglobin (MetHb). These changes begin at the periphery of the clot and then progress towards the center. In the late subacute phase (2-4 weeks), the RBCs lyse and MetHb is released from the intracellular into the extracellular space. In this stage the edema gradually dissolves. Later on, in the chronic phase (>4 weeks), the hematoma shrinks to finally form a small cavity, which is often slit-like. The cavity often contains ferritin- and hemosiderin-laden macrophages as long-standing markers of bleeding.

On CT, fresh blood clots typically appear as hyperdense lesions. Only in rare cases of extreme anemia or coagulation disorders, may acute hematomas also appear iso- or even hypodense. The density of blood clots then gradually diminishes, becoming slightly hypodense 2-4 weeks after hemorrhage. Typically, clots may appear isodense to brain 8-14 days after hemorrhage. Late subacute or chronic hematomas are usually hypodense and may approach cerebrospinal fluid (CSF) in attenuation.

On MR, the signal intensity depends on the sequence used, the predominant degradation product of hemoglobin, and whether the RBCs are still intact (Table 1).

Etiology of Nontraumatic Intracranial Hemorrhage by Age Group and Anatomic Location

Perinatal Hemorrhage

- Premature infants
  - Periventricular-intraventricular hemorrhage: Hypoxia may cause hypertension and subsequent rupture of vessels within the germinal matrix

Table 1. Computed tomography and magnetic resonance characteristics of intracranial hemorrhage[a]

Time	NECT	CECT	T1w	T2w	T2*w
Hyperacute (< 6 h)	Hyperdense		Iso	Hyper	Hypo
Acute (6 h-3 days)	Hyper		Iso	Hypo	Hypo
Early subacute (3-7 days)	Hyper/iso		Iso (center), hyper (rim)	Hypo	Hypo
Late subacute (1-4 weeks)	Iso/hypo	Rim enhancement	Hyper	Hyper	Hypo
Chronic (months-years)	Hypo		Hypo	Hypo	Hypo

CECT, Contrast-enhanced CT; *NECT*, non-enhanced computed tomography
[a]Density/signal intensity compared to cortex

  - Periventricular leukomalacia (PVL): Ischemic infarct causes coagulation necrosis of deep periventricular white matter; subsequent hemorrhage is found in up to 20% of patients
- Term infants
  - Traumatic delivery (scalp edema, subgaleal hemorrhage, cephalohematoma, subdural hematoma)
  - Hypoxic-ischemic injury (hemorrhagic transformation in deep gray nuclei, peri-rolandic hemorrhage)

Subarachnoid Hemorrhage

- Aneurysm
- Arterial dissection
- Angiogram-negative perimesencephalic hemorrhage
- Arteriovenous malformation
- Dural arteriovenous fistulae

Nontraumatic Subdural Hemorrhage

- Dural arteriovenous fistulae
- Aneurysm
- Moyamoya syndrome
- Dural metastases
- Coagulation defects

Intracerebral Hemorrhage in Elderly Adults

- Hypertensive intracerebral hemorrhage
  - Most common cause of nontraumatic intracerebral hemorrhage in adults
  - Typical locations: putamen/external capsule (60-65%), thalamus (15-20%), pons (5-10%), cerebellum (2-5%), hemispheric white matter (1-2%)
- Cerebral amyloid angiopathy
- Hemorrhagic infarction
- Coagulopathies
- Neoplasms

Intracerebral Hemorrhage in Young/Middle-Aged Adults

- Arteriovenous malformations
- Cavernous angioma
- Aneurysms
- Hemorrhagic infarction
- Venous infarction (thrombosis of dural sinus or cortical veins)
- Hypertensive encephalopathies (pre-eclampsia, renal failure, hemolytic-uremic syndrome)
- Drug abuse (e.g., cocaine)
- Neoplasms

Suggested Reading

Atlas SW (1996) Magnetic resonance imaging of the brain and spine. Lippincott Williams & Wilkins, Philadelphia

Krayenbuehl H (1982) Cerebral angiography. Thieme, Stuttgart-New York

Osborn AG (2004) Diagnostic imaging brain. WB Saunders, Philadelphia

Wiesmann M, Bruckmann H (2004) Magnetic resonance imaging of subarachnoid hemorrhage. RoFo 176:500-5005 [German]

Demyelinating Diseases - I

Kelly K. Koeller

Department of Radiology, Mayo Clinic, Rochester, MN, USA

The oligodendrocyte, predominantly found in the white matter of the brain, is the cell responsible for the production of myelin. As a general rule, demyelinating diseases result from either attacks on this cell or failure of the cell to regenerate under normal conditions. Consequently, a focal or diffuse loss of myelin occurs. Multiple sclerosis (MS) is the prototypical white matter disease. Many other diseases may mimic its appearance on imaging studies. While not an exhaustive list, this review highlights the important imaging manifestations of these demyelinating diseases that allow more specific diagnosis.

Multiple Sclerosis

Despite the more than 170 years that have passed since the first clinical features of MS were recognized, by Carswell and Cruveilhier in 1837, much of the demyelinating process remains poorly understood. There is a growing body of evidence suggesting that the disease is autoimmune in nature, although genetic factors, i.e., an allele on chromosome 6, have also been identified. Prior infection from Epstein-Barr virus or cytomegalovirus may also play a role. There is a frequent association of MS with many other autoimmune conditions, including Graves' disease, myasthenia gravis, Crohn's disease, and systemic lupus erythematosus.

The disease is more prevalent in cooler climates, with an incidence of about 1 per 1,000 in the United States and northern European countries. The vast majority (95%) of afflicted patients are between the ages of 18 and 50 years and it is the second most common disabling disease of young adults. Only acquired immune deficiency syndrome (AIDS) is more common. Most (60%) MS patients are female [1].

Typical clinical presenting symptoms include paresthesia, numbness, diplopia, weakness, gait disturbance, and burning sensations. About 7% of patients present with symptoms related to spinal cord involvement. Hemiparesis, constipation, urinary retention, and incontinence are typical features. Seizure activity occurs in about 5%. Uthoff's phenomenon, the worsening of symptoms when the patient is exposed to warm temperatures, has long been recognized as a feature of the disease and once was used as a provocative clinical test. MS is very rarely seen in children, especially before puberty. It has been noted that MS patients often experience an exacerbation of symptoms in the first 6 months post-partum. Interestingly, the rate of attacks appears to decrease during the second and third trimester of pregnancy. Detection of oligoclonal gammopathy on cerebrospinal fluid examination is an important laboratory finding but is not always present [2].

Optic neuritis, characterized clinically by retrobulbar pain, a central monocular loss of vision, and an afferent papillary defect (Marcus-Gunn pupil) is especially important as a clinical hallmark for MS. The likelihood of a female patient with optic neuritis having MS either at the time of presentation or sometime in the future is 74%. While the diagnosis is best substantiated by clinical inspection, magnetic resonance imaging (MRI) remains valuable in directing therapy. When two or more MS-like lesions are noted, intravenous corticosteroid therapy is advocated [3].

The clinical criteria (known as the McDonald criteria) required to establish the diagnosis are complex and require strict implementation to be effective [4]. In relapsing-remitting MS, the most common type overall, two distinctly different clinical "attacks" from two different lesions in the central nervous system are required to make the diagnosis. Each attack must last at least 24 h and the onset of the attacks must be separated by at least 30 days [4].

The second most common form of MS is the progressive form, subdivided into primary and secondary subtypes [5]. In the primary progressive form, which affects about 10-15% of the MS patient population, the clinical presentation is marked by a slow onset without the distinct attacks that are typical for the relapsing-remitting form [6]. In the secondary progressive form, the patient presents initially in the relapsing-remitting form with later transformation into progressively worsening disability as a result of individual clinical relapses.

About 10% of MS patients present with a "clinically isolated syndrome", also known as a "monosymptomatic attack". Patients with this form have one or two episodes of characteristic symptoms, followed by complete recovery to their neurologic baseline. By its very nature, it is clearly an unusual form of MS and some authorities question whether it is truly part of the MS family or a distinct clinicopathologic disease.

Several variants of MS have been identified. An especially aggressive form, known as acute fulminant MS of the Marburg type, manifests with a rapidly progressive neurologic deterioration from severe axonal loss, leading to death within just a few months [7]. Another variant, neuromyelitis optica (NMO), also known as Devic disease, is characterized by both visual and myelopathic symptoms because of simultaneous or sequential involvement of the optic nerve and spinal cord. Recent investigations have identified a specific serum antibody biomarker, NMO-IgG, for the target antigen, aquaporin 4, that distinguishes NMO from MS [8]. It is hypothesized that autoantibodies from peripheral B cells bind to aquaporin 4 along the endothelial surface and activate an inflammatory demyelination and necrosis [9]. Baló concentric sclerosis is a variant form characterized by alternating concentric bands of demyelination and normal myelination, noted not only histologically but also by MRI [10].

Pathologically, MS is an inflammatory process, with microglial infiltration combined with perivascular cuffing of lymphocytes marking the acute phase of MS plaque formation. In this phase, the oligodendrocyte is most affected by these changes, resulting in the overall loss of myelin. Together with focal hypercellularity, this characterizes the "sclerose en plaque", as it was originally called by Cruveilhier, which has a predilection for the periventricular zone. When the plaque enters the inactive phase, complete myelin loss and gliosis predominate while the inflammatory changes seen in the acute phase subside. Destruction of axons also ensues, with resultant parenchymal loss and atrophy.

Magnetic resonance imaging is the imaging modality of choice for the evaluation of patients suspected of having MS and is an essential tool in assessing the natural course of the disease as well as the effects of treatment. MRI frequently identifies many lesions that are not suspected from clinical examination [11]. Small focal hyperintense lesions, particularly in a periventricular distribution, with relatively less mass effect for the size of the lesion characterize the disease on T2-weighted images [12]. Many MS lesions are ovoid in shape with their long axis perpendicular to the ventricular wall. This pattern corresponds to the pathway of periventricular white matter vessels and constitutes a pathologic feature referred to as Dawson's finger [13]. An especially important location for MS plaques is the corpus callosum-septum pellucidum interface. The presence of lesions at this site carries increased specificity for the diagnosis of MS [14]. Fluid-attenuated inversion recovery (FLAIR) imaging is particularly helpful in identifying periventricular lesions, although lesions of the brainstem and cerebellum may be less obvious with this technique [15, 16]. Magnetization transfer imaging, especially on post-contrast imaging, is recommended for its higher contrast-to-noise ratio and has been advocated for the detection of disease in a patient with normal-appearing white matter on pre-contrast imaging [17, 18].

Specific MRI manifestations of the disease have now been recognized as fulfilling the "dissemination in space" and "dissemination in time" components of the clinical McDonald criteria. For dissemination in space, at least three of these four MRI features must be identified: one contrast-enhancing lesion or nine T2-hyperintense lesions if there is no contrast-enhancing lesion; at least one infratentorial lesion; at least one juxtacortical lesion; and at least three periventricular lesions. To fulfill dissemination in time, follow-up MRI after the initial examination is required and must show either a new contrast-enhancing lesion or a new T2 hyperintense lesion that was not evident on the initial study. Follow-up imaging is recommended at 3 months after the initial scan [17].

On initial inspection, the imaging appearance of some large plaques may mimic that of a brain tumor. Closer evaluation will reveal the relative lack of mass effect expected given the size of these "tumefactive" MS plaques, which provides a valuable clue to the correct diagnosis of demyelinating disease [19]. Distinction between plaques in the active phase and plaques in the chronic phase can be made with contrast-enhanced MRI, as active plaques enhance whereas chronic plaques do not [12, 20]. The enhancement correlates with the presence of inflammatory cells [12].

In long-standing disease, cerebral atrophy with prominent ventriculomegaly and sulcal enlargement is commonly noted on MR studies. These features appear to be more common in patients with the secondary progressive form of the disease than in patients with the relapsing-remitting form [21]. Assessment of cerebral atrophy, through subjective measurement of corpus callosum volume or third ventricle width or by computer-aided techniques, correlates better with clinical disability than the number of lesions on T2-weighted images [21, 22]. Advanced MRI techniques are expected to more precisely characterize the nature of the MS plaque and hold the promise of better assessing the effects of therapy. Magnetization transfer imaging has shown differences in magnetization transfer between MS plaques and other white matter lesions, such as those of senescence [23]. On MR spectroscopy, a decreased peak of *N*-acetyl aspartate (NAA), a decreased NAA:creatine ratio, and an increased choline:creatine ratio have been seen in active and in chronic plaques, although the incidence varies among the different clinical types of the disease. Increased amounts of choline, lipids, lactic acid, and inositol have also been variably reported and highlight the dynamic nature of the MS plaque [24, 25]. Recently, MR perfusion studies have shown regions of decreased perfusion, believed to represent areas of hemodynamic and microvascular abnormality, in areas of normal-appearing white matter on T2-weighted MR images.

In general, spinal cord MS plaques tend to involve one or two vertebral body segments, compared to transverse myelitis, which is usually more diffuse and often extends over more than four vertebral bodies. MS plaques are frequently wedge-shaped and have a predilection for the dorsal columns. In contrast, transverse myelitis usually manifests with more central spinal-cord involvement. Most (60%) patients with spinal-cord MS plaques have brain lesions as well.

Despite all of these imaging features, it is important to emphasize two "truths" about MS. First, the MS plaque is a dynamic entity, not only fluctuating between an active phase and a chronic phase but also showing remyelination, inflammatory changes, gliosis, and demyelination at any given time. Second, the diagnosis of MS is still only established by clinical correlation. None of the imaging presentations, either alone or in combination, described previously are pathognomonic. The diagnosis of MS carries a tremendous emotional undercurrent for the patient. With this in mind, the radiologist should strictly avoid labeling a patient as "having MS" in a radiological report in the absence of clinical confirmation.

White Matter Disease from Viral Infection

Acute Disseminated Encephalomyelitis

Acute disseminated encephalomyelitis (ADEM) is another demyelinating disease. It is typically seen after patients have been vaccinated or in those who report having had a viral infection 1-3 weeks before the onset of neurologic symptoms, which vary from mild (headache and meningeal signs) to severe (neurologic deficits and coma). In contrast to MS, ADEM is nearly always a monophasic illness and children are more commonly affected. Since ADEM is a diagnosis of exclusion, long-term follow-up is required to completely exclude MS. Most (80%) patients have a good prognosis but in 10-20% there is a persistent neurologic deficit; rarely, the disease can result in death. It is believed that ADEM represents a delayed hypersensitivity autoimmune response that triggers perivenous demyelination in immunocompetent patients. No virus or bacteria has ever been isolated in any patient with ADEM on autopsy examination. A rare hyperacute aggressive form, acute hemorrhagic leukoencephalitis, may occur in children and is usually fatal, secondary to brain herniation.

On computed tomography (CT), ADEM may not be detected or it may have an ill-defined nonspecific hypoattenuation. On MRI, the lesions of ADEM are frequently asymmetric, varying in size and number, with little or no mass effect, a hallmark feature of a demyelinating process. The lesions usually do not enhance on post-contrast studies. Occasionally, the lesions involve the optic nerve or spinal cord, similar to MS [26].

Progressive Multifocal Leukoencephalopathy

Progressive multifocal leukoencephalopathy (PML) is overwhelmingly a disease of the immunocompromised patient and most (55-85%) cases are related to AIDS. There is a wide age range of involvement, with the peak age of presentation in the sixth decade. The disease is caused by reactivation of a papovavirus (JC virus) that selectively attacks the oligodendrocyte, leading to demyelination. In contrast to patients with ADEM, untreated patients with PML have an extremely poor prognosis, with death common in the first 6 months following establishment of the diagnosis. Highly active anti-retroviral therapy (HAART) has markedly decreased the incidence of this disease and has even led to apparent complete resolution of lesions on imaging studies.

Like ADEM, the lesions of PML are characterized by little mass effect or enhancement. Most involve the subcortical white matter and deep cortical layers of the parieto-occipital or frontal white matter, although gray matter and posterior fossa lesions are also common, occurring in up to 50% of cases. PML lesions tend to be more confluent in their appearance than ADEM lesions. Scalloping of the lateral margin of the lesion at the gray matter-white matter junction is common. Occasionally, the lesions contain hemorrhage [27]. Development of mass effect and temporary enhancement in the early phase of HAART has been linked to prolonged survival [28].

Human Immunodeficiency Virus Encephalopathy

Human immunodeficiency virus (HIV) encephalopathy results from direct infection of the brain by the virus itself. Most patients are severely immunocompromised at the time of onset and exhibit psychomotor slowing, impaired mental status, and memory difficulties. Histologically, demyelination and vacuolation with axonal loss are noted, along with occasional microglial nodules. Mild cerebral atrophy is the first and sometimes only imaging feature of the disease, which is also known as AIDS dementia complex, HIV dementia, and HIV-associated dementia complex. Involvement of the central white matter, basal ganglia, and thalamus is characteristic. Typically, bilaterally symmetric abnormal T2 hyperintensity in the basal ganglia and small focal areas in the periventricular regions are noted on T2-weighted MR images. Regression of these findings has been seen following institution of HAART [29].

White Matter Disease from Toxic Imbalance

Chronic Alcohol Ingestion and Its Consequences

Chronic alcohol ingestion predominantly causes atrophy that involves the entire cerebral hemisphere and the superior cerebellar vermis. Two diseases are important consequences of this initial process. Selective demyelination and necrosis of the corpus callosum in patients with chronic alcohol ingestion is known as Marchiafava-Bignami disease. It was originally described by two Italian physicians who documented the disease in a cohort of poorly nourished patients who died from the effects of consuming too much Italian red wine. This disease can be seen in many different populations and from many different alcoholic agents. It has even been reported in poorly nourished non-drinkers. The necrotic zones are especially well visualized as abnormal hyperintense foci on sagittal T2-weighted images. In surviving patients, atrophy of the corpus callosum can be seen [30].

Wernicke encephalopathy is another potential complication of chronic alcohol ingestion. Initially, there is intracellular swelling, which is followed by necrosis in the medial thalamic nuclei and mamillary bodies. Patients typically present with ophthalmoplegia, ataxia, and confusion. Intravenous thiamine is the treatment of choice. If untreated, the disease progresses to severe amnesia, psychosis, and is often fatal. Abnormal T2 hyperintensity within the medial portions of the thalami, periaqueductal gray matter, and mamillary bodies is the hallmark imaging feature of this disease. Post-contrast T1-weighted images are recommended for patients with known chronic alcoholic consumption, as these may reveal abnormal enhancement of the mamillary bodies in the absence of an abnormal T2 signal [31].

Osmotic Myelinolysis

Formerly called "central pontine myelinolysis", the term "osmotic myelinolysis" was proposed a few years ago to emphasize that the source of the disease is a rapid intravascular osmotic change that causes endothelial injury, most prevalent in the regions where the gray matter and white matter are most closely apposed – the central portion of the pons. The end result of this endothelial injury is demyelination. Clinical symptoms usually include acute mental status changes, lethargy, dysphagia, and progressive quadriparesis. Once thought to be uniformly fatal, it is now known that this is not necessarily true and a return to a normal imaging appearance and clinical status may be seen over a variable period of time. The classic imaging appearance of osmotic myelinolysis is hypoattenuation on CT and T1 and T2 prolongation on MRI within the center of the pons and distinctive sparing of the pontine periphery, occasionally producing a classic "trident-shaped" appearance [32]. Extrapontine involvement may be noted in about 10% of cases and usually involves the basal ganglia and others locations within the brain [33].

White Matter Disease Associated with Radiation Therapy and Chemotherapy

Radiation Injury and Necrosis

The spectrum of radiation injury to the brain is broad. Three distinct categories of disease are noted: acute radiation injury, early delayed radiation injury, and late radiation injury. In acute radiation injury, clinical changes present very shortly after the initiation of radiation therapy. Transient encephalopathic symptoms are typical, generally mild, and respond to oral steroid therapy. No CT or MR findings are seen in patients with this form of injury. Early delayed radiation injury produces demyelination within the white matter at least 2 months from the start of radiation therapy. Lesions predominate in the white matter, basal ganglia, and cerebral peduncles. Late radiation injury has three different forms: focal radiation necrosis, diffuse radiation injury, and necrotizing leukoencephalopathy. While the first two usually occur 6-12 months from the start of therapy, the last entity manifests at least 3 months after the onset of therapy. Distinguishing radiation necrosis from recurrent malignant brain tumor, such as glioblastoma multiforme, is frequently impossible using conventional MRI. Both lesions may have mass effect, surrounding vasogenic edema, and enhance on contrast-enhanced studies. Metabolic imaging (e.g., positron emission tomography) may facilitate differentiating between the two diseases, as radiation necrosis is iso- to hypometabolic while recurrent high-grade tumors are typically hypermetabolic. MR spectroscopy (MRS) may also be useful, as radiation necrosis frequently shows a characteristic lactic acid peak and near-normal peaks for NAA and choline, while recurrent high-grade gliomas typically show elevated choline levels compared to NAA without or with elevated lactic acid levels. Perfusion imaging can identify the areas of increased blood flow associated with tumor recurrence whereas radiation necrosis is not expected to contain any increased blood flow [34].

Diffuse radiation injury is characterized by white matter changes that are "geographic" in nature, i.e., the areas of abnormal signal intensity or attenuation are limited to regions of the brain that conform to the radiation portal. This can produce striking differences between the involved zones and the spared surrounding white matter. The involved territories are often symmetric and do not enhance on post-contrast studies.

While originally reported in children with leukemia, diffuse necrotizing leukoencephalopathy has also been observed following treatment for many other malignancies in children and in adults. The disease may occur following chemotherapy alone but the incidence of disease is highest when chemotherapy is combined with radiation therapy. Both the histologic findings and imaging features bear resemblance to those of radiation necrosis. Axonal swelling, demyelination, coagulation necrosis, and gliosis dominate the histologic picture. Diffuse white matter changes, with hypoattenuation on CT and T1 and T2 prolongation on MRI, are common and often involve an entire hemisphere [35].

Mineralizing Microangiopathy

In children with cancer who have been treated with chemotherapy either alone or in combination with radiation therapy, deposits of calcium in and around small penetrating blood vessels of the deep brain lead to local areas of necrosis. This process is termed mineralizing microangiopathy and is the most common neuroradiologic abnormality noted in this group of patients. The disease has a predilection for the basal ganglia, especially the putamen, and, more rarely, the cerebral cortex. On CT and MR, evidence of cortical atrophy and abnormal attenuation/signal intensity changes within the white matter are commonly noted. Of all chemotherapeutic agents, methotrexate is the one classically associated with mineralizing microangiopathy. Patients younger than 5 years of age who have meningeal leukemia and have received high-dose methotrexate therapy are at greatest risk of developing this complication [36].

Vascular Causes of White Matter Disease

Posterior Reversible Encephalopathy Syndrome

Under normal circumstances, cerebral perfusion pressure is maintained at a relatively constant level by autoregulation, a physiologic mechanism that compensates for wide changes in systemic blood pressure. Hypertensive encephalopathy is believed to result from a loss of normal autoregulation, with competing regions of vasodilatation and vasoconstriction. The vessels of the posterior cerebral circulation, which have less sympathetic innervation than those of the anterior circulation, are unable to vasoconstrict in a normal manner and bear the brunt of these vascular changes. Reversible vasogenic edema is the result and it is associated with visual field deficits, as well as headaches, somnolence, and an overall impaired mental status. The term posterior reversible encephalopathy syndrome (PRES) has been popularized in the literature to describe this constellation of features. The disease is frequently seen in patients with renal failure, eclampsia, chemotherapy, or who have received immunosuppressive therapy, such as cyclosporine A and FK-506 (tacrolimus).

On MR studies, bilaterally symmetric abnormal T2 hyperintensity is most commonly seen in the distribution of the posterior circulation, although other sites including the frontal lobes and corpus callosum may be noted as well. Diffusion-weighted imaging (DWI) may be normal or show restricted water diffusion. This technique may be helpful to identify those regions that will progress to true infarction, with DWI hyperintensity and apparent diffusion coefficient (ADC) values that are normal or slightly elevated [37]. Perfusion studies reported in the literature indicate normal to increased perfusion in these zones. Biopsy findings of these regions show histologic evidence of white matter edema. Following treatment, the lesions resolve and the involved sites return to normal signal intensity [38].

Ischemia and Vascular Disease

Small focal lesions of T2 hyperintensity are quite common in the white matter of adult patients. The lesions are not associated with mass effect, do not enhance, and are typically isointense compared to normal white matter on T1-weighted images. Histologic examination of biopsied tissue reveals a spectrum of findings, including gliosis, loss of myelination, and areas of ischemia. The lesions tend to be located in the periventricular white matter, centrum semiovale, and optic radiations. In contrast to MS, they do not involve the corpus callosum, an important distinguishing feature. Since the lesions are so ubiquitous and appear to be a part of "normal" aging, various terms have been proposed: senescent white matter changes or disease, deep white matter ischemia, leukoariosis, etc. In general, the more numerous the lesions, the more likely it is that the patient will have cognitive problems or difficulties with neuropsychologic testing. However, it is not possible to predict a particular patient's status based on the imaging appearance alone. Hence, the diagnosis of Binswanger dementia should be avoided unless substantiated with clinical criteria.

In adult patients between 30 and 50 years of age, the presence of periventricular and subcortical lesions in a patient with a family history of similarly affected relatives should raise the possibility of cerebral autosomal dominant arteriopathy with subcortical infarcts and leukoencephalopathy (CADASIL). A defect in the notch3 gene on the long arm of chromosome 19 has been identified and apparently evokes an angiopathy affecting small and medium-sized vessels. Most lesions occur in the frontal and temporal lobes and less commonly in the thalamus, basal ganglia, internal and external capsules, and brain stem [39, 40].

Many other conditions and diseases are associated with small vessel injury within the brain and commonly involve the white matter as small focal areas of abnormal T2 hyperintensity. These include autoimmune disease, particularly systemic lupus erythematosus, Behçet disease, and giant cell arteritis, as well as arteritis associated with drug use (e.g., methamphetamine and heroin), radiation injury, and malignancy.

Dysmyelinating and Metabolic Diseases

The number of inherited metabolic white matter diseases that are identified continues to expand yearly but so does our understanding of them. Most will appear in childhood, especially in infancy, and many are transmitted in an autosomal recessive fashion. Imaging features in these diseases are rarely pathognomonic and practically all patients will require biochemical analysis of their blood, urine, and skin to establish the diagnosis. From a pathophysiologic basis, these disorders are categorized based on the cellular organelle in which metabolism is altered. Lysosomal disorders, or "storage disorders", are a clinically heterogeneous group of diseases caused by an enzyme deficiency that results in the accumulation of phospholipids, glycolipids, mucopolysaccharides, or glycoprotein, all of which interfere with myelin production. Peroxisomal disorders are caused by an enzyme deficiency within peroxisomes, an organelle that is particularly common in oligodendrocytes. In these conditions, normal lipid metabolism is altered, with the accumulation of very long-chain fatty acids. The mitochondrial disorders are a clinically heterogeneous group of diseases that result in spongy degeneration of myelin in various locations and also frequently involve muscles. Amino- and organic-acid disorders are very rare; their clinical presentation is dependent upon which organic acid or amino acid is involved. Special types of leukodystrophies compose the last group. These represent diseases that are associated with macrocrania (Canavan disease, Alexander disease) or sudanophilic deposits noted on histologic examination (Cockayne disease, Pelizaeus-Merzbacher disease) [41].

Diseases that tend to first involve the "central" white matter are Krabbe disease, x-linked adrenoleukodystrophy, and other peroxisomal disorders, metachromatic leukodystrophy, and Pelizaeus-Merzbacher disease, whereas Alexander disease, Canavan disease, and Cockayne disease tend to first affect the peripheral white matter. Diseases that involve gray matter in addition to the white matter involvement include mitochondrial disorders and the mucopolysaccharidoses. If hemorrhage is seen within a white matter lesion on an imaging study, it should provoke consideration of a diagnosis other than an inherited metabolic disorder.

References

1. Hauser SL (1994) Multiple sclerosis and other demyelinating disease. In: Isselbacher KJ, Graunwald E, Wilson JD et al (eds) Harrison's principle of internal medicine. McGraw-Hill, New York, pp 2287-2295
2. Farlow MR, Bonine JM (1993) Clinical and neuropathological features of multiple sclerosis. Neuroradiol Clin North Am 3:213-228
3. Trobe JD (1994) High-dose corticosteroid regimen retards development of multiple sclerosis in optic neuritis treatment trial. Arch Ophthalmol 112:35-36
4. McDonald WI, Compston A, Edan G et al (2001) Recommended diagnostic criteria for multiple sclerosis: guidelines from the international panel on the diagnosis of multiple sclerosis. Ann Neurol 50:121-127
5. Grossman RI, McGowan JC (1998) Perspective of multiple sclerosis. AJNR Am J Neuroradiol 19:1251-1265
6. Wolinsky JS (2003) The diagnosis of primary progressive multiple sclerosis. J Neurol Sci 206:145-152
7. Niebler G, Harris T, Davis T, Roos K (1992) Fulminant multiple sclerosis. AJNR Am J Neuroradiol 13:1547-1551
8. Matiello M, Jacob A, Wingerchuk D, Weinshenker B (2007) Neuromyelitis optica. Curr Opin Neurol 20:255-260
9. Jacob A, Matiello M, Wingerchuk D et al (2007) Neuromyelitis optica: changing concepts. J Neuroimmunol 187:126-138
10. Gharagozloo AM, Poe LB, Collins GH (1994) Antemortem diagnosis of Balo concentric sclerosis: correlative MR imaging and pathologic features. Radiology 191:817-819
11. Barkhof F, Scheltens P, Frequin ST et al (1992) Relapsing-remitting multiple sclerosis: sequential enhanced MR imaging vs clinical findings in determining disease activity. AJR Am J Roentgenol 159:1041-1047
12. Nesbit GM, Forbes GS, Scheithauer BW et al (1991) Multiple sclerosis: histopathologic and MR and/or CT correlation in 37 cases at biopsy and three cases at autopsy. Radiology 180:467-474
13. Horowitz AL, Kaplan RD, Grewe G et al (1989) The ovoid lesion: a new MR observation in patients with multiple sclerosis. AJNR Am J Neuroradiol 10:303-305
14. Gean-Marton AD, Vezina LG, Marton KI et al (1991) Abnormal corpus callosum: a sensitive and specific indicator of multiple sclerosis. Radiology 180:215-221
15. Hashemi RH, Bradley WG, Chen D-Y et al (1995) Suspected multiple sclerosis: MR imaging with a thin-section fast FLAIR pulse sequence. Radiology 196:505-510
16. Stevenson V, Parker G, Barker G et al (2000) Variations in T1 and T2 relaxation times of normal appearing white matter and lesions in multiple sclerosis. J Neurol Sci 178:81-87
17. Simon J, Li D, Traboulsee A et al (2006) Standardized MR imaging protocol for multiple sclerosis: consortium of MS centers consensus guidelines. AJNR Am J Neuroradiol 27:455-461
18. Miller D, Thompson AJ, Filippi M (2003) Magnetic resonance studies of abnormalities in the normal appearing white matter and grey matter in multiple sclerosis. J Neurol 250:1407-1419
19. Dagher AP, Smirniotopoulous JG (1996) Tumefactive demyelinating lesions. Neuroradiology 38:560-565
20. Grossman RI, Gonzalez-Scarano F, Atlas SW et al (1986) Multiple sclerosis: gadolinium enhancement in MR imaging. Radiology 161:721-725
21. Ge Y, Grossman RI, Udupa JK et al (2000) Brain atrophy in relapsing-remitting multiple sclerosis and secondary progressive multiple sclerosis: longitudinal quantitative analysis. Radiology 214:665-670
22. Dietemann JL, Beigelman C, Rumbach L et al (1988) Multiple sclerosis and corpus callosum atrophy: relationship of MRI findings to clinical data. Neuroradiology 30:478-480
23. Mehta RC, Pike GB, Enzmann DR (1996) Measure of magnetization transfer in multiple sclerosis demyelinating plaques, white matter ischemic lesions, and edema. AJNR Am J Neuroradiol 17:1051-1055
24. Grossman RI, Lenkinski RE, Ramer KN et al (1992) MR proton spectroscopy in multiple sclerosis. AJNR Am J Neuroradiol 13:1535-1543
25. Falini A, Calabrese G, Filippi M et al G (1998) Benign versus secondary-progressive multiple sclerosis: the potential role of proton MR spectroscopy in defining the nature of disability. AJNR Am J Neuroradiol 19:223-229
26. Singh S, Alexander M, Korah IP (1999) Acute disseminated encephalomyelitis: MR imaging features. AJR Am J Roentgenol 173:1101-1107
27. Whiteman M, Post MJ, Berger JR et al (1993) Progressive multifocal leukoencephalopathy in 47 HIV-seropositive patients: neuroimaging with clinical and pathologic correlation. Radiology 187:233-240
28. Thurner M, Post M, Rieger A et al (2001) Initial and follow-up MR imaging findings in AIDS-related progressive multifocal leukoencephalopathy treated with highly active antiretroviral therapy. AJNR Am J Neuroradiol 22:977-984
29. McArthur JC, Sacktor N, Seines O (1999) Human immunodeficiency virus-associated dementia. Semin Neurol 19:105-111
30. Izquierdo G, Quesada MA, Chacon J, Martel J (1992) Neuroradiologic abnormalities in Marchiafava-Bignami disease of benign evolution. Eur J Radiol 15:71-74
31. Zuccoli G, Galluci M, Capellades J et al (2007) Wernicke encephalopathy: MR findings at clinical presentation in twenty-six alcoholic and nonalcoholic patients. AJNR Am J Neuroradiol 28:1328-1331
32. Ruzek, KA, Campeau N, Miller G (2004) Early diagnosis of central pontine myelinolysis with diffusion-weighted imaging. AJNR Am J Neuroradiol 25:210-213
33. Miller GM, Baker HL, Okazaki H, Whisnant JP (1988) Central pontine myelinolysis and its imitators: MR findings. Radiology 168:795-802
34. Cha S (2006) Update on brain tumor imaging: from anatomy to physiology. AJNR Am J Neuroradiol 27:475-487

35. Chan Y, Leung S, King AD et al (1999) Late radiation injury to the temporal lobes: morphologic evaluation at MR imaging. Radiology 213:800-807
36. Davis P, Hoffman JJ, Pearl G, Braun I (1986) CT evaluation of effects of cranial radiation therapy in children. AJR Am J Roentgenol 147:587-592
37. Covarrubias D, Luetmer P, Campeau N (2002) Posterior reversible encephalopathy syndrome: prognostic utility of quantitative diffusion-weighted MR images. AJNR Am J Neuroradiol 23:1038-1048
38. Post JD, Beauchamp NJ (1998) Reversible intracerebral pathologic entities mediated by vascular autoregulatory dysfunction. Radiographics 18:353-367
39. Yousry TA, Seelos K, Mayer M et al (1999) Characteristic MR lesion pattern and correlation of T1 and T2 lesion volume with neurologic and neuropsychological findings in cerebral autosomal dominant arteriopathy with subcortical infarcts and leukoencephalopathy (CADASIL). AJNR Am J Neuroradiol 20:91-100
40. van dem Boom R, Lesnick Oberstein S, van den Berg-Huysmans A et al (2006) Cerebral autosomal dominant arteriopathy with subcortical infarcts and leukoencephalopathy: MR imaging changes and apolipoportein E genotype. AJNR Am J Neuroradiol 27:359-362
41. Kendall BE (1992) Disorders of lysosomes, peroxisomes, and mitochondria. AJNR Am J Neuroradiol 13:621-653

Demyelinating Diseases - II

Mark A. van Buchem

Department of Radiology, Leiden University Medical Center, Leiden, The Netherlands

Introduction: Myelin in Health and Disease

Myelin is an important component of the nervous system. It is a fatty substance made up of lipids and proteins and its high concentration in the white matter of the brain is responsible for that region's characteristic whitish color. Myelin is the main component of the sheaths that envelop axons in their trajectory from the neuronal cell body to the synapses. The functions of myelin are: (a) preventing short-circuiting (and thus cross-talk) between axons by providing an insulating layer of high electrical resistance between neighboring axons, and (b) increasing the speed of signal conduction along axons. Myelin is produced in the central nervous system by oligodendrocytes and in the peripheral nervous system by Schwann cells. The myelin sheaths enveloping axons are flat extensions of oligodendrocytes or Schwann cells that spiral around an axon to form concentric lamellae. Along the course of an individual axon multiple lamellae are found. These are separated from each other by short, unmyelinated stretches known as the nodes of Ranvier. Action potentials are propagated along axons by jumping from one node of Ranvier to the next. One oligodendrocyte can support as many as 60 different axons. Given this high number of lamellae supported by a single oligodendrocyte and since there is a continuous turnover of myelin in the brain, it is not surprising that oligodendrocytes are characterized by a high metabolic demand. Contrary to what is generally believed, oligodendrocytes and myelin are not restricted to the brain's white matter; they are also present in the gray matter, but in much lower concentrations.

Myelin disorders are usually subdivided in two main categories: demyelinating and dysmyelinating diseases. In demyelinating disorders, the myelin is initially normal, whereas in dysmyelinating disorders it is abnormal from the beginning due to genetic and enzymatic defects. The prevalence of demyelinating disorders is much higher than that of dysmyelinating diseases, and the former are the focus of this chapter.

Demyelinating disorders are a heterogeneous group of diseases. What they have in common could be described as "central white matter disease", in which myelin loss exceeds axonal loss. Numerous pathomechanisms have been identified in the different types of demyelinating diseases. These mechanisms include viral infection, allergic responses, primarily vascular disorders, and toxic effects. The different assaults can affect oligodendrocytes selectively, or they can be less specific with respect to target and thus damage other types of brain cells too. In addition to resulting from direct damage to oligodendrocytes, demyelination can be secondary to axonal damage, through a process known as Wallerian degeneration. Since myelin is present in gray and white matter, and demyelinating diseases can affect components of the brain other than myelin, it is not surprising that demyelinating diseases not only involve white matter but are also observed in gray matter.

The result of demyelinating diseases is the thinning or even focal disappearance of the myelin sheath of axons. Such changes will affect signal propagation in affected axons; depending on their location, this can lead to a host of neurologic and psychiatric symptoms. Moreover, these symptoms are not always static. When demyelination arises from the death of oligodendrocytes, new, immature oligodendrocytes can be recruited from the surrounding intact tissue and migrate to the demyelinating area. There, these cells differentiate into mature oligodendrocytes and start, more or less successfully, developing myelin sheaths for the still present but barren parts of the affected axons. This process of remyelination can improve the conduction of action potentials along axons and ultimately results in the regression of symptoms.

In the following, the classification of demyelinating disorders is described, with a few diseases discussed in greater detail.

Primary Demyelination

Demyelinating disorders can be primary or secondary (Table 1). In primary disorders, the cause of the disease is incompletely understood, whereas in secondary disorders the trigger that causes the disease is known. The quintessential primary demyelinating disease is multiple sclerosis (MS).

Table 1. Classification of white matter diseases. From [1]

I. Demyelinating diseases	
a. Primary demyelinating diseases	Multiple sclerosis
b. Secondary demyelinating diseases	*Allergic* Acute disseminated encephalomyelitis (ADEM) *Viral* Progressive multifocal leukoencephalopathy (PML) HIV-associated encephalitis Subacute sclerosing panencephalitis *Vascular* Binswanger disease Cerebral autosomal dominant arteriopathy with subcortical infarcts and leukoencephalopathy (CADASIL) Postanoxic encephalopathy Reversible posterior leukoencephalopathy *Metabolic* Osmotic demyelination *Toxic* Alcohol Radiation Marchiafava-Bignami disease Disseminated necrotizing leukoencephalopathy Drugs: chemotherapy and recreational drugs Toxins (triethyl tin, lead, mercury) *Traumatic* Diffuse axonal injury
II. Dysmyelinating disorders	Alexander's disease Krabbe's disease Sudanophilic leukodystrophy Pelizaeus-Merzbacher disease Canavan's disease Metachromatic leukodystrophy Adrenoleukodystrophy

A striking feature of MS is its prevalence with respect to distance from the equator: in both the southern and northern hemisphere, the prevalence of MS increases in populations living at increasing latitudes. This observation suggests an important role for environmental factors in disease pathogenesis; a role for infective agents has been suggested. In addition, genetic factors may be of importance; recent estimates of disease susceptibility as determined by genetic factors are as high as 40%. Regardless of the primary trigger of the disease and the factors that modulate its course, the result is that MS appears to be an autoimmune disease. A chronic inflammatory process with some remarkable features characterizes the pathology of MS: inflammatory changes comprising infiltrates of lymphocytes and plasma cells tending to occur around blood vessels, and especially veins; focal, punched-out areas of remarkable myelin loss, often with relatively intact axons and neurons (and thus the absence of Wallerian degeneration in tracts passing through demyelinated areas); multiplicity of lesions, with the coexistence of lesions of different histological age; coexistence of remyelinated lesions and lesions in which remyelination has failed; coexistence of focal lesions (plaques) and more diffuse, subtle, microscopic changes characterized by demyelination and gliosis.

The course of the disease is as heterogeneous as its pathological features. However, based on the clinical course, three forms of the disease have been identified: relapsing remitting (70%), progressive (20%; further subdivided in primary and secondary progressive), and monosymptomatic (10%). In addition, some rare variants of the disease are described: Devic's disease (neuromyelitis optica), Balo's disease (concentric sclerosis), Schilder's disease (diffuse sclerosis), and Marburg's variant of MS.

The heterogeneous pathological and clinical features of MS account for its diverse radiological manifestations. These are best appreciated with magnetic resonance imaging (MRI), whereas CT plays no role in the work-up of presumed MS patients. On MRI, the visible manifestations of MS are plaques, "dirty white matter", and atrophy.

Plaques represent well-defined, focal areas of disease; they can be isolated or, in more advanced disease stages, coalescent. The histological composition of these plaques can be highly variable. In early stages, they contain edema with very little other changes, whereas in late, burnt-out stages the plaques are severely demyelinated and show severe axonal loss. Chronic lesions may show signs of more or less successful remyelination. Early lesions may be associated with a leaky blood-brain barrier, whereas this is not observed with old lesions. Whatever their histological composition, MS plaques invariably have a high signal intensity on T2- and proton-density (PD)-weighted images. T1-weighted images, however, despite being considerably less sensitive to the presence of plaques, can, to a certain extent, better reflect their histological heterogeneity. MS plaques that display low signal intensity on T1-weighted images ("black holes") have been associated with more severe tissue destruction than those that are iso-intense on T1. FLAIR images, being a combination of T1 and T2 weighting, may show hyper-, iso-, and hypointense MS plaques based on variations in their T1 values. Still, the majority of MS lesions are hyperintense on FLAIR. FLAIR images are particularly useful in detecting lesions at the interface of brain parenchyma and CSF spaces, such as periventricular and cortical lesions. It is especially those lesions at the callosal-septal interface, which have been reported to have 93% sensitivity and 98% specificity in differentiating MS from vascular disease, that are easy to miss on T2-weighted images but easy to detect on FLAIR images. The enhancement pattern of plaques is variable too. Breakdown of the blood-brain barrier is characteristic of new lesions. Initially, the enhancement pattern is mostly nodular; later, this may evolve to a ring or arc pattern. Leaking of the blood-brain barrier is a temporary phenomenon in MS plaques, usually residing after 2-8 weeks (although enhancement of a plaque can be observed for 6 months or more). Although MS plaques characteristically show no mass effect, this does occur on occasion and may even suggest the presence of a high-grade intra-axial brain tumor. This condition is known as tumefactive MS. MS plaques can occur everywhere in the brain but sites of predilection are the periventricular area, corpus callosum, subcortical region, optic nerve and optic pathways, posterior fossa, and the cervical part of the spinal cord.

In advanced cases of MS, subtle, ill-defined areas of increased signal intensity can be observed on T2- and PD-weighted images as well as FLAIR images. These changes are often referred to as "dirty white matter" and probably reflect more widespread areas of less severe demyelination and gliosis. Similar histological changes are probably also responsible for abnormalities in the white and gray matter of MS patients that were not detected by conventional MRI but instead required quantitative MRI techniques, such as MR spectroscopy, magnetization transfer imaging, diffusion-weighted imaging, and T1-relaxation time measurements. Finally, atrophy of the brain and spinal cord can be observed in MS, mostly in advanced cases.

MRI plays an important role in the diagnostic work-up of patients in whom the diagnosis MS is considered. According to the widely used McDonald criteria for MS, patients can be labeled on clinical and para-clinical grounds as having "MS", "possible MS", and "not MS". Without a fitting clinical picture, the diagnosis MS cannot be made during life, but a solid part of the McDonald criteria is based on MRI findings. According to these criteria (Tables 2 and 3), the following MRI findings help to confirm the diagnosis of MS: multiplicity of hyperintense lesions on T2, enhancement, location (infratentorial, juxtacortical, and periventricular), dissemination in space, dissemination in time (Table 3). Dissemination in time is of particular interest, since it helps to differentiate MS from monophasic demyelinating diseases such as acute disseminated encephalomyelitis. Apart from providing evidence for the diagnosis MS, MRI is also used to exclude other explanations for the symptoms.

Table 2. Multiple sclerosis: definitions. From [3]

Magnetic resonance imaging must identify three out of the four criteria:
- One enhancing or nine T2 hyperintense non-enhancing lesions
- One or more infratentorial lesions
- One or more juxtacortical lesions
- Three or more periventricular lesions

Table 3. MS: criteria for dissemination of lesions in time. From [3]

1. Enhancing lesion demonstrated in a scan done at least 3 months after clinical attack at another site
2. In absence of an enhancing lesion at 3 months, follow-up scan after an additional 3 months showing enhancing lesion or new hyperintense lesion on T2

Secondary Demyelination

Infectious and post-infectious diseases

Viral infections of the brain can be categorized into those that are limited to the meninges, limited to the gray matter, limited to the white matter, and present in gray and white matter. The viruses with a specific affinity for the white matter are the JC virus and HIV.

The JC virus can give rise to *progressive multifocal leukoencephalopathy* (PML). This disease is the result of the infection of oligodendrocytes by the virus, and it is usually observed in immunocompromised patients. PML has a rapid course that often results in death after 6-12 months. Histologically, areas of demyelination are observed in the white matter, involving the subcortical U-fibers, and sparing the gray matter of the cortex and basal ganglia. On MRI, PML lesions have a high signal intensity on T2- and PD-weighted images and on FLAIR, but their signal intensity is low on T1-weighted images. Enhancement, mass effect, and involvement of gray matter are not the rule, but may be observed. Lesions can be solitary, multi-focal, or confluent.

HIV can infect the brain tissue directly and thus give rise to a progressive dementia complex that is also known as AIDS encephalopathy. This disorder is clinically characterized by a subcortical dementia, with cognitive, motor, and behavioral deficits. Pathologically, mild or severe inflammatory changes, myelin pallor, and atrophy are observed. The disease is usually widespread and tends to be most severe in subcortical cerebral structures, the white matter and basal ganglia in particular. MRI shows atrophy and widespread areas of high signal intensity in the white matter and basal ganglia on T2- and PD-weighted as well as on FLAIR images. The white matter changes may be symmetric or asymmetric, focal or diffuse. No enhancement or mass effect is observed. Cortical gray matter is usually spared.

While *acute disseminated encephalomyelitis* (ADEM) is also triggered by viruses, unlike PML and AIDS encephalopathy, it is not directly caused by viral invasion of the brain but rather through an allergic-type cell-mediated immune response due to cross-reaction with a viral protein. Infections with Epstein-Barr virus, cytomegalovirus (CMV) or *Mycoplasma pneumoniae*, among others, can give rise to ADEM. Vaccinations are another known trigger. Pathologically, the disease is characterized by perivenous cellular infiltrates that are surrounded by reactive microglia and demyelination. Axons in these lesions are preserved relative to myelin loss. Typically, symptoms of ADEM appear following a latent interval from the onset of the infectious disease or immunization that ranges from 2 to 14 days. The onset is sudden, with progression that rarely takes more than a few days. The illness typically starts with fever, headache, and meningeal signs and is followed within a day by focal neurologic deficits. Usually, patients recover completely from the disease, but significant sequelae occur in about 20%, and a fatal course is observed incidentally. Radiologically, lesions display high signal intensity on T2- and PD-weighted images and on FLAIR images. The lesions tend to be large and multiple, typically do not show mass effect, and may show enhancement. They can occur in the cerebral hemispheres, infratentorial structures, optic nerve, and in the spinal cord. Although primarily a white matter disorder, extension into the gray matter occurs. The clinical and radiologic symptoms of ADEM are not unlike a single episode of MS. However, unlike MS, ADEM is typically a monophasic disease, without progression or relapses.

Vascular

Demyelination and other white matter changes can also be the result of vascular diseases. Several mechanisms can be involved. In the *posterior reversible encephalopathy syndrome* (PRES), white matter abnormalities are the result of hyperperfusion and leakage of the blood-brain barrier, both of which occur when the autoregulation capacity of the posterior circulation is no longer able to accommodate sudden changes in blood pressure. This situation has been described in a variety of conditions, such as acute hypertensive crises, (pre)eclampsia, renal failure, and in patients using immunosuppressive agents such as cyclosporin A. On MRI, lesions with high signal intensity can be observed on T2- and PD-weighted and FLAIR images. The lesions are restricted to the parietal and occipital gray and subcortical white matter and usually occur bilaterally. If the patient's blood pressure is lowered or immunosuppressive drugs are discontinued, the clinical and radiologic symptoms usually regress.

In *postanoxic encephalopathy*, the initial trigger is an anoxic episode that is followed by coma. During that episode, myelin antigens are presumed to be exposed, which leads to an allergic demyelination. The typical clinical picture is the gradual deterioration of a patient who initially recovered from the anoxic episode. Deterioration typically occurs over a period of 2 weeks and progresses to coma and death. On MRI, high signal intensity on T2- and PD-weighted and FLAIR images is observed throughout the white matter. On diffusion-weighted images evidence of cytotoxic edema can be found.

Small vessel disease is another cause of demyelination in the brain. Narrowing of the lumina of arterioles and small arteries and loss of the capacity of these vessels to dilate can give rise to a situation in which there is insufficient oxygen to maintain the normal composition of brain tissue but enough to prevent infarction. This in turn gives rise to microscopic changes that have been described as incomplete infarction, and which are characterized by demyelination, gliosis, and microscopic areas of tissue loss. Several conditions can affect small arteries and lead to this condition, such as cerebral amyloid angiopathy, cerebral autosomal dominant arteriopathy with subcortical infarcts and leukoencephalopathy (CADASIL), and hypertension- or hyperinsulinism-related lipohyalinosis. Radiologic manifestations of these diseases comprise symmetric white matter hyperintensities without mass effect on T2- and PD-weighted and FLAIR images.

Toxic and Osmotic Effects

A host of toxins can affect the white matter (Table 1). The regional sensitivity of brain tissue for toxins differs with the toxin, but white matter lesions are often part of the radiologic manifestations of toxin-induced brain damage. In general, lesions have high signal intensity on T2- and PD-weighted and FLAIR images.

Three white matter disorders can be encountered in alcoholics: osmotic demyelination (central pontine myelinolysis), Marchiafava-Bignami syndrome, and Wernicke's encephalopathy. *Osmotic demyelination* is typically observed in malnourished alcoholic patients in whom serum sodium is low upon admission to the hospital but this is rapidly corrected during hospitalization. The sudden osmotic changes that ensue are presumed to give rise to subacute demyelination without an inflammatory response. Typically, the pons is affected, but extrapontine structures, such as thalamus, putamen, caudate nuclei, internal, external, and extreme capsules, claustrum, amygdala, and cerebellum, may also be involved. These areas display high signal intensity on T2- and PD-weighted and FLAIR images.

Marchiafava-Bignami disease is considered to be a variant of extrapontine myelinolysis and is also observed in chronic alcoholics with nutritional deficiencies. In this syndrome, demyelination and necrosis occur in the corpus callosum, giving rise to sudden encephalopathy in alcoholic patients. On MRI, the corpus callosum shows an area of high signal on T2- and PD-weighted and FLAIR images. During the acute stage, there is swelling and cytotoxic edema.

Thiamine deficiency in chronic alcoholics is responsible for *Wernicke's encephalopathy*. This disease is clinically characterized by severe memory impairment with anterograde amnesia. Pathologically, demyelination, axonal loss, hemorrhage, edema (in the acute phase), and atrophy (in the chronic phase) are found. These changes have particular sites of predilection: the mamillary bodies, hypothalamic nuclei surrounding the third ventricle, periventricular parts of the thalamus, the periaquaductal gray matter, the colliculi, fornices, and inferior olives. High signal intensity on T2- and PD-weighted and FLAIR images as well as atrophy can be observed in these structures.

References

1. Grossman RI, Yousem DM (2003) Neuroradiology – the requisites, 2nd edn. Mosby, Philadelphia
2. Graham DI, Lantos PL (2002) Greenfield's Neuropathology, 7th edn. Arnold, London
3. McDonald WI, Compston A, Edan G et al (2001) Recommended diagnostic criteria for multiple sclerosis: guidelines from the International Panel on the Diagnosis of Multiple Sclerosis. Ann Neurol 50:121-127

Imaging the Effects of Systemic Metabolic Diseases on the Brain

Mauricio Castillo

Department of Radiology, University of North Carolina at Chapel Hill, Chapel Hill, NC, USA

Introduction

This short review addresses the most important and common metabolic disorders that result in abnormal neuroimaging studies in clinical practice. In these cases, the patient's medical history is of the utmost importance, as imaging findings may be relatively nonspecific. This chapter concentrates on disorders that produce somewhat specific brain findings and thus are amenable to diagnosis by the radiologist. Most of these disorders affect the gray matter. Diffuse and focal involvement of the gray matter is generally secondary to ischemia (focal cortical involvement may be seen with seizures) and is not addressed here. Instead, the focus here is on abnormalities involving the subcortical gray matter.

Liver Failure and Parenteral Nutrition

Hepatic insufficiency leads to abnormalities on brain magnetic resonance imaging (MRI). A T1-weighted image shows increased signal intensity in the caudate nucleus, tectum (particularly the inferior colliculi), globus pallidus, putamen, subthalamic nucleus, red nucleus, adenohypophysis, and substantia nigra [1] (Fig. 1). The abnormalities are bilateral, symmetrical, and of homogenous signal intensity (Table 1). There are no corresponding abnormalities on T2-weighted images nor is there contrast enhancement, while CT scans are normal. The MRI findings are believed to be due to the increased amounts of manganese (Mn) and other factors that lead to short relaxation times (Table 2). Increased plasma levels of Mn may be found in patients with chronic liver failure, those receiving long-term parenteral nutrition, and those with occupational toxicity [2]. Approximately 95% of Mn is excreted in the bile. Mn is involved in enzymatic cell cycles, including those of superoxide dismutase and glutamine synthetase. It reaches the brain by erythrocytes and, bound to transferrin or albumin, by plasma. The half-life of Mn in the blood is 10-42 days but when it reaches the brain it may remain there for longer periods of time. Astrocytes have specific transport systems for Mn, which in the brain is neurotoxic, resulting in striatal dopamine

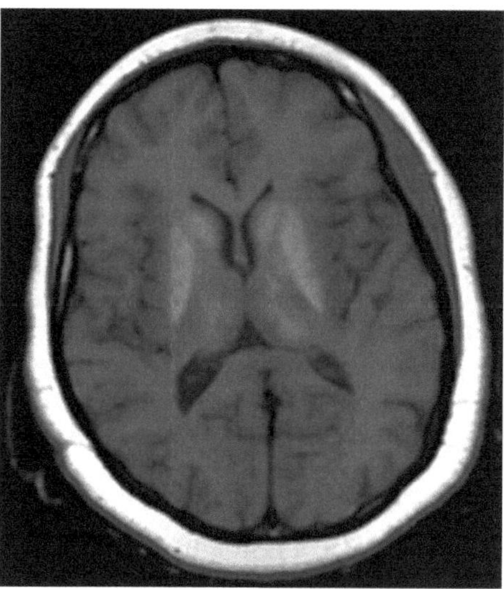

Fig. 1. Liver failure. Axial non-contrast T1-weighted image shows high signal intensity bilaterally and symmetrically in the basal ganglia and perhaps even the thalami. This is believed to be due to manganese deposition, which shortens T1 relaxation

Table 1. Differential diagnosis of common bilateral and unilateral T1 hyperintensity in the basal ganglia

Bilateral	Unilateral
Calcifications	Calcifications
Hemorrhage	Hemorrhage
Liver failure	Hyperglycemia
Parenteral nutrition	Sydenham chorea
Neurofibromatosis type 1	

Table 2. Causes of T1 hyperintensity in the basal ganglia of patients with chronic hepatic failure and other conditions

Chronic liver failure	Other conditions
Increased concentrations of manganese	Hemorrhage and calcifications
Overabundance of lipofuscin in mitochondria, endoplasmic reticulum, and Alzheimer's type II astrocytes	Hyperviscosity and chronic ischemia
Spongiform changes and myelin vacuolization	Reactive astrocytosis, demyelination, Wallerian degeneration

depletion, NMDA exitotoxicity, and oxidative stress.[2] Mn plays a role in the development of hepatic encephalopathy, which is characterized by pyramidal and extrapyramidal dysfunction, brisk tendon reflexes, and tremors. The concentration of Mn in the pallidus of cirrhotic patients is three times higher than in controls [3]. The frequency of MRI abnormalities in the brains of cirrhotic patients is approximately 73% [3].

Long-term total parenteral nutrition results in increased T1 signal intensity in the same regions. These solutions are rich in Mn and lead to the development of neurological symptoms. Once parenteral nutrition is discontinued, the MRI abnormalities may revert to normal [4]. The amount of time required for these abnormalities to resolve is not clear, but most do so within one year after the cessation of parenteral nutrition [5]. In one patient, T1 hyperintensity developed in the adenohypophysis and dorsal brainstem three months after the initiation of total parenteral nutrition and reverted to normal four months after treatment was discontinued.[6]. Similar findings were noted in patients following liver transplantation [2].

Liver failure brings an increased proliferation of Alzheimer's type II astrocytes in the affected brain regions. The etiology for the proliferation of these cells may be hyperammonemia. The cells are characterized by cytoplasmic hypertrophy and increased water content; the latter may decrease magnetization transfer by virtue of protein dilution. Proton magnetic resonance spectroscopy (MRS) of the brain may also show abnormalities in patients with liver failure. Studies have shown that MRS also may be able to show abnormalities in patients with subclinical and clinical hepatic encephalopathy [7]. These abnormalities include reduced levels of choline (Cho), reduced levels of myoinositol (Myo), and increased levels of glutamine. In patients with Wilson disease, MRS may be able to distinguish between portal-systemic encephalopathy and primary neurodegeneration by virtue of demonstrating low *N*-acetyl aspartate (NAA) in the latter [8]. MRS may also be helpful in assessing the effects of treatment in patients with hepatic encephalopathy [9].

Repeated episodes of hepatic failure may lead to the development of acquired (non-Wilsonian) hepatocerebral degeneration. The clinical symptoms are permanent and death commonly follows. Imaging studies of these patients no longer show the typical T1 hyperintensities in the basal ganglia described above for chronic hepatic encephalopathy. Instead, there is T2 signal intensity, particularly in the middle cerebral peduncles [10]. These zones correspond to spongiform myelinolytic changes, most likely the sequelae of ischemia.

Wilson Disease

Wilson disease (WD) is a genetic disorder of copper metabolism that is characterized by the failure to incorporate copper into ceruloplasmin in the liver, the failure of the liver to excrete copper into the bile, and the toxic accumulation of copper in multiple organs [9]. The defect has been mapped to chromosome 13q14.3. In addition, concentrations of other heavy metals, such as zinc, iron, silver, and aluminum, are increased. Most affected children (10-13 years) present with hepatic failure while most adults with WD present with neurological symptoms. The accumulation of copper within Descemet's membrane (in the cornea) results in Kayser-Fleischer rings, and within the lens in the rare "sunflower" cataracts. Pathologically, there is cell loss and cavitation in the lentiform nucleus. Copper concentrations at these sites are markedly increased. Other involved regions include the thalamus, subthalamus, red nucleus, substantia nigra, dentate nucleus, and brainstem. Microscopically, there are large cells with small nuclei (termed Opalski cells). The brain becomes diffusely atrophic.

MRI shows abnormalities even in the absence of clinical neurological findings. The paramagnetic effects of copper are visible by MRI only in untreated patients [11, 12]. Basal ganglia lesions are most often bilateral and symmetrical. The putamina shows a striking increase in T2 signal intensity. This is present to a lesser degree in other deep gray-matter structures. Thalamic lesions are often seen but the dorsomedial nuclei are typically spared. White-matter tracts, including the dentatothalamic, corticospinal, and pontocerebellar tracts, are commonly involved. The claustrum may show high T2 signal intensity (Fig. 2a). The midbrain is bright on T2-weighted images and FLAIR images, with relative sparing of its deep nuclei, giving rise to the "panda" sign [9] (Fig. 2b). Copper results in T1 and T2 shortening; thus, the imaging findings in WD are probably secondary to spongy degeneration, cavitation, neuronal loss, and reactive astrocytosis. There is a correlation between the clinical and the MRI findings. An abnormal-appearing striatum correlates with pseudoparkinsonism; an abnormal dentatothalamic tract, with cerebellar signs; and an abnormal pontocerebellar tract, with pseudoparkinsonism [13]. The presence of portosystemic shunting may correlate with abnormalities seen in the globus pallidus. The abnormal T2 signal intensity may improve after copper-trapping therapy [14]. MRS shows that NAA/Cr and Cho/Cr ratios are lower in WD patients than in controls [8]. In addition, patients with WD and portosystemic shunting have lower Myo/Cr than patients with WD and no portosystemic shunting.

Thrombotic Thrombocytopenic Purpura

This disorder is characterized by thrombocytopenia, microangiopathic anemia, and neurological symptoms. It results in a widespread thrombosis of small vessels [15] and is clinically indistinguishable from (and probably related to) hemolytic-uremic syndrome. Neurological symptoms are more pronounced in thrombotic thrombocytopenic purpura (TTP) than in hemolytic-uremic syndrome. In TTP patients, there is an anomaly in the cir-

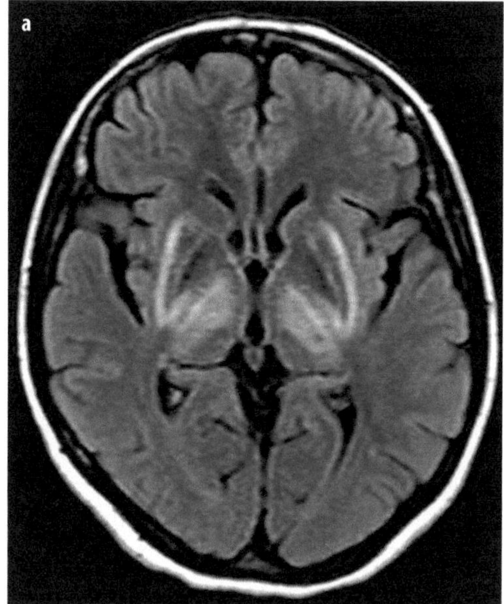

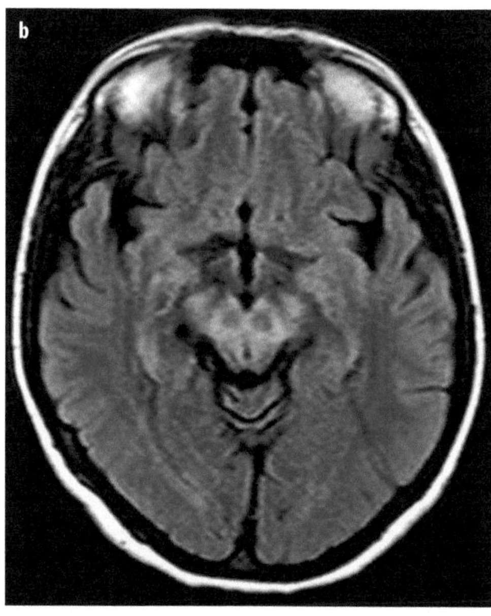

Fig. 2 a, b. Wilson disease. **a** Axial FLAIR image demonstrates high signal intensity in the thalami and outer aspects of the putamina. **b** The midbrain also shows high signal surrounding the dark red nuclei and substantiae nigra, giving rise to the "panda" sign

culation of platelet adhesion factors. Skin and mucosal purpura are typical and occur early on. The neurological symptoms are fatigue, confusion, headache, and abnormal vision and language. The imaging findings of TTP and hemolytic-uremic syndrome are similar and are often reported together. There may be small and disseminate brain hemorrhages [15]. No large vessel occlusions are seen. Small infarctions involving the basal ganglia and thalamus occur in about 50% of patients. Scattered multi-focal and confluent lesions involving the cortex and underlying white matter are common. These abnormalities show high T2 signal intensity [14] and are similar to the lesions seen in posterior reversible encephelopathy syndrome [16]. They may resolve or go on to become permanent infarctions. Some will show evidence of laminar necrosis, which is seen as fine linear areas of increased T1 signal intensity in the deep cortex. The frontal lobes may also be involved. To the best of our knowledge, at the time of this writing, there are no reports regarding the utility of other advanced imaging modalities in this entity.

Hypercalcemic Disorders Resulting in Brain Calcifications

Hypothyroidism may lead to intellectual deterioration, calcium deposition in the brain, and enlargement of the pituitary gland. Central hypothyroidism may be either an isolated defect or part of panhypopituitarism. Longstanding untreated hypothyroidism may result in enlargement of the pituitary gland [17]. This, in turn, may compress the optic chiasm, producing visual symptoms; these, however, are rarely the presenting clinical symptoms. Circulating thyroid hormones have a negative feedback on the gland. If an inadequate amount of thyroid hormones are being produced by the adenohypophysis, the serum level of thyroid stimulating hormone (produced by the hypothalamus) will increase, resulting in hyperplasia of the thyrotropin-releasing cells (also called thyrotrophs). Treatment with hormone replacement results in a reduction in the size of the pituitary gland and in an improvement of the symptoms. Hypothyroidism is said to be a rare cause of basal ganglia calcifications [18], which are found in many adults and are marked in up to 2% of the population. Since the majority of these individuals are normal, the presence of basal ganglia calcifications cannot be used as a marker for systemic disorders. While the majority of such calcifications are idiopathic and of no clinical significance, cerebellar calcifications are strongly associated with hypothyroidism [18].

Carbon Monoxide Intoxication

Carbon monoxide (CO) intoxication results in nearly 6,000 accidental and suicide deaths in the USA each year [19] The most common causes of increased CO levels are the burning of gasoline, kerosene, wood, coal, and, recently, propane. Individuals working in enclosed spaces ("warehouse workers headache") are particularly prone to acute CO intoxication. The incidence of CO intoxication is higher during the winter. The affinity of hemoglobin for CO is 200-250 times higher than for carbon dioxide. CO affects the cytochrome oxidase system, impairs the release of oxygen in tissues, and results in brain lipid peroxidation. Although symptoms tend to occur early, their severity has no correlation with the blood levels of CO. Early symptoms include headache, impaired vigilance, and abnormal audition and vision. Severe symptoms are nausea, vomiting, seizures, syncope, coma, and death.

Classic findings such as "cherry red" mucosa are rare. CO has two effects on the brain: (1) it binds to regions that have a high oxygen demand (selective vulnerability mechanism). such as the globus pallidus; (2) it binds to normal iron-containing structures such as the substantia nigra [19]. It is also possible that systemic hypotension contributes, or in some cases is mostly responsible for, the brain lesions. MRI and CT show lesions confined mostly to the globus pallidus. These lesions are of low CT density and of high signal intensity on T2-weighted, FLAIR, and diffusion-weighted images (Fig. 3). The lesions are not hemorrhagic. If the patient survives, diffuse brain atrophy may ensue.

Glycol-Related Intoxication

Ethylene glycol is a compound found in automobile antifreeze, hydraulic fluid, and industrial solvents, and is a common cause of poisoning and suicide deaths [20]. Related compounds, such as diethylene glycol and propylene glycol, are also toxic. These two latter compounds have been used to contaminate medications such as acetaminophen and have resulted in toxic epidemics in Haiti, India, and Nigeria [21]. After the ingestion of ethylene glycol, metabolic acidosis ensues, resulting in kidney damage, due to the accumulation of calcium and oxalate crystals in urine, and in acute renal failure, which secondarily affects the CNS. A typical clinical symptom of ethylene glycol poisoning is blindness. In one patient with ethylene glycol intoxication, emergency CT of the head showed only a subdural hematoma, which was probably post-trauma and not related directly to the effects of the toxin [22]. Patients who have ingested antifreeze solution show abnormal increased T2 signal intensity in the putamen, globus pallidus, caudate nucleus, and thalamus (Fig. 4). No hemorrhages are present. The clinical manifestations related to intoxication with diethylene glycol and propylene glycol include fever, vomiting, diarrhea, cough, abdominal pain, altered mentation, dyspnea, and acute renal failure.

Methanol Intoxication

Methanol (methyl alcohol) is used in the production of antifreeze solution, in illegal drinks (as a substitute for ethanol), and in poor-quality cologne [23]. Following the ingestion of methanol there is latent period of 1-72 h; thereafter, metabolic acidosis and cortical blindness ensue. Other symptoms are parkinsonism, inebriation, headache, dizziness, seizures, and coma [24]. Methanol and its byproducts (formaldehyde and formic acid) are toxic to the CNS. Putaminal hemorrhagic necrosis is a typical histological feature. CT shows the putamina to be of low density, swollen, and containing small hemorrhages. MRI shows the affected regions to be of either low or high T1 signal intensity as well as hyperintense on T2-weighted images. In some patients, there is also cortical necrosis, particularly in the paramedian aspects of the frontal lobes [23]. This finding results in high T2 signal intensity in the affected cortex. The cerebellum and occipital regions are typically spared. Optic atrophy may be seen, but the signal intensity in these structures remains within normal limits. The white matter may be diffusely edematous.

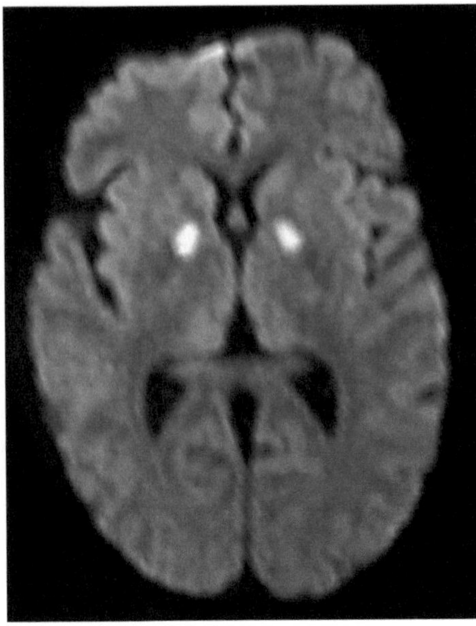

Fig. 3. Carbon monoxide intoxication. Axial diffusion-weighted image shows high signal intensity (which was restricted on the corresponding ADC map, not shown) in the globus pallidi

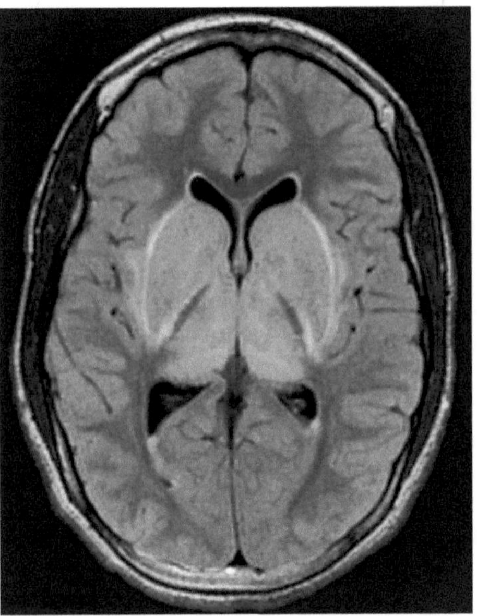

Fig. 4. Ethylene glycol intoxication. Axial FLAIR image in an autistic child who drank antifreeze fluid. There is swelling and high signal intensity in the basal ganglia and thalami

Inhalant Intoxication

Inhaling solvents, volatile substances, and glue vapors result in a transient euphoric state. Inhalant abusers are usually teenagers. The most commonly abused substances are listed in Table 3 [25].

The fumes of a substance may be inhaled directly or by placing them in a bag or soaked in a rag. After an initial euphoric state, drowsiness and sleep ensue. The lipophilic nature of inhalants explains their high affinity for the lipid-laden brain. Suffocation, aspiration, and dangerous behavior are common causes of death. The neuropathologic and imaging features of toluene abuse ("spray heads") are well known [26]. Chronic toluene abuse results in cognitive impairment, cerebellar ataxia, tremor, and anosmia. MRI shows diffuse cerebral, cerebellar, and brainstem atrophy. T2-weighted imaging shows an abnormal increase in the signal intensity of the white matter, which reflects underlying gliosis. Hypointensity in the basal ganglia and thalamus is seen on both T1- and T2-weighted images and is believed to be the result of iron deposition (a non-specific finding appreciable in many degenerative brain disorders). Interestingly, it has been suggested that the partitioning of toluene into the lipid membranes of cells in the brain may be responsible for this finding [26]. Other reported MRI findings in toluene abuse include loss of cerebral and cerebellar gray-white matter discrimination, scattered foci of abnormal signal intensity in white matter, thinning of the corpus callosum, and generalized atrophy [27].

Nitrous Oxide

The effects of nitrous oxide (NO) on the CNS have been documented [28]. NO is commonly used in dental anesthesia and as a propellant in containers of certain foods, such as whipped cream. In contrast to other inhalants, NO is not readily available to children and teenagers and its abuse is more common in the adult population. NO causes damage by irreversibly oxidizing vitamin B12. On a chronic basis, this results in the formation of abnormal substrates for fatty acid synthesis, which are eventually incorporated into the formation of myelin. The clinical manifestations of chronic NO toxicity are thus identical to those of vitamin B12 deficiency. There is involvement of the posterior columns of the spinal cord beginning at the thoracic level. This eventually leads to subacute spinal cord degeneration. T2-weighted images may show an abnormally increased signal intensity that is generally confined to the posterior columns [28]. Following appropriate therapy, this abnormality may resolve completely. Some patients also develop a peripheral neuropathy.

Table 3. Commonly abused inhalants

Aerosols	Liquids
Paint	Model building glue and contact cement
Butane	Gasoline
Cooking sprays	Lacquers
Cosmetics and toiletries	Dry cleaning fluids
Nitrous oxide	Typewriter correction fluid
	Lighter fluids

Disorders Related to Ethanol Abuse

Sequelae of alcohol abuse include direct toxicity, dangerous behavior leading to cerebral and spinal trauma, nutritional abnormalities (including vitamin deficiencies), and teratogenicity (including the fetal-alcohol syndrome). Chronic alcohol consumption results in ataxia and lower limb incoordination that correlates well with cerebellar atrophy, which is present in over 60% of alcoholics [29]. There is shrinkage of the folia, particularly in the superior vermis, which reflects a loss of Purkinje cells. Alcoholic myelopathy and peripheral neuropathy are probably related to a thiamine deficiency. Other disorders associated with alcoholism are central pontine myelinolysis and the Marchiafava-Bignami syndrome.

The acute symptoms of the Wernicke-Korsakoff syndrome (WK) include lethargy, confusion, altered memory, nystagmus, ophthalmoplegia, and ataxia [30]. Although WK is mostly seen in alcoholics, other related conditions include anorexia, protracted vomiting secondary to chemotherapy, digitalis toxicity, gastric plication procedures, starvation, and AIDS. The common underlying factor in all of these conditions is a thiamine deficiency. Following treatment, the patient may develop chronic memory problems (Korsakoff psychosis). Thiamine metabolism plays a role in brain glucose oxidation and in membrane permeability to chlorine ions. There is little natural reserve of thiamine, therefore its deficiency manifests early. Cerebral lactic acidosis also occurs early. Glutamate (an excitatory amino acid) is found in high concentrations in thiamine-depleted brain regions [30]. Acutely, there is vascular dilatation and endothelial swelling, mostly involving small arteries. Neuronal damage and swelling of astrocytes lead to ischemia of the mamillary bodies, dorsomedial thalamic nuclei, pulvinars, walls of the third ventricle, peri-ueductal gray matter, colliculi, third cranial nerve nuclei, inferior olives, and superior cerebellar vermis. On T2-weighted images, all of these regions show abnormal high signal intensity [31]. These findings are typical and, in the correct clinical situation, enable the diagnosis of acute Wernicke encephalopathy. Contrast enhancement of the mamillary bodies may be seen and is pathognomic of this condition. Hemorrhage is only found in about 20% of autopsy cases and is not usually seen on imaging studies [32]. It should be noted, however, that an absence of the imaging abnormalities mentioned above does not exclude the diagnosis of Wernicke encephalopathy [33]. CT is of no utility in these patients. In the chronic stage of thiamine deficiency, vascular damage is no longer present. There is diffuse brain atrophy that is more prominent at the level of the fornices and mamillary bodies.

Marchiafava-Bignami (MB) is a rare disorder seen in chronic alcoholics. Although it was initially described in drinkers of Italian red wine, it may be seen in persons ingesting other type of alcoholic beverages. There is cystic necrosis of the corpus callosum, particularly in its genu and body [29]. Similar lesions may be observed in the optic chiasm, anterior commissure, centrum semiovale, and brachium pontis. Histologically, there is demyelination with relative axonal preservation similar to that seen in patients with cyanide or CO poisoning. MRI shows that the anterior region of the corpus callosum is of low T1 and high T2 signal intensities [34]. Areas of abnormal increased T2 signal intensity may also be seen in the centrum semiovale [34]. MB is a diffuse brain disorder that is not restricted to the corpus callosum.

Disorders of Sodium Imbalance (Osmotic Myelinolysis)

Sodium imbalance may result in diffuse injury (hyponatremic encephalopathy) or focal lesions (osmotic myelinolysis). Chronic symptoms are anorexia, apathy, weakness, muscle cramps, nausea, vomiting, and headache [35]. Acute symptoms include seizures, ataxia, and death. The clinical manifestations of hyponatremic encephalopathy are given in Table 4 [35].

The brain is the target organ and is responsible for the morbidity and mortality associated with sodium imbalance. Hyponatremia results from excess water and the inability of the kidneys to excrete, and from urinary loss of sodium ions. Abnormal secretion of anti-diuretic hormone (ADH) also results in hypervolemia, particularly when associated with the syndrome of inappropriate secretion of ADH. When plasma osmolality falls as a result of hyponatremia, cellular equilibrium is maintained by the excretion of intracellular solutes and dilution of the intracellular compartment by influx of water into the cells. Cellular damage occurs predominantly as a consequence of water influx. Brain swelling that is greater than 5% of brain volume results in significant morbidity and mortality [35]. In acute hyponatremic encephalopathy, most deaths are due to brain swelling and herniations. The majority of patients with hyponatremic encephalopathy have one or more of the following underlying conditions: post-operative state, polydipsia-hyponatremia syndrome, use of pharmacologic agents that interfere with the ability of the kidneys to excrete free water, congestive heart failure, or AIDS [35]. In addition to the damage induced by low sodium, most of these patients are hypoxic. However, correction of the hyponatremia may lead to other pathologic conditions, including cerebral demyelination lesions.

The most common cerebral demyelinating lesion associated with correction of hyponatremia is central pontine myelinolysis (CPM). CPM may occur as a consequence of primary hyponatremia, induced hyponatremia during a variety of treatments, hypernatremic states, hypoxic events, and severe liver disease [35]. Conditions leading to CPM are alcoholism, extensive burns, sepsis, Hodgkin's disease, and other tumors. Myelinolysis is probably not a sequela of hyponatremia but is secondary to its correction, in that rapid correction of hyponatremia increases the risk of developing myelinolysis. CPM generally ensues 2-3 days after the hyponatremic event. Over 85% of patients clinically suspected to have CPM show no imaging abnormalities [35]. Curiously, CPM is occasionally seen in normonatremic patients. Microscopically, CPM shows destruction of the myelin but relative preservation of the axons [36]. The lesion is symmetrical and almost always located in the midline of the basis pontis. Outside of the brainstem but within the posterior fossa, the cerebellar cortex is often affected. Unfortunately, this latter type of involvement has not been documented by imaging studies. About 10% of patients with CPM will have other lesions, mostly supratentorial in location. In the cerebral hemispheres, myelinolysis often involves the deep gray structures that are surrounded by white matter. The thalamus is commonly affected but other regions, such as cortical and subcortical regions, may be involved [36]. The lesions are well seen on MRI studies: CPM has low T1 and high T2 signal intensity. On axial views the lesion is rounded or triangular in shape, while on coronal views the lesion has a "Batman" sign configuration. The need for contrast enhancement is rare. Similar MRI features are found in myelinolysis affecting other brain regions. We have seen myelinolysis affecting the corpus callosum in a young post-partum female after rapid correction of hypernatremia. In addition to the above-mentioned findings, these lesions are of moderately increased signal on diffusion-weighted imaging. The prognosis of patients with CPM is variable; some patients die from the disease while others survive, improving either slowly or not at all.

Table 4. Clinical symptoms of hyponatremic encephalopathy

Early symptoms	Advanced symptoms	Severe symptoms
Anorexia, headache, nausea, vomiting, muscle cramps, weakness	Impaired responses to verbal commands and pain, bizarre behavior, hallucinations, obtundation, respiratory distress	Decortication, bradycardia, hyper- or hypotension, altered temperature regulation, seizures, respiratory arrest, coma

Pantothenate Kinase Deficiency (Hallervorden-Spatz Disease)

Pantothenate kinase deficiency (PANK2) is related to iron overload and degenerative brain disease. It is linked to an abnormality in chromosome 20p12.3-p13. Large amounts of iron are deposited in the globus pallidus and pars reticulata of the substantia nigra [37]. Iron deposition leads to axonal swelling and decreased myelination. Microscopy demonstrates the presence of abnormal, spherical bodies that contain superoxide dismutase and are believed to be typical for PANK2. Eventually, these regions of the brain are destroyed. Patients with PANK2 suffer from dystonia, muscle rigidity, hyperreflexia, and choreoathetosis. Mental retardation is variable and death occurs 1-2 years after the diagnosis. Since the laboratory findings are non-specific, the combination of clinical symptoms and imaging findings are used to establish a diagnosis. The CT findings are also non-specific, whereas MRI is the method of choice. Initially, only hypointensity (more pronounced on T2- than on T1-weighted images) is seen in the globus pallidus. When gliosis ensues, the globus pallidus becomes hyperintense on T2-weighted images but remains surrounded by hypointensity [37, 38] (Fig. 5). This represents the "eye of the tiger" sign and is said to be characteristic for PANK2.

Hyperglycemia

Hyperglycemia also has adverse affects on the CNS. It may lead to increases in cerebral lactic acid, which can damage the brain primarily or worsen the outcome of patients with underlying infarctions. A typical manifestation of hyperglycemia, and at times the initial one, is hemichorea-hemiballism (HH). The clinical manifestation of HH are random and fast jerking motions in the distal extremities (chorea) as well as violent flinging and kicking, mainly involving the proximal joints (ballismus) [39]. In these patients, CT shows a high density conforming to one lentiform nucleus and the head of the ipsilateral caudate nucleus. These regions are of increased signal intensity on T1-weighted images while T2-weighted images are normal (Fig. 6). Occasionally, the ipsilateral cerebral peduncle also shows T1 hyperintensity in its anteromedial region [39]. Hemorrhage and/or calcifications have not been reported in HH and the findings are thought be due to the presence of gemistocytes. MRS obtained from the region of T1 signal intensity abnormality demonstrates elevated lactic acid and decreased Cr. These features have been interpreted as a consequence of energy depletion, leading to neuronal malfunction. Although the above-described MR abnormalities are fairly typical for HH, they were also noted in a patient with lupus erythematosus and chorea [40].

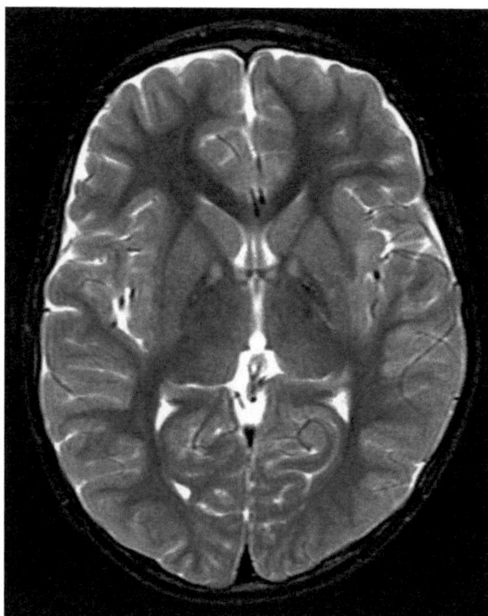

Fig. 5. Pantothenate kinase deficiency. Axial T2-weighted image shows low signal in the medial globus pallidi surrounding focal regions of high signal intensity ("eye of the tiger" sign)

Amyloidosis

A detailed review of this complex entity is beyond the scope of this chapter. Amyloidosis is a group of disorders that may result in systemic or local manifestations. Amyloid is mostly composed of fibrils arranged in a cross-beta pleated fashion [41]. These fibrils are responsible for amyloid's birefringence under polarized light microscopy. Amyloid is an insoluble compound that is deposited in the organ in which it is produced. The second component that makes up amyloid (b-component) is a protein that is identical in all types of amyloid. Amyloid A is seen in inflammatory processes and in senile amyloidosis. Amyloid AL has a light chain from immunoglobulin M and is commonly found in patients with multiple myeloma. In the brain, amyloid infiltrates neurons as well as the media and adventitia of blood vessel walls. The frontal, parietal, occipital, and temporal lobes are affected. Amyloid weakens the walls of vessels and may promote the formation of micro-aneurysms. These features are thought to be responsible for the common brain

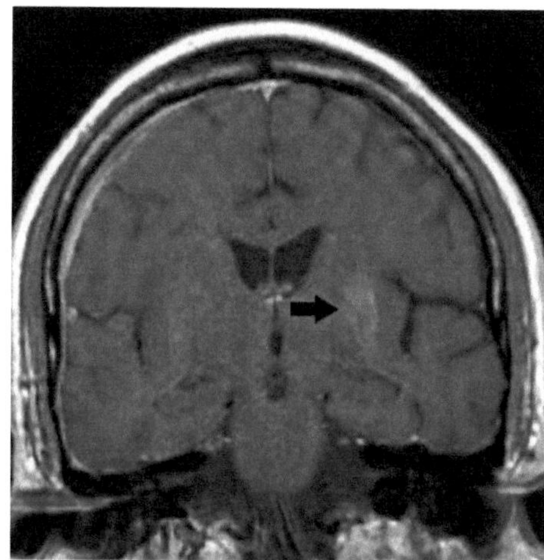

Fig. 6. Hyperglycemia. Coronal T1-weighted image shows high signal intensity (*arrow*) in the left basal ganglia in a patient with contralateral hemiballismus hemichorea

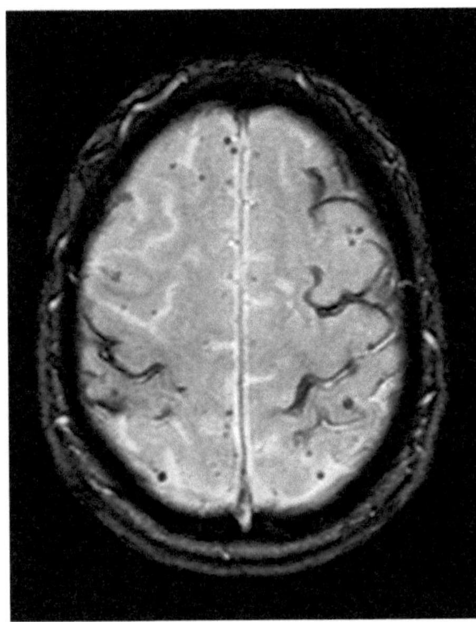

Fig. 7. Pial amyloidosis. Axial gradient-echo image shows superficial siderosis due to repeated subarachnoid hemorrhages in a patient with amyloidosis. (Courtesy of Dr. J. Grimme, Oregon, USA)

hematomas occurring in these patients. Senile amyloidosis is not uncommon after 80 years of life. Amyloidosis accounts for 5-10% of intracerebral hemorrhages in elderly individuals [41]. Other cerebral manifestations of amyloidosis are recurrent transient neurological events, rapidly progressing dementia, and mass-like lesions (amyloidomas). Brain amyloidomas are often isolated and not associated with systemic forms of the disease. Amyloid-related cerebral hemorrhages tend to be cortical or subcortical in location. The hematomas are large and often multi-focal. Their locations may be mirror-like in the two hemispheres. Amyloidomas are found in the parenchyma, choroid plexi, Gasserian ganglion, spine, pituitary gland, orbits, larynx, and tongue. They manifest as non-specific, non-enhancing masses. Correct diagnosis is made by biopsy. Amyloidosis may also result in cerebral microhemorrhages, mostly located in the peripheral white and gray matter (those that are due to systemic hypertension are commonly found in the deep gray matter). Additionally, amyloidosis involving the leptomeningeal blood vessels can cause repeated subarachnoid hemorrhages, with subsequent superficial siderosis (Fig. 7).

References

1. Etsuo I, Shinichi H, Narumi Y et al (1991) Portal-systemic encephalopathy: presence of basal ganglia lesions with high signal intensity on MR images. Radiology 179:551-555
2. Krieger D, Krieger S, Jansen O et al (1995) Manganese and chronic hepatic encephalopathy. Lancet 346:270-274
3. Pomier-Layrargues G, Spahr L, Butterworth RF (1995) Increased manganese concentrations in pallidum of cirrhotic patients. Lancet 345:735
4. Fell JM, Reynolds AP, Meadows N et al (1996) Manganese toxicity in children receiving long-term parenteral nutrition. Lancet 347:1218-1221
5. Mirowitz SA, Westrich TJ (1992) Basal ganglial signal intensity alterations: reversal after discontinuation of parenteral manganese administration. Radiology 185:535-536
6. Okamoto K, Ito J, Furusawa T et al (1998) Reversible hyperintensity of the anterior pituitary gland on T1-weighted MR images in a patient receiving temporary parenteral nutrition. AJNR Am J Neuroradiol 19:1287-1289
7. Ross BD, Jacobson S, Villamil F et al (1994) Subclinical hepatic encephalopathy: proton MR spectroscopic abnormalities. Radiology 193:457-463
8. Van Den Heuvel AG, Van der Grond J, Van Rooij LG et al (1997) Differentiation between portal-systemic encephalopathy and neurodegenerative disorders in patients with Wilson disease: H-1 MR spectroscopy. Radiology 203:539-543
9. Lee J, Lacomis D, Comu S et al (1998) Acquired hepatocerebral degeneration: MR and pathologic findings. AJNR Am J Neuroradiol 19:485-487
10. Albernaz VS, Castillo M, Mukherji SK et al (1997) Facies to remember, No. 11, Part I: The challenge. Int J Neuroradiol 3:206-217
11. Magalhaes AC, Caramelli P, Menezes JR et al (1994) Wilson's disease: MRI with clinical correlation. Neuroradiology 36:97-100
12. King AD, Walshe JM, Kendall BE et al (1996) Cranial MR imaging in Wilson's disease. AJR Am J Roentgenol 167:1579-1584
13. van Wassenaer-van Hall HN, van den Heuvel AG, Algra A et al (1996) Wilson disease: findings at MR imaging and CT of the brain with clinical correlation. Radiology 198:531-536
14. Engelbrecht V, Schlaug G, Hefter H et al (1995) MRI of the brain in Wilson disease: T2 signal loss under therapy. J Comput Assist Tomogr 19(4):635-638
15. Moore KR, Osborn AG, Townsend JJ et al (1997) The imaging and pathologic spectrum of hemolytic-uremic syndrome-thrombotic thrombocytopenic purpura (HUS-TTP Syndrome). Int J Neuroradiol 3:147-159
16. Okada J, Yoshikawa K, Matsuo H et al (1991) Reversible MRI and CT findings in uremic encephalopathy. Neuroradiology 33:524-526
17. Shimono T, Hatabu H, Kasagi K et al (1999) Rapid progression of pituitary hyperplasia in humans with primary hypothyroidism: demonstration with MR imaging. Radiology 213:383-388
18. Burke JW, Williamson BR, Hurst RW (1998) "Idiopathic" cerebellar calcifications: association with hypothyroidism. Radiology 167:533-536
19. Wesley EE, Moorehead B, Haponik EF (1995) Emergency evaluation and management of 30 patients with carbon monoxide poisoning. Am J Med 98:145-155
20. Roberts J (2000) Ethylene glycol intoxication and multiple trauma. Emerg Med 32:8
21. O'Brien KL, Selanikio JD, Hecdivert C et al (1998) Epidemic of pediatric deaths from acute renal failure caused by diethylene glycol poisoning. JAMA 279:1175-1180
22. Nau T, Seitz H, Kapral S et al (1999) Ethylene glycol poisoning and brain injury – a dangerous combination. Anasthesiologie 34:318-320
23. Tayfun C, Kurtaran HK, Bulakbasi N et al (1999) Cerebral and orbital magnetic resonance imaging findings in methyl alcohol intoxication. Int J Neuroradiol 5:145-150
24. Kuteifan K, Oesterle H, Tajahmady T et al (1998) Necrosis and haemorrhage of the putamen in methanol poisoning shown on MRI. Neuroradiology 40:158-160
25. Committee on Substance Abuse and Committee on Native American Child Health (1996) Inhalant abuse. Pediatrics 97:420-423
26. Unger E, Alexander A, Fritz, T et al (1994) Toluene abuse: physical basis for hypointensity of the basal ganglia on T2-weighted MR images. Radiology 193:473-476

27. Xiong L, Matthes JD, Li J, Jinkins JR (1993) MR imaging of "spray heads": toluene abuse via aerosol paint inhalation. AJNR Am J Neuroradiol 14:1195-1199
28. Pema PJ, Horak HA, Wyatt RH (1998) Myelopathy caused by nitrous oxide toxicity. AJNR Am J Neuroradiol 19:894-896
29. Harper C, Bitterworth R (1997) Nutritional and metabolic disorders. In: Graham DI, Lantos PL (eds) Greenfield's Neuropathology, 6th ed. Arnold, London, pp 613-615
30. Brody BA (1996) The Wernicke-Korsakoff syndrome. Int J Neuroradiol 2:216-230
31. Gallucci M, Bozzao A, Splendiani A et al (1990) Wernicke encephalopathy: MR findings in five patients. AJNR Am J Neuroradiol 11:887-892
32. Victor M (1990) MR in the diagnosis of Wernicke-Korsakoff syndrome. AJNR Am J Neuroradiol 11:895-896
33. Antunez E, Estruch R, Cardenal C et al (1998) Usefulness of CT and MR imaging in the diagnosis of acute Wernicke's Encephalopathy. AJR Am J Roentgenol 171:1131-1137
34. Ishii K, Ikejiri Y, Sasaki M et al (1999) Regional cerebral glucose metabolism and blood flow in a patient with Marchiafava-Bignami disease. AJNR Am J Neuroradiol 20:1249-1251
35. Fraser CL, Arieff AI (1997) Epidemiology, pathophysiology, and management of hyponatremic encephalopathy. Am J Med 102:67-77
36. Laureno R, Karp BI (1997) Myelinolysis after correction of hyponatremia. Ann Intern Med 126:57-62
37. Berg D, Hoggenmuller U, Hofmann E et al (2000) The basal ganglia in haemochromatosis. Neuroradiology 42:9-13
38. Hermann W, Reuter M, Barthel H et al (2000) Diagnosis of Hallervorden-Spatz disease using MRI, I-123-beta-CIT-SPECT and I-123-IBZM-SPECT. Eur Neurol 43:187-188
39. Shan DE, Ho DM, Chang C et al (1998) Hemichorea-hemiballism: an explanation for MR signal changes. AJNR Am J Neuroradiol 19:863-870
40. Kashihara K, Nakashima S, Kohira I et al (1998) Hyperintense basal ganglia on T1-weighted MR images in a patient with central nervous system Lupus and Chorea. AJNR Am J Neuroradiol 19:284-286
41. Castillo M, Mukherji SK (1998) Pits, patches, and protuberances: No. 10, Part I. The challenge. Int J Neuroradiol 4:349-356

Degenerative Brain Disease

Marco Essig

Department of Radiology, German Cancer Research Center, Heidelberg, Germany

Introduction

With the increase in the mean age of the populations of many countries, neurodegenerative diseases are becoming increasingly important. Of particular urgency is their early diagnosis, to allow for early therapeutic intervention since neurodegeneration begins long before the patient experiences any symptoms. In fact, it can be months or years before the clinical symptoms become obvious. The sensitivity of imaging in its ability to detect even small changes in the brain may be of vital importance in this scenario. Nonetheless, although the radiological evaluation of neurodegenerative diseases has improved markedly with the introduction of modern magnetic resonance imaging (MRI) techniques, the differential diagnosis between the different diseases remains a challenge. For this reason, a detailed understanding of the normal aging changes in the brain is needed to correctly interpret a patient's clinical findings and laboratory test results.

Aging Brain

In the normal aging brain, there are changes in iron content, brain volume, and the amount of white matter. The extent of these changes varies and is influenced by a large number of factors, including lifestyle, blood pressure, and diabetes. Normally, normal physiological changes cannot be differentiated from early pathological ones. However, to be able to detect the latter, the neuroradiologist should be well-acquainted with the normal findings.

Several studies have shown that there is an increase in cerebral iron deposition with age, although the cause is poorly understood. MRI is a sensitive method to visualize iron deposition in the brain, mainly in the basal ganglia. Taking into account that a higher field strength yields more sensitive iron detection (Fig. 1), subjects ≤70 years or younger should be further evaluated for neurodegenerative disease if there is a strongly diminished

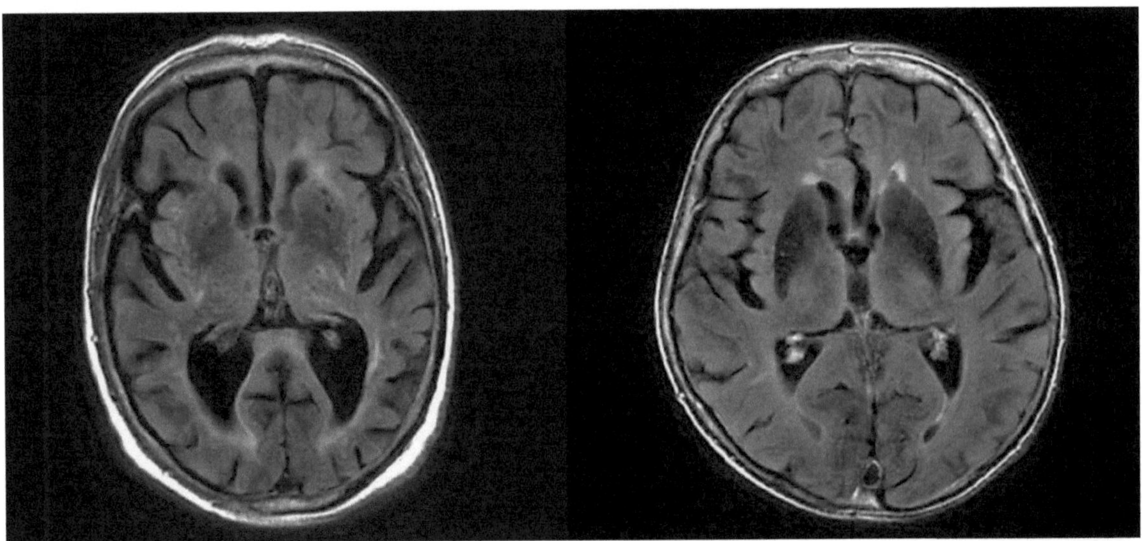

Fig. 1. *Left* Normal iron deposition in a patient with global cerebral atrophy (72 years of age and cogonitive impairment) on 3T-FLAIR MRI. The image on the right is from a patient (69 years old, 3T FLAIR MRI) with mental decline in the absence of atrophic changes. However, as seen in this image, the signal in the putamen is substantially reduced, which is suspicious for iron deposition and therefore the presence of a neurodegenerative disease

T2 signal in the basal ganglia, which is suggestive of pathologic iron deposition.

Focal or even diffuse white matter hyperintensities are common findings in the elderly population. They increase with age and are described to be more common in patients with dementia. To decide whether the hyperintensities are within the normal range or are pathologic is not possible in the majority of cases. The hyperintensities should be described as punctate, patchy, or confluent (Fig. 2). Some may be attributed to Virchow-Robin spaces.

Risk factors for an increased number of white-matter hyperintensities are hypertension, diabetes, and previous treatments. Pathologically, they represent arteriosclerotic atrophic demyelination in combination with dilated vascular spaces. The corpus callosum is normally not affected – in contrast to what is seen in inflammatory diseases. The changes can be visualized without the need for enhancement.

To better categorize these findings, diffusion imaging may be helpful in differentiating between acute, subacute, and chronic changes.

Volumetric changes of the brain also correlate with age. The brain achieves its maximum weight during the third decade of life, with a gradually decline of brain volume thereafter. MRI provides a volumetric tool to assess these changes as early indicators of neurodegenerative disease. A widening of the sylvian fissure, the basal cisterns, and, later, the interhemispheric fissures with associated widening of the ventricles occurs after the age of 65-70. The normal atrophic changes usually affect the frontal lobes first, followed by the parietal lobes with consecutive enlargement of the lateral ventricles, but sparing the temporal horns. A change in the temporal horns is therefore a sensitive marker of neurodegenerative disease (Fig. 3).

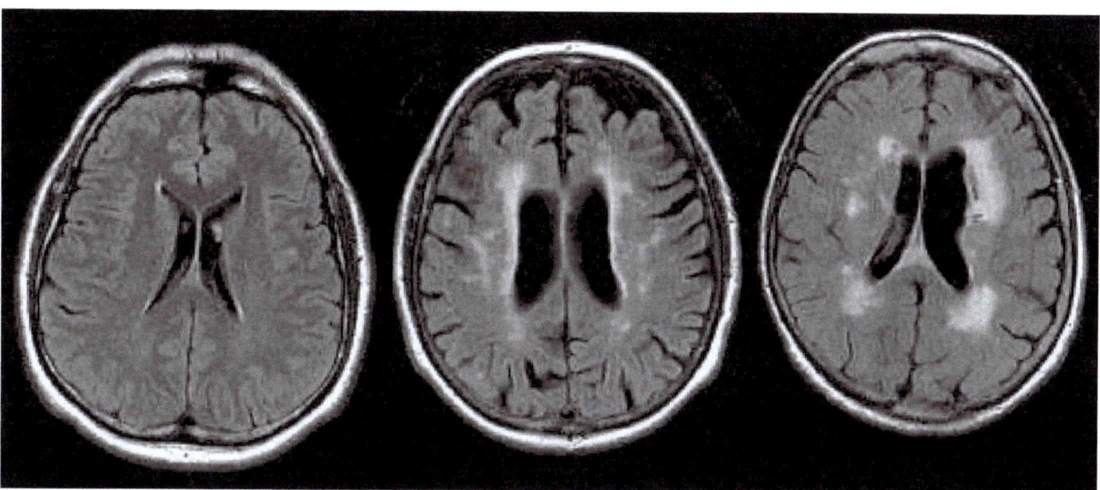

Fig. 2. White-matter hyperintensities on routine FLAIR imaging in three subjects, each 70 years of age. *Left* A normal finding is shown, with only solitary lesions; *middle* a mixed stage with solitary and partially confluent lesions; *right* major confluent lesions mixed with macroangiopathic changes indicative of hydrocephalus ex vacuo

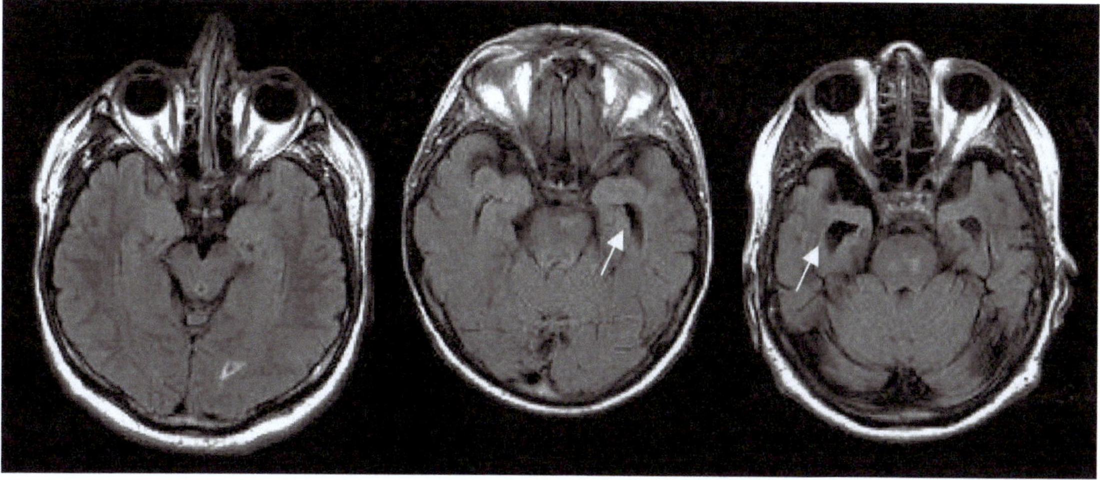

Fig. 3. Normal finding (*left*) and increasing atrophy of the temporal lobes with consecutive widening of the temporal horns (*arrows*) of the lateral ventricles (all three subjects 71 years of age)

Neurodegenerative Diseases

There are quite a large number of neurodegenerative diseases, and they can be divided into those with dementia as the primary symptom and those in which movement disorders caused by neurodegeneration are most prominent. There are also some diseases that feature both symptoms (Fig. 4). Table 1 summarizes some of the typical imaging findings according to the system used in Orrison's textbook.

To rule out secondary causes, like tumors (Fig. 5), normal-pressure hydrocephalus (Fig. 6), or other diseases, a neuroimaging study is mandatory in patients with mental decline or acquired movement disorders.

Dementia

Alzheimer's Disease

Approximately two-thirds of all neurodegenerative illnesses of later life are Alzheimer's disease (AD). The prevalence of dementia rises from <5% in individuals <75 years of age to about 10% in those between 80 and 84 years of age. After age 85, the incidence is approximately 20%, while after age 90 it is 40%. Typically, AD is of insidious onset, progressing over a timeframe of years during which there is a decline in a broad range of neuropsychological domains, such as memory, executive functions and attention, language, and praxia, leaving the patient in a helpless, severely demented state unable to perform even the simple activities of daily living. The preclinical phase of AD is characterized by mild cognitive deficits that exceed the age-related cognitive decline but which are not severe enough to be labeled dementia. Clinical and epidemiological evidence indicate that this syndrome – generally referred to as

Table 1. Diseases and associated MRI findings

Disease	MRI Findings
Alzheimer's disease	Nonspecific Atrophy with preferential medial temporal involvement Normal signal intensity in basal ganglia
Normal pressure hydrocephalus	Ventricular enlargement Normal outer CSF spaces Stretching of corpus callosum Signal void in aqueduct on PD and FLAIR
Creutzfeldt-Jakob disease	Non specific atrophic changes Rapidly progressive Symmetric T2 hyperintensities in striatum and thalamus
Pick's disease	Frontal/temporal atrophy
Parkinson's disease	Nonspecific atrophy Decreased width of pars compacta
Multi-system atrophies	Premature T2 hypointensity in striatum
Huntington's disease	Atrophy of caudate and putamen → globus pallidus
Wilson's disease	T2 Hyperintensities in putamen, thalami, and brain stem Mild generalized atrophy
Amyotrphic lateral sclerosis	Intermediate and T2 hyperintensities in intracranial corticospinal tracts
Leigh's disease	Symmetric T2 hyperintensities in globus pallidus, putamen, and caudate Signal abnormalities in periventricular white matter and periaqueductal gray matter

PD, Proton-density-weighted imaging; *FLAIR*, fluid-attenuated inversion recovery

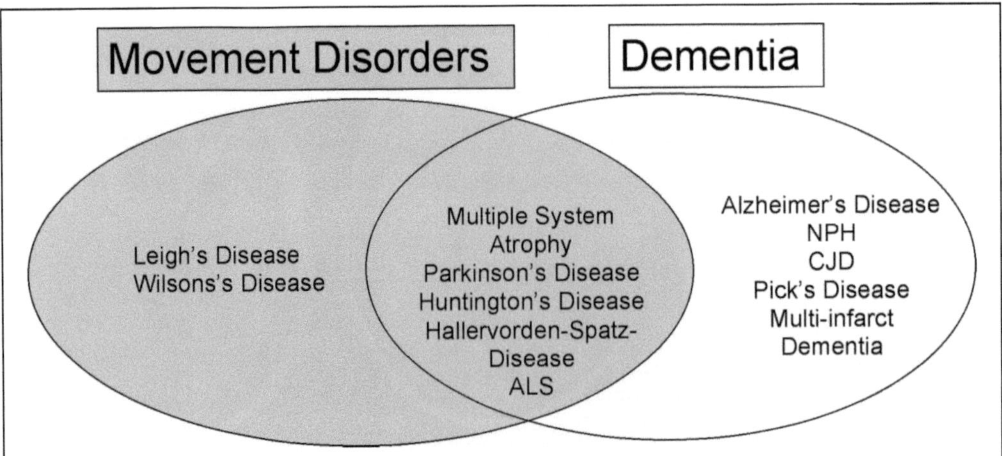

Fig. 4. The neurodegenerative diseases causing movement disorders and/or dementia. Most of the former also present with dementia and vice versa. The most common diseases are Alzheimer's disease, multi-infarct dementia, and Parkinson's disease. *ALS*, Amyotrophic lateral sclerosis; *CJD*, Creutzfeldt-Jakob disease; *NPH*, normal pressure hydrocephalus

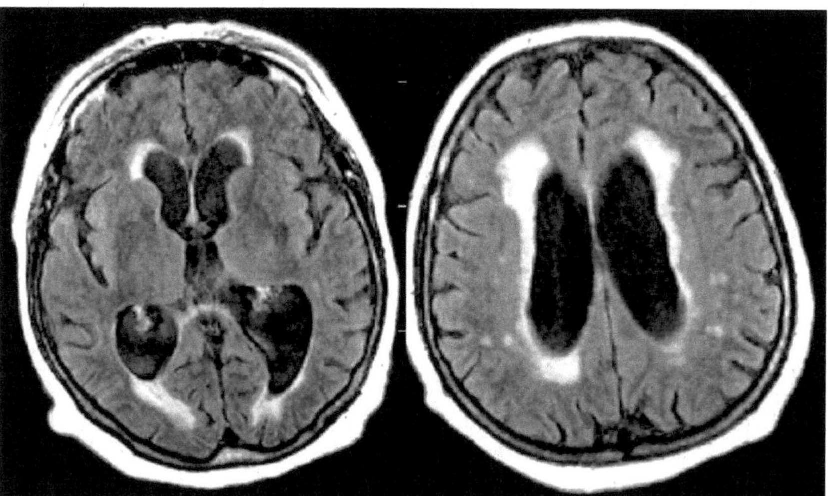

Fig. 5. FLAIR MRI in a patient with normal pressure hydrocephalus. Typical findings are the enlargement of the lateral and the third ventricle and the normal size of the cortical CSF spaces. Note also the CSF diapedisis via the ependymal tissue

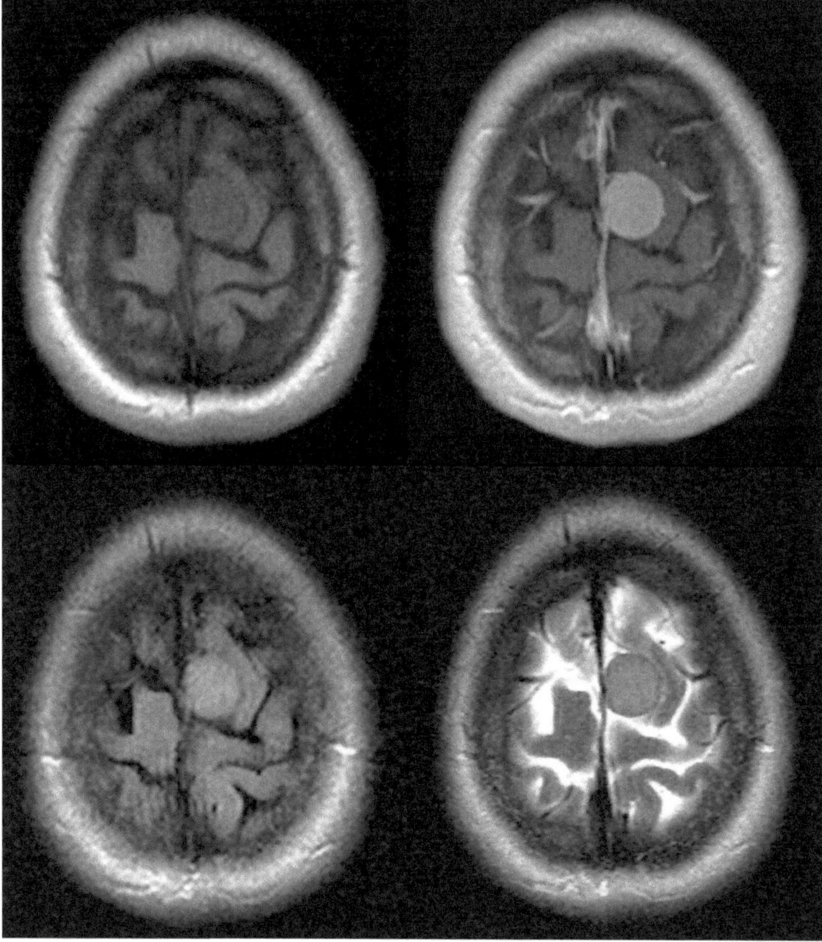

Fig. 6. Meningioma as an incidental finding in a patient with mental decline. Although the meningioma is small in this case, a frontal location may influence the patient's mnestic performance substantially

mild cognitive impairment (MCI) – remains subtle for a long time before the threshold of dementia is reached. This conclusion corresponds to the high prevalence of MCI even in the "young" old. It is assumed that MCI syndrome is associated with a strongly increased risk of dementia, especially of AD.

In the past few years, the use of neuroimaging in the diagnostic work-up of individuals suffering from mental decline has increased. Both computed tomography (CT) and MRI are performed to rule out secondary dementias (i.e., somatic disorders other than neurodegenerative diseases) or concomitant conditions that may be associated with the dementing disorder (Figs. 5, 6). This includes, in particular, the diagnosis of treatable conditions such as chronic subdural hematoma, tumors, infections, or normal pressure hydrocephalus, as well as the exclusion of concomitant neurovascular changes.

The accurate diagnosis and prognosis of the subtle changes that occur in the early stages of dementia, including investigations of the underlying pathophysiology, is not only of great importance to the patient but it is also essential for the development of new therapeutic concepts, including preventive strategies. The different pathological processes that produce cerebral dysfunction at a cellular level also produce macroscopic effects that may be detected with imaging. Thus, structural neuroimaging plays an important role, and is regarded as a major part of the investigation of a patient's mental decline. In addition to structural analyses, functional neuroimaging methods allow an even more detailed view into the pathophysiologic changes associated with the development of dementia.

Previous studies revealed the presence of clinically relevant imaging findings in 1-10% of patients with mental decline. About the same percentage was reported for the work-up of demented patients (n = 432), with 4% having an actual lesion. In the series of Hejl et al., significant findings occurred in about 3% of submitted cases (Fig. 2). The percentage of cerebrovascular findings was even higher. Volumetric MRI demonstrated the early diagnostic value of volume reductions in the parahippocampal gyrus and hippocampus as predictive sites of entorhinal and limbic atrophic change, respectively. Within the MCI group, volume reduction of the right parahippocampal gyrus was significantly associated with global cognitive impairment. These findings confirm the hypothesis that initial cerebral changes in MCI primarily involve the entorhinal area and the parahippocampal gyrus. The integrity of the hippocampus is consistent with this hypothesis since hippocampal changes would only be expected at a later timepoint, namely in the limbic stage.

In MRI, the technical requirements for volumetric analysis are ≤3-mm slices oriented parallel to the medial temporal lobe and skilfull handling of the calliper.

In different studies in which volumetric analyses were used, sensitivities of up to 95% in differentiating AD patients from controls were achieved, with a specificity of up to 90%.

The prognostic significance of hippocampal atrophy in MCI is still under investigation. However, based on the evidence from quantitative MRI studies, it seems likely that hippocampal or parahippocampal atrophy is already present before the onset of dementia and dramatically increases with the conversion to clinically apparent disease.

In order to be able to diagnose a mental decline as AD or to predict the disease, the process needs to be differentiated from other forms of dementia, especially from *frontotemporal lobar degeneration* (Pick's disease). The clinical criteria of frontal dementia were described by Neary et al., who also differentiated frontal and temporal atrophy as supportive diagnostic features for frontotemporal dementia; however, the absence of one or the other does not rule out the diagnosis. Asymmetric, predominantly left-sided perisylvian atrophy characterizes progressive nonfluent aphasia and asymmetric anterior temporal lobe atrophy is diagnostic of AD. With progression of the disease and over time, atrophy becomes more widespread in Pick's disease and AD but usually remains asymmetric in the latter. Galton et al. used MRI to assess frontotemporal dementia in patients with semantic dementia and the frontal variant of frontotemporal dementia (fvFTD). In a study consisting of 30 patients with AD, 17 with semantic dementia, 13 with fvFTD, and 18 controls, the authors used a new visual scale based on atrophy of the temporal pole, the parahippocampal gyrus, and the lateral temporal gyri that could be helpful in distinguishing AD from semantic dementia. In the semantic dementia group, there was significantly more atrophy in all these regions in both hemispheres. Boccardi et al. used a discriminant function on a set of AD and FTD patients, showing that inclusion of the asymmetry values obtained for the frontal and temporal regions could separate FTD from AD with 90% sensitivity and 93% specificity. They concluded that a pattern of atrophy is more useful than atrophy of single regions in the differential diagnosis. Chan et al. showed that, in addition to asymmetry, a marked anterior to posterior gradient of atrophy within the temporal lobe is also suggestive of FTD rather than AD.

Vascular dementia is the second most common cause of dementia, following AD. A diagnosis of vascular dementia consists of a decline in memory and intellectual ability that causes impaired functioning in daily living, associated with evidence of cerebrovascular disease, as demonstrated by either history or clinical examination and brain imaging. Therefore, modern neuroimaging techniques are required for confirmation of cerebrovascular disease in vascular dementia, providing information about the topography and severity of the vascular lesions. Both CT and MRI are suitable in the diagnostic workup of vascular lesions, with a clear advantage for MRI. The absence of vascular lesions on brain CT or MRI rules out probable vascular dementia and represents the most important element to distinguish it from AD. Since there are no CT or MR findings that are pathognomonic of vascular dementia, correlation with clinical evidence is mandatory. The sensitivity of MRI in evaluating vascular pathologies (Fig. 2) has not only boosted research into, and clinical recognition of vascular dementia, it has also aided tremendously in distinguishing between AD and other forms of dementia, especially vascular forms. However, there may well be overlap syndromes between the two disorders, and operational definitions for "mixed" dementia, indicating the presence of both AD and vascular dementia, are still lacking.

Creutzfeld Jakob Disease

Creutzfeldt-Jakob disease (CJD) is a very rare and incurable degenerative neurological disorder that is ultimately fatal. Among the types of transmissible spongiform encephalopathies found in humans, CJD is the most common. It is caused by prions, but can also be acquired genetically through a genetic mutation (5-10% of cases).

CJD is suspected when there are typical clinical symptoms and signs, such as rapidly progressing dementia with myoclonus. Further investigation can include MRI. although imaging is unspecific in the majority of cases. Unspecific atrophy and, in some patients, symmetric bilateral high signal intensity in the caudate nucleus and putamen bilaterally on T2- or FLAIR-weighted images may be seen.

Movement Disorders

Parkinson's Disease

In this degenerative disorder of the CNS, the sufferer's motor skills and speech are often impaired. Parkinson's disease (PD) is characterized by muscle rigidity, tremor, a slowing of physical movement (bradykinesia) and, in extreme cases, a loss of physical movement (akinesia). Secondary symptoms may include high-level *cognitive dysfunction* and subtle language problems. PD occurs in chronic and progressive forms. The idiopathic form, also referred to as paralysis agitans, is a common, progressive disorder that appears spontaneously in individuals between the ages of 50 and 80.

Imaging studies often show unspecific atrophy that in most of patients is diffuse. On high-resolution scanning, a decreased width of the pars compacta or a decreased definition of the gap between the pars reticularis and the red nucleus can be found. The underlying mechanism is increased iron deposition in the pars compacta.

Multiple System Atrophy

Several systems are involved in this collection of diseases. The associated cell degeneration causes problems with movement, balance, and automatic functions of the body, such as bladder control; the presence of pyramidal sign; and PD-like symptoms. There are no specific imaging findings in this group of diseases.

Wilson's Disease (Hepatolenticular Degeneration)

This is one of the few movement disorders in which there is a specific imaging finding. On T2-weighted MRI, prominent hyperintensities in the putamen, thalami, brain stem, and the dentate nuclei have been reported. Within the putaminal hypointensities, irregular areas of reduced signal may be present. These focal iron depositions may represent a susceptibility artifact. The deposition of copper causes the same finding.

Amyotrophic Lateral Sclerosis (ALS)

This progressive, usually fatal, neurodegenerative disease is caused by the degeneration of motor neurons, i.e., the nerve cells in the CNS that control voluntary muscle movement. While the diagnosis of ALS is made on the basis of clinical findings, imaging is used to exclude treatable causes of the symptoms, such as syringomyelia. Typical ALS findings on MRI are abnormal high signal intensities along the corticospinal motor tracts. Those changes can only be found along the intracranial portion of the tracts down to the pons. Along the spinal cord, only atrophic changes are observed.

Conclusions

The number of cases of neurodegenerative diseases is expected to increase during the coming decades. It is therefore important to understand the pathophysiologic changes that manifest as imaging alterations as early as possible in the disease process. In order to best serve society, clinicians need to recognize that imaging can play an important role in the early diagnosis of neurodegenerative diseases and may also allow the monitoring of treatment. While the assessment of atrophic changes is well established in AD, the most likely future use of imaging will be the identification of patients at risk for neurodegenerative diseases. For imaging, this will mean focusing on those areas that are affected earliest in the disease, i.e., the entorhinal cortex and hippocampus, using high-resolution structural or functional MRI techniques. With the ability to rapidly acquire high-contrast, high spatial resolution, three-dimensional brain images, a number of laboratories are experimenting with sophisticated brain-mapping algorithms. This process allows an individual MRI to be compared to an "average" or "ideal" brain, thus enabling the detection of anatomical differences at one point in time as well as changes in anatomical structure over repeated observations.

Suggested Reading

Aging

Busse A, Bischkopf J, Riedel-Heller SG, Angermeyer MC (2003) Mild cognitive impairment: prevalence and incidence according to different diagnostic criteria. Br J Psychiatry 182:449-454

Jack CR Jr, Petersen RC, Xu YC et al (1999) Prediction of AD with MRI-based hippocampal volume in mild cognitive impairment. Neurology 52:1397-1403

Petersen RC, Smith GE Waring SC et al (1997) Aging, memory, and mild cognitive impairment. Int Psychogeriatr (Suppl) 9:65-69

Ritchie K, Arteron S, Touchon J (2001) Classification criteria for mild cognitive impairment – a population-based validation study. Neurology 56:37-42

Imaging in Degenerative Brain Diseases

Ball MJ, Fisman M, Hachinski V et al (1985) A new definition of Alzheimer's disease: a hippocampal dementia. Lancet 1(8419):14-16

Boccardi M, Laakso MP, Bresciani L et al (2003) The MRI pattern of frontal and temporal brain atrophy in fronto-temporal dementia. Neurobiol Aging 24:95-103

Braak H, Braak E, Bohl J (1993) Staging of Alzheimer-related cortical destruction. Eur Neurol 33:403-408

Chan D, Fox NC, Jenkins R et al (2001) Rates of global and regional cerebral atrophy in AD and frontotemporal dementia. Neurology 57:1756-1763

Convit A, de Leon MJ, Tarshish C et al (1997) Specific hippocampal volume reductions in individuals at risk for Alzheimer's disease. Neurobiol Aging 18:131-138

Erkinjuntti T (2002) Diagnosis and management of vascular cognitive impairment and dementia. J Neural Transm Suppl 63:91-109

Galton CJ, Gomez-AnsonB, Antoun N et al (2001) Temporal lobe rating scale: application to Alzheimer's disease and frontotemporal dementia. J Neurol Neurosurg Psychiatry 70:165-173

Giesel FL, Hahn HK, Thomann PA et al (2006) Temporal horn index and volume of medial temporal lobe atrophy using a new semiautomated method for rapid and precise assessment. Am J Neuroradiol 27(7):1454-1458

Jack CR, Petersen RC, Xu YC et al (1998) Medial temporal atrophy on MRI in normal aging and very mild AD. Neurology 51:993-999

Jack CR, Petersen RC, Xu Y et al (2000) Rates of hippocampal atrophy correlate with change in clinical status in aging and AD. Neurology 55:484-489

Johnson S, Saykin A, Baxter L et al (2000) The relationship between fMRI activation and cerebral atrophy: comparison of normal aging and Alzheimer disease. Neuroimage 11:179-187

Kato T, Knopman D, Liu H (2001) Dissociation of regional activation in mild AD during visual encoding. Neurology 57:812-816

Kaye JA, Swihart T, Howieson D et al (1997) Volume loss of the hippocampus and temporal lobe in healthy elderly persons destined to develop dementia. Neurology 48:1297-1304

Laakso MP, Partanen K, Lehtovirta M et al (1995) MRI of amygdala fails to diagnose early Alzheimer's disease. Neuroreport 6:2414-2418

Laakso MP, Soininen H, Partanen K et al (1998) MRI of the hippocampus in Alzheimer's disease: sensitivity, specificity, and analysis of the incorrectly classified subjects. Neurobiol Aging 19:23-31

Massoud F, Devi G, Moroney JT et al (2000) The role of routine laboratory studies and neuroimaging in the diagnosis of dementia: a clinicopathological study. J Am Geriat Soc 48:1204-1210

Neary D, Snowden J, Mann D (2005) Frontotemporal dementia. Lancet Neurol 4:771-780

Pantel J, Kratz B, Essig M, Schröder J (2003) Parahippocampal volume deficits in subjects with aging-associated cognitive decline. Am J Psychiatry 160:379-382

Pantel J, Schönknecht P, Essig M et al (2002) Progressive medial temporal lobe changes in Alzheimer's disease revealed by quantitative MRI: potential use for monitoring of drug-related changes. Drug Dev Res 56:51-56

Prvulovic D, Hubl D, Sack A et al (2002) Functional imaging of visuospatial processing in Alzheimer's disease. Neuroimage 17:1403-1414

Roman GC, Erkinjuntti T, Wallin A et al (2002) Subcortical ischaemic vascular dementia. Lancet Neurol 1:426-436

Rombouts S, Barkhof F, Veltman D et al (2000) Functional MR imaging in Alzheimer's disease during memory encoding. AJNR Am J Neuroradiol 21:1869-1875

Saykin A, Flashman L, Frutiger S et al (1999) Neuroanatomic substrates of semantic memory impairment in Alzheimer's disease: patterns of functional MRI activation. J Int Neuropsychol Soc 5:377-392

Small S, Perera G, Delapaz R et al (1999) Differential regional dysfunction of the hippocampal formation among elderly with memory decline and Alzheimer's disease. Ann Neurol 45:466-472

Soininen HS, Partanen K, Pitkänen A et al (1994) Volumetric MRI analysis of the amygdala and the hippocampus in subject with age-associated memory impairment: correlation to visual and verbal memory. Neurology 44:1660-1668

Visser PJ, Scheltens P, Verhey FRJ et al (1999) Medial temporal lobe atrophy and memory dysfunction as predictors for dementia in subjects with mild cognitive impairment. J Neurol 246:477-485

Whitwell J, Jack CR (2005) Comparison between Alzheimer Disease, frontotemporal lobar degeneration and normal aging with brain imaging. Top Magn Reson Imaging 16:409-426

Neuroradiological Diagnosis of Craniocerebral Trauma: Current Concepts

Paul M. Parizel[1], C. Douglas Phillips[2]

[1] Department of Radiology, University of Antwerp, Antwerp, Belgium

[2] Department of Radiology, University of Virginia Health System, Charlottesville, VA, USA

Imaging Techniques

Plain Skull Films

When computed tomography (CT) scanning is available, plain skull films contribute little or no additional information in the clinical management of the acute trauma patient. Traditionally, X-ray films of the skull have been used to detect skull fractures, intracranial mass effect ("pineal shift"), air-fluid levels, foreign objects (metal, glass, projectile fragments, etc.). However, the diagnostic yield of plain X-ray films is low because there is poor correlation between skull fractures and intracranial injury. The old saying has never been truer: "it doesn't matter if the shell is cracked, only if the egg is scrambled".

Computed Tomography

Computed tomography is the initial imaging study of choice in acute craniocerebral trauma. It is a rapid and accurate technique. CT is also the diagnostic study of choice for the remainder of the acute patient evaluation: spine trauma, blunt chest trauma, and abdominal trauma. With the advent of multi-detector CT (MDCT), the exams can be performed very rapidly, and is also compatible with almost all medical devices. The availability of CT scanning has dramatically improved the survival of patients with epidural or subdural hematomas. CT scanning is used for the detection of:

- Hemorrhage: intra-axial and extra-axial, including subarachnoid blood
- Mass effect and edema; brain herniations
- Fractures, displaced bone fragments
- Foreign bodies

The CT examination should start with an AP and lateral scout image, which could be used as a digital radiograph to detect fractures. The non-contrast CT scan is performed with contiguous axial sections (slice thickness: 2.5-5 mm) from the base of the skull to the vertex; alternatively, a helical technique can be used and is preferred by many. Our preference is to use helical technique, acquiring very thin slices (0.625 mm) and reconstructing thicker sections for review (2.5-5 mm). The data can then be retrospectively reconstructed for the temporal bone, the orbits, or other purposes if requested. With modern PACS and the widespread use of stack reading of the images at a workstation, CT images of the head can easily be viewed in multiple window settings:

- Brain parenchyma window (L: 40 HU; W: 80-120 HU).
- Bone window (L: 500 HU; W: 2000-4000); any applicable edge-enhancement algorithm can be used to improve the depiction of subtle fractures.
- Blood or subdural window (L: 70-100 HU; W: 150-300); for the detection of a potentially thin layer of acute hemorrhage against the dense calvarium.

When fractures of the temporal bone, orbit, or maxillofacial structures are suspected, the acquired scan data can be reprocessed with very thin slices in different orientations to improve the yield. MDCT techniques also allow rapid acquisition of the cervical spine in patients with major trauma, when a spine-clearance CT may be requested. Helical (MDCT) scanning with coronal reformatting can be used as an alternative to direct coronal views when the patient cannot tolerate hyperextension of the neck. CT angiography (CTA) can be used in addition to the initial diagnostic CT to evaluate suspected traumatic vascular injuries. We have also used CT perfusion studies in the setting of altered intracranial perfusion during the post-trauma period or during vasospasm. The limitations of CT are its insensitivity to small cortical or non-hemorrhagic lesions, notably adjacent to bone, diffuse axonal injury (which may go unnoticed on CT), and early ischemia, which may accompany trauma and elevated intracranial pressure.

Magnetic Resonance Imaging

Magnetic resonance imaging (MRI) is the preferred technique in the evaluation of subacute and chronic brain injuries. Any patient in whom CT does not explain the clinical findings can benefit from MRI. It has the highest sensitivity in detecting parenchymal lesions, and is particularly useful for evaluating lesions in the posterior fossa or near the skull base (difficult to see on CT due to beam-hardening artifacts), diffuse axonal injury due to shearing stresses, and cortical contusions. Important limitations include the relative insensitivity for the detection of subarachnoid hemorrhage, cortical bone injury, and small bone fragments. Despite these limitations, some centers have begun to employ MRI earlier in the management of the traumatized patient. MRI perfusion and diffusion studies allow the assessment of viable brain in the setting of altered cerebral perfusion.

A reasonable standard imaging protocol consists of:

1. Axial fast-spin-echo (FSE) T2-weighted images.
2. Axial fluid attenuated inversion recovery (FLAIR) T2-weighted images for the detection of edema, or gliosis and encephalomalacia.
3. Axial and/or coronal gradient-echo (GE) or T2*-weighted images with a short TE (15-35 ms) for the detection of hemorrhagic foci (e.g., in diffuse axonal injury), or, if the imaging platform supports the sequence, a susceptibility-weighted acquisition to detect small foci of hemorrhage.
4. Sagittal spin-echo (SE) or GE T1-weighted scans for the detection of cortical contusions or post-traumatic encephalomalacia in the anterior and inferior parts of the frontal lobes, and the anterior temporal lobes.
5. Diffusion-weighted echo-planar imaging (EPI) in the acute phase.

It is important to note that routine MRI studies in the traumatized patient population are probably without good indication. The technology is best utilized to evaluate patients in whom the CT study does not adequately explain the clinical situation. Studies have been published in which a real contribution of MRI in the diagnosis of acute traumatic brain injury could not be documented.

Scalp and Skull Lesions

Scalp and skull lesions are commonly observed in head trauma. Scalp lacerations occur when the scalp is crushed or lacerated against the underlying bone. They heal well because of the generous blood supply – this also explains why scalp wounds bleed profusely. Scalp wounds must be carefully examined to exclude foreign bodies or depressed bone fragments. CT scanning is the preferred imaging technique for showing soft-tissue swelling of the scalp. When the integrity of the skin is disrupted, a scalp hematoma may contain small amounts of air. CT not only shows the scalp lesions, but also the associated intracranial abnormalities. The major importance of these injuries may be in their providing evidence of the site of direct cranial impact, and the close scrutiny of the underlying brain.

Caput succedaneum, subgaleal hematoma, subgaleal hygroma, and cephalohematoma are commonly confused. They are discussed together in Table 1, which provides a comparative summary of the distinct features of these entities.

A detailed discussion of skull fractures is beyond the scope of this presentation, but a limited discussion of facial injuries follows. Facial injuries are not uncommon accompaniments to central nervous system (CNS) trauma. Head trauma may result in intracranial injuries, which are often the critical injuries in the immediate trauma setting. However, major facial trauma may be a serious cause of morbidity and mortality in this patient group, particularly due to respiratory problems. Major morbidity in this patient group may result from facial injuries in the subacute period. The injuries that lead to considerable patient morbidity include orbital trauma, central skull base and temporal bone fractures with resulting injury to cranial nerves, vascular structures, and the adjacent soft-tissue structures, as well as the obvious deformity and loss of function that may result.

The era of MDCT has led to a significant alteration in the acute imaging of these patients. Quite simply, the rapidity of CT scanning – with very thin sections and the ability to perform multi-planar reconstruction (MPR) images that equal the quality of directly acquired images in the sagittal or coronal planes – has led many services to perform the entire evaluation of a trauma patient (CNS, abdomen, pelvis, spine, and the detailed evaluation of facial trauma) in one setting. We have adopted a series of trauma protocols for patient evaluation that

Table 1. Overview of scalp lesions

Lesion type	Caput succedaneum	Subgaleal hematoma (extracranial subdural hematoma)	Subgaleal hygroma	Cephalo-hematoma (extracranial epidural hematoma)
Occurrence	After normal vaginal delivery	After head trauma (or after birth)	Birth trauma (forceps delivery)	Birth trauma (skull fracture during birth)
Location	Superficial to the galea aponeurotica	Beneath the galea aponeurotica	Beneath the galea aponeurotica	Subperiosteal (flat skull bones)
Composition	Edema (with microscopic hemorrhages)	Venous blood	Cerebrospinal fluid	Subperiosteal hemorrhage
Clinical presentation	Pitting edema	Diffusely spreading, firm fluctuating mass	–	Well-defined, focal, firm mass
Skull fracture		Yes or no	Yes	Yes
Crosses suture lines?	Yes	Yes	Yes	No

simplify the plan for imaging in this patient group. The initial exam is an unenhanced CT of the brain, with the scan beginning at the level of the midface or mandible (depending on the injuries noted) followed quickly by the requested abdominal, chest, or pelvic examination, as required by the trauma service. In the setting of major trauma, the examination then addresses the cervical spine or other affected spinal segments. The cervical spine CT may accompany the initial head and face CT exam. If the cervical spine CT is performed during contrast infusion, the exam serves as a very adequate vascular screening for traumatic vascular injury. In cases in which the patient has significant injuries and minimal time to spend in the CT suite, it is easy to obtain very high quality examinations of the lumbar or thoracic spine from reformatted data from the abdominal, chest, or pelvic CT study.

We prefer to initially categorize injuries to the facial skeleton according to the presence or absence of involvement of the pterygoid plates. Fracture of the pterygoid plates results in dissociation of the facial skeleton and the skull. These fractures were first examined in detail by the French surgeon LeFort. His rather gruesome investigation involved blunt trauma to the midface of cadavers, with subsequent investigation of the patterns of fracture. LeFort categorized three different levels of fracture, a system still used to large extent to this day. LeFort I injuries result in a “floating palate”, with the fracture plane below the level of the orbital rim, which allows mobility of the inferior maxilla in relation to the remainder of the midface. LeFort II injuries result in dissociation of the palate and the inferior orbital rim on the involved side. The fracture involves the medial and lateral maxilla but will permit displacement of the inferior orbital rim if traction is applied to the palate. LeFort III fractures result in dissociation of the entire midface in relation to the skull, and the superior fracture plane involves the root of the nasal bone. We have found that axial, coronal, and particularly sagittal CT images allow excellent assessment of these fractures. There are other fairly common patterns of facial injury, easily characterized by CT examination. The “tripod” or zygomaticomaxillary fracture accompanies an angular blow to the midface, typically in proximity to the zygomaticomaxillary suture. The injury results in fractures of the zygomatic arch, the anterior wall of the maxilla, and the posterolateral wall of the maxilla. Isolated orbit fractures, fractures of the orbital rims, nasal bones, zygomatic arch, maxillary and mandibular alveolus, and mandible may be seen. There is also wide acceptance of the value of 3D images in the review of these injuries. The ease with which these exams can be post-processed has led to an increase in their use in the acute trauma setting.

Investigation of facial fractures should include careful review of the important skull-base foramina and of the soft-tissue structures of the midface. Evaluation of the orbital soft tissues is critical with injury in this region. Particular attention should be paid to the carotid and the optic canals. Involvement of either of these foramina may lead to the need for surgical management or to additional investigations.

Temporal bone fractures are beyond the scope of this review but can be divided into longitudinal or transverse fractures, depending upon the fracture orientation in relation to the axis of the temporal bone. Many of these fractures are complex, with orientation in both the longitudinal and transverse planes. Longitudinal fractures are more commonly associated with ossicular involvement and hearing loss, and transverse fractures are more commonly associated with facial nerve injury; however, there is considerable overlap. Previously, with single-slice CT devices, questionable involvement of the skull base led to re-scanning this region with thin slices, and thus with a larger cumulative radiation dose to the patient. In the era of MDCT, very often the initial data set can be reformatted and will prove adequate to thoroughly evaluate the temporal bone. Nonetheless, whenever the question is raised as to the possibility of temporal bone fracture, it is inherent in our responsibility to insure that the examination is adequate to answer the question.

Intracranial Hypertension and Cerebral Herniations

Severe brain swelling or large intracranial mass lesions (e.g., hemorrhage) may cause displacement of brain tissue. The cranial cavity is divided into anatomic compartments based on the bony ridges and dural septa (falx cerebri and tentorium cerebelli). The three major compartments contain: (1) the right cerebral hemisphere, (2) the left cerebral hemisphere, and (3) the posterior fossa structures. The falx and the tentorium protect the brain against excessive motion but also limit the amount of compensatory shift and displacement that develops in response to increased intracranial pressure (ICP). When the pressure in one of the dural compartments increases beyond the physiological compensatory mechanisms, increased ICP or intracranial hypertension occurs and a pressure gradient ensues. This leads to a displacement of brain, cerebrospinal fluid (CSF) and blood vessels from one cranial compartment to another and a cerebral herniation follows.

Cerebral herniations are the most common secondary effect of an expanding intracranial mass. They can be due to an intra-axial process (e.g., intracerebral contusion or hematoma, edema, tumor) or an extra-axial mass (e.g., epidural or subdural hematoma). The subarachnoid spaces and basal cisterns become obliterated, hydrocephalus develops, vascular compression results in brain ischemia, and compression of vital brain tissue causes profound neurological deficits. Therefore, early detection of brain herniation can be of major clinical importance in patient management.

Six types of brain herniation can be distinguished. They are discussed in Table 2.

Table 2. Cerebral herniation types

Type of cerebral herniation	Subfalcial (cingulate)	Tonsillar	Descending transtentorial	Ascending trans-tentorial	Uncal	External
Definition	Medial displacement of cingulate gyrus under inferior free margin of the falx	Inferior displacement of cerebellar tonsil(s) through foramen magnum	Downward shift of diencephalon, mesencephalon, and upper brainstem	Superior displacement of the vermis through the tentorial incisura	Herniation of medial temporal lobe through tentorial notch	Brain tissue extrudes externally through a skull defect
Cause	Supratentorial mass (e.g. epidural and subdural hematomas, hemispheric mass lesion)	Posterior fossa mass lesions or supratentorial mass effect	Increasing supratentorial mass effect	Posterior fossa mass lesion (tumor)	Temporal lobe mass lesion, e.g., focal hematoma	Increased ICP associated with a traumatic or surgical skull defect
Imaging	Mass lesion Bowing of falx Compression of ipsilateral lateral ventricle Contralateral ventricle enlarges due to obstruction of the foramen of Monro	Downward displacement of cerebellar tonsils below the level of the foramen magnum Obliteration of the cisterna magna	Obliteration of peri-mesencephalic cisterns with complete plugging of tentorial incisura Downward shift of pineal calcification Brainstem is foreshortened (sagittal plane) and compressed (axial plane)	4th ventricle becomes obliterated Effacement of the superior cerebellar and quadrigeminal cisterns	Obliteration of the suprasellar cistern Shift of mesence-phalon to opposite side Widening of ipsi-lateral CPA cistern Obstructive hydrocephalus (due to aqueductal obstruction)	Extracranial displacement of brain tissue Bone defect can be observed on CT
Compression of vascular structures	Anterior cerebral artery infarction (pericallosal and callosomarginal arteries)	Posterior inferior cerebellar artery infarction	Posterior cerebral artery compression leads to occipital lobe ischemia or infarction	Superior cerebral artery compression may result in cerebellar infarction	Compression of the contralateral posterior cerebral artery against the tentorial edge	Venous obstruction may result in venous infarction (propensity to hemorrhage)

Extra-axial Lesions

Four types of extra-axial hemorrhage can be considered: epidural, subdural, subarachnoid, and intraventricular.

Epidural and Subdural Hemorrhage

These extra-axial hemorrhages are discussed together and are compared in Table 3. The finding of a unilateral low-density hemisphere associated with acute subdural hematoma in children who have trauma has merited the term "big black brain", which signifies the potential for unilateral infarction unique in this patient population. This finding carries an ominous prognosis.

Traumatic Subarachnoid Hemorrhage

Traumatic subarachnoid hemorrhage (SAH) represents a significant finding in the acutely traumatized patient. Outcomes are worse in patients with head trauma and traumatic SAH. Several etiologic mechanisms have been proposed: (1) superficial cerebral contusion with leakage of blood into the subarachnoid space; (2) direct injury to leptomeningeal vessels; (3) intraventricular hemorrhage with reflux through the 4th ventricular foramina into the subarachnoid space. The real significance of traumatic SAH is somewhat controversial. It may be only a marker for a more serious traumatic brain injury, or it may lead to secondary deleterious effects, such as vasospasm and ischemia.

Non-contrast CT is the preferred imaging technique for detection of acute traumatic SAH, with a reported accuracy of 90-95%. Traumatic SAH is most often focal, often over the convexities, and lying within one or two gyri. It can be found overlying a site of cortical bruising or subjacent to a subdural hematoma. Blood in the interpeduncular fossa is a reliable indicator of SAH. Diffuse spread of SAH throughout all the subarachnoid spaces is less common in head trauma and merits consideration of another etiology of hemorrhage, such as a ruptured aneurysm. SAH is usually most apparent on presentation CT scans and resolves over the following days.

MRI is less useful for the detection of acute traumatic SAH. The higher oxygen tension (pO_2) in the subarachnoid space slows the transformation of oxyhemoglobin ($Hb\text{-}O_2$) to paramagnetic breakdown products such as de-

Table 3. Epidural vs. subdural hematoma

Epidural hematoma (EDH)	Subdural hematoma (SDH)
Often on coup side	Often on contre-coup side
Associated with skull fracture in ±90% of cases	No consistent relationship with skull fractures
Does not cross suture lines	Consistently cross suture lines
Not limited by falx or tentorium (may extend from supra- to infratentorial or across midline)	limited by falx and tentorium (confined to supra- or infratentorial compartment, does not cross midline)
Origin: – Arterial (majority, due to tearing of one or more branches of the meningeal arteries, most commonly the middle meningeal artery) – Venous (minority, due to laceration of a dural venous sinus, e.g., along the sphenoparietal sinus)	Origin: – Venous, due to laceration of superficial bridging cortical veins
Medical emergency	May be chronic
Magnitude of the mass effect caused by EDH is directly related to the size of the extracerebral collection	Magnitude of the mass effect caused by subdural hematoma is more often associated with underlying parenchymal injury
CT is preferred imaging technique because: – Rapid accessibility – Shows both the hemorrhage and the skull fracture	CT will diagnose many SDH
MRI can be useful for: – Detection of parenchymal repercussions (edema, mass effect, herniations)	MRI is preferred imaging technique because: – It is more sensitive than CT, especially in the detection of isodense SDHs (may be difficult to see on CT), or thin SDHs – Better definition of multi-compartmental nature of SDHs

oxyhemoglobin (Hb) and methemoglobin (Hb-OH). Recent evidence suggests that FLAIR sequences are more useful than SE or turbo spin-echo TSE sequences in the detection of SAH. Nevertheless, in most centers, CT scanning remains the method of choice for the detection of SAH in the acute phase.

Intraventricular Hemorrhage

Traumatic intraventricular hemorrhage (IVH) can occur as a result of tearing of subependymal veins, which line the ventricular cavities. Most commonly affected are the subependymal veins on the ventral surface of the corpus callosum and along the fornix and septum pellucidum. Rupture of an intracerebral hemorrhage into the adjacent ventricle can also cause IVH. The single cell layer that forms the ependymal lining of the ventricles does not constitute a significant barrier to the extension of an intraparenchymal bleed. Finally, IVH may be due to reflux of SAH through the 4th ventricular foramina of Luschka and Magendie. Traumatic IVH seems to be associated with a poor outcome, although the outcome is likely to be ultimately determined by the associated injuries, which in most cases led to the IVH.

CT or MRI studies of trauma patients may reveal a horizontally sedimented blood-CSF level, more common in the occipital horns. Even a small amount of IVH is well seen on CT. When the intraventricular thrombus matures, clot retraction occurs and a hyperdense intraventricular blood clot is observed adjacent to the intraventricular CSF. Signal intensities on MRI of IVH will vary depending on its age, presence or absence of clotting, and whether or not erythrocyte lysis has occurred.

Intra-axial Lesions

Post-traumatic Cerebral Edema

Post-traumatic cerebral edema with intracranial hypertension is a life-threatening secondary traumatic brain lesion. It starts immediately after injury, but massive edema usually takes 24-48 h to develop. It can be associated with intra-axial or extra-axial lesions. Unilateral swelling of a cerebral hemisphere is most often secondary to an ipsilateral subdural or epidural hematoma.

Cerebral edema leads to compression of the intracranial blood vessels, thereby causing underperfusion and ischemia of the edematous region or hemisphere(s). If the intracranial pressure is not relieved, the brain will gradually herniate through the tentorial incisure and/or the foramen magnum (see Table 2). This results in compression of the brainstem, with depression of breathing and cardiac function and, eventually, death. Cerebral edema is more common in children than in adults; in children, brain swelling may be the only identifiable feature of head injury.

CT scanning is quite sensitive for the detection of hyperacute cerebral edema, nearly as sensitive as MRI. Early imaging findings in diffuse cerebral edema include: decreased cerebral attenuation values; diminished gray-white matter differentiation; increased density of the falx and tentorium (due to vascular stasis, associated subdural hematoma, SAH, or both); downward bowing of the tentorial leaflets due to a supratentorial mass effect; effacement of the cortical sulci of the cerebral surface; and obliteration of the subarachnoid cisterns near the skull base, particularly the suprasellar, quadrigeminal plate and ambient cisterns. The cerebellum may appear relatively hyperdense: this is the so-called white cerebellum sign.

Edema associated with intracerebral hemorrhagic contusions often increases dramatically during the days following the acute event. Therefore, it is not unusual for the initial CT scan to show no or only limited edema, and for the follow-up examination to reveal massive perilesional edema and associated mass effect.

Cerebral Contusion and Hematoma

The term "cerebral contusion" is used to indicate (punctate) hemorrhages within the brain parenchyma. Contusions are often multiple and located near the surface of the brain; associated SAH is a common finding. Traumatic cerebral contusions are most often encountered supratentorially. They are caused when the brain hits either irregularities of the inner skull table or dural folds (falx, tentorium). Sites of predilection include the anterior and inferior frontal lobes, anterior and inferior temporal lobes, and the gyri around the sylvian fissure. Contusions are much less frequent in the cerebellar hemispheres, which are protected by the smooth inner surface of the thick occipital bone.

The term "cerebral hematoma" refers to a well-circumscribed parenchymal hemorrhage. Cerebral hematomas tend to be located in the deeper parts of the brain. Delayed development of a post-traumatic intracerebral hemorrhage is not uncommon and should be suspected when the patient's neurological condition is worsening. As the hematoma matures and the clot retracts, it becomes surrounded by a hypodense rim of edema; a hemorrhagic sedimentation level may develop. Cerebral hematomas can spontaneously decompress into the ventricles, thereby causing IVH. In trauma patients, a deep hematoma may be found along with one or more cortical contusions.

In acceleration or deceleration brain injuries, intraparenchymal bleeding sites can be categorized as "coup" or "contre-coup" injuries. "Coup injury" occurs at the site of primary impact, which is identified by the associated scalp injuries or skull fractures. Epidural hematoma or contusion or laceration of the brain surface often occurs at the site of a fracture, especially if it is depressed. "Contre-coup" injury arises on the opposite side. Hemorrhagic cerebral contusions are more common at the contre-coup side, although both coup and contre-coup injuries can be hemorrhagic.

A severe impact on the stationary head (e.g., a blow with a blunt object) results in skull fractures but generally does not cause contre-coup contusions. This is because in these cases the head does not accelerate or decelerate, and there is no brain lag. This knowledge is useful in distinguishing head injuries due to falls from those due to blows.

On CT images, acute intraparenchymal hemorrhagic contusions are recognized as patchy, ill-defined frontal or temporal low-density lesions, often containing small, hyperdense, punctate foci of petechial hemorrhage. Lesions may not be seen on an initial CT scan and follow-up scans are indispensable when the patient's clinical condition deteriorates. Over the next few days, as the clot retracts, the hemorrhagic area becomes surrounded by a rim of edematous brain. After surgical decompression of an epidural or subdural hematoma, hemorrhagic contusions may become more apparent. The phenomenon of delayed traumatic intracranial hemorrhage can be quite significant and likely reflects the alteration in perfusion of contused brain when the intracranial pressure is altered, either by surgical decompression or medical management. Over time, CT density values decrease as thrombolysis progresses; this may cause the affected area to become almost isodense with the surrounding normal brain tissue. The perilesional edema diminishes. A resolving hematoma may enhance in a ring-like pattern after intravenous contrast administration. In this stage of evolution, differentiation from an infarct or tumor may be extremely difficult.

On MRI, the appearance of intraparenchymal hemorrhage is extremely complex. Imaging findings are determined by many parameters, such as: age, location and size of the hematoma; pulse sequence; magnetic field strength; presence or absence of continued bleeding; local tissue pH; and oxygen tension (pO_2). The MRI appearance of intracerebral hemorrhage follows the evolution as described in Table 4.

Diffuse Axonal Injury (Shearing Injury of the White Matter)

Even with a closed-head injury, the brain can suffer severe damage by shearing injuries caused by acceleration, deceleration, or rotational forces. The lesions are determined by the magnitude of rotational acceleration and the difference in density and rigidity between two adjacent tissues, especially gray and white matter. Clinically, diffuse axonal injury (DAI) is characterized in the acute phase by impairment or complete loss of consciousness from the moment of impact. A typical example is the "uppercut" in boxing, which induces a sudden linear and rotational acceleration of the skull, causing a sudden loss of consciousness. Less severe hemispheric DAI can cause loss of telencephalic functions: decreased attention span, memory loss, concentration difficulties, lower IQ, headaches, seizures, less stress resistance, and behavioral changes. DAI lesions can be found in the following sites of predilection (in decreasing order of frequency):

1. The hemispheric gray-white matter junction is the most common location for DAI, because the peripheral location increases the vulnerability to trauma and because of the abrupt change in tissue density between the gray and white matter. The frontal and parietal lobes are most frequently involved.
2. The corpus callosum is the second most common location for DAI shearing lesions. The splenium is more commonly affected because of its closer proximity to the falx.
3. Basal ganglia and internal capsule shearing injuries.

Table 4. Sequential signal intensity changes of intracranial hemorrhage on MRI (1.5 T)

	Hyperacute hemorrhage	Acute hemorrhage	Early subacute hemorrhage	Late subacute hemorrhage	Chronic hemorrhage
What happens	Blood leaves the vascular system (extravasation)	Deoxygenation with formation of deoxy-Hb	Clot retraction and oxidation of deoxy-Hb to met-Hb	Cell lysis (membrane disruption)	Macrophages digest clot
Time frame	<12 h	Hours-days (weeks in center of hematoma)	A few days	4-7 days to 1 month	Weeks-years
Red blood cells	Intact erythrocytes	Intact, but hypoxic erythrocytes	Still intact, severely hypoxic (solution of lysed cells)	Lysis	Gone; encephalomalacia with proteinaceous fluid
State of hb	Intracelluar oxy-Hb (HbO_2)	Intracellular deoxy-Hb (Hb) (first at periphery of clot)	Intracellular met-Hb (HbOH)	Extracellular met-Hb (HbOH)	Hemosiderin (insoluble) and ferritin (water soluble)
Oxidation state	Ferrous (Fe2+) No unpaired e-	Ferrous (Fe2+) 4 unpaired e-	Ferric (Fe3+) 5 unpaired e-	Ferric (Fe3+) 5 unpaired e-	Ferric (Fe3+) 2,000×5 unpaired e-
Magnetic properties	diamagnetic (c <0)	Paramagnetic (c >0)	Paramagnetic (c >0)	Paramagnetic (c >0)	FeOOH is superparamagnetic
SI on T1-weighted images	≈ or ↓	≈ (or ↓) (no PEDD interaction)	↑↑ (PEDD interaction)	↑↑ (PEDD interaction)	≈ (or ↓) (no PEDD interaction)
SI on T2-weighted images	↑ (high water content)	↓ T2 PRE (susceptibility effect)	↓↓ T2 PRE (susceptibility effect)	↑↑ No T2 PRE	↓↓ T2 PRE (susceptibility effect)

Hb, Hemoglobin; *e-*, electrons; *FeOOH*, ferric oxyhydroxide; ↑, increased SI relative to normal gray matter; ↓, decreased SI relative to normal gray matter; *PRE*, proton relaxation enhancement; *PEDD*, proton-electron dipole-dipole interaction

4. Brainstem and mesencephalon shearing lesions are only observed with more severe injuries; they are always associated with multiple hemorrhages in the deep white matter and the corpus callosum. Most commonly involved is the dorsolateral quadrant of rostral brainstem adjacent to the superior cerebellar peduncle. Differential diagnosis includes Duret hemorrhage of the brainstem in transtentorial herniation.
5. Cerebellar shearing injuries are infrequent.

The neuroradiological diagnosis of DAI is difficult. In the acute phase, a non-contrast CT scan may reveal small, punctate petechial hemorrhages, intraventricular blood (shearing of subependymal veins), and peri-mesencephalic subarachnoid hemorrhage. However, CT scanning underestimates DAI lesions, because non-hemorrhagic lesions are difficult to identify. Therefore, when a patient's neurological or psychiatric status is worse than predicted from the CT findings, MRI must be performed as it is far more sensitive in detecting DAI lesions. FLAIR sequences are useful for the detection of non-hemorrhagic lesions and areas of gliosis. GE sequences are used to detect the susceptibility effects of hemosiderin.

Ischemia and Infarction

Post-traumatic ischemia and infarction are common complications in patients with craniocerebral trauma. The causes are listed in Table 5.

Table 5. Etiology of post-traumatic ischemia and infarction

Vasospasm secondary to:
– Subarachnoid hemorrhage
– Direct vessel injury (laceration)
Extrinsic compression of a blood vessel by:
– Cerebral herniation (see Table 2)
– Extra-axial mass (e.g. EDH, SDH)
Hypoxia/anoxia
Thrombosis/distal embolisation secondary to:
– Vascular dissection
– Fat embolization due to long bone fracture

Post-traumatic Sequelae

Encephalomalacia and Gliosis

If trauma to the brain has been focal (e.g., cerebral contusions and hematomas), localized encephalomalacia (intraparenchymal tissue loss) may result. Areas of encephalomalacia are often surrounded by a rim of gliosis. Findings on CT scans include one or more lucent areas of tissue loss; focal dilatation of the ventricle nearest to the traumatic lesion is common. On MRI, encephalomalacia and gliosis are of high signal intensity on T2-weighted images and are indistinguishable. Moreover, a GE sequence is of value to detect hemosiderin deposition. Frank cavitation, referred to by the neuropathologist as macrocystic encephalomalacia, may occur in areas of cerebral injury. This cavitation will be apparent on FLAIR images as regions of low signal intensity invariably surrounded by areas of increased T2 signal intensity, representing the areas of microcystic change in the adjacent injured brain.

Atrophy and Ventricular Enlargement

More diffuse trauma can result in generalized atrophy of one or both hemispheres, with enlargement of the sulci and ventricles. Post-traumatic atrophy is observed as diffuse, non-focal enlargement of the intracranial CSF spaces. Diffuse ventricular enlargement can be due to communicating hydrocephalus (e.g., decreased CSF absorption due to adhesions in the subarachnoid space after SAH or meningitis). Focal ventricular enlargement is most often secondary to central tissue loss (ex vacuo).

Vascular Injuries

Carotid Artery-Cavernous Sinus Fistula

Traumatic carotid artery-cavernous sinus fistula (CCF) is caused by a wall defect in the cavernous portion of the internal carotid artery (ICA), thus allowing a direct communication with the adjacent cavernous sinus. The increased arterial inflow into the cavernous sinus leads to dilatation of the superior ophthalmic vein, the facial veins, and the internal jugular vein. Clinical findings include pulsating exophthalmos, chemosis, conjunctival edema, restricted ocular mobility, and persistent bruit. The most common CT and MRI findings are widening of the affected cavernous sinus (convex lateral margin), and dilatation of the superior ophthalmic vein. Magnetic resonance angiography can be used to demonstrate the venous widening.

Post-traumatic Aneurysms

Post-traumatic aneurysms are infrequent complications of head trauma. The most common locations include the cervical, petrous, and cavernous ICA. The distal anterior and middle cerebral arteries are less commonly affected. Basal skull fractures, penetrating injuries, or shearing stress (e.g., against a dural margin) are the primary causes of post-traumatic cerebral aneurysms.

Traumatic Vascular Dissection

Vascular dissections are caused by the development of a hematoma within the intima; this results in splitting of the vessel wall and thus a false lumen within the media. Vascular dissection may lead to luminal occlusion or distal embolization. Dissections most commonly occur in the ICA (60%) or vertebral artery (20%); involvement of both arteries is seen in up to 10% of cases. Traumatic dissection can be caused by blunt or, less frequently, penetrating trauma to the neck. In cases of "spontaneous" dissection, there is often a non-recalled or trivial trauma in the history; if not, a primary arterial disease should be considered. The neuroradiological diagnosis can be established by different techniques:

- Catheter angiography shows a flame-like or radish tail-like tapering of the vessel lumen.
- Duplex Doppler ultrasound is being increasingly used for the diagnosis of intimal dissections.
- Spiral CT scans of the neck with surface rendering and maximum intensity projection (MIP) reconstructions can be used as an alternative to catheter angiography.
- MRI should include an axial T1-weighted sequence through the upper neck and skull. These images must be carefully studied to detect a crescentic area of high signal intensity, which represents the subintimal hematoma in the wall of the ICA. Findings can be confirmed by magnetic resonance angiography.

CSF Leaks and Pneumocephalus

A post-traumatic CSF leak occurs arises from a combination of a dural tear and a bone fracture. Thus, it can be the result of penetrating trauma (bullet wounds, stabbing) or blunt trauma (with skull-base fractures). CSF leakage into the paranasal sinuses or nasal cavity is associated with fractures of the anterior cranial fossa: ethmoid, posterior wall of the frontal sinus, planum sphenoidale, or cribriform plate. CSF leakage into the middle ear is associated with fractures of the floor of the middle cranial fossa, extending into the tegmen tympani. Otorrhea only occurs if the tympanic membrane is perforated or ruptured. If the tympanic membrane is intact, the CSF drains via the Eustachian tube into the rhinopharynx, and rhinorrhea occurs. High-resolution CT images of the skull base and petrous bones with thin sections and bone algorithm images are useful for precise localization of the fracture(s). The presence of intracranial air bubbles (pneumocephalus) is an ominous finding.

Infections

In non-penetrating head trauma, meningitis can occur as the result of an open calvarial fracture, a skull-base fracture, or a post-operative craniotomy defect. Meningitis may progress to cerebritis and brain abscess. If the abscess ruptures into the ventricular system, ventriculitis will develop. Ventriculitis and meningitis are frequently followed by obstructive hydrocephalus. In penetrating head trauma, infection is caused by debris (scalp, hair, foreign material) that is carried into the brain by a projectile.

Diabetes Insipidus

Pituitary dysfunction, especially diabetes insipidus, can occur as a result of trauma. Transient diabetes insipidus usually develops within the first week after trauma and is probably due to a contusion of the neurohypophysis. Permanent diabetes insipidus indicates structural damage to the pituitary gland, the pituitary stalk, or the neurosecretory nuclei of the hypothalamus. One should look for fractures involving the floor of the sella, hemorrhage within the neurohypophysis, transection or laceration of the pituitary stalk, petechial hemorrhages in the hypothalamus, and elevated intracranial pressure. Delayed-onset diabetes insipidus arises months after trauma and should suggest optochiasmatic arachnoiditis.

CT scanning should be used to exclude hemorrhages in the suprasellar region or skull-base fractures extending into the sellar floor. MRI shows an absence of the normal hyperintense signal in the posterior pituitary lobe.

Leptomeningeal Cysts

Leptomeningeal cysts are rare complications of pediatric skull fractures. Herniation of the leptomeninges through the skull fracture and associated dural tear prevent normal healing of the fracture margins. The systolic-diastolic pulsation of the brain and CSF produces fracture diastasis. The result is a calvarial defect, which usually becomes visible 3-5 months after injury. Leptomeningeal cysts are also known as "growing fractures", because of their tendency to increase in size over time. On plain X-ray films, a skull defect with indistinct, scalloped margins is seen. On CT scans, a CSF density cyst adjacent to or in the skull is observed. The cyst is caused by subarachnoid fluid that becomes trapped in the herniated tissue, probably secondary to arachnoidal adhesions. On MRI, the cyst is isointense with CSF and communicates with the subarachnoid space. Frequently, there is an underlying area of encephalomalacia due to compression of the cerebral cortex by the cyst.

Suggested Reading

Armin SS, Colohan AR, Zhang JH (2006) Traumatic subarachnoid hemorrhage: our current understanding and its evolution over the past half century. Neurol Res 28(4):445-452

Atzema C, Mower WR, Hoffman JR; National Emergency X-Radiography Utilization Study (NEXUS) II Group (2006) Prevalence and prognosis of traumatic intraventricular hemorrhage in patients with blunt head trauma. J Trauma 60(5):1010-1017

Duhaime AC, Durham S (2007) Traumatic brain injury in infants: the phenomenon of subdural hemorrhage with hemispheric hypodensity ("Big Black Brain"). Prog Brain Res 161:293-302

Fiser SM, Johnson SB, Fortune JB (1998) Resource utilization in traumatic brain injury: the role of magnetic resonance imaging. Am Surg 64(11):1088-1093

Gentry LR (2002) Head trauma. In: Atlas SW (ed) Magnetic resonance imaging of the brain and spine, 3rd edn. Lippincott-Raven, Philadelphia, pp 1059-1098

Gentry LR (ed) (1991) Current concepts in imaging of craniofacial trauma. Neuroimaging Clinics of North America. WB Saunders, Philadelphia

Ghysen D, Özsarlak Ö, van den Hauwe L et al (2000) Maxillo-facial trauma. J Belge Radiol/Belg Tijdschr Radiol (JBR/BTR) 83:181-192

Haydel MJ, Preston CA, Mills TJ et al (2000) Indications for computed tomography in patients with minor head injury. N Engl J Med 343:100-105

Kido DK, Cox C, Hamill RW et al (1992) Traumatic brain injuries: predictive usefulness of CT. Radiology 182:777-781

Lipper MH, Kishore PR, Girevendulis AK et al (1979) Delayed intracranial hematoma in patients with severe head injury. Radiology 133(3 Pt 1):645-649

Makkat S, Vandevenne JE, Parizel PM, De Schepper AM (2001) Multiple growing fractures and cerebral venous anomaly after penetrating injuries: delayed diagnosis in a battered child. Pediatr Radiol 31:381-383

Parizel PM, Ceulemans B, Laridon A, Jorens PG (2003) Cortical hypoxic-ischemic brain damage in shaken baby syndrome: value of diffusion-weighted MRI. Pediatr Radiol 33:868-871

Parizel PM, Makkat S, Jorens PG et al (2002) Brainstem hemorrhage in descending transtentorial herniation (Duret hemorrhage). Intensive Care Med 28(1):85-88

Parizel PM, Makkat S, Van Miert E et al (2001) Intracranial hemorrhage: principles of CT and MRI interpretation (review). Eur Radiol 11(9): 1770-1783

Parizel PM, Özsarlak Ö (1999) Imaging of craniocerebral trauma. European Society of Neuroradiology & Lasion Europe (CD-ROM teaching file containing 4000 images, part of the educational program of the European Society of Neuroradiology)

Parizel PM, Ozsarlak Ö, Van Goethem JW et al (1998) Imaging findings in diffuse axonal injury after closed head trauma. Eur Radiol 8(6):960-965

Nontraumatic Neuroemergencies - I

Patrick A. Brouwer

Department of Nuclear Medicine, Leiden University Medical Center, Leiden, The Netherlands

Introduction

The nontraumatic neuroemergencies comprise a large spectrum of diseases varying from ischemic stroke to infection, from subarachnoid hemorrhage to tumors, and from metabolic disease to disc herniation. The various vascular causes will be discussed below.

Patients with vascular causes of neuroemergencies may present with neurological deficit, acute headache, seizures, loss of vision, or worsening of a known clinical picture (e.g., dementia). The clinical history and complaints at presentation most often point to the underlying cause, but there is some overlap between the diseases.

Intracranial Aneurysm

The intracranial berry aneurysm has a prevalence of about 6% but is variable around the world. The percentage of patients suffering from a subarachnoid hemorrhage (SAH) is therefore also largely dependent on the geographical distribution. Risk factors for SAH are numerous but some manageable factors, such as smoking, cocaine and alcohol abuse, oral contraceptives, and hypertension, are known.

The patient suffering a SAH is generally very ill, may have lost consciousness, and will afterwards describe the headache as "the worst headache of my life". About one-third of SAH patients will die before reaching the hospital and a further 10-20% will succumb later due to complications including vasospasm or severe neurological deficit.

Imaging of the SAH patient should consist of a non-contrast CT scan, showing the hemorrhage, and subsequent computed tomography angiography (CTA). 3D reconstruction of the CTA images will facilitate the decision regarding the treatment of choice, i.e., endovascular coiling or surgery. Additional digital subtraction angiography (DSA) is only warranted if the CTA is of limited quality. The value of magnetic resonance angiography (MRA) is not yet clear; it has, however, proven to be useful in the follow-up of patients with coiled or incidental aneurysms.

Arterial Dissection

Patients with intracranial arterial dissection may present with either acute focal neurological deficit due to loss of perfusion or with a subarachnoid hemorrhage. In the latter case, clinical distinction from an aneurysmal SAH is difficult. The initial imaging modality of choice is CT scanning, which allows a hemorrhage to be ruled out. Additionally, a CTA can be performed to visualize the vascular tree and help to obtain a diagnosis. A dissection can be recognized by either vessel enlargement, vessel narrowing, or absence of the vessel. In some cases, additional imaging with DSA is needed. In larger vessels, magnetic resonance imaging (MRI) using T1 spin echo sequences with fat saturation may show intramural thrombus.

In many patients, the dissection occurs at locations near the dural folds (e.g., the tentorium and falx), in which case it is considered to be either traumatic or due to repetitive stress, although it may also have appeared spontaneously. Underlying diseases, e.g. fibromuscular dysplasia. Marfan syndrome, and Ehlers-Danlos syndrome, have to be ruled out. Treatment is often based on sacrificing the artery by means of coils or glue.

Venous Thrombosis

Venous (or sinus) thrombosis has numerous underlying causes and very often a nonspecific presentation. Consequently, imaging plays a central role in the diagnosis. Headache and gradually worsening neurological symptoms are common. Venous stroke may be accompanied by hemorrhages in regions that are atypical for arterial causes. This is the result of the limited possibilities for drainage and therefore swelling of the brain, especially in the case of cortical vein thrombosis.

The vast list of differential diagnoses makes initial CT imaging the method of choice in most centers. Additional MR/MRA can be performed when the suspicion of venous thrombosis is raised, or if the CT remains inconclusive. The sequences of choice for confirmation will be gradient-echo-based. Treatment regimens vary between centers but both anti-coagulation and endovascular therapy are employed.

Ischemic Stroke

Arterial emboli, arterial thrombosis at a site of a pre-existing stenosis, or a complication of surgery or endovascular procedures, are the most frequent causes of ischemic stroke. With the increasing age of the populations of many countries, the number of stroke cases will steadily increase. Since the functional outcome is directly related to the time to treatment, it is clear that a swift diagnosis is necessary. Treatment is based on the imaging findings and may consist of intravenous recombinant tissue plasminogen activator (rtPA) or intra-arterial thrombolysis, thrombosuction, or thrombodestruction. The latter can be combined with stenting of a stenosis if necessary.

Imaging in the acute phase is directed at excluding hemorrhage, proving ischemia, and showing salvable tissue. The latter can be done by perfusion studies and is, with the newer multi-slice CT-scanners, common practice. Diffusion-weighted MR sequences are capable of showing ischemia and can be used to follow the (lack of) effect of treatment.

Dural Arteriovenous Fistula

Patients with a dural arteriovenous fistula (dAVF) may present with a bruit that is pulsatile and very often diminishes or resolves with local compression of, e.g., the occipital artery. A more emergent presentation is chymosis and proptosis or acute mental deterioration (dementia).

A dAVF is the result of a fistulous connection of an artery to a dural venous structure. Most fistulas are found on the transverse sinus, but they can be located anywhere from the superior sagittal sinus to the cavernous sinus. If the fistula causes blood to run in a retrograde fashion in the cortical veins, it is called a "cortical venous reflux." This finding is a reason for treatment since it is an indicator for increased risk of intracerebral hemorrhage or infarction.

In such patients, a CT/CTA might be helpful in showing congested veins. MR and MRA may show the vascular disturbance caused by engorgement of the cortical veins. Edema and impressive white-matter changes may be present on T2 (or FLAIR) weighted images. To obtain a good understanding of the dynamics of the disease and for treatment planning, a DSA should be performed. Treatment is aimed at the closure of the fistulous connection(s).

Arteriovenous Malformation

Arteriovenous malformations (AVMs) are disturbances in the normal capillary network of the vessels in the brain. There is a direct communication of the arterioles with the venules. The resulting high flow can create flow-related aneurysms, venous pouches, and steal phenomena. The major risk of AVMs lies in the potential for intracerebral hemorrhage, but patients may also present with seizures or mass effects.

The anatomy of the AVM nidus and the surrounding tissue can be visualized by MRI. For treatment planning and an understanding of the dynamics, DSA is necessary. Treatment may consist of surgery, endovascular embolization, radiosurgery, or a combination of these three modalities.

Giant Aneurysms

A giant aneurysm is different from a berry aneurysm in its etiology. The former is considered to be a defect in the vessel wall, with subsequent growth due to progressive thrombosis of the entering blood. At a later stage, the vasa vasorum may start to bleed intermittently, due to growth of the wall, which confers an onion-skin-like layered aspect to the lesion due to blood of different ages in the aneurysm. Calcification in the wall is common and may, in conjunction with the location, be a key to the diagnosis. Imaging can be done with CT and MRI but it is not uncommon to mistake a giant aneurysm for a tumor. CTA and MRA can make the distinction but 3D-DSA is the gold standard. DSA is also used for to plan treatment, which might consist of surgery or endovascular occlusion.

Arterial Dolichoectasia (Serpentine Aneurysm)

An arterial dolichoectasia is considered to be a segmental mural disease and is characterized by an increase in vessel diameter and length. This might be due to atherosclerosis or a dissection, either of which can cause an inflow of blood between the layers of the vessel wall. This disease is often found in the vertebrobasilar region but can also occur in the middle cerebral and internal carotid arteries. The atherosclerotic variant usually shows a luminal thrombus that is sometimes mistaken for a giant aneurysm. This thrombus is in direct contact with the blood and may be the cause of transient ischemic attacks in these patients. Other complaints are mostly related to mass effects, especially in the region of the brainstem. Treatment may consist of occlusion or stenting of the diseased segment.

Perimesencephalic Hemorrhage

Patients with a perimesencephalic bleed (PMH) present with the signs of a SAH but tend to be in better clinical condition, without loss of consciousness. The diagnosis is made by CT/CTA. In PMH, the blood is located around the mesencephalon and will not be in the distal sylvian fissure or in the ventricles. The amount of blood can be huge, but the spread does not change. PMH is considered to be due to a venous rupture, a conclusion supported by the fact that venous variations are present in these patients. The recurrence rate is believed to be 0 and the clinical outcome is excellent.

Suggested Reading

Biondi A, Jean B, Vivas E et al (2006) Giant and large peripheral cerebral aneurysms: etiopathologic considerations, endovascular treatment, and long-term follow-up. AJNR Am J Neuroradiol 27(8):1685-1692

Flemming KD, Wiebers DO, Brown RD Jr et al (2004) Prospective risk of hemorrhage in patients with vertebrobasilar nonsaccular intracranial aneurysm. J Neurosurg 101(1):82-87

Khandelwal N, Agarwal A, Kochhar R et al (2006) Comparison of CT venography with MR venography in cerebral sinovenous thrombosis. AJR Am J Roentgenol 187(6):1637-1643

Köhrmann M, Jüttler E, Huttner HB et al (2007) Acute stroke imaging for thrombolytic therapy – an update. Cerebrovasc Dis 24(2-3):161-169

Lubicz B, Levivier M, François O et al (2007) Sixty-four-row multisection CT angiography for detection and evaluation of ruptured intracranial aneurysms: interobserver and intertechnique reproducibility. AJNR Am J Neuroradiol 28(10):1949-1955

Pelkonen O, Tikkakoski T, Pyhtinen J, Sotaniemi K (2004) Cerebral CT and MRI findings in cervicocephalic artery dissection. Acta Radiol 45(3):259-265

van Dijk JM, Willinsky RA (2003) Venous congestive encephalopathy related to cranial dural arteriovenous fistulas. Neuroimaging Clin N Am 13(1):55-72

van Gijn J, Rinkel GJ (2001) Subarachnoid haemorrhage: diagnosis, causes and management. Brain 124(Pt 2):249-278

Warren DJ, Hoggard N, Walton L et al (2001) Cerebral arteriovenous malformations: comparison of novel magnetic resonance angiographic techniques and conventional catheter angiography. Neurosurgery 48(5):973-82; discussion 982-983

Nontraumatic Neuroemergencies - II

John R. Hesselink

Department of Radiology, University of California, San Diego Medical Center, San Diego, CA, USA

Several clinical presentations require emergent neuroimaging to determine the cause of the neurological deficit and to institute appropriate therapy. Time is critical because neurons that are lost cannot be replaced. Generally, the clinical symptoms are due to ischemia, compression, or destruction of neural elements. The two primary imaging modalities for the central nervous system (CNS) are computed tomography (CT) and magnetic resonance imaging (MRI). CT is fast and can readily visualize fractures, hemorrhage, and foreign bodies. Otherwise, in patients who can cooperate for the longer imaging study, MRI provides better contrast resolution and has higher specificity for most CNS diseases. The five major categories of nontraumatic neuroemergencies are discussed below.

Acute Focal Neurological Deficit

Arterial Thrombosis/Occlusion

Thrombotic strokes may occur abruptly but the clinical picture often shows gradual worsening over the first few hours. Primary causes of arterial thrombosis include atherosclerosis, hypercoagulable states, arteritis, and dissection. Secondary compromise of vascular structures can result from traumatic injury, intracranial mass effect, neoplastic encasement, meningeal processes, and vasospasm (Fig. 1).

Arterial Embolus

Embolic strokes characteristically have a very abrupt onset. After a number of hours, there may be sudden improvement in symptoms as the embolus lyses and travels more distally. The source of the embolus is usually either the heart (patients with atrial fibrillation or previous myocardial infarction) or ulcerated plaques at the carotid bifurcation in the neck.

Arterial Dissection

Relatively minor trauma is sufficient to cause a dissection, or it can be spontaneous. The magnetic resonance angiogram (MRA) may demonstrate complete occlusion or only narrowing of the arterial lumen. Spin-echo images, especially T1-weighted with fat suppression, should

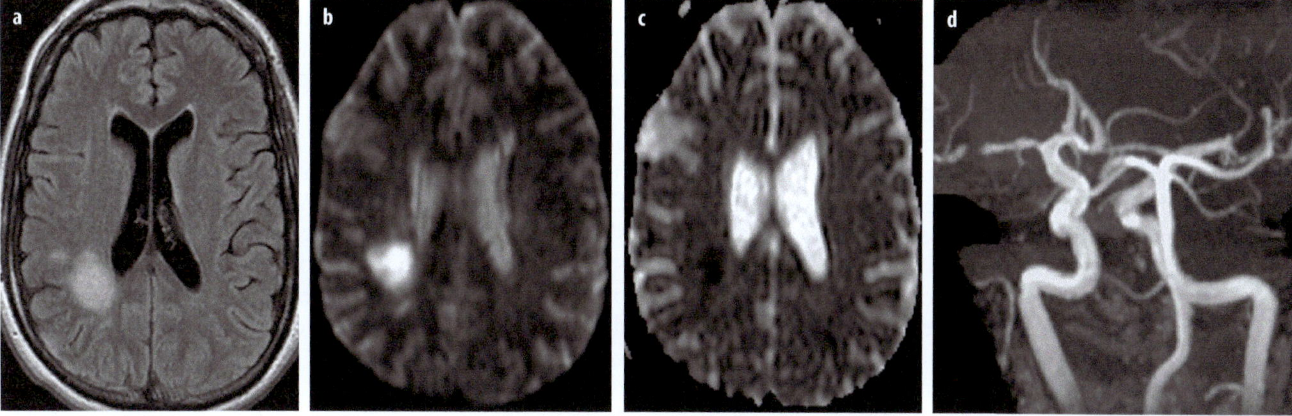

Fig. 1 a-d. Acute cerebral infarct secondary to a right MCA stenosis. **a** Axial fluid-attenuated inversion recovery (FLAIR) image shows focal hyperintensity in the deep white matter of the right parietal lobe, causing slide mass effect on the lateral ventricle. **b, c** Restricted diffusion on the diffusion-weighted imaging (DWI) (**b**) is confirmed by hypointensity on the apparent diffusion coefficient (ADC) map (**c**). **d** Magnetic resonance (MR) angiogram reveals a high-grade stenosis of the right middle cerebral artery

also be obtained because they are very sensitive for detecting the intramural hemorrhage. The typical appearance of an oval-shaped hyperintensity with an eccentrically placed flow void may be more convincing evidence for a dissection than the MRA. The MRA is very useful for following a dissection to look for recanalization of a complete occlusion, resolution of the vascular compromise caused by the intramural thrombus, or development of a pseudoaneurysm [1].

Brain Hemorrhage

Localized hemorrhages into the brain may present with a focal neurological deficit. Most of these are caused by vascular malformations. The four types of vascular lesions include AV malformation, cavernous angioma, capillary telangiectasia, and venous malformation. AV malformations are more likely to present acutely. Hemorrhage into tumors or infarct is not uncommon, but patients usually have symptoms related to the underlying lesion. Hypertensive hemorrhages are often large and deep within the brain and produce more global neurological deficits.

Hypotension/Hypoxia

Hypotension can be cardiac in origin or result from blood volume loss or septic shock. Anoxia/hypoxia events are usually related to respiratory compromise from severe lung disease, perinatal problems, near drowning, high altitude, carbon monoxide inhalation, or CNS-mediated effects.

Venous/Sinus Occlusion

Thrombosis of the cerebral venous sinuses has multiple etiologies, including hypercoagulable states, pregnancy, sepsis, dehydration, paranasal sinus infection, and neoplastic invasion. Occlusion of the venous sinuses results in cerebral venous engorgement, brain swelling, and increased intracranial pressure. If the thrombosis extends retrograde and involves the cortical veins, secondary cerebral infarction can occur.

Acute thrombus is hyperdense on CT and may be detected within one of the major sinuses or cortical veins. The other classic sign is the "empty delta" sign due to non-filling of the superior sagittal sinus on a contrast scan. Nonetheless, MR is far superior for diagnosing abnormalities of the cerebral veins and sinuses. Normally, the dural sinuses have sufficient flow to exhibit a flow void. If that flow void is missing or if the sinuses are hyperintense, thrombosis should be suspected. One must be careful to exclude the possibility of any in-flow enhancement effect. The diagnosis must be confirmed with gradient-echo techniques or MRA. Phase-contrast and Gd-enhanced time-of-flight MRA are the preferred techniques because they are not adversely affected by intraluminal clot [2].

Associated parenchymal infarcts are found in the areas of venous abnormalities, and the infarcts are often hemorrhagic because arterial perfusion is maintained to the damaged tissue. In cases of superior sagittal sinus thrombosis, the infarcts are typically bilateral and in a parasagittal location.

Cortical Mass Lesion

Any lesion that irritates the cortical neurons can be a source of seizures. Neoplasia, encephalitis, meningitis, abscess, and hemorrhage are the more common causes of new onset seizures.

Worst Headache of Life

Subarachnoid Hemorrhage

The incidence of congenital aneurysms in the general population is about 1-2%. Clinically, a ruptured aneurysm presents as sudden onset of severe headache. In cases of subarachnoid hemorrhages, the most common aneurysms are posterior communicating, 38%; anterior communicating, 36%; and middle cerebral, 21%. These three locations account for 95% of all ruptured aneurysms. The basilar artery accounts for only 2.8% and posterior fossa aneurysms are even less common.

The CT scan is important, firstly, to document the subarachnoid hemorrhage and to assess the amount of blood in the cisterns (Fig. 2). Detection of subarachnoid blood is very dependent on how early the scan is obtained. If the scan is obtained within 4-5 days, the detection rate is very high. Secondly, CT helps localize the site of the aneurysm based on the distribution of blood within the cisterns. If conventional angiography is not available or is not planned immediately, CT angiography is very good for detecting and characterizing intracranial aneurysms. Thirdly, the CT is important to evaluate complicating factors such as cerebral hematoma, ventricular rupture, hydrocephalus, cerebral infarction, impending uncal herniation, and re-bleed.

Conventional MRI sequences are very insensitive for detecting subarachnoid hemorrhage. Clots within cisterns can be detected but, in general, MRI is not the procedure of choice in the work-up of patients with subarachnoid hemorrhage. Due to the flow void phenomenon, aneurysms about the circle of Willis can be identified on spin-echo MRI [3]. With fluid-attenuated inversion recovery (FLAIR) sequences, the cerebrospinal fluid (CSF) is dark, so that subarachnoid hemorrhage can be seen more easily. These sequences may be helpful for detecting subarachnoid blood in the posterior fossa, where CT has difficulty [4].

Acute Meningitis

Bacterial meningitis is an infection of the pia and arachnoid and adjacent cerebrospinal fluid. The most common

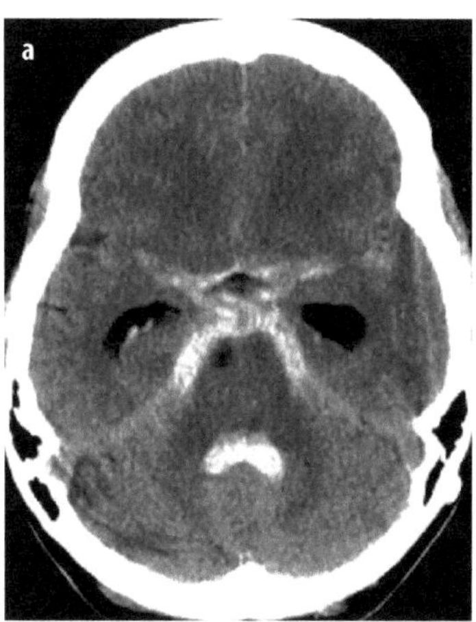
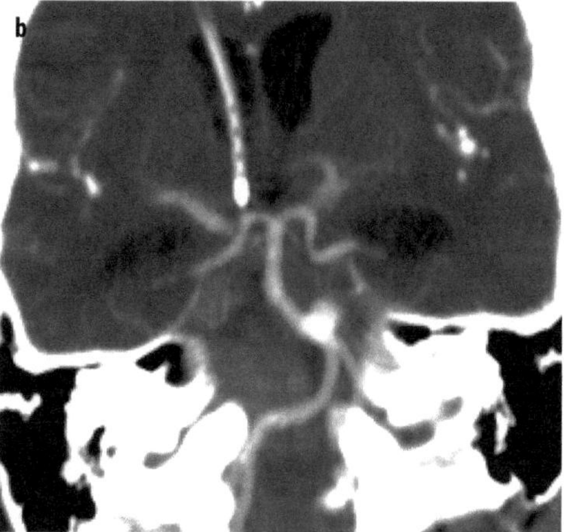
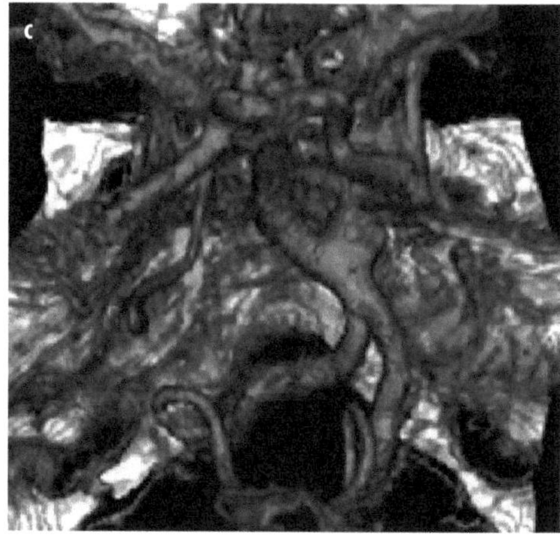

Fig. 2 a-c. Subarachnoid hemorrhage due to basilar aneurysm. **a** Axial CT scan reveals acute blood in the basal cisterns and fourth ventricle. Temporal horn dilatation indicates hydrocephalus. **b,c** CT angiography and a surface-shaded reconstruction demonstrate a wide-necked aneurysm at the left vertebrobasilar junction

organisms are *Hemophilus influenza, Neisseria meningitides (Meningococcus)*, and *Streptococcus pneumoniae.* Patients present with fever, headache, seizures, altered consciousness, and neck stiffness. The overall mortality ranges from 5 to 15% for *H. influenza* an meningococcal meningitis and as high as 30% with streptococcal meningitis. In addition, persistent neurological deficits are found in 10% of children after *H. influenza* meningitis and in 30% of patients with streptococcal meningitis.

The ability of nonenhanced MR to image meningitis is extremely limited, and in the majority of patients the findings are normal or show mild hydrocephalus. In severe cases, the basal cisterns may be completely obliterated, with high signal intensity replacing the normal CSF signal on FLAIR images. Intermediate signal intensity may be seen in the basal cisterns on T1-weighted images in these patients. Meningeal enhancement often is not present, unless a chronic infection develops [5].

Fungal organisms can start as a meningitis or cerebral abscess, or can invade directly from an extracranial compartment. Coccidioidomycosis is endemic to the central valley regions of California and desert areas of the southwestern United States. Infection occurs by inhalation of dust from soil usually heavily infected with arthrospores. Primary coccidioidomycosis, a pulmonary infection, is followed by dissemination in only about 0.2% of immunocompetent patients. CNS involvement most often represents meningitis, but cerebral abscess and granuloma formation can also occur [6]. Other fungal infections are primarily found in immunocompromised hosts.

Migraine

Migraine headaches can be severe and unrelenting. At presentation, the severity of the headache may raise the clinical question of possible subarachnoid hemorrhage or acute meningitis. Also, patients with known migraine may develop atypical headaches.

Acute/Increasing Confusion and Obtundation

Obstructive Hydrocephalus

Acute obstructive hydrocephalus is caused by compression of the ventricular system to the point of obstructing the outflow of CSF. The common locations of blockage are at the foramina of Monroe, the cerebral aqueduct, and the outlets of the fourth ventricle. Possible causes include tumor, abscess, ventriculitis, and hemorrhage. Brain injury or cerebral infarction with massive vasogenic edema can also cause obstructive hydrocephalus.

Brain Stem or Basal Ganglia Hemorrhage

Most large deep hemorrhages in the brain are associated with hypertension. The criteria for hypertensive hemorrhage include a hypertensive patient, 60 years of age or older, and a basal ganglia or thalamic location of the hemorrhage. CT or MR scan is the procedure of choice for evaluating these patients. Arteriography is necessary only if one of these criteria is missing. Hypertensive hemorrhages are often large and devastating. Since they are deep hemorrhages and near ventricular surfaces, ventricular rupture is common. One-half of hypertensive hemorrhages occur in the putamen; the thalamus is affected in 25%; pons and brainstem in 10%, cerebellum in 10%, and cerebral hemispheres in 5%.

Brain Herniation

As with hydrocephalus, any large mass lesion or process with prominent vasogenic edema can produce brain herniation. With large frontal or parietal lesions, subfalcine herniation is common. Also, any large hemispheric lesion can result in medial migration of the temporal lobe and subsequent inferior herniation through the tentorial incisura. Subfalcine herniation can compress the ipsilateral anterior cerebral artery, leading to brain infarction, whereas temporal lobe herniation commonly compresses the contralateral posterior cerebral artery, causing an occipital infarct. Diffuse brain swelling or posterior fossa masses can result in herniation of the cerebellar tonsils and brain stem inferiorly through the foramen magnum.

Encephalitis

Encephalitis refers to a diffuse parenchymal inflammation of the brain. Patients with acute encephalitis of the non-herpetic type present with signs and symptoms similar to those of meningitis but with the added features of any combination of convulsions, delirium, altered consciousness, aphasia, hemiparesis, ataxia, ocular palsies, and facial weakness. The major causative agents are arthropod-borne arboviruses (Eastern and Western equine encephalitis, St. Louis encephalitis, California viral encephalitis). Eastern equine encephalitis is the most serious but, fortunately, also the least frequent of the arbovirus infections. The enteroviruses, such as Coxsackie virus and echoviruses, can produce meningoencephalitis, but mild aseptic meningitis is more common with these organisms. MR reveals hyperintensity on T2-weighted scans within the cortical areas of involvement, associated with subcortical edema and mass effect.

Herpes simplex is the commonest and gravest form of acute encephalitis with a 30-70% fatality and equally high morbidity. It is almost always caused by type 1 herpesvirus except in neonates, in whom type 2 herpesvirus predominates. Symptoms may reflect the propensity to involve the inferomedial frontal and temporal lobes, i.e., hallucinations, seizures, personality changes, and aphasia. MRI demonstrates positive findings in viral encephalitis as soon as 2 days after symptoms, more quickly and definitively than CT. Early involvement of the limbic system and temporal lobes is characteristic of herpes simplex encephalitis. The cortical abnormalities are first noted as ill-defined areas of high signal on T2-weighted scans, usually beginning unilaterally but progressing to become bilateral. Edema, mass effect, and gyral enhancement may also be present [7].

Meningitis

As described above, in addition to severe headache, patients with acute meningitis commonly present with fever, seizures, altered consciousness, and neck stiffness. Most of these cases are bacterial in origin, but tuberculosis and fungal infections can also present acutely (Fig. 3).

Metabolic/Toxic Disorders

Whenever a patient presents to the emergency department, the possibility of ingestion of drugs or other toxic substances must be considered. The narcotics and sedatives generally produce respiratory depression, which can lead to global cerebral hypoxia. Some toxic agents specifically target the basal ganglia or the white matter. In diabetic patients, the possibility of an insulin overdose and hypoglycemia must be considered. Cocaine and metamphetamine also cause vasospasm, so these patients may present with an acute focal neurological deficit.

Acute/Progressive Visual Deficit

Monocular Deficit

Monocular visual loss can be caused by anything anterior to the optic chiasm that blocks light from the retina or compresses the optic nerve. Ocular diseases, such as retinal detachment and ocular hemorrhage, are generally first evaluated by direct visualization with fundoscopy or by ultrasound. A mass compressing the optic nerve or causing severe proptosis can cause a visual deficit. Severe proptosis and stretching of the optic nerve can compromise the arterial supply to the nerve. Finally, intrinsic optic nerve lesions, such as tumors, ischemia, and inflam-

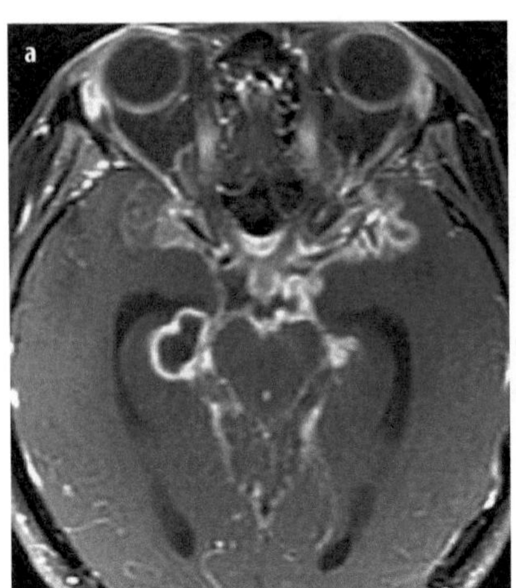

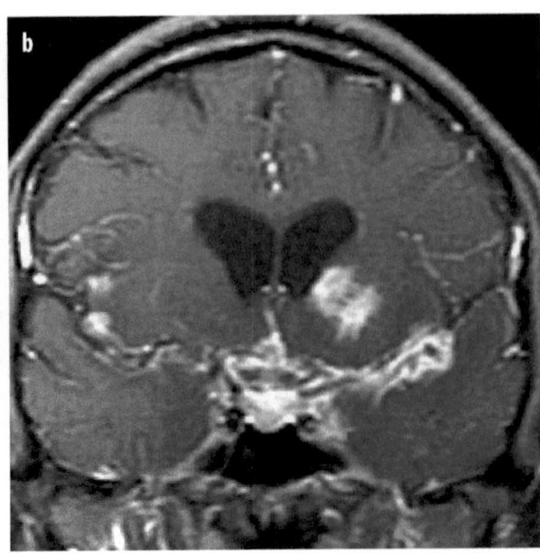

Fig. 3 a, b. Tuberculous meningitis. Axial (**a**) and coronal (**b**) Gd-enhanced T1-weighted images show diffuse meningeal enhancement in the suprasellar, Sylvian, and perimesencephalic cisterns. An enhancing mass is also present in the left basal ganglia

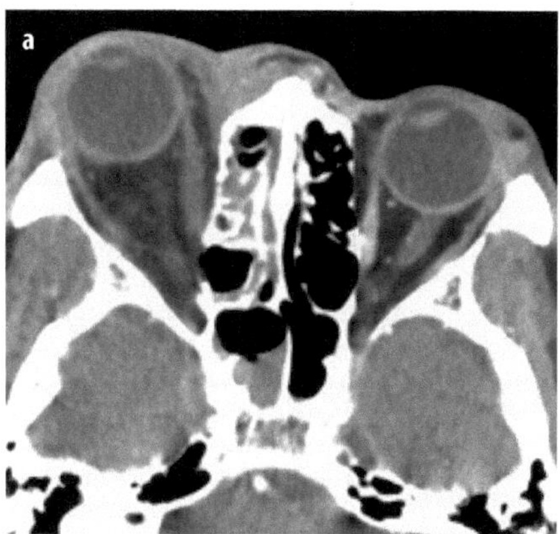
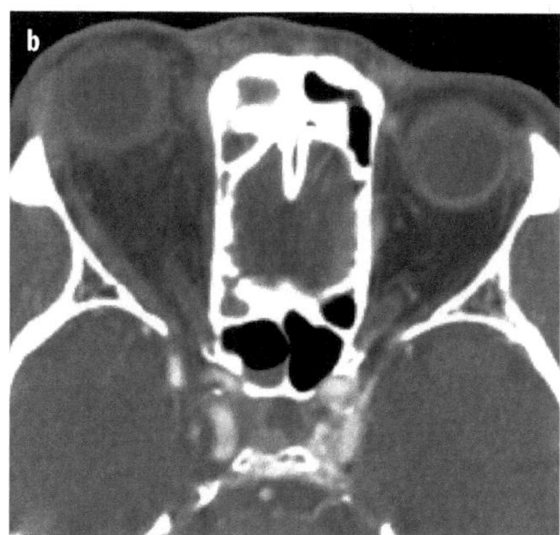
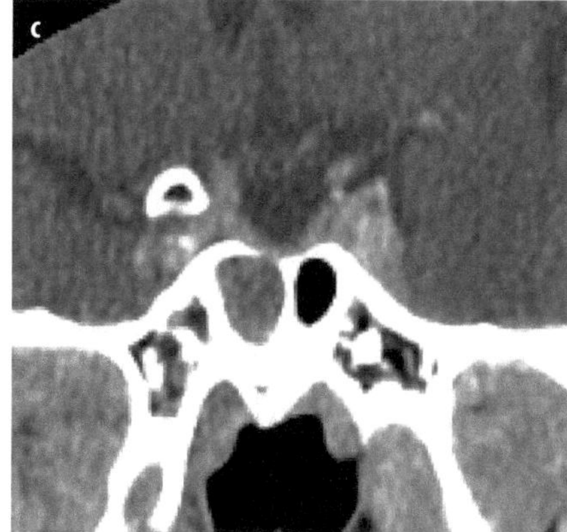

Fig. 4 a-c. Aspergillosis with cavernous sinus thrombosis. Contrast-enhanced CT scans. **a** The right ethmoid and sphenoid air cells are partially opacified; right proptosis is present, and abnormal soft tissue has infiltrated the extraconal and intraconal compartments and the preceptal tissues. Axial (**b**) and coronal (**c**) bscans show no enhancement of the right cavernous sinus, due to septic thrombosis

mation, are other causes of visual loss. Intraorbital diseases are evaluated equally well by CT or MRI (Fig. 4). For intracranial disease, MRI is the imaging procedure of choice.

Bitemporal Hemianopsia

This visual deficit is caused by chiasmatic compression, usually by a mass in the suprasellar cisterns. Differential diagnosis includes all tumors and inflammatory conditions that can occur in the suprasellar region.

Homonymous Hemianopsia

The most common cause of a homonymous hemianopsia is ischemia in the distribution of the posterior cerebral artery that supplies the calcarine cortex of the occipital lobe. Also, mass lesions can compress the geniculate ganglion or the optic radiations in the temporal-occipital region.

Acute/Progressive Myelopathy

Epidural Hemorrhage

Most epidural hemorrhages are post-traumatic or post-operative. Also, patients who are anticoagulated are at greater risk for epidural hemorrhage. The introduction or presence of an epidural catheter also increases the risk of both hemorrhage and infection.

Epidural Abscess

Most epidural abscesses are associated with diskitis or osteomyelitis; however, isolated infections of the epidural space can occur. The diagnosis of epidural abscess can be a challenge for both the clinician and radiologist. Patients may present with back pain or radicular pain. Fever and leukocytosis may be mild. Early diagnosis and prompt therapy are critical for favorable patient outcomes.

The imaging findings can be quite subtle on plain T1- and T2-weighted images. During the cellulitis stage, the first sign of infection is thickening of the epidural tissues, which are initially isointense on T1-weighted images and moderately hyperintense on T2-weighted images. When liquefaction occurs, the abscess cavity becomes hypointense and more hyperintense on T1- and T2-weighted images, respectively. Detection of the infectious process is easier on Gd-enhanced scans. The inflamed tissues (phlegmon) are very vascular and enhance with gadolinium. On both the T2-weighted images and the enhanced T1-weighted images, fat suppression increases the contrast between the infectious process and normal tissues. The abscess cavity does not enhance. It appears as a linear or elongated region of hypointensity surrounded by the enhancing cellulitis on sagittal images and as an oval configuration on axial images [8] (Fig. 5).

Tumor

Epidural tumor usually extends from the spine. The vast majority of spine tumors are metastases, with the common primaries being lung, breast, and prostate. Occasionally, the epidural space may be directly seeded by lymphoma or leukemia.

Patients with spinal cord tumors and other intradural tumors (schwannoma and meningioma) may present with a progressive myelopathy.

Inflammatory Diseases

Several demyelinating diseases are associated with a transverse myelitis and acute myelopathy. In addition to classic multiple sclerosis, post-viral syndromes and Guillain-Barré are in the differential diagnosis. In HIV patients, the two primaries diseases to consider are epidural abscess and CMV polyradiculopathy.

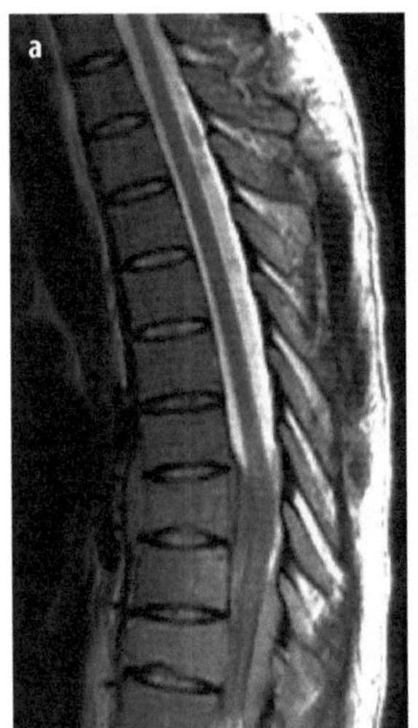

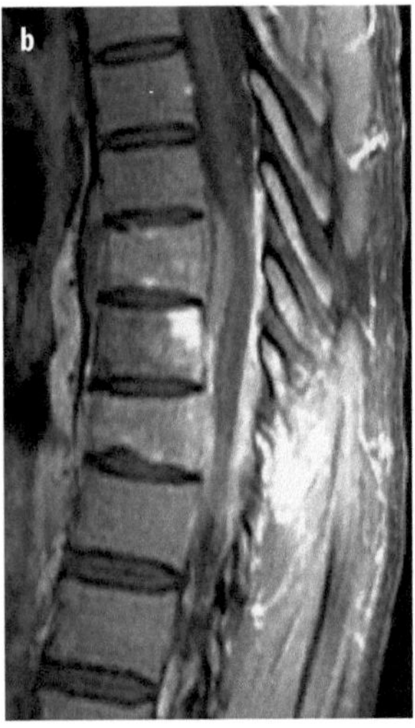

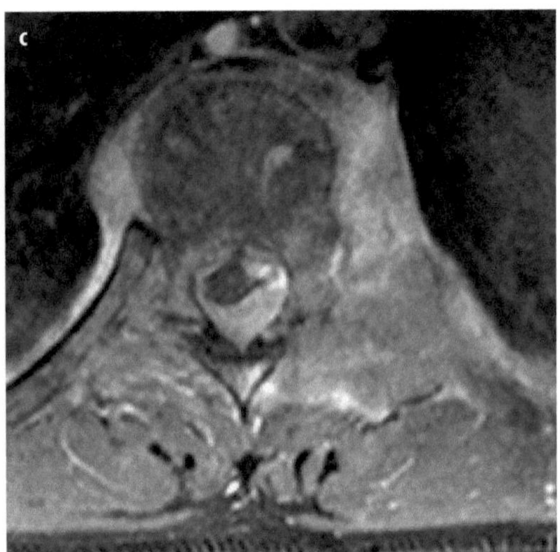

Fig. 5 a-c. Epidural spinal lymphoma. **a** Sagittal T2-weighted image shows epidural mass compressing the thecal sac. Sagittal (**b**) and axial (**c**) Gd-enhanced T1-weighted scans reveal enhancing epidural and paraspinal masses, as well as involvement of three lower thoracic vertebrae

Ischemia

Spinal cord ischemia is rare. It is usually associated with spinal and paraspinal tumors or surgical procedures on the spine and aorta that may compromise the blood supply to the cord.

Cervical or Thoracic Disk Extrusion

Disk extrusions in the cervical and thoracic spine, if sufficiently large, can compress the spinal cord and produce a myelopathy. Accompanying cord edema can exacerbate the problem. Emergent laminectomy and diskectomy may be necessary to relieve the cord compression.

References

1. Levy C, Laissy JP, Raveau V et al (1994) Carotid and vertebral artery dissections: three-dimensional time-of-flight MR angiography and MR imaging versus conventional angiography. Radiology 190:97
2. Lee SK, terBrugge KG (2003) Cerebral venous thrombosis in adults: the role of imaging evaluation and management. Neuroimag Clin N Am 13:139-152
3. Chepuri NB, Perl II J, Masaryk TJ, Turski PA (2006) Aneurysms and central nervous system vascular malformations. In: Edelman, Hesselink, Zlatkin, Crues (eds), Clinical magnetic resonance imaging. 3rd edn. Saunders-Elsevier, Philadelphia, pp 1414-1453
4. Noguchi K, Ogawa T, Inugami A et al (1995) Acute subarachnoid hemorrhage: MR imaging with fluid-attenuated inversion recovery pulse sequences. Radiology 196:773-777
5. Kanamalla US, Ibarra RA, Jinkins JR (2000) Imaging of cranial meningitis and ventriculitis, Neuroimaging Clin N Am 10:309-332
6. Karampekios S, Hesselink JR (2006) Infectious and inflammatory diseases. In: Edelman, Hesselink, Zlatkin, Crues (eds) Clinical magnetic resonance imaging. 3rd edn. Saunders-Elsevier, Philadelphia, pp 1248-1286
7. Sämann PG, Schlege J, Müller G et al (2003) Serial proton MR spectroscopy and diffusion imaging findings in HIV-related herpes simplex encephalitis. AJNR Am J Neuroradiol 24:2015-2019
8. Khan SH, Hussain MS, Grieber RW, Hettingh S (2003) Comparison of primary and secondary spinal epidural abscesses: a retrospective analysis of 29 cases. Surg Neurol 59:28-33

Imaging Approaches to the Epileptic Patient

Richard A. Bronen[1], Linda J. Bagley[2]

[1] Yale University School of Medicine, New Haven, CT, USA

[2] Department of Radiology, Hospital of the University of Pennsylvania, Philadelphia, PA, USA

Epilepsy and Neuroimaging

Seizures are the result of excessive and abnormal electrical discharges from the cortical neurons. Epilepsy, the condition of spontaneously recurring seizures, is quite common, affecting approximately 0.4-1% of the population. The epilepsy syndromes can be categorized into localized, or partial, and generalized. Generalized seizures originate from both cerebral hemispheres simultaneously. Partial seizures are generated from a localized area of the brain. These can be further divided into complex partial, with loss of consciousness, and simple partial, without loss of consciousness. Partial seizures can secondarily generalize by spread from one area to another. Seizure classification has therapeutic and prognostic values that help in the care of patients with epilepsy.

Epilepsy is a potentially psychosocially devastating and even life-threatening disorder. While many advances have been made in the medical therapy of epilepsy, many cases, between 15 and 30%, remain medically intractable. Medically intractable epilepsy is a social, economic, and medical burden to both the individual and the general community. Surgical therapies are appropriate for certain patients and include lesional resections, temporal lobectomies, selective amygdalohippocampectomies, callosotomies, hemispherectomies, and subpial transections. With the increasing use of surgical management, the role of neuroimaging has increased in importance. The main purposes of neuroimaging in epilepsy patients are to identify underlying structural abnormalities that require specific treatment (usually surgery) and to aid in formulating a syndromic or etiologic diagnosis. Magnetic resonance imaging (MRI), with its excellent spatial resolution, soft tissue contrast, and multi-planar capabilities, is the primary imaging modality for this purpose. Phased-array surface-coil imaging, MR spectroscopy, MR perfusion-weighted imaging, functional MRI, single-photon emission computed tomography (SPECT), positron emission tomography (PET), and, in some cases, angiography may also aid in this regard. In patients with medically refractory epilepsy, the sensitivity of MRI in identifying epileptogenic substrates has been reported to be between 82 and 86%. In patients with idiopathic generalized epilepsy, however, MRI has not been shown to be useful. The major utility of computed tomography (CT) scanning is in the initial evaluation of seizures, particularly in a trauma or emergent setting or when associated with focal neurologic signs or fever.

In surgical candidates, MRI plays a crucial role not only in identifying the anatomic location of a substrate, but also in demonstrating the relationship of the lesion to the eloquent regions of the brain. Correlation and concordance of the MRI-identified substrate with clinical and electrophysiologic findings are essential to avoid false-positive localization of the epileptogenic substrate. In those instances in which the MRI findings and noninvasive electrophysiologic data are concordant, invasive electroencephalograpic evaluation can be avoided.

The diagnostic potential of MRI depends on the population being imaged. Published guidelines indicate that nonemergent MRI should always be performed in patients with epilepsy, with the exception of those with primary idiopathic generalized epilepsy. Patients with febrile seizures and those with primary idiopathic generalized epilepsy do not routinely need to be imaged, unless there are complicating factors. One should also keep in mind that the sensitivity of MRI is high for patients with intractable partial epilepsy and relatively low for those with new onset of seizures.

MRI can also prognosticate the post-operative seizure control of epileptogenic substrates. Post-operative seizure control depends on the identification of the substrate by MRI and the characteristics of the MRI-identified abnormality.

Lastly, in the post-operative setting, MRI can identify surgical complications as well as causes for the failure of surgical treatment, such as a recurrent or residual lesion.

Imaging Features of Epileptogenic Substrates

The substrates underlying localization-related, or partial, epilepsy can be categorized into the following groups: hippocampal sclerosis, malformations of cortical development, neoplasms, vascular abnormalities, gliosis, and miscellaneous abnormalities. Each category can be defined by a number of unifying parameters. These parameters include mechanism of action, etiology, treatment options, and surgical outcome.

Hippocampal Sclerosis

Hippocampal sclerosis is the most common epileptogenic substrate, and is characterized by gliosis and neuronal loss. After anterior temporal lobectomy, 67% of patients with hippocampal sclerosis are seizure free. In hippocampal sclerosis, the two major MRI findings are atrophy and abnormal T2 hyperintensity. Secondary findings include loss of hippocampal head interdigitations, loss of internal architecture, atrophy of the ipsilateral fornix and mammillary body, atrophy of the collateral white matter between the hippocampus and collateral sulcus, dilatation of the ipsilateral temporal horn, and temporal-lobe volume loss (Fig. 1). By qualitative assessment, MRI has a sensitivity in the range of 80-90% for the detection of hippocampal sclerosis. Quantitative methods such as hippocampal volumetry and T2 relaxometry increase the sensitivity to 90-95% in patients with surgically intractable epilepsy. These quantitative methods can be particularly useful when hippocampal sclerosis is present bilaterally and without obvious T2 signal changes, which occurs in 10-20% of patients. This can help to lateralize the source of the seizures. Dual pathology is a term used when hippocampal sclerosis coexists with another epileptogenic substrate, as occurs in 8-22% of surgical epilepsy patients. The most frequent epileptogenic substrate that coexists with hippocampal sclerosis is cortical dysgenesis. Combined hippocampectomy and lesionectomy may improve the surgical outcome in patients with dual pathology.

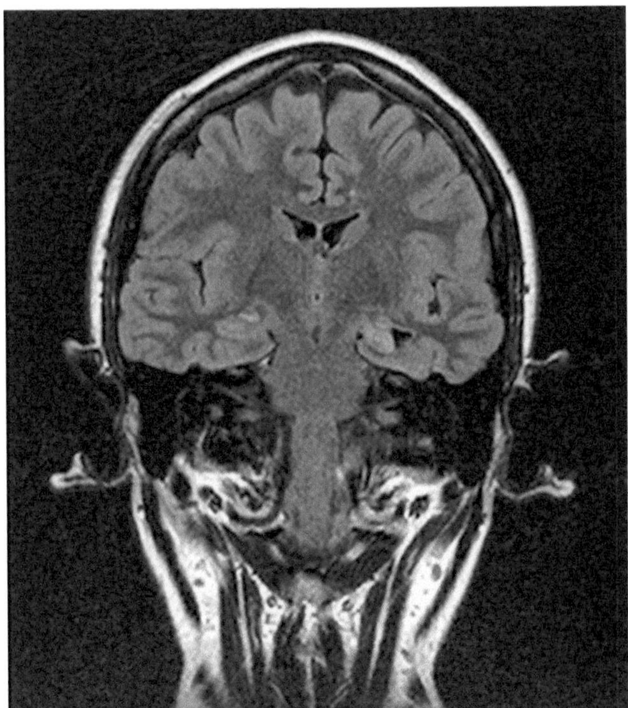

Fig. 1. Coronal FLAIR images demonstrate an atrophic left hippocampus with architectural distortion and increased signal intensity. There is dilatation of the ipsilateral temporal horn

Malformations of Cortical Development

Malformations of cortical development (MCD) account for 10-50% of pediatric epilepsy cases and 4-25% of adult cases. MRI has resulted in the increased recognition of developmental malformations as causes of epilepsy in children and young adults. The most widely used classification of MCD consists of four categories: (1) malformations due to abnormal neuronal and glial proliferation or apoptosis, (2) malformations due to abnormal neuronal migration, (3) malformations due to abnormal cortical organization, and (4) malformations of cortical development, not otherwise classified.

MRI findings seen in MCD are listed as follows:

- Cortical thickening
- Blurring of gray-white junction
- Irregularity of gray-white junction
- Increased gray-matter signal on T1-weighted images
- Macrogyria
- Mini-gyria (polymicrogyria)
- Paucity of gyri
- Sulcal cleft and cortical dimple
- Sulcal morphologic changes
- Radial bands of hyperintensity
- Transmantle gray matter
- Gray-matter heterotopia
- Band heterotopia

Malformations of cortical development are often intrinsically epileptogenic. The extent of the epileptogenic zone can be more extensive than the area of MRI abnormality. Furthermore, the epileptogenic zone may not correlate directly with the malformation but may in fact be at a distance from it. Invasive electrophysiologic studies (i.e., subdural and depth electrodes) are often used to ensure concordance in the pre-surgical evaluation of these malformations. Since many of them may be subtle, it is necessary to employ high-resolution imaging, which provides excellent visualization of the corticomedullary junction (Fig. 2).

Vascular Malformations

Vascular malformations, most typically cavernous hemangiomas, and – albeit to a lesser extent – arteriovenous malformations and dural arteriovenous fistulas serve as epileptogenic substrates in approximately 5% of epilepsy patients. Approximately 25-50% of patients with cavernous hemangiomas (also known as cavernous malformations or cavernomas) will have seizures (Fig. 3). Gradient echo sequences and angiographic imaging can aid in the detection and characterization of vascular abnormalities.

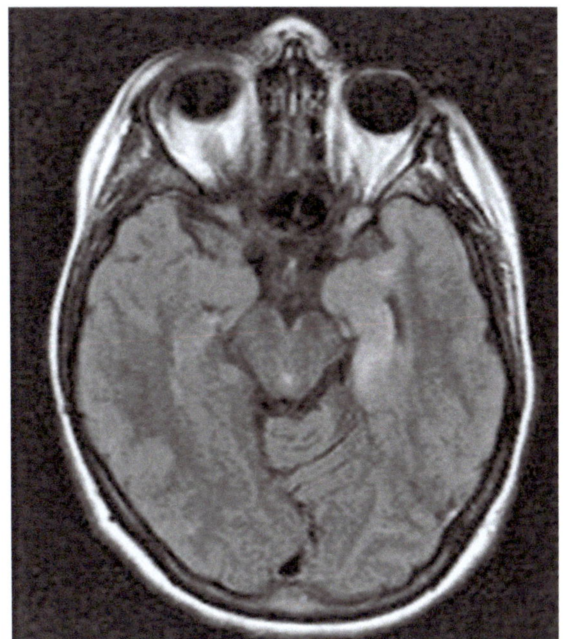

Fig. 2. Axial FLAIR images reveal cortical thickening and T2 hyperintensity within the left hippocampus

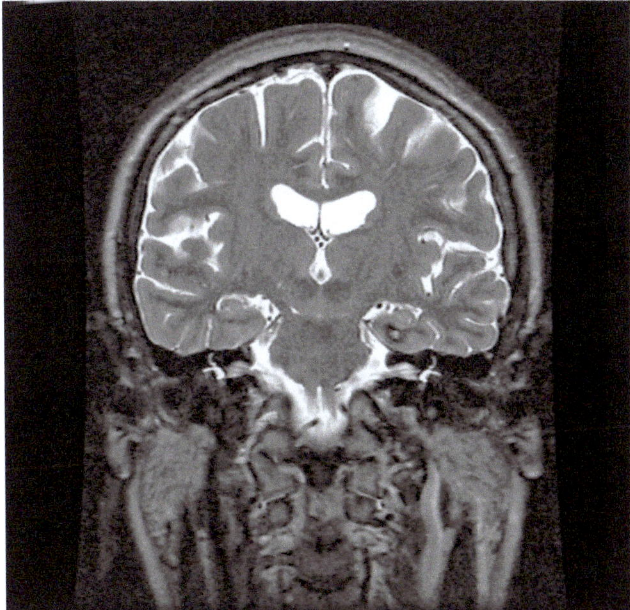

Fig. 3. Coronal T2-weighted images demonstrate a small focus of signal abnormality with surrounding hemosiderin ring in the medial left temporal lobe, just inferior to the hippocampus

Neoplasia

Brain neoplasms are the source of seizures in approximately 2-4 % of epileptic patients. Typically, tumors inducing medically intractable epilepsy are slow-growing, benign, cortical or juxtacortical lesions, such as gangliogliomas, pilocytic astrocytomas, low-grade astrocytomas or oligodendrogliomas, pleomorphic xanthoastrocytomas, and dysembryoplastic neuroepithelial tumors (Fig. 4). However, higher-grade primary neoplasms or metastases may be the source of new-onset seizures in older patients. Complete surgical resections of the lesions and adjacent cortex often result in significant seizure reduction or seizure-free outcomes.

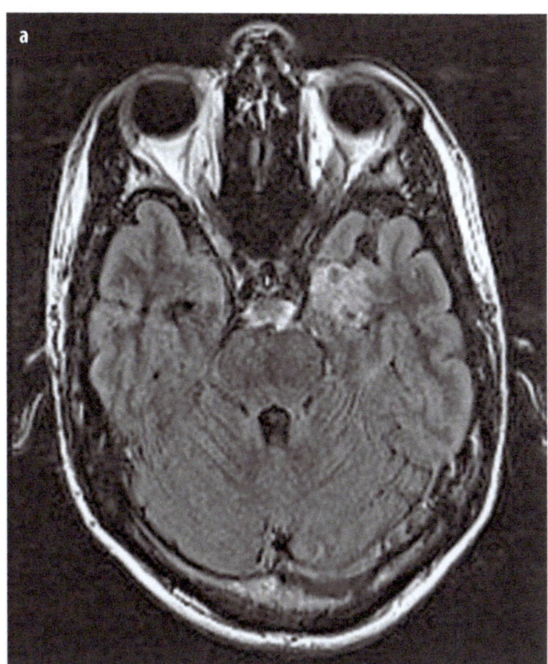

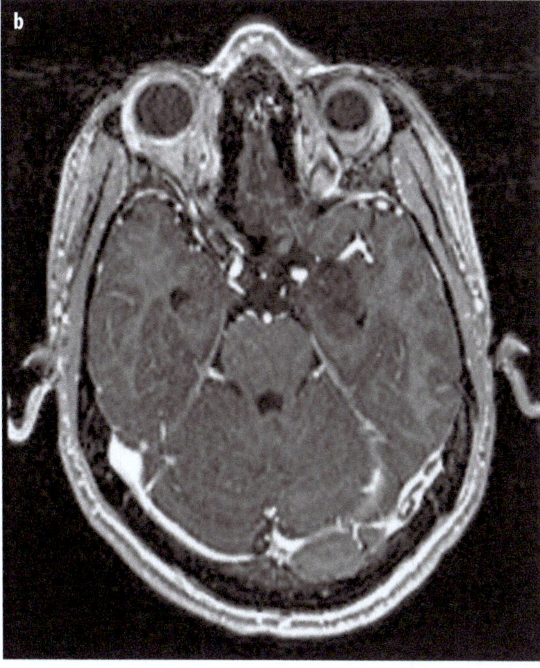

Fig. 4 a, b. Axial FLAIR (**a**) and gadolinium-enhanced T1-weighted (**b**) images demonstrate a non-enhancing, heterogeneous, cortically based T2 hyperintense lesion in the medial left temporal lobe, pathologically proven dysembryoplastic neuroepithelial tumor (DNET)

Gliosis

Regions of encephalomalacia, the sequelae of prior trauma, infection, and/or infarction, may also be the source of epileptiform discharges (Fig. 5). Imaging findings may include focal or diffuse brain atrophy, signal abnormalities, hemosiderin deposition, porencephaly, and irregular cystic cavities. Resultant seizure disorders are often medically and surgically intractable.

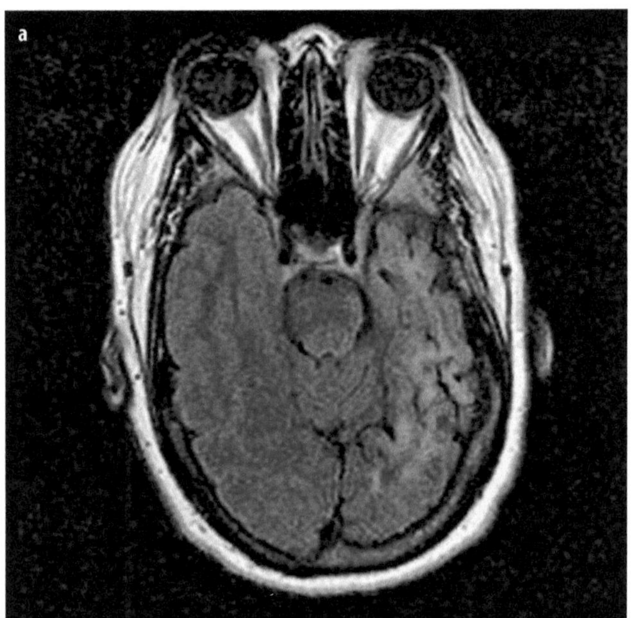

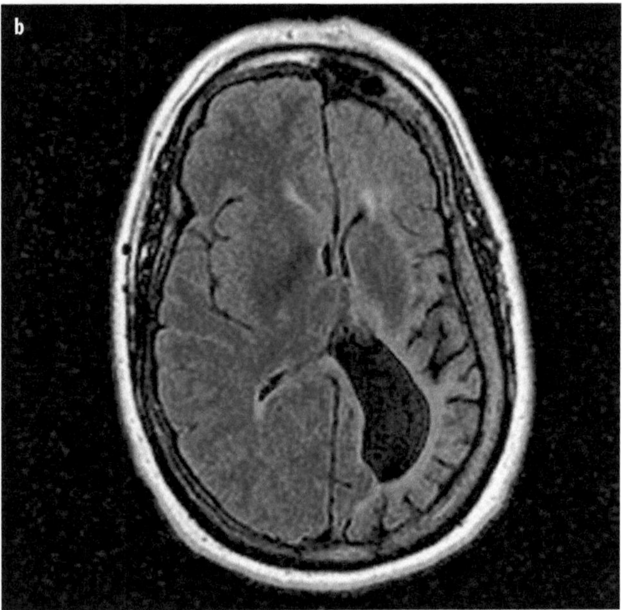

Fig. 5 a, b. Axial FLAIR images (**a**, **b**) obtained in a patient with a remote history of varicella encephalitis reveal extensive atrophy and signal abnormality within the left hemisphere, with ex-vacuo dilatation of the left lateral ventricle and thickening of the left calvarium

Paradigms of Magnetic Resonance Imaging

In order to arrive at appropriate recommendations for imaging protocols, one needs to account for a number of factors, including the population being imaged and the imaging characteristics of the possible substrates one is likely to encounter. Different substrates vary in their frequency depending on the age of the population imaged (Table 1). One must consider the substrates most likely to be evaluated and their unique imaging features. Lastly, when seeking an optimal protocol, one must consider the age-related changes in the imaging characteristics of the brain.

When evaluating patients <1.5 years of age, hippocampal sclerosis is not a consideration. Inversion recovery and fast spin echo-T2 weighted sequences can optimize distinction between gray and white matter in these patients. In neonates, infection and stroke may be diagnostic considerations. As above, after the age of 50 years, the frequency of neoplasm and stroke as underlying substrates for new onset seizures greatly increases. Hence, diffusion-weighted and gadolinium-enhanced images are necessary in these two patient groups.

Patients between the ages of 1.5 and 50 years are the group most likely to be evaluated for intractable partial epilepsy, and thus will have the highest yield for the detection of structural pathology by MRI. Due to the subtle nature of the imaging findings sometimes present in entities like hippocampal sclerosis and cortical dysplasia, routine MRI protocols are often inadequate for detection. Imaging parameters, such as image orientation, slice thickness, and pulse sequences, should be optimized in order to identify these substrates.

After the age of 1.5 years, hippocampal sclerosis becomes a major diagnostic consideration. When evaluating for hippocampal sclerosis, the coronal-oblique or cross sectional plane (perpendicular to the long axis of the hippocampus) is best for demonstrating relevant findings, as it depicts signal changes, atrophy, and abnormalities of internal architecture in the hippocampus. Fluid-attenuated inversion recovery (FLAIR) sequences are most sensitive for demonstrating hippocampal signal abnormality. The hippocampus is normally slightly hyperintense compared to gray matter on FLAIR sequences in some patients. Since this makes interpretation of hippocampal signal intensity difficult if one relies solely on the FLAIR images, we employ a combination of coronal FLAIR and coronal fast spin echo T2-weighted sequences for assessment. T1-weighted gradient volume acquisitions (SPGR or MP-RAGE) are excellent for evaluating the morphology of the hippocampus and developmental disorders. The raw data from these images can be reconstructed in any plane and aid in qualitative and volumetric analysis of the hippocampus.

Inversion recovery sequences can provide good corticomedullary contrast and information regarding morphology and signal abnormalities. Some epilepsy centers use spectroscopy and T2 relaxometry for additional evaluation of the hippocampus and medial temporal lobes. T2

Table 1. Causes of Epilepsy by Patient Age at Seizure Onset

Cause	Age at seizure onset (years)				
	0-2	3-20	21-40	41-60	>60
Metabolic abnormalities or inborn error of metabolism	X				
Cerebral anoxia	X				
Infection	X	X			
Congenital or developmental malformations	X	X			
Phacomatoses	X	X			
Hippocampal sclerosis		X			
Primary generalized seizures		X			
Vascular malformation		X	X		
Post-traumatic epilepsy		X	X	X	X
Tumor			X	X	X
Stroke				X	X

relaxometry obtained from multi-echo T2-weighted sequences is useful in cases in which the findings on visual analysis are equivocal or in lateralization of seizure focus when abnormalities are evident in both hippocampi.

Developmental malformations are very subtle abnormalities and can be missed easily if high-resolution imaging and sequences with good gray-white matter differentiation are not employed. Coronal T1-weighted gradient volume sequences (SPGR or MP-RAGE) with thin slice thickness (1–1.6 mm) can demonstrate subtle developmental malformations. FLAIR and T2-weighted sequences are recommended to assess for hyperintense signal changes in the subcortical and deep white matter (including radial bands) associated with MCD.

There are a number of additional measures that can be used to increase the yield for detecting MCD, including high-resolution imaging with phased-array coils, image registration and averaging, and high field magnets (>3T). Multiple phased-array surface coils centered over the suspected epileptogenic area provide high-resolution images with high signal to noise ratios. Grant et al. (1997) compared head and surface-coil imaging in 25 patients with medically refractory partial neocortical epilepsy. The imaging protocols employed included a coronal volumetric 3DFT gradient echo series and, in most cases, a fast spin echo or spin echo high-resolution T2-weighted sequence. Surface-coil images improved the detection and definition of focal cortical lesions in 64% of the patients studied. Additional foci of dysplasia were seen; polymicrogyria was distinguished from pachygyria; and areas of T2 signal abnormality were more confidently classified as neoplastic or non-neoplastic. Post-processing of the raw data from a 3D volume set can yield high-resolution 3D reformations, which can demonstrate cortical dysplasia, abnormal sulcal morphology, gray-white matter indistinctiveness, and the relationship of developmental abnormalities to the eloquent cortical regions. Quantitative analysis of gray and white matter, when compared with normal controls may show widespread developmental abnormalities. However, the location and extent of cortical dysplasia identified by MRI may not correlate with the seizure semiology or the electrophysiologic data.

Strategies for Interpretation

Successful MRI and its interpretation can be challenging because the abnormalities we seek to detect may be quite subtle. One must be able to differentiate normal variations from pathologic conditions.

Normal Variations Related to Gyral and Sulcal Configurations

One needs to be aware of normal gyral and sulcal variations to avoid misdiagnosis. Some of the common variations that can be mistaken for cortical dysplasia are:

- Cortex adjoining the superior temporal sulcus on the right side is usually slightly thicker than that of the left side.
- The gyri surrounding the calcarine sulcus usually indent the occipital horn (in an area known as the calcar avis), giving rise to the appearance of thickened gyri, which can be asymmetric.
- Normal undulations of the cortex may give the appearance of cortical thickening on cross-sectional images, if the gyrus is parallel to the cross-sectional plane. Dysplasia can be distinguished from this normal finding by observing cortical thickening on multiple images (usually at least three contiguous thin-section images) or confirming that cortical thickening is present in another plane.
- Perirolandic gray matter (see below).

The region of the perirolandic fissure is another potential source of confusion between normal findings and cortical dysplasia. On coronal images, there is often poorer visualization of the gray-matter thickness in the perirolandic fissure region than in the rest of the frontal lobes as well as poor distinction between gray and white matter. This variation appears to be due to a combination of factors, one of which is that the gray matter surrounding the rolandic fissure is normally thinner than the cortices in the rest of the brain. Another factor is that the frontal sulci and gyri anterior to the rolandic fissure (i.e., superior, middle, and inferior frontal gyri) are perpendicular to the coronal plane, allowing for good definition of their cross-sectional surfaces, while the rolandic fissure and adjacent gyri are parallel to the coronal plane, yielding partial volume effects with white matter. Due to the difficulty in interpreting this region on coronal images, reference to axial images should be obtained, especially since frontal-lobe epilepsy is secondary only to temporal-lobe epilepsy in terms of the most common regions of partial seizures.

Lastly, one should keep in mind that the signal characteristics of gray and white matter in the incompletely myelinated infant can be confusing and are a possible source of misinterpretation. For example, the myelinated optic radiations surrounded by unmyelinated white matter could be mistaken for gray matter and misdiagnosed as band heterotopia.

Hippocampal Asymmetry and Variations

Other potential sources for errors in interpretation can occur in the evaluation of the hippocampus. As previously discussed, the key features of hippocampal sclerosis are hippocampal asymmetry and signal hyperintensity on FLAIR imaging. Artificial hippocampal size asymmetry can be created by head rotation because the cross-sectional size of the hippocampus is greatest anteriorly (at its head) but progressively tapers on more posterior sections. Correct interpretation depends on accurate alignment of the patient's head in the scanner and on taking head rotation into account for determining hippocampal symmetry in those subjects who fail to be properly aligned . Caution is also advised when interpreting FLAIR sequence images. The signal intensity of the hippocampus on FLAIR sequences is slightly greater than the cortex in normal subjects; this may lead to a false diagnosis of bilateral hippocampal sclerosis in seizure patients. The configuration of the hippocampus can be quite variable and this can also result in difficulties with interpretation. The hippocampal body usually has an oval or round shape in the coronal plane. Infrequently, it may have a more vertical configuration, such that cortical dysgenesis maybe erroneously diagnosed. However, some reports in the literature suggest that a round- or vertical-shaped hippocampus may be due to a malformation related to epileptogenesis. In cases of corpus callosum agenesis or holoprosencephaly, there may be associated incomplete infolding of the cornu ammonis and dentate gyrus, which manifest as a vertically shaped hippocampus with a (shallow) medial cleft on coronal images.

Avoiding Pitfalls When Considering the Differential Diagnosis

Potential misinterpretations of imaging findings in seizure patients arise from a number of situations, in addition to the normal variations listed above. Transient lesions are perhaps the most troubling, because of the potential for in appropriately performing lesional resective surgery in a setting in which epileptogenesis is either widespread (e.g., Rasmussen's encephalitis) or outside the lesional area. Focal transient signal abnormalities in seizure patients appear to be the result of infections, toxic-metabolic abnormalities, or prolonged or frequent seizures. Post-ictal changes can present as focal or multi-focal hyperintense abnormalities of the cortex or hippocampus on long TR sequences and as reduced diffusion. While these latter findings may indicate ischemic changes, perfusion studies show increased rather than decreased blood flow associated with infarction. In Rasmussen's syndrome, the signal changes may not only be transient, but also move from location to location. Therefore, caution should be exercised in interpreting findings and in recommending invasive studies for actively seizing subjects. Morphologic and signal abnormalities are also reported in recurrent focal or febrile seizures in the hippocampus. Transient lesions may affect the splenium of the corpus callosum. This rare isolated focal lesion is seen in 0.5% of epilepsy patients, and is characterized by T2 hyperintensity, reduced diffusion, and lack of enhancement. The abnormality is thought to result from either frequent seizures or abrupt changes in anti-epileptic drug concentrations that, in turn, elevate arginine vasopressin, which has been suggested to cause cytotoxic edema in the splenium.

Differentiating neoplasms from either focal cortical dysplasia or hippocampal sclerosis may be problematic. Hyperintense signal changes on T2-weighted images in the subcortical white matter may be present in neoplasms and in focal cortical dysplasia (particularly balloon-cell focal cortical dysplasia). Surgical strategies may differ for these entities, especially if an epileptogenic lesion is located in an eloquent area of the cortex. Imaging findings suggestive of dysplasia rather than neoplasm include cortical thickening, the presence of a radial band extending from the lesion to the ventricle, and the homogenous appearance of subcortical white-matter hyperintensity. High-resolution imaging, perhaps with a magnet of high field strength or phased-array surface coils, may be helpful for demonstrating cortical thickening. A frontal-lobe location is more commonly seen in dysplasias, while a temporal-lobe location is more frequently associated with tumors. The presence of subependymal or multiple subcortical lesions should raise concerns of tuberous sclerosis.

In subjects with a hyperintense hippocampus on long TR images, one must distinguish tumor from hippocampal sclerosis. This is not particularly difficult if the hippocampus is ipsilaterally small, which is the cardinal finding in determining hippocampal sclerosis. However, the hippocampus is not always small in such cases. Findings suggestive of neoplasm include heterogeneous signal changes and extension of the signal changes beyond the hippocampus into the parahippocampal white matter.

In MCD, it is sometimes difficult to distinguish one malformation from another and from normal structures. Differentiating polymicrogyria from the pachygyria/agyria (lissencephaly) spectrum is especially challenging. Both entities demonstrate cortical thickening, which may be bilateral and may appear as smooth cortices (due to the "micro" gyri in polymicrogyria). One differentiating feature is the tendency for polymicrogyria to affect the sylvian fissure and to be associated with a cerebrospinal fluid (CSF) cleft. Sagittal images may be particularly useful – perisylvian polymicrogyria often results in a sylvian fissure that is continuous with the central sulcus, which is well-demonstrated in the parasagittal plane. Although polymicrogyria may be bilateral, it is not usually as diffuse as pachygyria. However, pachygyria may affect the brain regionally; for example, in the frontal lobes. Multiple microgyri can sometimes be visualized with the use of high-resolution imaging in patients with polymicrogyria.

The differential diagnosis for periventricular findings that are isointense with gray matter on T1-weighted images includes periventricular heterotopia, normal caudate nucleus, and subependymal tuberous sclerosis hamartomas. True gray matter follows the signal intensity of the cortex on all pulse sequences, not only T1-weighted sequences. Regarding the caudate nucleus, the head is easily identified, which then allows identification of the body and tail on subsequent slices and differentiation from heterotopia.

The asymmetric hemisphere may also be problematic, and hemi-megalencephaly is sometimes mistaken for the hemi-atrophic syndrome. In both entities, there is ventricular enlargement, one hemisphere is larger than the other, and there may be diffuse white-matter hyperintensity. However, the ventricular enlargement in hemi-atrophy is in the smaller hemisphere, while ventricular enlargement occurs in the larger hemisphere in hemi-megalencephaly. Unlike hemi-atrophy, hemi-megalencephaly is associated with cortical thickening, sulcal abnormalities, heterotopias, and radial bands.

An important pitfall to avoid relates to dual pathology (the presence of both an extra-hippocampal lesion and hippocampal sclerosis). Once an obvious lesion is found, one can easily neglect to scrutinize the hippocampus, especially if there are concordant electroclinical findings. Coincidental hippocampal sclerosis is not infrequent, particularly with developmental anomalies. It is often necessary to surgically remove both lesions in order to attain a seizure-free outcome.

A very rare cause of epilepsy is temporal-lobe encephalocele, which can be easily overlooked due to its extra-axial location. The basal temporal lobes should be closely examined for this entity, which must be distinguished from the normal protrusions of brain tissue occurring in this region (Fig. 6).

Additional Imaging Techniques

Multi-slice continuous arterial spin-labeled perfusion MRI has also been used in the study of patients with temporal-lobe epilepsy. In preliminary work, Wolf et al. (2001) found interictal asymmetries in the perfusion of the medial temporal lobes in these patients. The authors also reported a trend toward a correlation between the magnitude of perfusional asymmetry and a seizure-free surgical outcome.

Apparent diffusion coefficient maps and diffusion tensor imaging can identify abnormal diffusion at the epileptogenic foci in normal-appearing standard MRI studies. Abnormal magnetization transfer ratios in epilepsy patients with negative conventional MRI may detect and delineate the extent of occult MCD.

Currently, most candidates for epilepsy surgery undergo pre-operative Wada testing (cerebral angiography and intracarotid injections of amobarbitol followed by neuropsychological testing) in an effort to lateralize memory and language function and thereby minimize post-operative deficits. The role of functional MRI has been increasing in an attempt to replace this invasive procedure. Functional

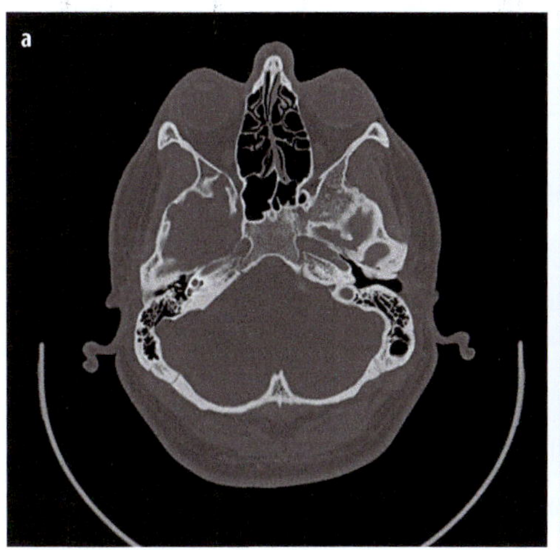

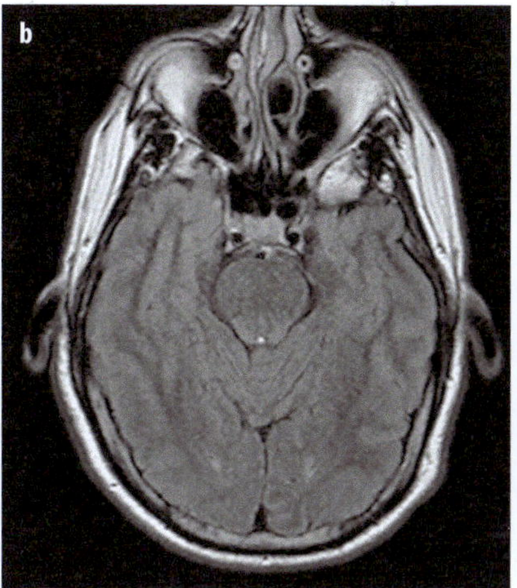

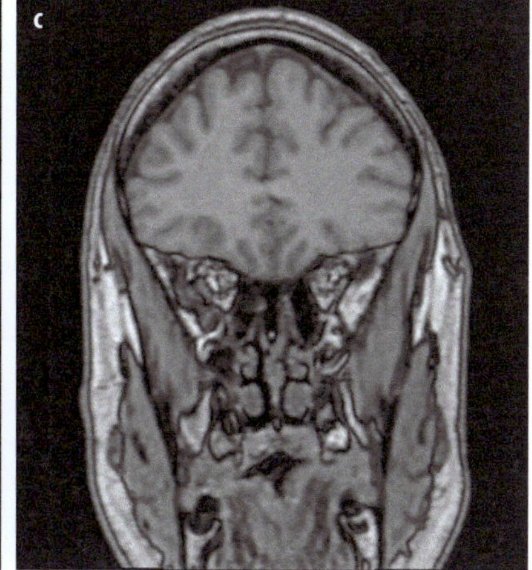

Fig. 6 a-c. **a** Axial CT scan demonstrates a small corticated defect in the right sphenoid wing. **b** Corresponding FLAIR image reveals brain tissue protruding through this defect. **c** Coronal T1-weighted gradient-echo image demonstrates the encephalocele inferior to the right orbit

MRI employs a blood oxygen level-dependent (BOLD) technique. Deoxyhemoglobin has para-magnetic effects, so that its presence results in T2 signal loss. Oxygenated hemoglobin has a minimally para-magnetic effect. Since levels of blood oxygenation are increased in areas of cortical activation, T2 signal loss due to the presence of deoxyhemoglobin is less pronounced in these activated areas. The BOLD technique has been used to localize visual and motor cortex and language centers. Efforts are on-going to improve localization of memory with functional MRI.

Proton magnetic resonance spectroscopy (MRS) compliments conventional MRI in improving our understanding of brain disorders, including epilepsy. Proton MRS provides metabolic information by determining the presence and levels of select neurochemicals. In patients with suspected mesial temporal sclerosis, small regions of interest, referred to as voxels, are placed over the medial temporal lobes. Reduced levels of *N*-acetyl aspartate (NAA), found primarily in axons and neurons, have been reported in the temporal lobe containing the seizure focus. Myo-inositol resonance, seen on short-echo MRS, has been associated with areas of gliosis and may be elevated in the temporal lobe ipsilateral to the seizure focus. Phosphorus (P-31) spectroscopy has been notable for demonstrating reduced levels of phosphocreatine and inorganic phosphate in the affected temporal lobe. Interictally, pH in the affected temporal lobe has been found to be elevated. Ictally, lactate levels are increased; hence, pH is decreased.

Nuclear medicine studies, such as PET and SPECT, provide physiologic information about the eleptogenic brain. PET studies use the radioisotope fludeoxyglucose (FDG) to measure glucose metabolism in neurons. Interictally, the temporal lobe ipsilateral to the seizure focus is hypometabolic (Fig. 7). The sensitivity of FDG-PET for identifying the abnormal temporal lobe in patients with partial epilepsy has been reported to be 70-91% (Grant et al., 1997). The sensitivity of this study for localizing the seizure focus is reduced in extra-temporal epilepsy, however. SPECT is performed with the radiotracer Tc99m HMPAO, which is distributed in the brain in proportion to regional blood flow. Interictally, the sensitivity of SPECT is much lower than that of PET. However, when Tc99m HMPAO is injected during a seizure, increased blood flow typically results in increased uptake of the radiotracer. The sensitivity of studies aimed at lateralizing the seizure focus has been reported to exceed 95%; however, it may be technically difficult to obtain an injection during seizure and requires dedicated resources in terms of audiovisual EEG monitoring and skilled personnel to obtain such high sensitivity.

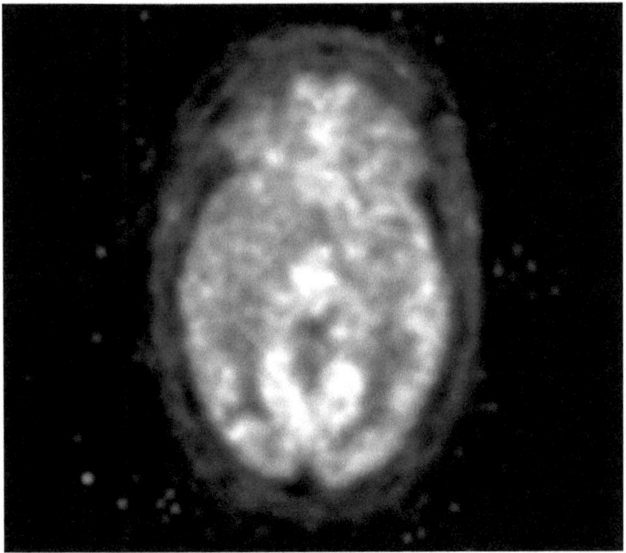

Fig. 7. Axial PET image reveals marked hypometabolism in the right temporal lobe

A Systematic Approach

Since many epileptogenic lesions are subtle and can be overlooked, a systematic approach is useful during the interpretation of imaging studies from a seizure patient. One approach that can be followed can be remembered by the mnemonic HIPPO SAGE (Table 2).

The hypothalamus should be reviewed to detect a hypothalamic hamartomas, particularly in children. These can be subtle and overlooked, especially if the patient does not present with gelastic seizures. Hippocampal size, symmetry, and signal abnormalities are assessed in the coronal plane to evaluate for hippocampal sclerosis. Since head rotation may lead to a false diagnosis of hippocampal atrophy, it is assessed based on the symmetry of the internal auditory canals and of the atria of the left lateral ventricles. If head rotation is present, assessment of hippocampal symmetry must be compensated for by comparing compatible coronal hippocampal sections (i.e., the right hippocampal section adjacent to the right internal auditory canal should be compared with lthe eft hippocampal section adjacent to the left internal auditory canal). Periventricular regions should be scrutinized for subependymal gray-matter heterotopias, which occur most commonly adjacent to the atria of lateral ventricles.

Table 2. Systematic evaluation of MRI scans of seizure patients

- Hippocampal size and signal abnormality; hypothalamic hamartoma
- Internal auditory canal and atrial asymmetry (assess for head rotation when evaluating for hippocampal atrophy)
- Periventricular heterotopia
- Peripheral abnormalities
- Obvious lesion: the identification of one pathology can cause hippocampal sclerosis to go undetected in patients with dual pathologies
- Sulcal morphologic abnormalities
- Atrophy
- Gray-matter thickening
- Encephalocele of the anterior temporal lobe

Gray matter should not be present inferiorlateral to the temporal horns and is abnormal. Because focal epilepsy is a cortical-based process, the periphery of the brain should be carefully scrutinized for developmental anomalies, atrophic processes, and small neoplasms or vascular malformations. We closely inspect the sulci and gyri for morphologic changes (which underlie developmental disorders), atrophic processes, gray-matter thickening, and indistinctness of the gray-white matter junction (associated with developmental disorders). The inferior aspect of the anterior temporal lobe is assessed to exclude a temporal lobe encephalocele, an extremely uncommon cause of epilepsy but one that is easily overlooked if not specifically searched for. Finally, we evaluate any obvious lesion in the brain and assess its characteristics. It may be an incidental finding, an epileptogenic substrate, or an additional lesion. If the neuroradiologist concentrates only on an obvious lesion, there is a chance that concurring hippocampal sclerosis will not be detected in those patients with dual pathologies.

Conclusions

Neuroimaging, in particular MRI, plays a critical role in the evaluation of the epileptic patient. The advanced MRI techniques, MRS, and nuclear medicine studies described above are often complementary and may be obtained in the pre-surgical evaluation of epilepsy patients. Used in conjunction with electroencephalographic data, video-EEG monitoring, and neuropsychologic testing, neuroimaging identifies epileptogenic substrates, predicts prognosis, and directs therapy.

Suggested Reading

Andermann F (1997) Brain structure and epilepsy: the impact of modern imaging. AJNR Am J Neuroradiol 18:302-306

Arroyo S, Freeman JM (1994) Epilepsy surgery in children: state of the art. Adv Pediatrics 41:53-81

Barkovich AJ, Kuzniecky RI, Jackson GD et al (2001) Classification system for malformation of cortical development: update 2001. Neurology 57:2168-2178

Bell GS, Sander JW (2001) The epidemiology of epilepsy: the size of the problem. Seizure 16:165-170

Berkovic SF, McIntosh AM, Kalnios RM et al (1995) Preoperative MRI predicts outcome of temporal lobectomy: an actuarial analysis. Neurology 45:1358-1363

Bernal B, Altman N (2003) Evidence-based medicine: neuroimaging of seizures. Neuroimaging Clin N Am 13:211-224

Bien CG, Widman G, Urbach H et al (2002) The natural history of Rasmussen's encephalitis. Brain 125:1751-1759

Bladin CF, Alexandrov AV, Bellavance A et al, for the Seizures after Stroke Study Group (2000) Seizures after stroke. Arch Neurol 57:1617-1622

Bronen RA (1992) Epilepsy: the role of MR imaging. AJR Am J Roentgenol 159:1165-1174

Bronen RA, Fulbright RK, Kim JH et al (1997) A systematic approach for interpreting MR images of the seizure patient. AJR Am J Roentgenol 169:241-247

Bronen RA, Fulbright RK, Spencer DD et al (1995) MR characteristics of neoplasms and vascular malformations associated with epilepsy. Magn Reson Imaging 13:1153-1162

Bronen RA, Fulbright RK, Spencer DD et al (1996) Refractory epilepsy: comparison of MR imaging, CT, and histopathologic findings in 117 patients. Radiology 201:97-105

Bronen RA, Knowlton R, Garwood M et al (2002) High resolution imaging in epilepsy. Epilepsia 43:11-18

Cendes F, Cook MJ, Watson C et al (1995) Frequency and characteristics of dual pathology in patients with lesional epilepsy. Neurology 45:2058-2064

Commission on Classification and Terminology of the International League against Epilepsy (1989) Proposal for revised classification of epilepsies and epileptic syndromes. Epilepsia 30:389-399

Commission on Neuroimaging of the International League against Epilepsy (1998) Guidelines for neuroimaging evaluation of patients with uncontrolled epilepsy considered for surgery. Epilepsia 39:1375-1376

Fisher RS, Stein A, Karis J (1997) Epilepsy for the neuroradiologist. AJNR Am J Neuroradiol 18:851-863

Frey LC (2003) Epidemiology of post-traumatic epilepsy: a critical review. Epilepsia 44(Suppl 10):11-17

Friedland R, Bronen R (1996) Magnetic resonance imaging of neoplastic, vascular, and indeterminate substrates. In: Cascino G, Jack CJ (eds) Neuroimaging in epilepsy: principles and practice. Butterworth-Heinemann, Newton (MA), pp 29-50

Grant PE, Barkovich AJ, Wald LL et al (1997) High-resolution surface-coil MR of cortical lesions in medically refractory epilepsy: a prospective study. AJNR Am J Neuroradiol 18:291-301

Jack CJ, Sharbrough FW, Cascino GD et al (1992) Magnetic resonance image-based hippocampal volumetry: correlation with outcome after temporal lobectomy. Ann Neurol 31:138-146

Li LM, Cendes F, Andermann F et al (1999) Surgical outcome in patients with epilepsy and dual pathology. Brain 122:799-805

Quigg M, Bertram EH, Jackson T, Laws E (1997) Volumetric magnetic resonance imaging evidence of bilateral hippocampal atrophy in mesial temporal lobe epilepsy. Epilepsia 38:588-594

Raymond AA, Fish DR, Sisodiya SM et al (1995) Abnormalities of gyration, heterotopias, tuberous sclerosis, focal cortical dysplasia, microdysgenesis, dysembryo-plastic neuroepithelial tumour and dysgenesis of the archicortex in epilepsy. Clinical, EEG and neuroimaging features in 100 adult patients. Brain 118:629-660

Rugg-Gunn FJ, Eriksson SH, Symms MR et al (2002) Diffusion tensor imaging in refractory epilepsy. Lancet 359:1748-1751

Rugg-Gunn FJ, Eriksson SH, Symms MR et al (2003) Magnetization transfer imaging in focal epilepsy. Neurology 60:1638-1645

Spencer D (1999) Classifying the epilepsies by substrate. Clin Neurosci 19942:104-109

Wolf RL, Alsop DC, French JA et al (2001) Detection of mesial temporal lobe hypoperfusion in patients with temporal lobe epilepsy using multislice arterial spin labeled perfusion MRI. AJNR Am J Neuroradiol 22:1334-1341

Yoo SY CK, Song IC, Han MH et al (2002) Apparent diffusion coefficient value of the hippocampus in patients with hippocampal sclerosis and in healthy volunteers. AJNR Am J Neuroradiol 23:809-812

Cerebral Infections

David Mikulis[1], Stephan Wetzel[2]

[1] Department of Medical Imaging, The University Health Network, The Toronto Western Hospital, Toronto, ON, Canada
[2] Neuroradiologie, Universitätsspital, Basel, Switzerland

Introduction

The broad categories of infectious diseases that affect the brain continue to present diagnostic challenges. Although imaging patterns of disease are well-established, overlap between categories can occur. For example, the differentiation of cycticercosis, a parasitic infection, from a tuberculous abscess, a bacterial infection, can be difficult. Additional challenges are posed by the increasing probability of encountering nonendemic pathogens secondary to the "globalization" of infections brought on by the expansion of international travel, transportation, and immigration. Furthermore, increasing numbers of individuals are undergoing treatments and therapies that compromise the immune system, leading to altered host responses that no longer express the expected patterns of tissue injury.

Imaging plays a central role in the detection and differentiation of cerebral infections, with conventional magnetic resonance imaging (MRI) serving as the modality of choice by virtue of its superior tissue contrast. This enables accurate "staging" of an infection and can provide an objective measure of treatment response. Functional MRI methods can also add useful information that increases diagnostic confidence. Perhaps the best example of this is the detection of restricted water diffusion in a ring-enhancing lesion, confirming the presence of an abscess. Proton magnetic resonance spectroscopy (MRS) has also shown utility in the detection of cerebral abscesses via detection of resonances derived from the by-products of bacterial metabolism.

In view of these considerations, this chapter will focus on each of the broad categories of infectious diseases that affect the brain and its coverings, with an emphasis on the pathophysiology since the evolving response of the host to the pathogen can provide clues to an accurate diagnosis. Alterations of the host response caused by the immunosupressed state can then be better understood. Certain atypical infectious agents will be mentioned when appropriate to highlight the need for awareness of the spectrum of pathogens that may be encountered in modern practice.

Cerebral Abscess

In the pre-antibiotic era, brain abscesses were most commonly caused by direct extension from infected paranasal sinuses. Now, the most common source is blood-borne bacterial seeding originating from infections elsewhere in the body. The abscess initially begins as a region of cerebral inflammation or cerebritis that progresses to form a pus-filled cavity with a fibroglial capsule. The typical abscess will have a relatively thin, smooth wall showing intense contrast enhancement on computed tomography (CT) or MRI. Edema in the adjacent white matter is common. The abscess wall can appear bright on T1-weighted images. This is thought to be the result of a T1 shortening effect related to constituents in white blood cells [1].

The critical imaging issue, however, revolves around the similarities between brain abscess and neoplastic diseases, especially metastases. Both commonly show ring enhancement following contrast administration. How then can they be distinguished? In general, the enhancing ring of an abscess is thin and quite smooth as opposed to a neoplasm, in which some irregularity or nodularity is present. The deepest portion of the abscess wall "pointing" to the ventricular system is typically thinner than other portions of the rim (Fig. 1). However, these features are not reliable as metastases can have "perfect" enhancing rims, and abscesses can often have irregular margins. Increases in diagnostic specificity can be gained through application of diffusion methods and MRS. Abscess cavities on MR diffusion imaging typically show restricted water movement similar to that seen with acute ischemic stroke (Fig. 2).

It has been theorized that decreased water diffusion is related to dead or dying white cells "absorbing" extracellular water, analogous to the proposed mechanism for ischemic neurons and glia in ischemic stroke. A direct relationship between cell density and the apparent diffusion coefficient (ADC) has been shown in abscess cavities [2]. The specificity of this finding, however, is diminished by the fact that metastases, composed of cells with high nuclear to cytoplasmic ratios or of cells that produce a large amount of proteinaceous material (mucin), can also show restricted water diffusion. A progressive increase in ADC

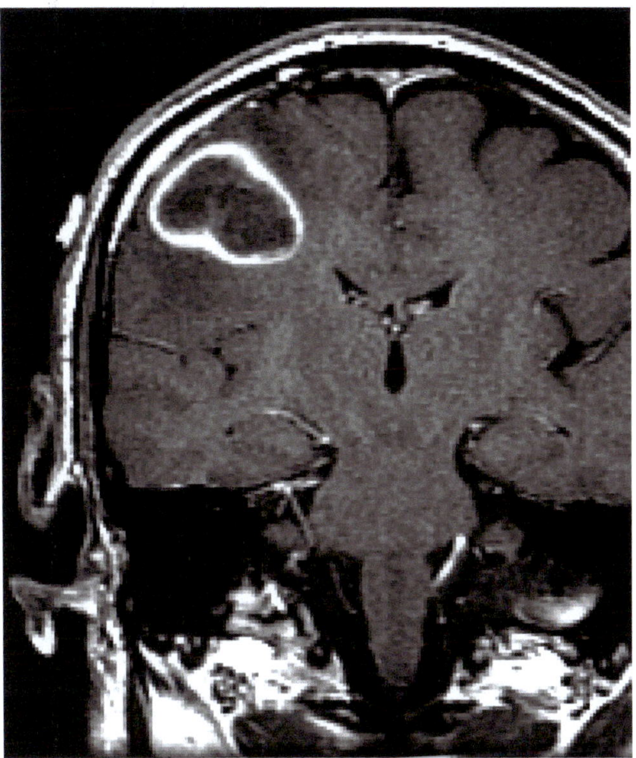

Fig. 1. Brain abscess showing smooth enhancing rim on this post-gadolinium T1 image. Note that the thinnest portion of the abscess wall "points" toward the ventricle

values in association with abscess shrinkage has been shown to reflect a positive response to antibiotic treatment. Return of restricted diffusion, however, has been correlated with the re-accumulation of pus [3].

Perhaps the most important contribution that MRS has made in the diagnosis of cerebral infections is the ability to detect bacteria based on their metabolic signatures. Certain by-products of bacterial metabolism are not seen in mammals in spectroscopically significant concentrations (millimolar range). Proton MRS is capable of detecting the distinct spectral peaks of some of these substances, such as succinate and acetate. However, pre-treatment with antibiotics prior to MRS may reduce these metabolites to undetectable levels. Amino acids, produced by proteases released by white cells as part of the inflammatory response, can also be detected. This is relevant since amino acids are not seen in large amounts in normal brain or other disease processes and may be present even if antibiotics have been administered. Table 1 lists these peaks and their resonant frequencies in parts per million (ppm).

While the expected utility of MRS in untreated patients is high, in modern practice, many patients are under-treated with antibiotics and the expected spectral peaks are often absent. If these peaks are visible, MRS offers the opportunity to monitor therapeutic efficacy. Declines in acetate and pyruvate one week after antibiotic treatment have been reported in patients with bacterial abscesses. This finding has been shown to correlate with positive clinical responses to treatment [4].

Table 1. Proton MRS metabolites in bacterial and fungal infections

Metabolite	Resonant frequency (ppm)
Broad amino-acid peak (valine, leucine, and isoleucine: all intracytosolic)[a]	0.9
Alanine[b]	1.4 and 1.6 doublet
Succinate	2.4
Acetate	1.9
Pyruvate	2.4
Trehalose	3.6-3.8

[a] Shows phase reversal (inverted peak) at TE = 135.
[b] Shows phase reversal at TE = 135; peak at 1.4 overlaps with peak of lactate doublet; can be seen in meningiomas and demyelination

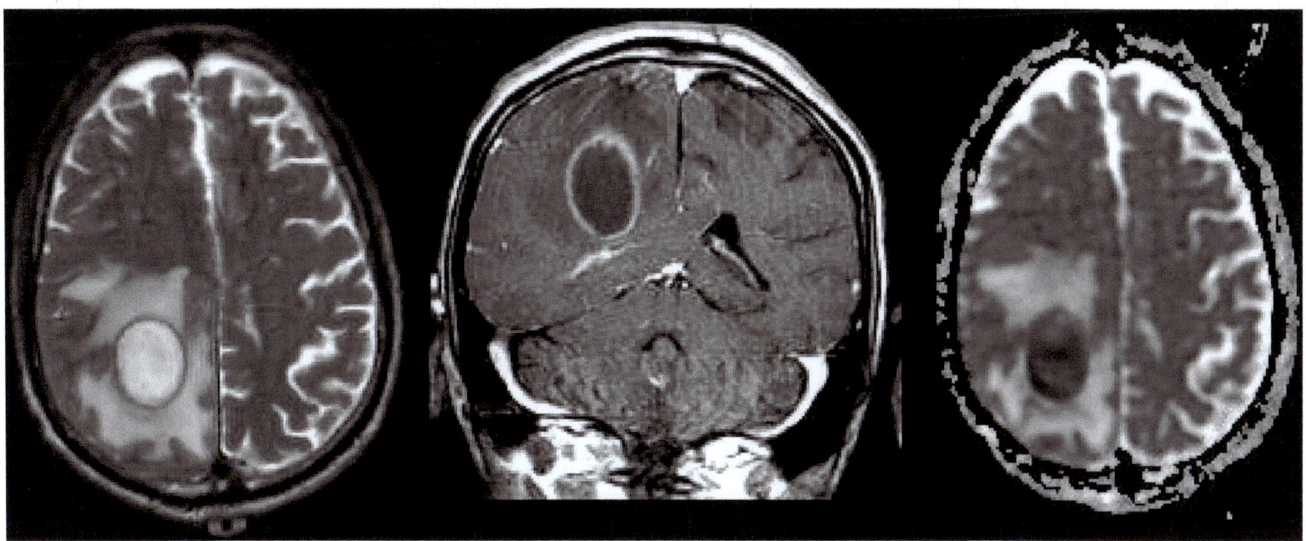

Fig. 2. Brain abscess. *From right to left*: T2, post-gadolinium T1, and apparent diffusion coefficient (ADC) map. Note the decreased signal in the abscess on ADC, indicating restricted diffusion

Tuberculoma/Tuberculous Abscess

Tuberculoma by definition is a parenchymal infection in which granulomas are found, whereas a tuberculous (TB) abscess contains pus but is devoid of granulomas and caseation. In either case, there may be ring enhancement. Tuberculomas usually have decreased T2 signal, whereas the TB abscess is bright on T2 and has a hypointense wall. Both tuberculoma and TB abscess can be surrounded by T2 bright edema in the adjacent brain.

There is some evidence that diffusion-weighted imaging (DWI) and ADC are normal in tuberculomas whereas restriction of water movement is seen in TB abscesses [5]. MRS has shown that there are differences between bacterial and mycobacterial brain abscesses. Although both can show elevations in lipid and lactate, mycobacterial infections show a conspicuous absence of the other bacterial metabolites indicated in Table 1 [6]. Tuberculomas may also show an elevated lipid peak related to caseation.

Fungal abscesses typically occur in immune-compromised patients but can present spontaneously in patients with no known immune deficiencies. These abscesses fail to display the typical characteristics of a bacterial abscess. Wall irregularity with multiple non-enhancing regions, i.e., features that mimic neoplastic disease, is dominant. In a series of 91 bacterial, 11 tuberculous, and eight fungal abscesses, only fungal abscesses (8/8) showed intracavitary projections arising from the wall [7]. Furthermore, the wall of the bacterial and tuberculous abscesses cavities showed restricted water diffusion, but the cavity of the fungal abscess showed increased water diffusion [7]. However, restricted, increased, and mixed patterns of water diffusion have also been reported [8]. From a MRS perspective, three important observations can be made: (1) only the bacterial abscesses demonstrated acetate or succinate, (2) the only metabolites in the TB abscesses were lipid and/or lactate, and (3) only the fungal abscesses showed peaks in the range of 3.6-3.8, considered to represent the disaccharide trehalose.

Meningitis

The diagnosis of bacterial meningitis is almost always based on clinical presentation. Patients will typically have high fever, signs of meningismus, and a rapidly decreasing level of consciousness. Imaging is usually performed to assess the status of the ventricles prior to lumbar puncture, since hydrocephalus is a relative contraindication to this procedure. CT can show evidence of increased attenuation in the basal cisterns and sulci due to high concentrations of inflammatory cells. This must not be confused with subarachnoid hemorrhage, as both can show increased attenuation in the basal cisterns [9]. Vessels in the subarachnoid space can become directly involved in the inflammatory process, with necrotizing panarteritis and septic thrombophlebitis causing ischemic injury to the brain. In addition, the inflammatory process can extend directly into the brain resulting in cerebritis. Hydrocephalus occurs in most patients resulting in increased intra-cranial pressure that further compromises blood flow. These secondary manifestations of the meningeal infection can be detected with diffusion imaging demonstrating the extent of acute cortical ischemic injury. However, direct brain infection causing cerebritis can have a similar appearance with evidence of restricted water movement [10]. We rarely perform MRI in the assessment of *acute* meningitis since all patients initially receive broad-spectrum antibiotics and imaging would not alter subsequent management.

Imaging does play a role in the detection and management of less fulminant forms of meningitis. TB meningitis, for example, can initially be quite indolent, with patients presenting with headache and cranial neuropathies. Untreated, the disease can progress rather suddenly with high mortality. Cerebrospinal fluid (CSF) analysis may show no growth of the bacillus, but there is usually an elevation in the white cell count and protein level. Pre-contrast MRI in these less fulminant forms can be normal, although -attenuated inversion recovery (FLAIR) images may show increased signal in the sulci when CSF protein is sufficiently elevated [11]. Gadolinium-enhanced acquisitions can show striking enhancement of the leptomeninges. Tuberculous pachymeningeal involvement also occurs [12].

Patients with immune deficiencies are also susceptible to TB meningitis, but fungal, viral, and treponemal forms of the disease must also be considered, including cryptococcal, varicella-zoster virus, cytomegalovirus, and neurosyphilis. Although these other agents and diseases can be associated with leptomeningeal enhancement [13, 14], they usually do not exhibit the intense diffuse and/or nodular pattern of enhancement in the basal cisterns that is seen with TB (Fig. 3).

Meningeal enhancement is uncommon in viral meningitis, with MRI appearing normal unless an encephalitic component develops, in which case there are signal changes in the parenchyma.

Encephalitis

Encephalitis can be divided into two groups (Table 2). In the first group, the virus is transmitted to humans via an insect vector (ticks and mosquitoes). Viruses in the second group infect the brain primarily. Brain inflammation can also occur as a complication of viral infections with measles, mumps, chicken pox, etc., or in autoimmune disorders such as multiple sclerosis or Rasmussen's encephalitis, but they will not be considered here. Although Creutzfeldt-Jacob disease (CJD) is due to a prion, which is not an infectious agent in the true sense, the behavior of this altered protein mimics an infection and is therefore included here.

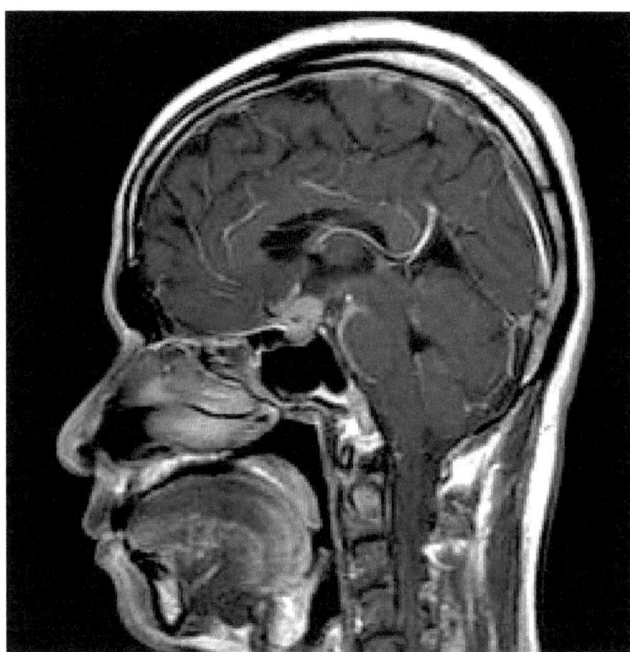

Fig. 3. Post-gadolinium T1 image showing nodular enhancement in the suprasellar cistern and diffuse leptomeningeal enhancement on the surface of the pons in a patient with tuberculous meningitis

Table 2. Group classification of brain viral infections

Group 1: arbovirus encephalitis	Group 2: primary infective
St. Louis	Herpes simplex
Japanese B	Cytomegalovirus
Equine	Epstein-Barr virus
Russian spring-summer	JC virus (progressive multifocal leukoencephalopathy)
Louping-ill	Rabies
Powassan	HIV (LAV/HTLV-III or AIDS virus)
Colorado tick fever	Subacute sclerosing panencephalitis[a]
California	Japanese encephalitis
West Nile	Nipah and Hendra virus (infects humans and animals; fruit bat source)

HIV, Human immunodeficiency virus; *LAV*, lymphadenopathy associated virus; *HTLV-III*, human T cell lymphotropic virus type III; *AIDS*, acquired immunodeficiency syndrome
[a]Reactivation of latent measles virus

In view of the number of viruses that can infect the brain, time and space limitations impose limits on the discussion presented herein. Emphasis will therefore be placed on adult herpes encephalitis, the most commonly encountered acute viral brain infection. However, West Nile encephalitis will also be discussed since it is a good example of the rapid spread of a nonendemic infection. Viral infections that occur in the setting of immunodeficient individuals will be discussed in a separate section.

Herpes Simplex Virus

Herpes simplex encephalitis is the most common sporadic viral infection in the western world [15]. The virus resides in the trigeminal ganglion and is usually benign except when it produces lesions in the oral mucosa. Rarely does the virus re-activate to produce encephalitis. In general terms, the disease should be considered in any patient presenting with acute changes in mental status and parenchymal signal abnormalities in the temporal lobe. Clinical outcome depends on early recognition and institution of antiviral treatment (acyclovir). CT images in the early stages of the infection are normal whereas MRI is capable of showing decreased T1- and increased T2-weighted intensity, involving the mesial temporal lobes and insular cortex (Fig. 4).

As the disease progresses, gadolinium enhancement can be seen, and the lesions may become hemorrhagic. Unilateral presentation is common. We have even observed re-development of the infection in the contralateral temporal lobe several months after successful treatment of an initial infection. DWI has shown evidence of both increased and decreased water mobility. Those areas of the parenchyma with restricted water movement, presumably representing cytotoxic edema, are often associated with lesions that have minimal T2 signal changes, while in those areas that show increased water movement, indicating vasogenic edema, there may be prominent increases in the T2 signal [16]. There is evidence that cytotoxic edema is present early in viral encephalitis, perhaps as a result of pre-morbid changes in the cell (swelling) as the virus takes over the cellular machinery [17-19]. Vasogenic edema appears later, as the cells rupture.

Alternatively, the infectious load may be the controlling factor. This concept is supported by findings observed in vitro with cells infected by West Nile virus (WNV) [20]. Cells exposed to a high infectious load become swollen and rupture due to extensive viral budding and loss of membrane integrity. High mobility group 1 (HMGB1) protein, a pro-inflammatory cytokine, is then released into the extracellular space. This protein is a pro-inflammatory cytokine that leads to inflammation and vasogenic edema in vivo. If the infectious load is low, delayed cell death occurs due to apoptosis. This model supports a similar temporal pattern of cytotoxic edema followed by vasogenic edema.

West Nile Virus

Prior to 1999, WNV was confined to Africa, the Middle East, and Asia. The first North American cases occurred in New York in 1999. The first Canadian case was reported in Ontario in 2001. The first European cases were reported in 1958 (two fatalities in Albania), Since that time, there have been few cases except for small outbreaks between 1996 and 2000 in Romania, Morocco, Tunisia, Italy, Russia, Israel, and France. A few cases are reported on a yearly basis in Romania [21, 22]. A larger

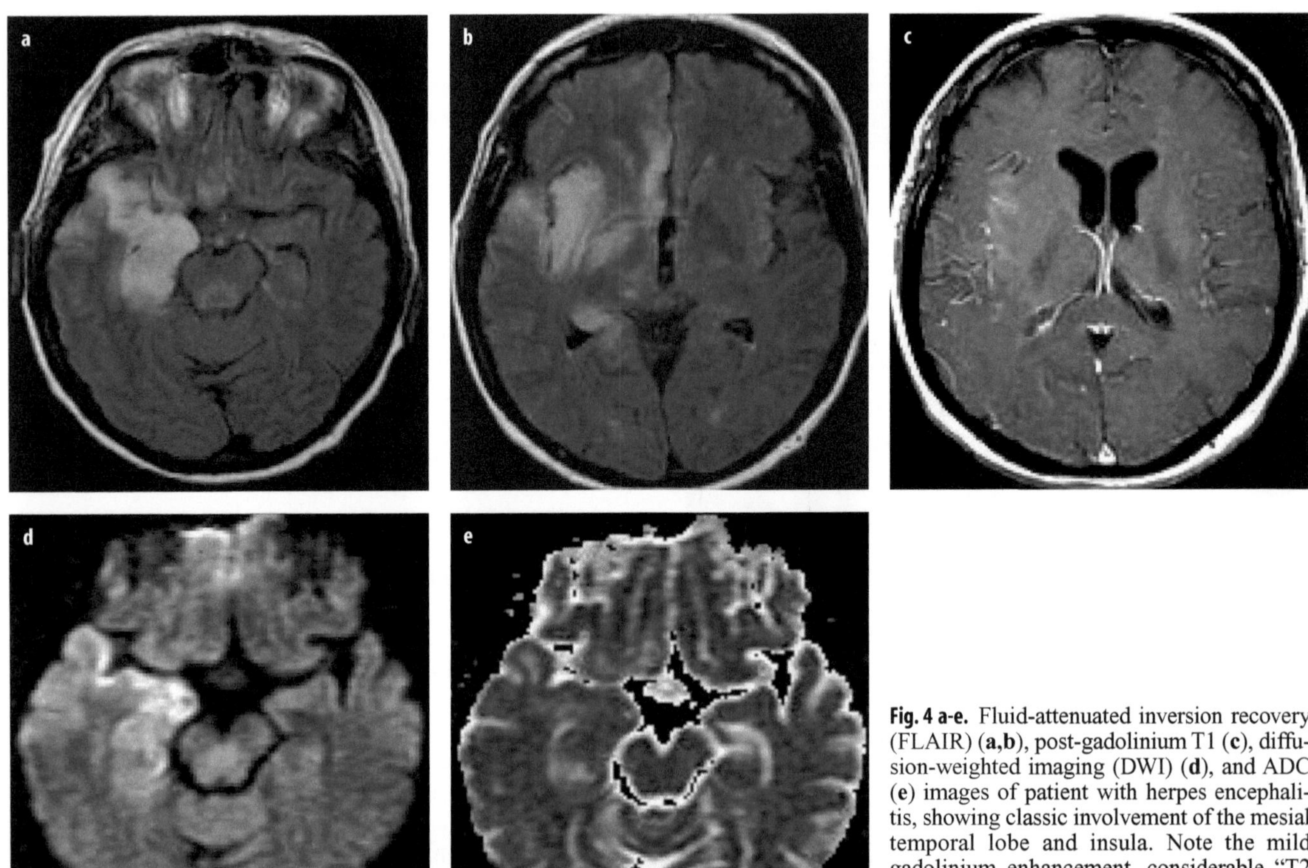

Fig. 4 a-e. Fluid-attenuated inversion recovery (FLAIR) (**a,b**), post-gadolinium T1 (**c**), diffusion-weighted imaging (DWI) (**d**), and ADC (**e**) images of patient with herpes encephalitis, showing classic involvement of the mesial temporal lobe and insula. Note the mild gadolinium enhancement, considerable "T2 shine-through" on DWI, and mixed pattern of water diffusion (increased in white matter and slightly decreased in cortex) on ADC

European outbreak is a significant concern. Fortunately, most WNV infections are mild, with no clinical symptoms. Approximately 20% of patients have a mild illness lasting 3-6 days and consisting of malaise, headache, anorexia, myalgia, nausea, vomiting, and/or rash. One in 150 patients develops severe neurological disease, consisting of meningitis and/or encephalitis. The pattern of central nervous system (CNS) involvement is very different from that seen with herpesvirus infections. WNV tends to involve the brainstem, cerebellum, and thalami. CT images are frequently normal but MRI shows an increased T2 signal with evidence of swelling within these structures. In contrast to herpesvirus infection, the neocortex is not usually involved.

Gadolinium enhancement is usually not present except in the setting of meningitis, in which case there is leptomeningeal enhancement. The spinal cord and cauda equina can also be affected. Some patients present with a myeloradiculopathy similar to that seen with Guillian-Barre syndrome. Enhancement of the pia along the spinal cord and cauda equina has been observed. Parenchymal signal changes can occur within the spinal cord. Pathologic changes in the spinal cord resemble those seen in poliomyelitis [23, 24]. We previously reported a case in which diffusion imaging during the early phase of the WNV infection showed marked restriction of water movement in the pons at a time when conventional sequences were normal. Later in the disease, water diffusion became markedly increased in the pons, supporting the concept that early viral infections are associated with restricted water diffusion in the infected tissue [17].

Little information is available concerning MRS and encephalitis. Acquiring diagnostic spectra from the temporal lobe, brainstem, cerebellum, and thalamus is challenging due to shimming problems that arise from tissues near the skull base. This is made even more difficult in uncooperative patients. The spectral similarities of encephalitis and brain tumors, in which there are elevations in choline and reductions in N-acetyl aspartic acid (NAA), have been reported [25]. However, there are no specific spectroscopic features diagnostic of encephalitis.

Prion Diseases

Scrapie, bovine spongiform encephalopathy, kuru, and CJD are examples of prion (from "proteinaceous" and "infectious") diseases causing spongiform encephalopathy.

Scrapie occurs in sheep and goats. Kuru is found in New Guinea tribes that practice cannibalism. Bovine spongiform encephalopathy has been linked with variant CJD, which occurs in people. In addition to this variant form, which is probably of greatest concern since it is propagated through food (eating contaminated beef), sporadic and familial forms also exist. These diseases have a common theme in that the responsible agent is thought to be a misfolded protein (the prion) that induces further misfolding of normal proteins into protease-resistant aggregates. These accumulate and cause progressive cerebral degeneration over a period of 3-6 months leading to death.

The most important neuropathologic feature from the neuroimaging standpoint is cytoplasmic vacuolization, which is most likely responsible for the decreases in water diffusion observed on MR diffusion imaging. Ultrastructurally, the cytoplasmic vacuoles contain a proliferation of membranes in a "labyrinth-like manner", explaining the restriction in water movement [26]. There is also extensive gliosis in areas of neuronal loss, perhaps explaining the elevations in T2 relaxation [27]. However, there is conflicting evidence showing that the T2 and ADC signal abnormalities correlate with sites of abnormal prion protein deposition, not the presence of vacuoles or gliosis [28]. These T2 and ADC abnormalities evolve as the disease progresses. It has been suggested that, in the initial phase of the disease, signal behavior is influenced by vacuoles in intact neurons, with diffusion imaging more sensitive than T2 or FLAIR images. Later in the disease, as neurons disappear and are replaced by tissue, ADC may normalize and the T2 abnormalities gain prominence [29]. Figure 5 demonstrates the multifocal cortical involvement typical of this disease.

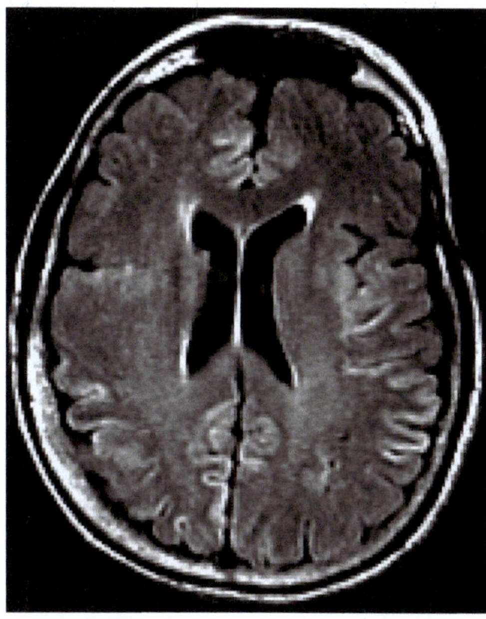

Fig. 5. FLAIR image in a patient with sporadic Creutzfeldt-Jacob disease. Multiple cortical "ribbons" with increased T2 signal are a characteristic feature

Table 3. MRI findings in human prion disease

T2 and FLAIR	Pattern 1: increased in striatum Pattern 2: increased in cortex (patchy)[a]
ADC	Decreased (may change with disease progression)
Post-gadolinium T1	No enhancement
MRS	Decreased NAA
Brain morphology	Atrophy develops as disease progresses
Pulvinar sign	Characteristic of variant CJD

FLAIR, Fluid-attenuated inversion recovery; *ADC*, apparent diffusion coefficient; *MRS*, proton magnetic resonance spectroscopy; *NAA*, N-acetyl aspartic acid; *CJD*, Creutzfeldt-Jacob disease
[a]Pattern 1 may evolve into or be coexistent with pattern 2

The pulvinar sign is thought to be a distinguishing feature of variant CJD, occurring in over 80% of cases [30]. However, pulvinar abnormalities have been reported in variant CJD [30, 31]. Table 3 summarizes the imaging findings observed in sporadic disease. There are few MRS studies in patients with prion disease. It appears that MRS can detect neuronal loss, showing areas of reduced NAA [32]. A general reduction in all metabolites has also been reported [33]. There are no specific metabolites unique to prion-mediated diseases.

Parasites

Parasitic infections of the brain typically affect individuals living in the undeveloped world and include cysticercosis, malaria, neuroschistosomiasis, paragonimiasis, angiostrongyliasis, hydatid disease, sparganosis, trypanosomiasis, and gnathostomiasis. Toxoplasmosis is also considered to be a parasitic disease but it is infective in immunocompromised hosts and is therefore discussed in the subsequent section. Since most parasitic infections of the CNS are rarely seen clinically, they will not be discussed. Cysticercosis however, is seen frequently enough to merit attention. The larval stage of the pork tapeworm (*Taenia solium*) can infect the human nervous system and cause neurocysticercosis. The larvae have a variable appearance on imaging depending on whether they: (1) are not under attack by host immune defenses (vesicular phase), (2) are under immune attack (colloidal/nodular phase), or (3) are dead (involutional phase). It must be kept in mind that the larvae can either infect the parenchyma directly or seed the CSF spaces, including the ventricles, sulci, and cisterns. The larvae typically form cysts with a central scolex. The cysts are thin walled with a small central solid component representing the scolex. We have even observed enhancement of the scolex following gadolinium administration. This finding is difficult to explain since it infers that some connection with the host blood supply must exist for the contrast agent to find its way to the parasite in the cyst (Fig. 6).

The cysts can be multi-loculated especially in the subarachnoid space, resulting in a "racemose" appearance. If

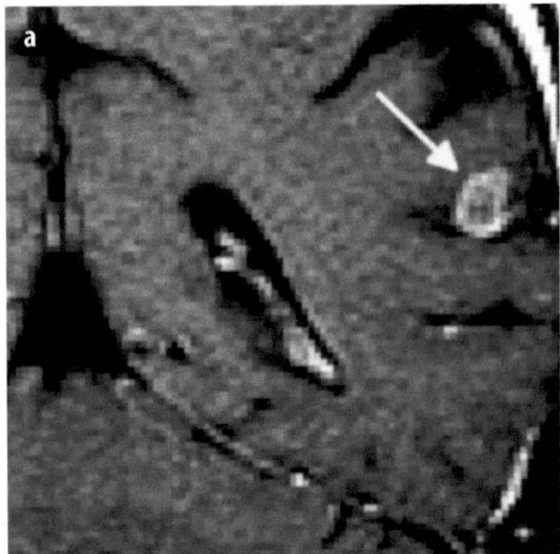

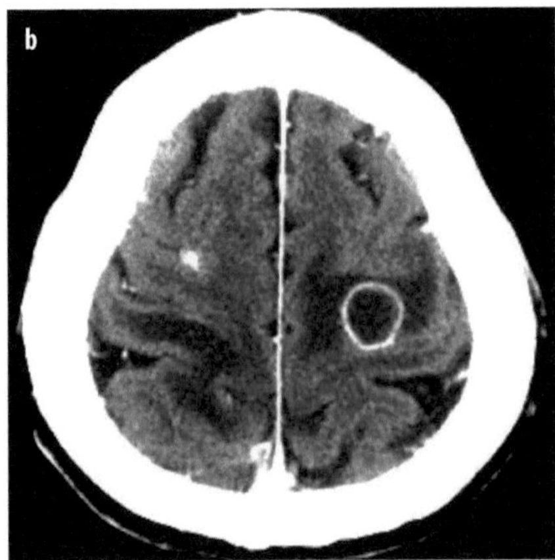

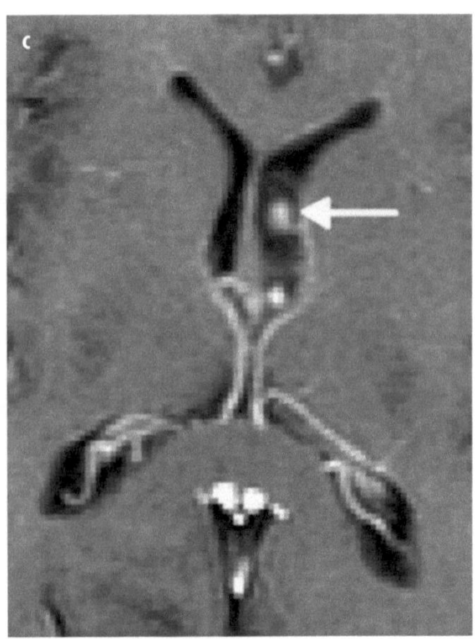

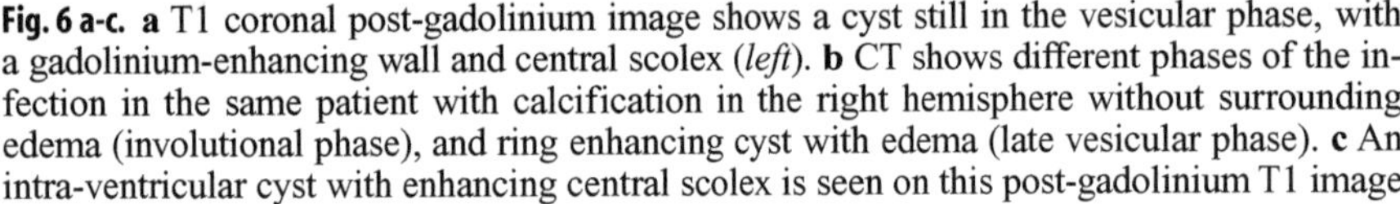

Fig. 6 a-c. **a** T1 coronal post-gadolinium image shows a cyst still in the vesicular phase, with a gadolinium-enhancing wall and central scolex (*left*). **b** CT shows different phases of the infection in the same patient with calcification in the right hemisphere without surrounding edema (involutional phase), and ring enhancing cyst with edema (late vesicular phase). **c** An intra-ventricular cyst with enhancing central scolex is seen on this post-gadolinium T1 image

the cysts are present in strategic locations of the ventricular system, obstructive hydrocephalus may ensue. Some ventricular cysts can even move into dependent locations based on the position of the head. When the cysts are viable, the intracystic fluid matches CSF on CT and on all MR pulse sequences, although some cysts may have a slightly different signal especially on FLAIR sequences. No adjacent edema is seen. The cysts have an average diameter of 0.5-1 cm but they can be much larger. When a host immune reaction is present (typically associated with seizures), the cyst wall thickens and enhances. There is edema in the adjacent parenchyma. In the final stages of the immune response, the cysts begin to disappear while nodular areas of enhancement remain. These areas eventually become densely calcified. The cysticerci in this intermediate phase can be difficult to distinguish from other nodular enhancing lesions. They may also be hypointense on T2-weighted images. A soft-tissue X-ray survey of the patient's muscles may reveal calcified cysticercal lesions, indicating the correct diagnosis.

Occasionally, even calcified lesions may show some adjacent edema and contrast enhancement, probably reflecting the continued host reaction to residual larval antigens. DWI does not play a significant role in establishing the presence of cysticerci, since the diagnosis is predominantly based on morphological characteristics alone. However, restricted diffusion has been reported within the scolex during the vesicular phase of the disease [34, 35]. MRS may play a significant role, especially in the nodular form of the disease, when the etiology is uncertain. Elevations in alanine, succinate, acetate, and amino acids, similar to the metabolites seen in bacterial infections, may be present. Significant pyruvate elevations have been also reported in cysticercus cysts and in hydatid cysts [36, 37]. Nodular cysticercus lesions can be hypointense on T2-weighted images and can appear virtually identical to tuberculomas. Since the latter show none of these metabolites, MRS should be helpful in distinguishing between them. However, additional MRS experience, especially with the nodular form of cysticercisis, is required to determine whether this observation can be reliably applied.

Infections in the Immunocompromised Patient

Infectious agents are opportunists and will take advantage of weaknesses in the host's immune system under a variety of conditions. How, and in what setting, these defects in the immune system appear will influence the type of organism that invades and the host response to it. Manipulation of the immune response in the setting of transplantation and the emergence of AIDS are examples of immune compromise that allow unusual infections to develop. Not only are immunocompromised patients prone to infections that are seen in normal hosts, but they also become infected quite commonly by agents that are easily controlled by the normal immune system. This section will focus on two of the most common agents that infect the immunocompromised patient: toxoplasma and JC virus. In addition, cryptococcal infection, encephalitis, and neurosyphilis will be briefly addressed.

Toxoplasma Infection

These infections tend to present as enlarging irregular mass lesions with perilesional edema, variable signal characteristics, and variable contrast enhancement. They can be difficult to distinguish from lymphoma, a significant diagnostic consideration in immune-compromised individuals. ADC values have been shown to be higher in toxoplasmosis than in lymphomas but there is considerable overlap [38, 39]. Toxoplasma have a predilection for the basal ganglia and any mass involving this structure in an immunocompromised individual should be considered to represent toxoplasmosis until proven otherwise especially since the infection is easily treatable (Fig. 7).

Multiple lesions are usually present and involvement of the frontal and parietal lobes is common. As opposed to other infectious agents, no specific or unique metabolite peaks are present in toxoplasmic lesions. In fact, MRS cannot reliably distinguish lymphoma from toxoplasmosis. If the host is deficient in inflammatory cells, as in bone marrow transplant recipients, fulminant infections, including toxoplasmosis, can occur and may show very little if any gadolinium enhancement [40]. In general, hemorrhage within a cerebral abscess is rare; however, there are reports of toxoplasmosis abscesses containing blood products and/or associated with parenchymal hemorrhages [41].

Progressive Multifocal Leukoencephalopathy

Infection with JC virus of oligodendrocytes in the immunocompromised host gives rise to PML. The disease typically involves only white matter structures and has the appearance of demyelinating lesions. There is very little or no contrast enhancement (Fig. 8).

Like multiple sclerosis, PML has a predilection for the middle cerebellar peduncles. Both increased and decreased water diffusion has been seen in these lesions. It has been suggested that ADC is reduced in early infections, indicating swelling of infected cells, but later increases as cells are lost and gliosis develops [42]. A decrease in the ADC is also observed at the advancing edge of the lesions [43]. Tissue injury tends to be more severe in patients with AIDS than in other immunocompromised hosts, most like-

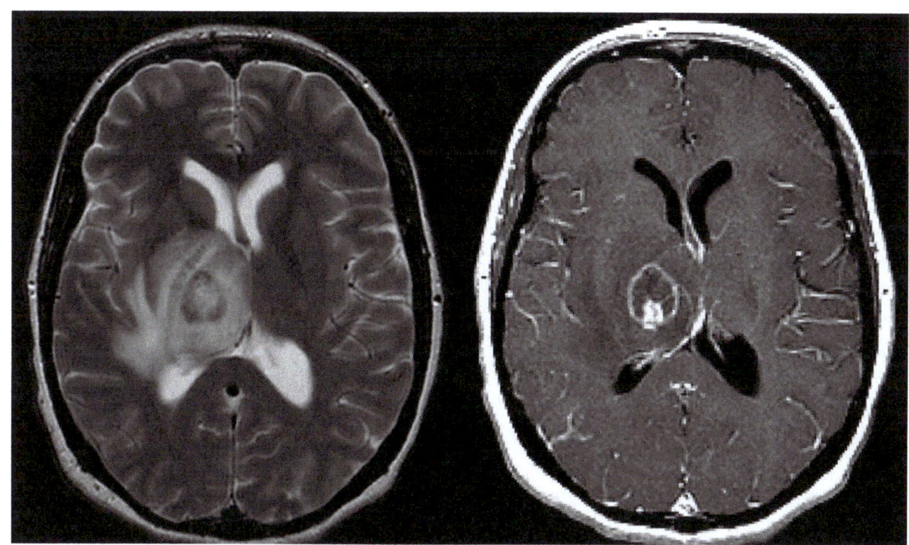

Fig. 7. T2 and T1 post-gadolinium images of a toxoplasmic abscess involving the basal ganglia

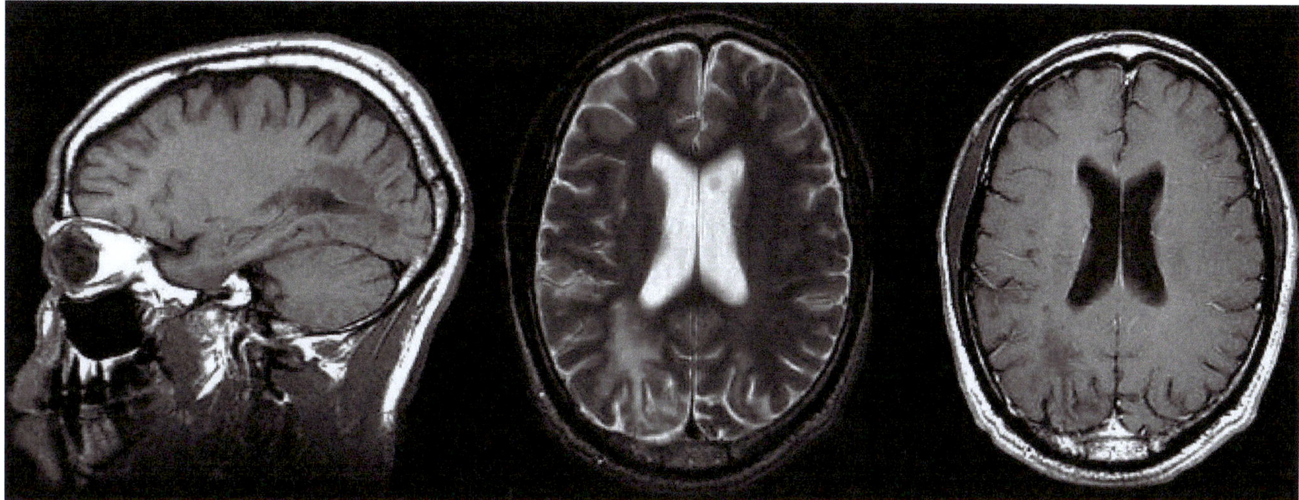

Fig. 8. Progressive multifocal leukoencephalopathy. *From left to right*: sagittal T1, axial T2, and post-gadolinium axial T1 images. Note the absence of a mass effect and the lack of gadolinium enhancement

ly because of co-existent injury from the human immunodeficiency virus (HIV). MRS shows a decrease in NAA that is usually greater than that seen with HIV encephalopathy alone. Elevated choline, lipid, and lactate with reduced NAA have been reported [44, 45]. No spectral peaks unique to this infection have been identified.

Cryptococcal Infection

Cryptococcal infections manifest as meningitis or mass lesions (cryptococcomas) in the CSF spaces or brain parenchyma. The typical infection is that of meningitis with spread into the Virchow-Robin spaces at the base of the brain into the basal ganglia. The enlarged spaces show increased T1 and T2 relaxation without contrast enhancement. However, enhancement in the meninges and in cryptococcomas can occur. Secretion of an external polysaccharide capsule by these yeast-like organisms gives rise to large gelatinous pseudocysts that can form in the ventricular system or subarachnoid space. Surprisingly, there is limited information concerning DWI and MRS in patients with these lesions. Increased water diffusion was described in one case report [46]. MRS findings include elevated lipids and low myo-inositol (a marker of gliosis) and NAA levels [47]. No distinctive resonances are present.

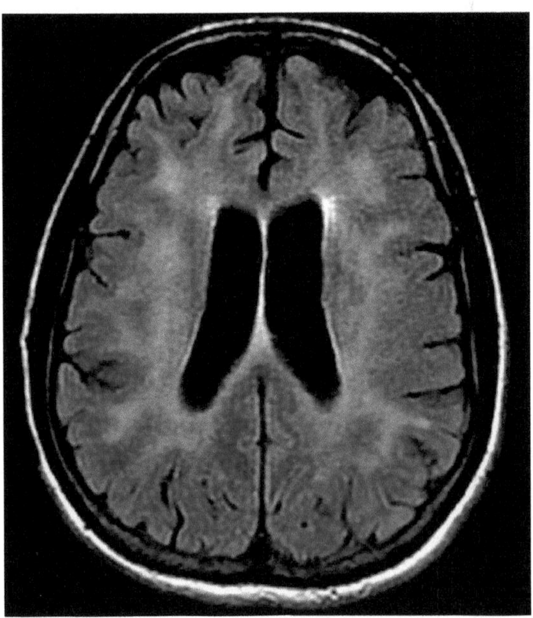

Fig. 9. HIV encephalitis. Axial FLAIR image shows patchy increased T2 signal in the white matter, accompanied by generalized cerebral atrophy

HIV Encephalitis

Infected macrophages that cross the blood-brain barrier to enter the CNS are the source of HIV in the brain. Direct neuronal infection, as seen in other viral encephalitides, is thought not to occur, although this has not been entirely ruled out. Since there is initial preservation of neurons, CNS symptoms consisting of dementia are delayed. It has been proposed that the pathogenesis of dementia proceeds along non-inflammatory and inflammatory pathways. In the non-inflammatory pathway, infection of the microglia inhibits the supportive function of these cells. Reduced levels of growth factors and impaired clearance of excitotoxic neurotransmitters lead to neuronal loss. The production of pro-inflammatory cytokines and the ensuing inflammatory process cause neuronal injury, directly leading to gliosis and brain atrophy [48]. MRI findings include white matter lesions and generalized cerebral atrophy (Fig. 9).

MRS shows a reduction in NAA, elevations in choline, and increased myo-inositol [49]. DWI is generally noncontributory. Diffusion tensor analysis has shown decreases in fractional anisotropy of the splenium of the corpus callosum in HIV-positive patients [50].

Neurosyphilis

Neurosyphilis is typically a meningovascular disease that produces meningeal inflammation as well as ischemic brain injury from vasculitis and vascular occlusion. The meninges may show enhancement following contrast administration. Occasionally, meningeal granulomas or "gummas" form. They are rare in the parenchyma but, when present, appear as enhancing nodules with increased T2 signal intensity surrounded by edema. Ischemic brain infarction can occur due to vascular compromise by the inflammatory process. In fact, significant vascular narrowing may be seen at angiography. There is a form of encephalitic involvement that is becoming increasingly recognized. On MRI, it mimics the appearance of herpes encephalitis, with increased T2 signal and mild swelling of the mesial temporal lobes [51]. This finding emphasizes the need to broaden the differential diagnosis of temporal lobe infections. The classical progression of neurosyphilis from meningeal to cerebrovascular to encephalitic phases over decades can be considerably foreshortened in immunocompromised patients. Diffusion imaging can help to establish evidence of acute ischemic injury to the brain parenchyma as a result of vascular compromise. The role of MRS is unclear, as there are no published studies of this disease.

Conclusions

Conventional MRI methods are the mainstay for evaluating patients with cerebral infections. The majority of these infections can be accurately assessed using a combination of clinical information and MRI patterns, supported by diffusion and MRS information. Those infections most commonly encountered in clinical practice have been highlighted here. Although not comprehensive, the information can be used as a framework for building a greater understanding of cerebral infections.

References

1. Haimes AB, Zimmerman RD, Morgello S et al (1989) MR imaging of brain abscesses. AJR Am J Roentgenol 152:1073-1085
2. Mishra AM, Gupta RK, Saksena S et al (2005) Biological correlates of diffusivity in brain abscess. Magn Reson Med 54:878-885
3. Duprez TP, Cosnard G, Hernalsteen D (2005) Diffusion-weighted monitoring of conservatively treated pyogenic brain abscesses: a marker for antibacterial treatment efficacy. AJNR Am J Neuroradiol 26:1296-1298 author reply 1300-1291
4. Dev R, Gupta RK, Poptani H et al (1998) Role of in vivo proton magnetic resonance spectroscopy in the diagnosis and management of brain abscesses. Neurosurgery 42:37-42
5. Basoglu OK, Savas R, Kitis O (2002) Conventional and diffusion-weighted MR imaging of intracranial tuberculomas. A case report. Acta Radiol 43:560-562
6. Gupta RK, Vatsal DK, Husain N et al (2001) Differentiation of tuberculous from pyogenic brain abscesses with in vivo proton MR spectroscopy and magnetization transfer MR imaging. AJNR Am J Neuroradiol 22:1503-1509
7. Luthra G, Parihar A, Nath K et al (2007) Comparative evaluation of fungal, tubercular, and pyogenic brain abscesses with conventional and diffusion MR imaging and proton MR spectroscopy. AJNR Am J Neuroradiol 28:1332-1338
8. Gaviani P, Schwartz RB, Hedley-Whyte ET et al (2005) Diffusion-weighted imaging of fungal cerebral infection. AJNR Am J Neuroradiol 26:1115-1121
9. Chatterjee T, Gowardman JR, Goh TD (2003) Pneumococcal meningitis masquerading as subarachnoid haemorrhage. Med J Aust 178:505-507
10. Tung GA, Rogg JM (2003) Diffusion-weighted imaging of cerebritis. AJNR Am J Neuroradiol 24:1110-1113
11. Kuwahara S, Kawada M, Uga S (2001) Cryptococcal meningoencephalitis presenting with an unusual magnetic resonance imaging appearance – case report. Neurol Med Chir (Tokyo) 41:517-521
12. Goyal M, Sharma A, Mishra NK, Gaikwad SB, Sharma MC (1997) Imaging appearance of pachymeningeal tuberculosis. AJR Am J Roentgenol 169:1421-1424
13. Erly WK, Bellon RJ, Seeger JF, Carmody RF (1999) MR imaging of acute coccidioidal meningitis. AJNR Am J Neuroradiol 20:509-514
14. Berkefeld J, Enzensberger W, Lanfermann H (1999) Cryptococcus meningoencephalitis in AIDS: parenchymal and meningeal forms. Neuroradiology 41:129-133
15. Lipkin WI (1997) European consensus on viral encephalitis. Lancet 349:299-300
16. Heiner L, Demaerel P (2003) Diffusion-weighted MR imaging findings in a patient with herpes simplex encephalitis. Eur J Radiol 45:195-198
17. Agid R, Ducreux D, Halliday WC et al (2003) MR diffusion-weighted imaging in a case of West Nile virus encephalitis. Neurology 61:1821-1823
18. Lim CC, Lee WL, Leo YS et al (2003) Late clinical and magnetic resonance imaging follow up of Nipah virus infection. J Neurol Neurosurg Psychiatry 74:131-133
19. Nolan MA, Craig ME, Lahra MM et al (2003) Survival after pulmonary edema due to enterovirus 71 encephalitis. Neurology 60:1651-1656
20. Chu JJ, Ng ML (2003) The mechanism of cell death during West Nile virus infection is dependent on initial infectious dose. J Gen Virol 84:3305-3314
21. Zeller HG, Schuffenecker I (2004) West Nile virus: an overview of its spread in Europe and the Mediterranean basin in contrast to its spread in the Americas. Eur J Clin Microbiol Infect Dis 23:147-156
22. Environmental Risk Analysis Program – Cornell University. Available at: http://environmentalrisk.cornell.edu/
23. Jeha LE, Sila CA, Lederman RJ et al (2003) West Nile virus infection: a new acute paralytic illness. Neurology 61:55-59
24. Kraushaar G, Patel R, Stoneham GW (2005) West Nile Virus: a case report with flaccid paralysis and cervical spinal cord: MR imaging findings. AJNR Am J Neuroradiol 26:26-29
25. Calli C, Ozel AA, Savas R et al (2002) Proton MR spectroscopy in the diagnosis and differentiation of encephalitis from other mimicking lesions. J Neuroradiol 29:23-28
26. Liberski PP, Gajdusek DC, Brown P (2002) How do neurons degenerate in prion diseases or transmissible spongiform encephalopathies (TSEs): neuronal autophagy revisited. Acta Neurobiol Exp (Wars) 62:141-147
27. Urbach H, Klisch J, Wolf HK et al (1998) MRI in sporadic Creutzfeldt-Jakob disease: correlation with clinical and neuropathological data. Neuroradiology 40:65-70
28. Haik S, Dormont D, Faucheux BA et al (2002) Prion protein deposits match magnetic resonance imaging signal abnormalities in Creutzfeldt-Jakob disease. Ann Neurol 51:797-799
29. Tschampa HJ, Murtz P, Flacke S et al (2003) Thalamic involvement in sporadic Creutzfeldt-Jakob disease: a diffusion-weighted MR imaging study. AJNR Am J Neuroradiol 24:908-915
30. Tschampa HJ, Zerr I, Urbach H (2007) Radiological assessment of Creutzfeldt-Jakob disease. Eur Radiol 17:1200-1211
31. Martindale J, Geschwind MD, De Armond S et al (2003) Sporadic Creutzfeldt-Jakob disease mimicking variant Creutzfeldt-Jakob disease. Arch Neurol 60:767-770
32. Pandya HG, Coley SC, Wilkinson ID, Griffiths PD (2003) Magnetic resonance spectroscopic abnormalities in sporadic and variant Creutzfeldt-Jakob disease. Clin Radiol 58:148-153
33. Lim CC, Tan K, Verma KK et al (2004) Combined diffusion-weighted and spectroscopic MR imaging in Creutzfeldt-Jakob disease. Magn Reson Imaging 22:625-629
34. Raffin LS, Bacheschi LA, Machado LR et al (2001) Diffusion-weighted MR imaging of cystic lesions of neurocysticercosis: a preliminary study. Arq Neuropsiquiatr 59:839-842
35. do Amaral LL, Ferreira RM, da Rocha AJ, Ferreira NP (2005) Neurocysticercosis: evaluation with advanced magnetic resonance techniques and atypical forms. Top Magn Reson Imaging 16:127-144
36. Chang KH, Song IC, Kim SH et al (1998) In vivo single-voxel proton MR spectroscopy in intracranial cystic masses. AJNR Am J Neuroradiol 19:401-405
37. Pandit S, Lin A, Gahbauer H et al (2001) MR spectroscopy in neurocysticercosis. J Comput Assist Tomogr 25:950-952
38. Camacho DL, Smith JK, Castillo M (2003) Differentiation of toxoplasmosis and lymphoma in AIDS patients by using apparent diffusion coefficients. AJNR Am J Neuroradiol 24:633-637
39. Schroeder PC, Post MJ, Oschatz E et al (2006) Analysis of the utility of diffusion-weighted MRI and apparent diffusion coefficient values in distinguishing central nervous system toxoplasmosis from lymphoma. Neuroradiology 48:715-720
40. Ionita C, Wasay M, Balos L, Bakshi R (2004) MR imaging in toxoplasmosis encephalitis after bone marrow transplantation: paucity of enhancement despite fulminant disease. AJNR Am J Neuroradiol 25:270-273
41. Chaudhari AB, Singh A, Jindal S, Poon TP (1989) Haemorrhage in cerebral toxoplasmosis. A report on a patient with the acquired immunodeficiency syndrome. S Afr Med J 76:272-274
42. Bergui M, Bradac GB, Oguz KK et al (2004) Progressive multifocal leukoencephalopathy: diffusion-weighted imaging and pathological correlations. Neuroradiology 46:22-25
43. da Pozzo S, Manara R, Tonello S, Carollo C (2006) Conventional and diffusion-weighted MRI in progressive multifocal leukoencephalopathy: new elements for identification and follow-up. Radiol Med (Torino) 111:971-977
44. Iranzo A, Moreno A, Pujol J et al (1999) Proton magnetic resonance spectroscopy pattern of progressive multifocal

leukoencephalopathy in AIDS. J Neurol Neurosurg Psychiatry 66:520-523

45. Hurley RA, Ernst T, Khalili K et al (2003) Identification of HIV-associated progressive multifocal leukoencephalopathy: magnetic resonance imaging and spectroscopy. J Neuropsychiatry Clin Neurosci 15:1-6
46. Ho TL, Lee HJ, Lee KW, Chen WL (2005) Diffusion-weighted and conventional magnetic resonance imaging in cerebral cryptococcoma. Acta Radiol 46:411-414
47. Kingsley PB, Shah TC, Woldenberg R (2006) Identification of diffuse and focal brain lesions by clinical magnetic resonance spectroscopy. NMR Biomed 19:435-462
48. Avison MJ, Nath A, Berger JR (2002) Understanding pathogenesis and treatment of HIV dementia: a role for magnetic resonance? Trends Neurosci 25:468-473
49. Yiannoutsos CT, Ernst T, Chang L et al (2004) Regional patterns of brain metabolites in AIDS dementia complex. Neuroimage 23:928-935
50. Wu Y, Storey P, Cohen BA et al (2006) Diffusion alterations in corpus callosum of patients with HIV. AJNR Am J Neuroradiol 27:656-660
51. Bash S, Hathout GM, Cohen S (2001) Mesiotemporal T2-weighted hyperintensity: neurosyphilis mimicking herpes encephalitis. AJNR Am J Neuroradiol 22:314-316

Mass Lesions of the Brain: A Differential Diagnostic Approach

Guido Wilms

Department of Radiology, University Hospitals K.U., Leuven, Belgium

Introduction

After careful examination of the computed tomography (CT) and magnetic resonance (MR) images of a patient with a cerebral mass lesion, the neuroradiologist aims at getting as close as possible to the final anatomopathological diagnosis. The final diagnostic proposition is the result of an intellectual process of stepwise examination of the radiological features, with quick exclusion of some impossible or improbable entities, comparison with images in his or her personal "database" accumulated through neuroradiological training, literature search, and experience. Together these allow a diagnosis or at least a ranking of possible tumors within the differential diagnostic list.

Pathognomonic Images

Some images, especially on MRI, are almost pathognomonic or are so typical in a certain clinical context that they can quickly be used to make or exclude a diagnosis [1, 2]: A colloid cyst of the third ventricle, a dermoid cyst and an epidermoid cyst, a lipoma, a hamartoma of the tuber cinereum in a patient with gelastic seizures, a dysplastic gangliocytoma of the cerebellum (Fig. 1), a cystic hemangioblastoma of the cerebellum with a strongly enhancing mural nodule in a patient with a known von Hippel Lindau disease, the giant cell astrocytoma in a patient with tuberous sclerosis presenting as an enhancing mass in the foramen of Monro in a patient with subependymal calcifications, many meningiomas with a broad implantation on the dura and with homogeneous enhancement and a dural tail, vestibular schwannomas extending within a funnel shaped widened internal auditory canal, etc. Nonetheless, one has to bear in mind that for all these lesions atypical forms exists too. Other less-typical tumors require more careful examination of the radiological features.

Distinction Between an Intra-axial and an Extra-axial Lesion

When dealing with a cerebral mass, the first step in the diagnosis and differential diagnosis is the distinction between an intra-axial and an extra-axial lesion, since extra-axial tumors tend to have pathological and prognostic characteristics different from those of intra-axial lesions [1]. Extra-axial lesions (Fig. 2) cause white matter buckling, expand the ipsilateral subarachnoid space, and can be surrounded by a CSF cleft or halo. Intra-axial lesions expand the cortex of the brain, do not widen subarachnoid spaces, and have a specific way of spreading into the brain.

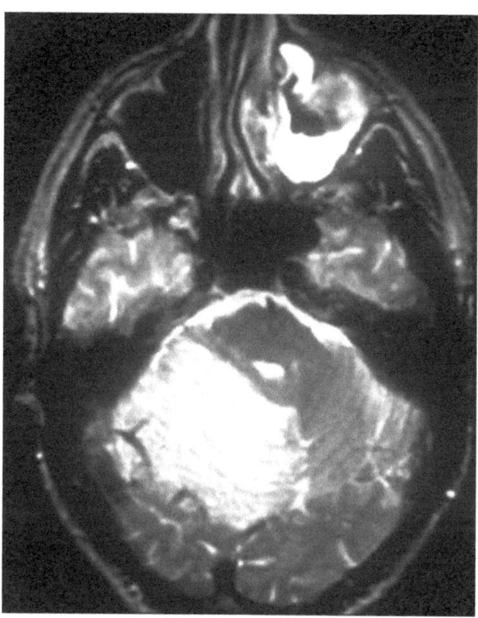

Fig. 1. Dysplastic gangliocytoma of the cerebellum. Transverse T2-weighted magnetic resonance (MR) image. The folia of the right cerebellar hemisphere are thickened and appear hyperintense. The brainstem is displaced and compressed

The Relative Incidence of Brain Tumors

The neuroradiologist must take into consideration the relative incidence of brain tumors [1]. In the extra-axial compartment, meningiomas and schwannomas account for more then 80% of the lesions. If metastases account

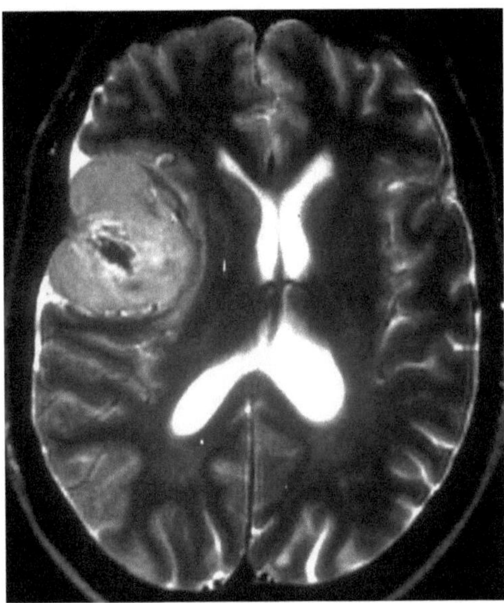

Fig. 2. Extra-axial tumor: convexity meningioma. Transverse T2-weighted MR image. The lesion has a broad implantation on the dura, causes widening of the ipsilateral cisterns, and white matter buckling

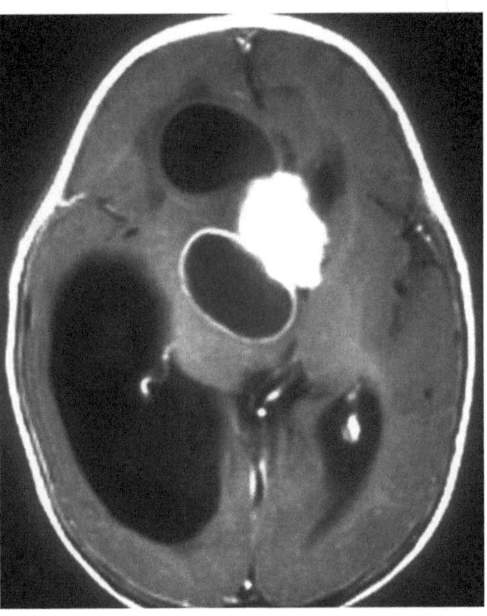

Fig. 3. Choroid plexus papilloma in a 1-year-old child. Transverse gadolinium-enhanced T1-weighted image. Mass with a solid and a ring-like enhancing component in the right lateral ventricle

for about 50% of all intra-axial lesions and half of them are solitary, the chance is 1 in 4 that a solitary enhancing brain mass is a metastasis. If gliomas account for 50% of all intrinsic brain tumors and 75% of them are malignant then 1 out of 5 lesions would be a malignant glioma. Therefore concluding that a lesion is a "malignant glioma or a metastasis" might be as good as guessing, without even looking at the images.

The Role of Patient Age

The incidence of a particular tumor has, of course, also much to do with the age of the patient [1]. As for other pathologies, children are not small adults. Specific tumours occur in children [3-5] under age 2, for example, choroid plexus papilloma (Fig. 3), anaplastic astrocytoma, and teratoma. In the first decade of childhood, medulloblastoma, ependymoma of the fourth ventricle, brainstem glioma, craniopharyngeoma, and hypothalamic glioma are found. Glioblastoma, meningioma, oligodendroglioma, pituitary adenoma, schwannoma, and metastases are almost exclusively seen in adults.

The CT or MR Characteristics of the Lesion

Once all these factors have been accounted for, the CT or MR characteristics, namely the CT density or the intensity of the lesion on MR have to be studied [2]. Most tumors are hypodense on CT and can be surrounded by hypodense edema. Meningiomas, however, are usually isodense or slightly hyperdense. Hypercellular tumors, such as lymphomas (Fig. 4a) or medulloblastomas can be hyperdense. Calcification is streaky or patchy in oligodendroglioma (Fig. 5a), can be punctate to dense in meningioma, or more sparse in ependymoma. Cystic components are seen in pilocytic astrocytoma, hemangioblastoma, ganglioglioma, but also in or near to meningioma and schwannoma.

The signal intensities of normal structures and of pathological findings on conventional T1- and T2-weighted MR images depend on many factors and therefore have to be carefully studied [6]. The amount of water, the proton density, the chemical structure and or/binding, the presence or absence of blood flow or CSF, calcification, fat, blood degradation products, melanin, etc., are all factors influencing the signal characteristics. Most tumoral lesions appear bright on T2-weighted images and dark on T1-weighted images [2]. In lesions with a cystic appearance , one can only state very confidently that the lesion is truly a cyst if it is exactly isointense to CSF on all routine sequences and if its signal is totally attenuated on fluid-attenuated inversion recovery (FLAIR) images (Fig. 6) [7].

A bright appearance on T1-weighted images and a dark appearance on T2-weighted images can be due to the presence of fat, such as in lipoma, dermoid cysts, or teratoma; melanin, such as in melanoma and metastasis of melanoma; mucin, in metastasis of mucinous adenocarcinoma of the gastrointestinal tract, such as sigmoid carcinoma (Fig. 7); colloid material in a colloid cyst and Rathke cleft cyst; and even calcification in oligodendroglioma (Fig. 5b).

A bright aspect on both T1 and T2-weighted images can be due to cholesterine in cholesterol granuloma or the

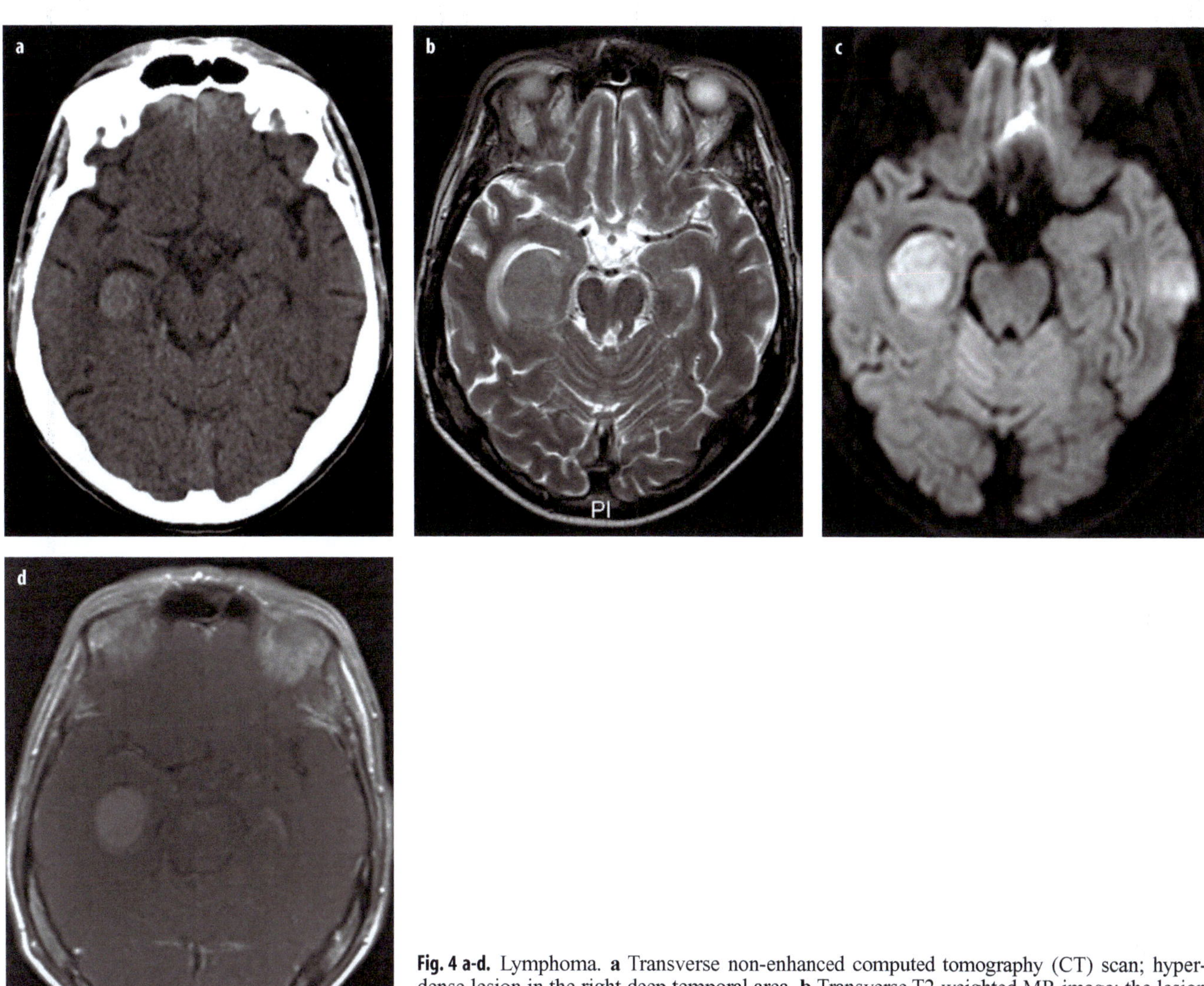

Fig. 4 a-d. Lymphoma. **a** Transverse non-enhanced computed tomography (CT) scan; hyperdense lesion in the right deep temporal area. **b** Transverse T2-weighted MR image: the lesion is homogeneously hypointense. **c** Transverse diffusion-weighted image; the lymphoma has restricted diffusion due to its hypercellularity. **d** Transverse gadolinium-enhanced T1-weighted image: homogeneous enhancement of the tumor

Fig. 5 a-c. Calcified oligodendroglioma. **a** Transverse non-enhanced CT scan; streaky calcifications in a right pre-rolandic mass. **b** Transverse T1-weighted image; some of the calcifications are hyperintense. **c** Transverse gadolinium-enhanced T1-weighted image shows patchy enhancement

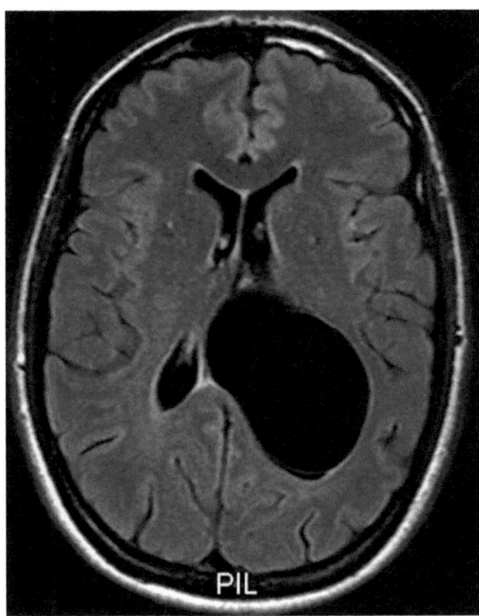

Fig. 6. Intraventricular cyst in the left lateral ventricle. Transverse fluid-attenuated inversion recovery (FLAIR) image: the content of the cyst is attenuated in the same way as the CSF in the ventricles

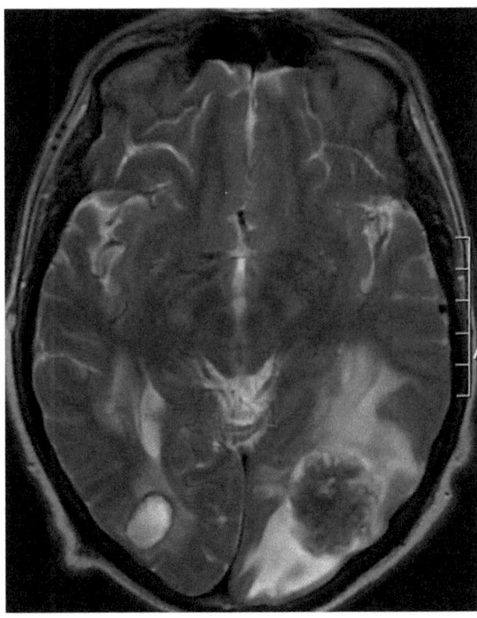

Fig. 7. Left occipital metastasis of coloncarcinoma. Transverse T2-weighted image: the metastasis is strongly hypointense on this T2-weighted sequence, as described in metastases of mucinous adenocarcinoma of the gastrointestinal tract

cystic component of craniopharyngioma, high protein content in tumoral cysts or the presence of methemoglobin in hemorrhagic neoplasms. Flow voids point to hypervascular tumors such as hemangioblastoma or some hypervascular metastases.

Calcification can appear as dark dots within a tumor, but some totally calcified meningiomas can be totally dark.

The Propensity for Calcification and Hemorrhage

Closely related to this, another differential diagnostic point is the propensity for calcification and hemorrhage. Oligodendrogliomas are the most likely intra-axial tumours to calcify (Fig. 5) [8], and calcification is detected in approximately 90% of these tumors. However, because astrocytomas occur more commonly and up to 20% of astrocytomas calcify, a calcified intra-axial lesion is statistically more likely to be an astrocytoma. Other lesions that commonly calcify are metastases, ependymoma, choroid plexus tumors, and extra-axial tumors, such as meningiomas, craniopharyngiomas, and chordomas. It should be kept in mind that calcium in these tumors is bound to macromolecules such that calcifications can have a short T1 (Fig. 5b).

Lesions that are most likely to hemorrhage include high-grade astrocytomas and oligodendroglioma as well as metastases from vascular primary tumors, particularly melanoma, renal cell carcinoma, and thyroid carcinoma [9].

The Location of the Lesion

The location of the tumor can suggest certain diagnoses. Glioblastoma is almost exclusively seen in the supratentorial araea, while a cystic pylocytic astrocytoma in childhood and hemangioblastomas are preferentially infratentorial [10]. A cerebellar mass in a patient over age 50 is likely to be a metastasis. A cortical lesion is likely to be a pleomorphic xanthoastrocytoma, ganglioglioma, or dysembroblastic neuroepithelial tumour (DNET) (Fig. 8) [11]; a corticomedullary lesion is most likely to be a metastasis or oligodendroglioma; and a deep periventricular lesion could be an astrocytoma, ependymoma or lymphoma, the latter more specifically if multiple (Fig. 4). Primary glial tumors arise deep in the white matter, away from the cortex.

Some tumors have a predilection for the suprasellar area. Besides the classical hypothalamic glioma, pilocytic astrocytoma, craniopharyngeoma and even germinoma can occur. In the pineal region, pineocytoma and pineoblastoma have to be differentiated from germinoma and even from tectal glioma. In patients with temporal lobe epilepsy, cystic lesions with an enhancing mural nodule in the uncus of the temporal lobe frequently correspond to ganglioglioma. Intraventricular tumors have a very specific differential diagnosis, varying even according to which specific ventricle the lesion is located in [12].

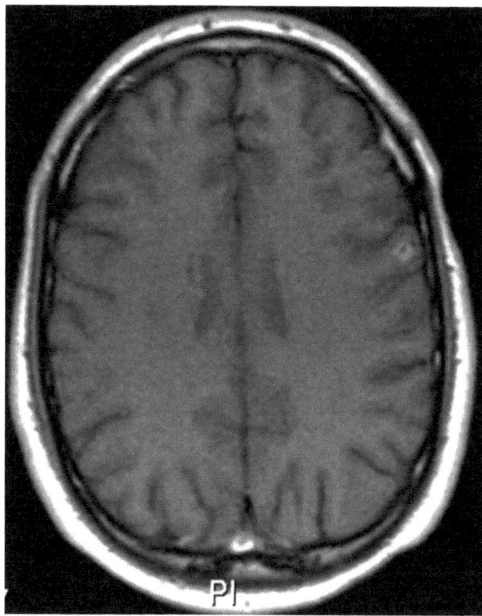

Fig. 8. Dysembryoplastic neuroepithelial tumor (DNET). Transverse gadolinium-enhanced T1-weighted image: cortical tumor in the left frontal lobe with some enhancement

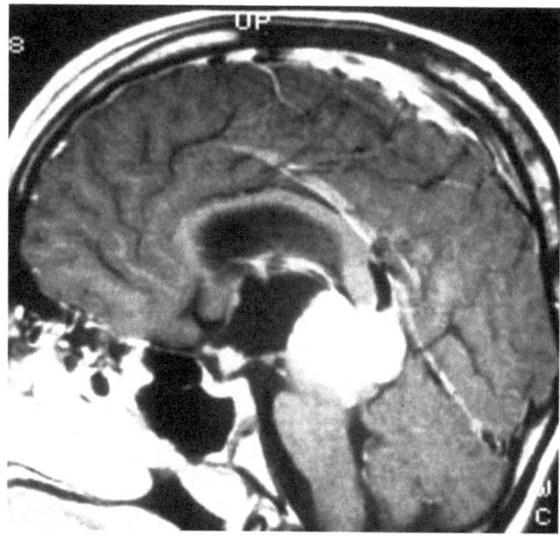

Fig. 10. Germinoma with infundibular seeding. Sagittal gadolinium-enhanced T1-weighted image: homogeneously enhancing mass in the pineal region. Second smaller nodule in the suprasellar area representing seeding to the infundibulum

The Extension and/or Spread of the Tumor

Another point to consider in the differential diagnosis is tumor extension and/or spread. Diffusely infiltrating astrocytomas spread along white matter tracts and as such do not respect the boundaries of the cerebral lobes. Glioblastoma of the corpus callosum shows a typical butterfly extension to the fontal or occipital lobes (Fig. 9). Ependymomas of the fourth ventricle in children tend to extend not only through the foramen of Magendie to the cisterna magna, but also through the lateral foramina of Lushka to the cerebellopontine angle. Oligodendroglioma typically shows a cortical extension. Primitive neuroectodermal tumours (PNET's) such as medulloblastomas and pineoblastoma tend to seed very quickly via the cerebrospinal fluid to the subarachnoid space, with formation of multiple tumoral nodules on the surface of the brain and spinal cord [13]. Germinoma of the pineal gland very specifically spreads to the hypophyseal infundibulum (Fig. 10); this location can even be the sole manifestation of the disease.

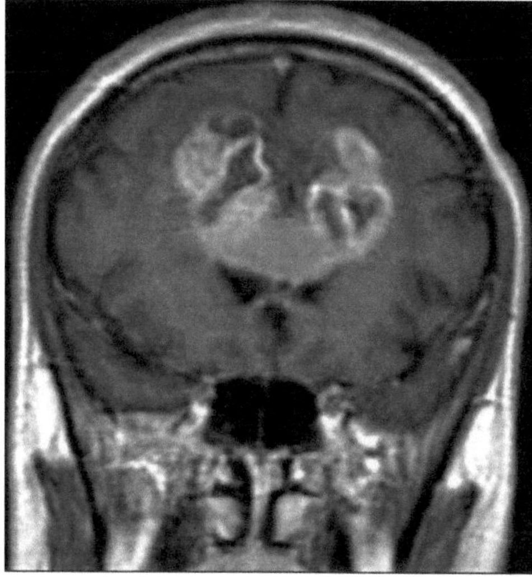

Fig. 9. Butterfly glioblastoma of the corpus callosum. Coronal gadolinium-enhanced T1-weighted image: inhomogeneously enhancing lesion in the corpus callosum with bilateral extension to the frontal white matter

Type and Degree of Contrast Enhancement

A major factor of interest is the type and degree of contrast enhancement [14]. In most meningiomas and acoustic schwannomas, enhancement is homogeneous, except for some intratumoral cystic areas, calcifications, or flow voids. Homogeneous enhancement can also be seen in nodular metastases at the corticomedullary junction, periventricular lymphoma (Fig. 4d), germinoma (Fig. 10) and other pineal gland tumors, pilocytic astrocytoma in the brainstem and the suprasellar area and in the solid part of cystic or fluid-secreting pilocytic astrocytomas or hemangioblastoma [10, 14]. The enhancement of oligodendroglioma tends to be patchier (Fig. 5c). High-grade primary tumors, exemplified by glioblastoma multiforme, are very anarchic, multilocular, thick-walled ring-enhancing masses (Fig. 11). The rings have a shaggy inner margin with a thick and irregular wall. Bridging septa may cross the necrotic cavities and nodular formations can be present on the septa.

Another typical pattern of enhancement is the ring-enhancing lesion [15]. It is typically seen in metastasis (Fig. 12) but also in glioblastoma and even in non-tumoral lesions such as abscess, multiple sclerosis, chronic hematoma, and a variety of infectious (Fig. 13) and inflammatory lesions.

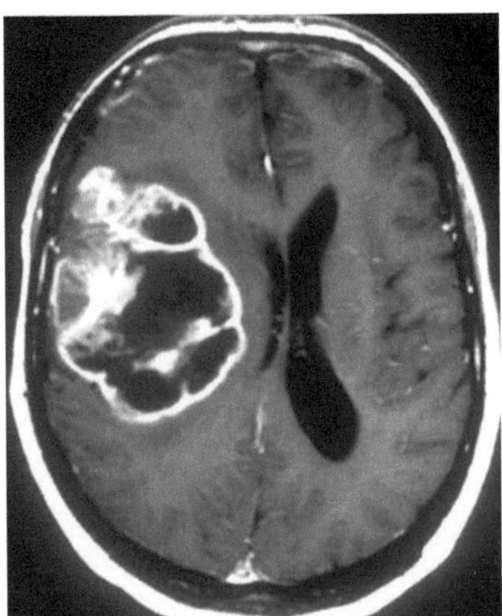

Fig. 11. Glioblastoma. Transverse gadolinium-enhanced T1-weighted image: multilocular mass with enhancing thick-walled rings and bridging septa with nodular formations

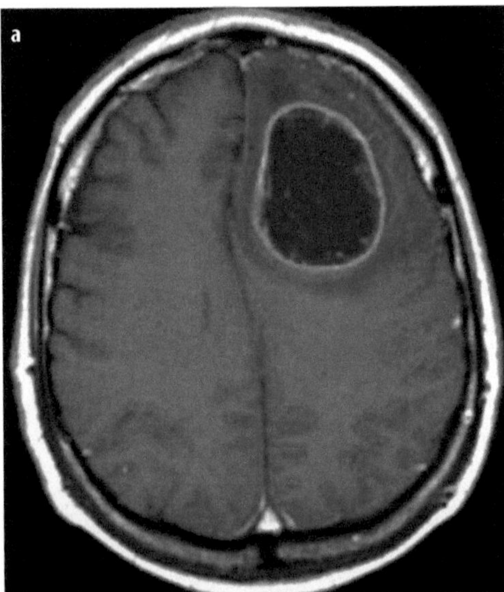

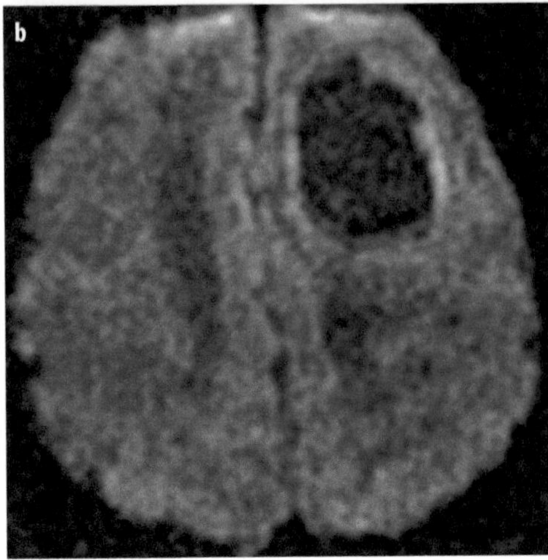

Fig. 12 a, b. Ring-enhancing metastasis. **a** Transverse gadolinium-enhanced T1-weighted image: left frontal ring-enhancing lesion. **b** Transverse diffusion-weighted image: no diffusion restriction

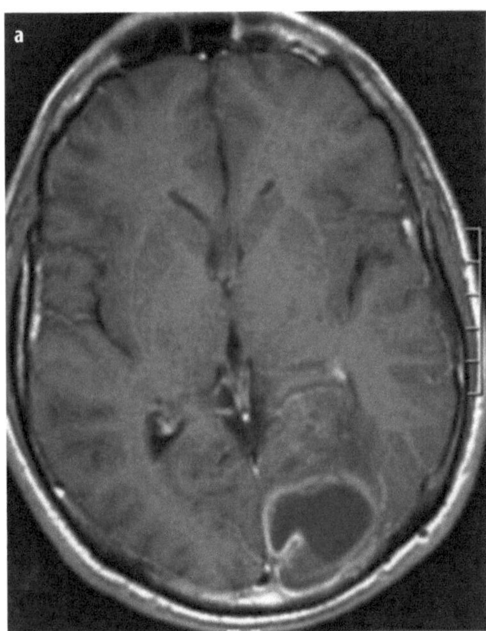

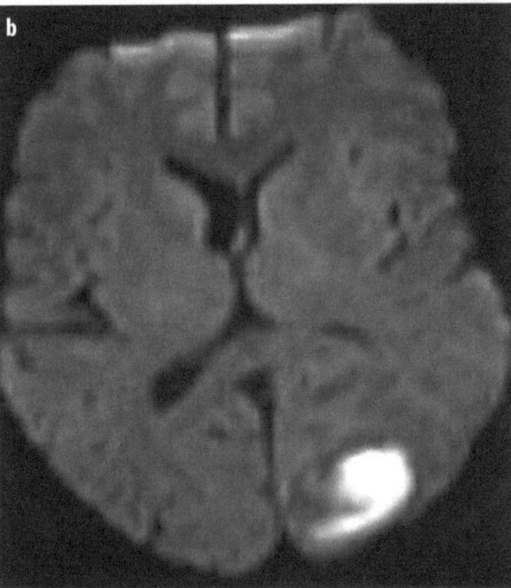

Fig. 13 a, b. Ring-enhancing abscess. **a** Transverse gadolinium-enhanced T1-weighted image; left occipital lesion with peripheral enhancement. **b** Transverse diffusion-weighted image; strong hyperintensity due to diffusion restriction of the pus in the abscess

The Basis of Contrast Enhancement of Brain Tumors: Value of Perfusion MR Imaging

Contrast enhancement in brain tumors is based not only on tumor's vascularity and/or angiogenesis but also on the breakdown of the blood-brain barrier. Extremes are the extra-axial meningioma, in which contrast enhancement only reflects the hypervascular character of the tumor, and pilocytic astroctoma of childhood, in which enhancement is due only to the breakdown of the blood-brain barrier. In most diffusely infiltrating astrocytomas, enhancement is due to a mixture of both. The timing of imaging after the infusion of contrast medium influences the relative contribution of each factor: earlier imaging illustrates the intravascular component, while later imaging reflects extravascular or interstitial enhancement.

Classically, it is said that with a higher degree of malignancy, contrast enhancement will increase. [16, 17]. During the evolution of a non-enhancing, diffusely infiltrating lesion, the appearance of contrast enhancement mostly is considered as a sign of anaplastic transformation of the tumor. Thus, contrast enhancement is considered essential in the diagnosis of malignancy of a new lesion, and in the diagnosis of malignant transformation of a previously benign one. Although these rules can usually be applied, important restrictions apply concerning the value of contrast enhancement in the grading of cerebral tumors. First of all, it has to be kept in mind that tumors extend beyond the area of contrast enhancement [18]. Consequently, removing the enhancing part of the tumor will not be enough to cure the patient. Furthermore, as paradoxical as it may seem, areas of maximal enhancement do not correspond to the areas of maximal malignancy. Therefore guiding of a biopsy with enhancement as the only criterion might give rise to incorrect grading of the lesion.

Non-enhancing tumors generally are considered as benign, meaning grade 2 for diffusely infiltrating astrocytomas; but at biopsy, up to 40% of non-enhancing tumors show signs of anaplastic transformation [19]. Moreover, it is known that several benign tumors show contrast enhancement. Also, in oligodendroglioma striking changes in contrast enhancement occur without any change in the degree of malignancy as determined at biopsy [8]. Finally breakdown of the blood-brain barrier and therefore the appearance of contrast enhancement can occur with radiation necrosis [20]. For all these reasons, contrast enhancement alone is insufficient for a diagnosis of malignancy.

Recently, perfusion MR was introduced as a means of assessing the vascularity of a lesion [21-25]. It has been shown that regional cerebral blood flow (rCBV) correlates well with tumor grade. Therefore, perfusion MR can be used to demonstrate angiogenesis in an enhancing and in a non-enhancing tumor. Perfusion MR will also indicate the optimal site for biopsy at the place of maximal angiogenesis, which indeed was proven not to correspond to areas of maximal enhancement. Furthermore, perfusion MR has proven that a non-enhancing astrocytoma with high rCBV has to be considered as high-grade (Fig. 14). Finally, perfusion MR can also be used to differentiate between tumor recurrence with high rCBV and radiation necrosis or other inflammatory changes after therapy that present with low rCBV.

Diffusion-weighted imaging (DWI) and, more specifically, the apparent diffusion coefficient (ADC) is another method used to grade diffusely infiltrating tumors [26]. ADC seems to correlate with tumor cellularity. Hence, lower ADC values are present in the solid portions of anaplastic gliomas, while non-enhancing brain gliomas with low ADCs are anaplastic. In strikingly hy-

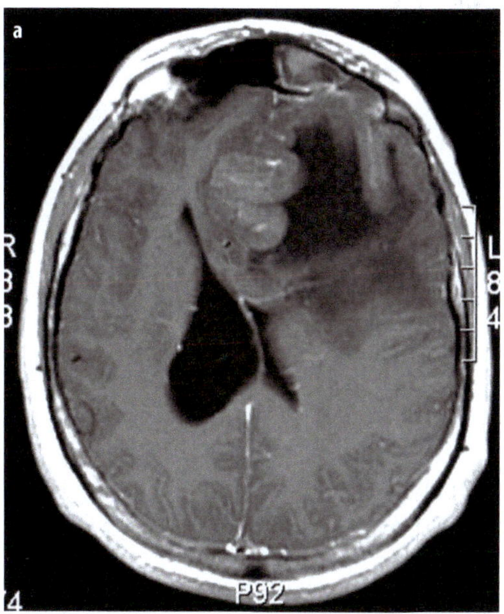

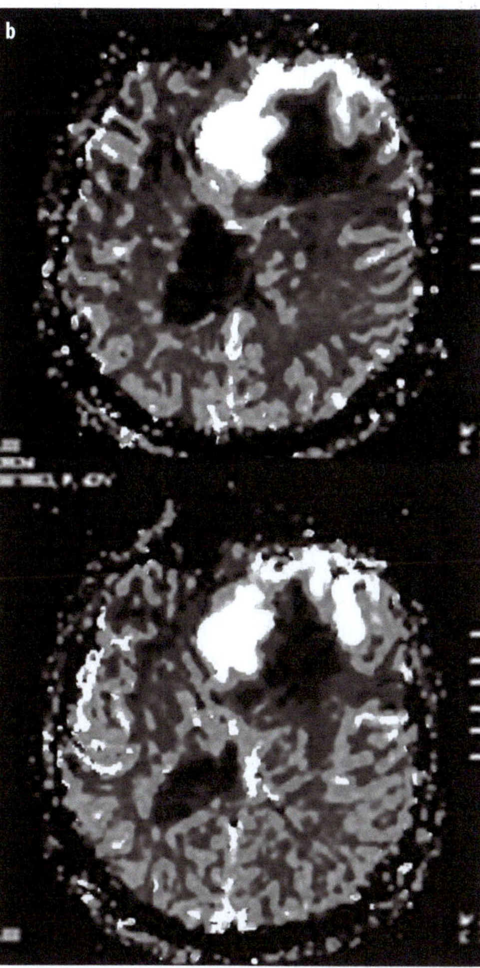

Fig. 14 a, b. Non-enhancing malignant tumor, proven by perfusion-weighted imaging. **a** Transverse gadolinium-enhanced T1-weighted image; huge mass in the left frontal lobe with central necrosis. There is only faint enhancement of the lesion. **b** Color-coded perfusion-weighted images; red color (white in the figure) corresponds to high rCBV. The rCBV of the tumor appears to be very high, pointing to angiogenesis. Oligodendroglioma grade III-V at biopsy

percellular tumors, such as lymphoma, the extremely low ADC is even reflected by the DWI hyperintensity (Fig. 4c) [27]. The hyperintensity of epidermoid cysts on DWI is probably due to a T2 shine-through effect [7, 15]. The main application of DWI in epidermoid cysts is the determination of postoperative residual pathological tissue [15].

Differential Diagnosis of Non-tumoral Lesions

Finally, it is important to note that, in the presence of a space-occupying lesion in the brain, the differential diagnosis has to include non-tumoral lesions, such as abscesses, radionecrosis, aneurysms, multiple sclerosis, infarction, etc. The clinical presentation of these lesions differs in each case and can be very confusing. Abscesses can appear as ring-enhancing lesions on contrast-enhanced MR. Here, DWI plays a major diagnostic role, since the presence of pus, bacteria, and cellular debris in the center of an abscess leads to strong restriction of diffusion, with very high signal on DWI, whereas in tumors, such as necrotic metastasis, no diffusion restriction is seen (Figs. 12, 13) [15]. In radionecrosis, conventional MR can show an enhancing mass lesion surrounded by edema, thus mimicking tumor recurrence. Here again, DWI can demonstrate the avascular nature of the enhancing mass, confirming the diagnosis of radionecrosis [28]. A differential diagnosis that considers aneurysms is most frequently necessary for lesions in the suprasellar area, where giant aneurysms can simulate an enhancing mass. Here the flow void on non-enhanced T1- and T2-weighted images and the increase in pulsation artifacts after gadolinium can be very helpful in the differential diagnosis. In the differential diagnosis of an enhancing infarction, the distribution within a vascular territory and the gyriform pattern of enhancement can give clues as to the right diagnosis [14]. Tumefactive demyelination can be very hard to differentiate from a necrotic tumor, especially in the absence of a history of MS. The "open ring sign" [29], manifesting as an incomplete ring in a ring-enhancing lesion, would be highly specific of demyelination. MR imaging of the spinal cord may demonstrate additional lesions to support the diagnosis.

References

1. Osborn AG, Blaser S, Salzman K (2004) Diagnostic imaging: Brain. Amirsys, Salt Lake City
2. Wilms G, Demaerel P, Sunaert S (2005) Intra-axial brain tumours. Eur Radiol 15(3):468-484
3. Kornreich L, Schwarz M, Karmazyn B et al (2005) Role of MRI in the management of children with diffuse pontine tumors: a study of 15 patients and review of the literature. Pediatr Radiol 35(9):872-879
4. Schneider JF, Viola A, Confort-Gouny S et al (2007) Infratentorial pediatric brain tumors: the value of new imaging modalities. J Neuroradiol 34(1):49-458
5. Tzika AA, Zarifi MK, Goumnerova L et al (2002) Neuroimaging in pediatric brain tumors: Gd-DTPA-enhanced, hemodynamic, and diffusion MR imaging compared with MR spectroscopic imaging. AJNR Am J Neuroradiol 23(2):322-333
6. Goraj B, Spiller M, Valsamis MP et al (1995) Determinants of signal intensity in MRI of human astrocytomas. Eur Radiol 5:74-82
7. Osborn AG, Preece MT (2006) Intracranial cysts: radiologic-pathologic correlation and imaging approach. Radiology 239(3):650-664
8. White ML, Zhang Y, Kirby P, Ryken TC (2005) Can tumor contrast enhancement be used as a criterion for differentiating tumor grades of oligodendrogliomas? AJNR Am J Neuroradiol 26(4):784-790
9. Carrier DA, Mawad ME, Kirkpatrick JB, Schmid MF (1994) Metastatic adenocarcinoma to the brain: MR with pathologic correlation. Am J Neuroradiol 15:155-159
10. Fulham MJ, Melisi JW, Nishimiya J et al (1993) Neuroimaging of juvenile pilocytic astrocytomas: an enigma. Radiology 189:221-225
11. Koeller KK, Henry JM (2001) From the archives of the AFIP: superficial gliomas: radiologic-pathologic correlation. Armed Forces Institute of Pathology. Radiographics 21(6):1533-1556
12. Jelinek J, Smirniotopoulos JG, Parisi JE, Kanzer M (1990) Lateral ventricular neoplasms of the brain: differential diagnosis based on clinical, CT, and MR findings. Am J Neuroradiol 11:567-574
13. Koeller KK, Rushing EJ (2003) From the archives of the AFIP: medulloblastoma: a comprehensive review with radiologic-pathologic correlation. Radiographics 23(6):1613-1637
14. Smirniotopoulos JG, Murphy FM, Rushing EJ et al (2007) Patterns of contrast enhancement in the brain and meninges. Radiographics 27(2):525-551
15. Stadnik TW, Demaerel P, Luypaert RR et al (2003) Imaging tutorial: differential diagnosis of bright lesions on diffusion-weighted MR images. Radiographics 23(1):e7
16. Asari S, Makabe T, Katayama S et al (1994) Assessment of the pathological grade of astrocytic gliomas using an MRI score. Neuroradiology 36:308-310
17. Dean BL, Drayer BP, Bird CR et al (1990) Gliomas: classification with MR imaging. Radiology 174:411-415
18. Cha S, Lupo JM, Chen MH et al (2007) Differentiation of glioblastoma multiforme and single brain metastasis by peak height and percentage of signal intensity recovery derived from dynamic susceptibility-weighted contrast-enhanced perfusion MR imaging. AJNR Am J Neuroradiol 28(6):1078-1084
19. Ginsberg LE, Fuller GN, Hashmi M et al (1998) The significance of lack of MR contrast enhancement of supratentorial brain tumors in adults: histopathological evaluation of a series. Surg Neurol 49(4):436-440
20. Sugahara T, Korogi Y, Tomiguchi S et al (2000) Posttherapeutic intraaxial brain tumor: the value of perfusion-sensitive contrast-enhanced MR imaging for differentiating tumor recurrence from nonneoplastic contrast-enhancing tissue. Am J Neuroradiol 21(5):901-909
21. Lev MH, Ozsunar Y, Henson JW et al (2004) Glial tumor grading and outcome prediction using dynamic spin-echo MR susceptibility mapping compared with conventional contrast-enhanced MR: confounding effect of elevated rCBV of oligodendroglimoas. Am J Neuroradiol 25(2):214-221
22. Al-Okaili RN, Krejza J, Wang S et al (2006) Advanced MR imaging techniques in the diagnosis of intraaxial brain tumors in adults. Radiographics 26(Suppl 1):S173-S189
23. Al-Okaili RN, Krejza J, Woo JH et al (2007) Intraaxial brain masses: MR imaging-based diagnostic strategy – initial experience. Radiology 243(2):539-550
24. Calli C, Kitis O, Yunten N et al (2006) Perfusion and diffusion MR imaging in enhancing malignant cerebral tumors. Eur J Radiol 58(3):394-403

25. Law M, Yang S, Babb JS et al (2004) Comparison of cerebral blood volume and vascular permeability from dynamic susceptibility contrast-enhanced perfusion MR imaging with glioma grade. Am J Neuroradiol 25(5):746-755
26. Hayashida Y, Hirai T, Morishita S et al (2006) Diffusion-weighted imaging of metastatic brain tumors: comparison with histologic type and tumor cellularity. AJNR Am J Neuroradiol 27(7):1419
27. Cotton F, Ongolo-Zogo P, Louis-Tisserand G et al (2006) Diffusion and perfusion MR imaging in cerebral lymphomas. Neuroradiol 33(4):220-228
28. Covarrubias DJ, Rosen BR, Lev MH (2004) Dynamic magnetic resonance perfusion imaging of brain tumors. Oncologist 9(5):528-537
29. Masdeu JC, Quinto C, Olivera C et al (2000) Open-ring imaging sign: highly specific for atypical brain demyelination. Neurology 54(7):1427-1433

MRI/MRS of Brain Tumors

Michael Brant-Zawadzki

Department of Radiology, Hoag Memorial Hospital, Newport Beach, CA, USA

The role of any imaging modality in the evaluation of brain tumors is first and foremost the detection of such a tumor when clinical suspicion exists. In addition, characterization of the tumor with respect to its localization helps in formulating management plans. Finally, to the degree that an imaging modality can help in presurgical (or other therapeutic) planning, the value of the modality increases.

The initial clinical evaluation of magnetic resonance imaging (MRI) rapidly documented the superior sensitivity of this modality compared to computed tomography (CT) for the demonstration of most intracranial neoplasms. This can be ascribed to two major reasons: (1) The artifacts associated with the CT scanning in the region of the posterior fossa and temporal lobes preclude accurate assessment of brain parenchyma in these regions. (2) The physics of CT, which rely on changes in electron density for differentiation of normal from abnormal tissue, are not as sophisticated as relaxation and other MRI parameters, which enable detection of tissue alteration. Only the presence of calcification is more sensitively detected by CT compared to MRI.

The basic parameters of T1 and T2 weighting as well as those of magnetic susceptibility effects aid in the initial characterization of the tumor. Certain tumors, such as lymphoma and mucinous adenocarcinoma, exhibit relatively low T2-weighted signal features due to the presence of specific components, including free radicals and mucin, respectively. High T1 signal is the hallmark of the methemoglobin component of hemorrhage within a tumor, which allows highly vascular tumors, such as melanoma, adenocarcinoma, or even glioblastoma, to be distinguished from more benign types of tumors. Occasionally, floccular calcification can produce T1 shortening of hydrogen nuclei at the surface of such calcified regions, thus mimicking hemorrhagic components.

Tumor location helps in the differential diagnosis from a purely anatomic perspective. The broadest categorization is between tumors of the intra-axial vs. the extra-axial space (the latter includes intraventricular, subarachnoid, and extraleptomeningeal processes). This differentiation is simple when the tumor is within brain substance; however, the distinction may be difficult in regions such as the cerebella pontine angles and even the skull base. The angle between the mass and the adjacent inner table of the cranium, the presence of vascular displacement, and menisci of the spinal fluid space are features that contribute to this distinction. Cerebellopontine angle tumors have a relatively limited differential, composed of the more common lesions such as acoustic neuromas, meningiomas, aneurysms of the vertebral basilar arterial branches, and neuromas of the glossopharyngeal nerve, as well as relatively less common lesions such as lipomas and arachnoid cysts. Focal localization of a tumor to the pineal region leads to a completely different differential diagnosis, starting with tumors of pineal origin, such as pinealomas, pineal blastomas, and tumors of the germ-cell layer, such as germinomas and teratomas, followed by the more atypical lesions originating in the cellular histology of the region including tumors of neural origin, such as neurocytoma, glial tumors, ependymoma, and even meningioma.

The ability of tumors to present on both sides of the brain's midline limits the differential diagnosis to lesions such as infiltrating tumors of the malignant glial variety, epidermoids that cross the midline through the subarachnoid space, dural tumors such as meningiomas and metastatic lesions to the dura of the interhemispheric falcine structure, as well as lymphoma, which can infiltrate brain tissues and obviously be multi-focal. Indeed, the presence of multiple foci of tumor provides an additional natural differentiating feature. Metastatic disease, lymphoma, as well as inflammatory and infectious processes that mimic neoplastic disease and vasculitis are in the differential. One must remember that even primary brain tumors typically seen in a single region can have a multi-centric variant (multi-centric glioblastoma, gliomatosis cerebri).

The development of paramagnetic contrast agents further expanded the diagnostic capabilities of MRI. Not only could typical insults associated with blood-brain barrier disruption be demonstrated by these contrast agents, but physiologic evaluation of perfusion and blood volume parameters became possible as well. Indeed, recent work has documented that cerebral blood volume and contrast permeability analysis within the tumor can help distinguish malignant tumors from more benign categories of tumor. Correlation with positron emission tomography (PET) scanning has verified the close relationship of tumor-tissue blood volume and tumor activity. Despite these advances in MR capabilities, persistent shortcomings include the inability to differentiate residual and/or recurrent tumor from post-radiation or other therapeutic brain damage. Further work both in physiologic blood pool agent imaging and magnetic resonance spectroscopy (MRS) may help overcome these limitations. MRS allows the analysis of specific metabolites within brain tissue. Tumors, especially primary brain tumors, can be evaluated based on their choline (a maker of cell membrane turnover) profile and by the loss of *N*-acetylaspartate (NAA, a neuronal marker).

It should be noted, however, that MRS is nonspecific. Any rapidly evolving process that involves membrane breakdown or turnover (including multiple sclerosis) can produce tumor-like spectra, with elevation of choline levels being the dominant feature, although the decrease in NAA is not as prominent in such processes unless there is associated depletion of neuronal cells. Also, diffusion-weighted imaging, which typically shows restricted diffusion and high signal on appropriately reconstructed images, can occasionally yield abnormal findings in highly cellular tumors such as lymphoma. These tumors may mimic ischemic insult and its restriction of diffusion due to the compartmentalization of intracellular water. Diffusion is also helpful in distinguishing necrotic tumor cavities from abscess cavities, the latter marked by very heavily proteinaceous components that restrict diffusion.

Other useful tools for distinguishing active neoplasm from other processes include the radionuclide modalities of PET and single photon emission computed tomography (SPECT). However, the findings are relatively nonspecific. For example, the high metabolic activity of brain tissue can mask tumor activity, resulting in a false-negative PET study for brain neoplasm. The increased blood volume of highly malignant tumors can be determined with PET and SPECT. Once a neoplasm has been detected, localized, and characterized, the additional advantages of MRI lie in the sphere of treatment planning. The three-dimensional capability of this technique allows much better delineation of tumor extent and the relationships of the tumor to eloquent brain structures. The availability of data in three dimensions makes post-processing of three dimensional images on commercially available workstations relatively straightforward. Furthermore, surface contouring of the scalp, brain, and internal structures produces a "virtual reality" for the neurosurgeon within which to plan treatment. Indeed, the ability to merge 3D MR angiographic data with segmented three-dimensional brain images can be coupled to robotic probes placed in the operating room. Coregistration of the image data with the patient in the operating room then allows real-time surgical decisions to be made based on the three dimensional MR images.

Glioblastoma multiforme defies any form of therapy because the tumor cannot be effectively treated locally. White-matter infiltration of tumor cells beyond the gadolinium-enhancing tumor mass is the rule. Studies have suggested that fluid-attenuated inversion recovery (FLAIR) sequences are most sensitive to tumor, and that proton MRS improves the specificity of tumor detection within and beyond FLAIR-positive zones. When conventional field radiation therapy is used, survival times historically are approximately 6-10 months for patients with recurrent disease. However, survival can be prolonged by targeting the "leading edge" zones, as defined by FLAIR and MRS, with boost stereotactic radiosurgery. Our experience suggests a survival advantage using FLAIR- or MRS-directed "leading edge" gamma-knife radiosurgery for patients with recurrent glioblastoma multiforme.

Development of dedicated intra-operative MR scanners to help the surgeon to operate in the MR environment itself is ongoing. This tool couples diagnosis and treatment much more intimately, in that imaging will guide the surgeon's hands to the best possible endpoint.

Suggested Reading

Baumgartner JE, Edwards MS (1992) Pineal tumors. Neurosurg Clin N Am 3(4):853-862

Blakeley JO, Grossman SA (2006) Management of pineal region tumors. Curr Treat Options Oncol 7(6):505-516

Bonneville F, Savatovsky J, Chiras J (2007) Imaging of cerebellopontine angle lesions: an update. Part 2: intraaxial lesions, skull base lesions that may invade the CPA region, and non-enhancing extraaxial lesions. Eur Radiol 17(11):2908-2920

Bradley WG, Waluch V, Yadley R, Wycoff R (1984) Comparison of CT and MR in 400 patients with suspected disease of the brain and cervical spinal cord. Radiology 152: 695-702

Brant-Zawadzki M, Badami JP, Mills CM et al (1984) Primary intracranial tumor imaging: a comparison of magnetic resonance and CT. Radiology 150: 435-440

Bydder GM, Steiner RE, Young IR et al (1982) Clinical NMR imaging of the brain; 140 cases. AJR Am J Roentgenol 139:215-236

Cha S (2004) Perfusion MR Imaging of brain tumors. Top Magn Reson Imaging 15(5):279-289

D'Angelo VA, Galarza M, Catapano D et al (2005) Lateral ventricle tumors: surgical strategies according to tumor origin and development – a series of 72 cases. Neurosurgery 56(1 Suppl):36-45

Fayed-Miguel N, Morales-Ramos H, Modrego-Prado PJ (2006) Magnetic resonance imaging with spectroscopy, perfusion and cerebral diffusion in the diagnosis of brain tumors. Rev Neurol 42(12):735-742

Hamid B, Harris C, Spiess J (2007) Metastatic adenocarcinoma in the cerebellopontine angle mimicking facial nerve Schwannoma. Am J Clin Oncol 30(5):556-557

Law M, Hamburger M, Johnson G et al (2004) Differentiating surgical from non-surgical lesions using perfusion MR imaging and proton MR spectroscopic imaging. Technol Cancer Res Treat 3(6):557-565

Lemort M, Canizares-Perez AC, Van der Stappen A, Kampouridis S (2007) Progess in magnetic resonance imaging of brain tumors. Curr Opin Neurol 19(6):616-622

Provenzale JM, Mukundan S, Barboriak DP (2006) Diffusion-weighted and perfusion MR imaging for brain tumor characterization and assessment of treatment response. Radiology 239(3):632-649

Rees J (2003) Advances in magnetic resonance imaging of brain tumors. Curr Opin Neurol 16(6):643-650

Young GS (2007) Advanced MRI of adult brain tumors. Neurol Clin 25(4):947-973

Young RJ, Knopp EA (2006) Brain MRI: tumor evaluation. J Magn Reson Imaging 24(4):709-724

Imaging of Central Nervous System Disease in Pediatrics

Tina Young Poussaint

Harvard Medical School and Department of Radiology, Division of Neuroradiology, Children's Hospital Boston, Boston, MA, USA

Introduction to Imaging Central Nervous System Disease in Pediatrics

Pediatric Neuroradiology, a radiologic discipline in which neuroimaging techniques are used to assess central nervous system (CNS) disease in the infant, child, and teenager, relies on: (1) an understanding of normal brain development and maturation from gestation through adolescence; (2) a technical mastery of the neuroimaging techniques that are used in evaluating brain diseases of childhood; (3) an overall grasp of the imaging features of numerous brain pathologies, both acquired and congenital; and (4) the ability to select the most appropriate modality or modalities in evaluating a suspected or diagnosed case of pediatric CNS disease.

This chapter presents an overview of the primary neuroimaging modalities currently used in evaluating pediatric brain disease; and a descriptive cataloguing of the various CNS diseases of childhood as well as the basic imaging features that inhere in each one. For additional detail, the reader is directed to in-depth textbooks on this subject [1].

Neuroimaging Techniques

Ultrasound

The utility of ultrasound (US) in detecting and managing neonatal disease in the preterm infant is well-established. This versatile modality has numerous advantages, including ready access, portability, real-time and multi-planar capabilities, and reproducible results. Moreover, it is a non-invasive, radiation-free procedure that can be performed at the bedside, in the intensive care unit, or on an intubated, ventilated baby following delivery. Improved graded Doppler techniques and high-resolution transducers now produce detailed mastoid and posterior fontanelle views that offer new insights into the structural and vascular abnormalities of the neonatal brain. US has also proven very useful in detecting intracerebral hemorrhages, such as intraventricular and periventricular hemorrhagic venous infarction, and for detecting hypoxic-ischemic changes [2]. In the neonate and young infant, US of the head is often used as an initial screening exam for conditions such as hydrocephalus. Brain US is used reliably to evaluate the full-term neonate, especially in circumstances in which the patient is too ill to withstand transport to the magnetic resonance imaging (MRI) suite, or when an MRI examination is not available immediately or at all [3]. If meticulous attention is paid to US technique, abnormalities found on US images may correlate well with abnormalities seen on MRI [3].

Computed Tomography

Computed tomography (CT) is the modality of choice for pediatric brain imaging in acute or emergent presentations. It is performed when US does not satisfy the clinical question, or when an acoustic window is not available. CT also is useful in detecting acute or subacute processes, such as intracranial hemorrhage, cerebral edema, hypoxic-ischemic injury, infarction, hydrocephalus/shunt dysfunction, neoplasm, or abnormal collections. With 3D reconstruction algorithms, CT effectively evaluates skull or facial abnormalities in patients with syndromes or craniosynostosis. CT is also useful in detecting intracranial calcifications such as tuberous sclerosis, TORCH (syphilis, rubella, cytomegalovirus, herpesvirus type 2, and human immunodeficiency virus) infection, and craniopharyngioma. CT is also the modality of choice for assessing the bones of the skull and face in the setting of trauma.

Magnetic Resonance Imaging

This technique is considered the modality of choice in evaluating the brain in patients of all ages. MRI provides superior anatomic detail, has multi-planar capabilities, shows high sensitivity in detecting brain pathology, and can provide functional and physiologic information about the brain. Among its vast capabilities, MRI is also incredibly useful in defining complex CNS anomalies such as disorders of dorsal induction (e.g., Chiari II malformation, cephaloceles) or ventral induction (e.g., holoprosencephaly, Dandy-Walker malformation). MRI also provides excellent contrast between gray matter and white matter, allowing the detection of disorders of cortical development. It can differentiate myelinated from unmyelinated white matter in the infant and is the modality of choice for evaluating encephaloclastic disorders and disorders of maturation (i.e., myelination and cortical maturation). MRI also demonstrates high sensitivity for anoxic injury to the brain arising from multiple causes.

Fetal MRI provides a morphological approach that aids in identifying CNS abnormalities in utero. The single-shot fast spin echo (FSE) technique, in particular, produces rapidly acquired images that can generate critical information about the fetus; these, in turn, may be used in counseling families about current and future pregnancies and may guide therapies after birth.

Advanced MRI Applications

Magnetic Resonance Diffusion

Diffusion-weighted imaging (DWI) uses strong diffusion gradients that generate images based upon differences in the rate of diffusion of water molecules. This technique is particularly sensitive to intracellular change [4,5], generating images that reflect the molecular translational motion (Brownian motion) of water within the section of the brain being studied. Once these images are produced, the rate of diffusion, or apparent diffusion coefficient (ADC), is calculated, effectively canceling out the T2 weighting of the echoplanar diffusion sequence. This provides a quantitative and reproducible evaluation of the diffusion changes, not only in areas that demonstrate abnormal T2 prolongation on conventional MRI, but also in areas of normal signal. The ADC varies according to the microstructural or physiologic state of a tissue. DWI may provide a more precise assessment of maturation based on ADC and anisotropy parameters. Clinical applications of DWI in children include the evaluation of brain maturation [6], the detection of early focal or diffuse ischemic injury or other acute injury, assessment of tumor cellularity and tumor response to therapies, traumatic brain injury, and infection [7].

Diffusion tensor imaging characterizes the rate and direction of white matter diffusion by providing visualization of fiber tract direction and integrity. This technique has been used to assess white matter fiber tracts in the immature brain, congenital disorders, acquired disorders of white matter, malformations of cortical development, effects of chemotherapy and radiation in patients with brain tumors, leukodystrophies, and hypoxic ischemic encephalopathy [8].

MR Spectroscopy

Proton nuclear magnetic resonance spectroscopy (MRS) provides additional complimentary metabolic information beyond standard anatomic MRI. Techniques include single voxel and multi-voxel MRS with 2D and 3D acquisitions. This technique allows the monitoring of important brain metabolites such as N-acetyl aspartate (NAA), creatine (Cr), choline (Cho), and lactate (Lac). NAA is found in normally functioning neurons; Cho and Cho-containing compounds are associated with cellular membranes; Cr compounds are indicators of cellular energetics; and Lac is a marker of anaerobic metabolism in hypoxic regions, tumors, and metabolic disease. Applications for MRS include brain development and maturation assessment, perinatal injury, metabolic and neurodegenerative disorders, detection of brain tumors, and response to therapy.

Functional MRI

Functional MRI (fMRI) is the term often applied to brain activation imaging wherein local or regional changes in cerebral blood flow that accompany stimulation or activation of sensory (e.g., visual, auditory), motor, or cognitive centers are displayed. This technique is also useful in identifying eloquent regions of the pediatric brain when surgical resection of a brain tumor is planned. The blood oxygenation level dependent (BOLD) technique, which gauges the level of oxygenation of hemoglobin during brain activity, is also utilized. Magnetic source imaging (MSI) integrates anatomic data from conventional MRI with electrophysiological data from magnetoencephalography, which measures magnetic fields associated with intracellular current flows within neurons. These fMRI techniques may guide the surgical approach to brain tumors as well as aid in treatment planning for epilepsy patients who are surgical candidates [9].

MR Perfusion

As an adjunct to conventional MRI, magnetic resonance perfusion imaging is currently being used to evaluate cerebral perfusion dynamics by analyzing hemodynamic parameters, including relative cerebral blood volume, relative cerebral blood flow, and transit time. The techniques used to perform perfusion imaging include T2*-weighted dynamic susceptibility, arterial spin labeling techniques, and T1-weighted dynamic contrast-enhanced perfusion techniques. Magnetic resonance perfusion techniques use either exogenous tracer agents such as paramagnetic contrast material, or endogenous tracer agents, such as magnetically labeled blood (arterial water). Clinical applications include pediatric stroke, brain tumors, and perinatal hypoxic-ischemic encephalopathy.

Nuclear Medicine

Molecular imaging includes modalities such as single photon emission computed tomography (SPECT) and positron emission tomography (PET). These techniques are most often applied in patients with brain tumors and epilepsy.

Specific Categories of Disease

Hypoxic/Ischemic Encephalopathy

Clinical presentation depends on the severity and duration of the insult and on the gestational age of the patient.

The Premature Infant

Hemodynamic alterations in premature infants frequently result in brain injuries, such as germinal matrix hemorrhage (GMH), intraventricular hemorrhage (IVH), periventricular hemorrhagic infarction (PVHI), post-hemorrhagic hydrocephalus, periventricular leukomalacia (PVL), and cerebellar infarction and atrophy. White matter injury secondary to PVL is considered the most significant sequela of prematurity and can be cystic or diffuse. US is useful in detecting GMH/IVH and cystic PVL; however, MRI is superior to US in detecting diffuse white matter injury with non-cystic or necrotic changes, delayed myelination, and thinning of the corpus callosum.

The Term Infant

In the term neonate, hypoxic-ischemic encephalopathy (HIE) is the main cause of brain injury. Brain damage in HIE is selective, depending on the relative energy requirements of given areas of the brain at various stages of brain maturation. Mild to moderate hypotension will result in cortical injury involving intravascular boundary zones, known as "watershed areas", situated between either the anterior and middle cerebral arteries or between the middle and posterior cerebral arteries. Profound hypotension results in injury to the lateral thalami, posterior putamina, hippocampi, and corticospinal tracts, all metabolically active regions. Combined patterns (i.e., partial prolonged plus profound HIE) are also common. DWI is the modality of choice for detecting these injuries; determining the pattern, extent, and severity of injury; and aiding in clinical management of these children. Early edema, necrosis, or infarction in the acute and subacute phase may be detected. MRS has been used in infants with perinatal asphyxia. MRS studies that demonstrate higher lactate-choline ratios in basal ganglia and thalami are generally predictive of poor clinical outcomes [10]. This technique is frequently combined with conventional MRI and DWI to predict neonatal outcomes. Significant perinatal hypoglycemia in the neonate can result in diffuse brain damage within the parieto-occipital white matter and cortex of the brain, as evidenced by restricted diffusion on MRI.

Occlusive Neurovascular Disease and Sequelae

Occlusive neurovascular disease in the child may be arterial or venous in origin and typically results in focal or multi-focal lesions distributed within the occluded vessel or vessels. Arterial occlusive disease may be partial or complete because of stenosis, thrombosis, or embolization. The result may be ischemic infarction or hemorrhagic infarction followed by atrophy. Arterial occlusive disease may occur as a prenatal or perinatal event (emboli of placental origin or from involuting fetal vessels), as a complication of infection (e.g., meningitis), with congenital heart disease, or from a hypercoagulopathy. Other causes include trauma (e.g., dissection), moyamoya, and metabolic disorders (e.g., mitochondrial cytopathies). Vascular occlusive disease may occur as a complication of meningitis, heart disease, or sickle cell disease. Other causes include hypercoagulable prothrombotic states, moyamoya syndrome, vasculitis, migraine, and metabolic disorders (e.g., mitochondrial cytopathies). Conditions commonly associated with cortical or dural venous sinus occlusive disease include infection, dehydration, perinatal encephalopathy, cyanotic congenital heart disease, leukemia (l-asparaginase therapy), polycythemia (newborn), other hypercoagulable states, disseminated intravascular coagulopathy (DIC), oral contraceptives, and trauma. MRI is sensitive and specific in the acute and subacute phases for ischemic infarction, hemorrhagic infarction, and venous thrombosis. Magnetic resonance angiography (MRA) or CT angiography (CTA) contribute to the diagnosis of arterial or venous occlusion and clarify the need for cerebral angiography, particularly when anticoagulation or thrombolysis is being considered.

Intracranial Hemorrhage and Vascular Diseases

Acute spontaneous intracranial hemorrhage is readily diagnosed by CT. MRI, however, provides better specificity beyond the acute phases. Vascular malformations producing intracranial hemorrhage in childhood include arteriovenous malformations (AVM), cavernous malformations, developmental venous anomalies, and telangiectasias. Aneurysms are very rare in childhood, but may be congenital, associated with a syndrome (e.g., Turner syndrome), or related to trauma or infection (e.g., mycotic aneurysm). Vein of Galen malformations are subclassified as choroidal or mural types. They often present in infants with congestive heart failure or hydrocephalus, respectively. Neoplastic malformations or neovascularity rarely produce an acute hemorrhage, although hemorrhage due to coagulopathy is sometimes seen concomitantly with hemophilia, leukemia, idiopathic thrombocytopenic purpura (ITP), and DIC. Hyperintensive hemorrhage is also rare in childhood but should be ruled out in the child with elevated blood pressure and encephalopathy. Susceptibility-weighted MRI has been demonstrated as sensitive to the detection of blood products in a variety of hemorrhagic lesions [11].

Head and neck vascular anomalies of childhood include hemangiomas and vascular malformations (e.g., AVM, lymphatic, venous). These often involve the head and neck region or the paraspinal region and are definitively evaluated by MRI for management. Hemangiomas of the face can be associated with posterior fossa malformations, arterial anomalies, cardiac anomalies, eye anomalies, and sternal clefting or supraumbilical raphe [12].

Infection

Congenital infections of the CNS, which usually occur via the transplacental route, can affect the developing nervous system. Depending on the fetal age at the time of insult, manifestations of infection may vary. Congenital infections include, but are not limited to toxoplasmosis and TORCH. Infections contracted during the first two trimesters may result in congenital malformations, while those occurring in the third trimester typically manifest as destructive lesions. On neuroimaging, the chronic sequelae of congenital infections include disorders of cortical development, calcifications, hydrocephalus, atrophy, demyelination, and porencephaly. Cytomegalovirus and HIV are discussed below.

Cytomegalovirus

Of the TORCH infections, cytomegalovirus (CMV) is the most common. Clinical presentation includes developmental delay, microcephaly, seizures, hearing problems, and chorioretinitis. The extent of damage to the CNS depends upon the timing of the infection. Infections occurring during the first half of the second trimester can result in lissencephaly, hypoplastic cerebellum, delayed myelination, significant ventriculomegaly, and periventricular calcifications. Insults that take place in the middle of the second trimester will result in polymicrogyria, less ventriculomegaly, and, on occasion, cerebellar hypoplasia. Infections occurring near the end of pregnancy will have normal gyral patterns, but mild ventricular dilatation, periventricular or subcortical leukomalacia, scattered periventricular calcification, or hemorrhage. CT studies of patients with CMV infections may show calcification, volume loss, ventricular dilatation, porencephaly, encephalomalacia and cerebellar hypoplasia. MRI better demonstrates the disorders of cortical development, gliosis, and delayed myelination.

Human Immunodeficiency Virus

Human immunodeficiency virus (HIV) type 1 is the etiologic agent of the acquired immunodeficiency syndrome (AIDS). It is an RNA retrovirus with a long incubation period (slow virus) and is associated with persistent and chronic infections, including slowly progressive CNS disease [13]. HIV infections in childhood most commonly result from maternal transmission to the fetus. When contracted congenitally, HIV is usually asymptomatic at birth, but signs and symptoms of CNS generally develop during the first year of life, typically presenting in children as developmental delay [14]. The virus produces a wide disease spectrum, with AIDS being the most severe form. HIV infects T4 helper cells resulting in opportunistic infections (e.g., *Pneumocystis jiroveci*, CMV, candida, herpes, and toxoplasmosis) or in neoplasia (e.g., lymphoma or Kaposi sarcoma). Two types of CNS involvement have been described: (1) CNS dysfunction directly or indirectly related to the retrovirus; and (2) secondary CNS complications or sequelae from immunosuppression (AIDS) or other AIDS-related conditions. Neuropathologic findings of HIV meningoencephalitis include glial and microglial nodules in the basal ganglia, brainstem, and white matter along with multinucleated giant cells; perivascular calcifications especially in the basal ganglia (i.e., the putamen and globus pallidus); and perivascular inflammation with demyelination. Neuroimaging demonstrates varying degrees of atrophy with resultant, prominent subarachnoid spaces and ventricles. Calcifications may be present bilaterally and symmetrically in the basal ganglia, subcortical white matter (most commonly in the frontal lobes), and occasionally in the cerebellum. Among children whose HIV infection was vertically acquired or who were exposed to the virus in the neonatal period and developed severe immune suppression, an increased incidence of cerebrovascular disease consisting of aneurysms and infarction is not uncommon.

Meningitis, and its sequelae or complications, are best evaluated with MRI. This includes subdural effusion, cerebral infarction, ventriculitis, hydrocephalus, abscess, or empyema. Subdural empyema and intracerebral abscesses usually demonstrate restricted diffusion on MRI [15]. These conditions are most often precipitated by suppurative bacterial infections (e.g., group B streptococcal, gram-negative, pneumococcal), and less commonly by granulomatous infections (e.g., TB, fungal, parasitic). Recurrent infectious or noninfectious meningitis may require investigation for a parameningeal focus (e.g., sinus or mastoid infection, dermal sinus, primitive neurenteric connection, CSF leak after trauma, dermoid-epidermoid). Brain abscess or empyema may be associated with a sinus infection, trauma, surgery, sepsis, the immunocompromised state, or uncorrected cyanotic congenital heart disease.

Infectious or post-infectious encephalitis is usually viral or post-viral in origin. The latter includes acute disseminated encephalomyelitis (ADEM). MRI is more sensitive than CT in demonstrating encephalitis and ADEM. Cysticercosis is a common cause of encephalitis with focal seizures in childhood. Calcification may not be present on CT at initial presentation.

For infections of the spinal column, MRI of the spine is often needed for definitive diagnosis and for treatment follow-up. MRI with gadolinium is the procedure of choice for evaluating spinal neuraxis infections.

Neoplastic Diseases

The classification of CNS tumors is primarily based on pathological criteria. Anatomic predilection and corresponding clinical signs provide other measures for classifying intracranial tumors in childhood, including cerebral hemispheric tumors, tumors about the third ventricle, and posterior fossa tumors [16]. Deep or hemispheric cerebral tumors of childhood include astrocytoma (e.g., pilocytic), choroid plexus papilloma, ganglioglioma, other glial tumors, and embryonic tumors (e.g., primitive neuroectodermal tumor, PNET). Tumors that develop around the third ventricle (i.e., the suprasellar or pineal regions) are frequently encountered in childhood. These lesions include optic glioma, craniopharyngioma, and germ cell tumors (i.e., germinoma, teratoma). Common posterior fossa tumors of childhood include medulloblastoma, cerebellar astrocytoma, brainstem glioma, and ependymoma. Rare intracranial tumors include sarcomas, meningeal tumors, and metastatic disease. Parameningeal tumors are those that arise extradurally and often directly invade the CNS. Common parameningeal tumors of childhood include neuroblastoma, histiocytosis, rhabdomyosarcoma, other sarcomas, PNET, leukemia, lymphoma, angiofibroma, and plexiform neurofibroma.

MRI is the procedure of choice for making an accurate diagnosis, developing a comprehensive treatment plan, evaluating disease progression, and assessing tumor response to treatment and its effects. Furthermore, the superior sensitivity of MRI makes it the definitive procedure for detecting tumors that are often occult to CT or US, particularly in unexplained focal seizure disorders, unexplained hydrocephalus, unexplained neuroendocrine disorders, and for cervicomedullary junction tumors and leptomeningeal neoplastic processes. MRI is also an important adjunct to CT in the evaluation of parameningeal or extradural tumors that encroach upon or invade the CNS. Craniospinal MRI with gadolinium enhancement is important for assessing tumor seeding, especially in medulloblastoma, germ cell tumors, and malignant glial tumors. Although MRI is sensitive to treatment effects, functional or metabolic imaging (e.g., SPECT, PET, MRS) may add specificity in differentiating radionecrosis from tumor progression.

Posterior reversible leukoencephalopathy (PRES) is an uncommon but serious complication of treatment in children with cancer, reported predominantly in patients with leukemia and non-Hodgkin lymphoma. These patients typically have risk factors such as hypertension, which, in the setting of prolonged exposure to remission induction chemotherapy and/or tacrolimus, may predispose them to PRES [17]. In addition, PRES may be seen with cyclosporine A therapy after transplantation. These lesions generally develop in the posterior parietal and occipital lobes and have increased diffusion relative to normal brain; in children, the anterior border-zone regions between the anterior cerebral artery and middle cerebral artery are frequently involved [7]. Atypical features in one series included restricted diffusion in 37.7% of 111 cases of PRES and hemorrhage in 17.1% of cases. The atypical manifestations do not correlate with edema severity [18].

Neoplastic diseases of the spine and spinal neuraxis may also be classified anatomically as extradural, intradural, or intramedullary. Extradural tumors may be relatively benign (e.g., aneurysmal bone cyst, osteoid osteoma, osteochondroma), or relatively malignant and invasive (e.g., neuroblastoma, PNET, sarcoma, histiocytosis). Bone scan imaging may provide superior sensitivity in detecting multiple lesions. Common intradural extramedullary neoplasms of childhood include schwannoma, neurofibroma, and seeding. Astrocytoma and ependymoma make up the majority of intramedullary tumors in children and are often associated with cysts or hydrosyringomyelia. Although CT may be indicated for single-level lesions (e.g., osteoid osteoma), MRI is recommended for the definitive evaluation of all spinal column and spinal neuraxis tumors. Spinal MRI is particularly indicated in children with atypical scoliosis when hydrosyringomyelia is demonstrated and a developmental cause (e.g., Chiari I malformation) must be distinguished from a neoplastic cause (e.g., astrocytoma) [19].

Congenital and Developmental Abnormalities

A review of the wide spectrum of congenital abnormalities is beyond the scope of this chapter; however, congenital abnormalities include anomalies of the corpus callosum, malformations of the cerebral cortical development, holoprosencephalies, Chiari malformations, Dandy Walker complex, non-syndromic and syndromic craniosynostosis/craniofacial anomalies, and chromosomal anomalies (e.g., Down syndrome, trisomies 13 and 18, fragile X syndrome) [1].

Malformations of cortical development have recently been updated by Barkovich et al. [1], whose classification is based on the point at which the earliest abnormal step occurs. Malformations with abnormal cell proliferation, migration, and organization are thus classified as arising from abnormal neuronal and glial proliferation or apoptosis. These include, but are not limited to, microcephaly, microlissencephaly, cortical hamartomas of tuberous sclerosis, cortical dysplasia with balloon cells, hemimegalencephaly and neoplasias with associated disordered cortex (e.g., dysembryoplastic neuroepithelial tumor, ganglioglioma, and gangliocytoma). Malformations that develop secondary to abnormal migration and organization are classified as arising from abnormal neuronal and cortical organization. These include, but are not limited to, lissencephaly/subcortical band heterotopia spectrum ; heterotopia (e.g., subependymal, subcortical, and marginal glioneuronal); polymicrogyria and schizencephaly ;and malformations secondary to metabolic disorders (e.g., mitochondrial, pyruvate, and peroxisomal disorders) [1].

Advanced imaging techniques such as diffusion tensor imaging have also been used to characterize white matter tracts in congenital brain malformations [8].

In spine disorders of the neural tube, closure can result in skin-covered abnormalities, such as lipomyelomeningocele or diastematomyelia, or open defects such as myelomeningocele. Although US is the initial screening procedure of choice for spinal neuraxis malformations in the fetus and in young infants, MRI is the definitive modality for diagnosis, surgical planning, and follow-up. CT is only occasionally needed in patients with metallic spinal instrumentation, since such artifacts often compromise MRI quality. Non-enhanced spinal CT, however, is often used for evaluating bony anatomy.

Metabolic and Neurodegenerative Disorders

Metabolic disorders, also known as inborn errors of metabolism, normally result from defects in single gene that code for enzymes facilitating conversion of one substance into another. Problems typically arise when substances toxic to the brain or which interfere with normal function accumulate, or when the ability to synthesize essential compounds is reduced or compromised. These disorders may manifest as non-specific clinical symptoms, such as seizures, spasticity, ataxia, movement disorder, or developmental delay.

Neurodegenerative disorders present clinically as progressive neurologic impairment in the absence of a CNS tumor or another identifiable process (e.g., infection). MRI is used to evaluate the disease extent and anatomic distribution. Additionally, MRS can provide specific metabolic characterization of some of these disorders. The final diagnosis is usually clinical, involving metabolic testing or biopsy of brain or muscle. Numerous classifications of metabolic and degenerative disorders have been described [1] and are beyond the scope of this chapter. Based on neuroimaging characteristics, these disorders can be classified as involving gray matter only, involving white matter only, or as involving a combination of gray and white matter.

Disorders primarily involving cortical gray matter include storage diseases arising from lysosomal enzyme defects such as lipidoses (e.g., GM1 gangliosidosis, neuronal ceroid lipofuscinoses) and mucolipidoses. Disorders primarily involving the corpus striatum (i.e., caudate and putamen) include mitochondrial disorders (e.g., Leigh disease, MELAS), organic acidopathies, and aminoacidopathies (e.g., glutaric aciduria), Wilson's disease, juvenile Huntington's disease, hypoxic-ischemic injury, and hypoglycemic injury. Disorders primarily involving the globus pallidus include Hallervorden-Spatz disease, methylmalonic acidemia, hyperbilirubinemia (i.e., kernicterus), and toxic exposure (e.g., carbon dioxide, manganese). Disorders primarily involving the white matter are known as leukoencephalopathies and include the peroxisomal disorders (e.g., adrenoleukodystrophies), the lysosomal leukodystrophies (e.g., metachromatic, globoid cell), and other white matter diseases (e.g., Pelizaeus-Merzbacher, Canavan, Alexander, and Cockayne diseases).

Certain metabolic disorders involve both gray and white matter. These are generally distinguished by: (1) the presence of cortical gray matter that is involved with normal bones *and* evidence of cortical dysgenesis (e.g., Fukyama congenital muscular dystrophy and Walker-Warburg syndrome); (2) the presence of cortical gray matter *only* and no evidence of cortical dysgenesis (e.g., Alpers and Menkes diseases); or (3) the presence of cortical gray matter that is involved with abnormal bones (e.g.,mucopolysaccharidoses, lipid storage, and peroxismal disorders). If deep gray matter is involved, the differential diagnosis depends on the nuclei involved.

Trauma

Pediatric head trauma is one of the leading causes of injury in childhood, with head injury a leading cause of mortality and morbidity in children [20].

Because CT can be rapidly delivered and is widely available and inexpensive, it remains the modality of choice for cranial imaging in acute trauma. Moreover, CT can accommodate life support equipment, traction, and monitoring devices and is easy to obtain in most pediatric emergency room and intensive care settings. It is especially useful in detecting acute or subacute hemorrhage, scalp injury, and pneumocephalus as well as other neurosurgically significant lesions, such as hydrocephalus, midline shift, masses and mass effect, ischemia, and herniation, all of which require rapid detection for proper management. CT is also helpful in diagnosing and evaluating linear skull fractures located outside of the scanning plane as well as depressed, basilar skull, and facial fractures. Limitations of CT center on the presence of beam-hardening streak artifact in the posterior fossa; patient motion; the effects of partial volume averaging; and poor detection and assessment of small extra-axial hematomas as well as the sequelae of head trauma, conditions that are better evaluated with MRI.

MR provides multi-planar capability and superior sensitivity in assessing the anatomy and function of the injured pediatric brain. MR with diffusion is the modality of choice for hypoxic-ischemic injury. On diffusion imaging, the measurement of lesion volume in a single series provides the strongest correlation with a score of sub-acute on a modified Rankin scale at discharge [21]. MRI is often reserved for circumstances in which neurologic deficits persist and the CT is negative or nonspecific (e.g., non-hemorrhagic lesions such as brainstem infarction, white matter shear injury, cortical contusion, gliosis, and microcystic encephalomalacia). MRI is often more specific than CT for hemorrhage beyond the acute or subacute stage. In evaluating the trauma patient, the use of susceptibility-weighted imaging (SWI), a 3D gradient echo MRI technique that offers high spatial resolution, has resulted in improved sensitivity in detecting blood products as well as hemorrhagic lesions [11]. Neurologic disability in children correlates with SWI studies that show the number and volume of hemorrhagic diffuse axonal injury (DAI) lesions and reduced levels of NAA [22]. In children with atypical intracranial hemorrhage (hemorrhage out of proportion to the history of trauma), MRI is also useful in detecting the existing vascular malformation, showing a hemorrhagic neoplasm, or suggesting child abuse, especially when there are hemorrhages of various ages.

In birth trauma, extracranial hemorrhage can include caput succedaneum, subgaleal hemorrhage, and cephalohematoma, as well as skull injury and intracranial injury, which can occur during delivery secondary to cephalopelvic disproportion, breech presentation, or from instrumentation involving forceps or vacuum extraction [20].

Owing to a softer and thinner calvarium, infants and young children (<5 years) are more susceptible to fractures than are older children and adults. CT or plain film is used for diagnosis. Leptomeningeal cyst is a unique lesion in pediatric patients that occurs as a delayed complication in approximately 0.05% to 1.6% of infants and children with skull fracture [23].

Beyond the acute phase when extra-axial and intra-axial hemorrhages (e.g., contusions, DAI, intracerebral hematomas) typically present, patients with traumatic injury may also develop sequelae that include vascular injury (e.g., arterial dissections, venous occlusions, and carotid-cavernous fistula), diffuse cerebral edema, hydrocephalus, hypoxic-ischemic injury, developmental delay, post-traumatic seizures, cognitive deficits, encephalomalacia, infection, cranial nerve injury, and pituitary/hypothalamic injury.

Child abuse is a global problem, with head trauma the leading cause of morbidity and mortality in abused children younger than 2 years of age. Non-accidental injury should be suspected in the infant or young child who presents with no history of injury; when there is a discrepancy between the explanation and nature of lesions; if there are injuries of various ages or multiple injuries; in associated retinal hemorrhages are detected; and/or if there is a change or inconsistency in the history, delay in medical care, repeated injuries, or overall poor care [24]. MRI is the modality of choice for determining the sequelae of injury that present as extra-axial hemorrhage, brain contusion, shear injury, and infarction. In addition, DWI has demonstrated increased sensitivity in the early detection of injury in children with non-accidental head trauma [25]. Patterns of involvement can be diffuse or localized to the parieto-occipital regions. MRI is more sensitive than CT or US in the detection of small hematomas and non-acute hematomas because of its multi-planar capabilities and lack of artifacts from the adjacent calvarium. Subdural collections may have areas of different density, intensity characteristics and levels, loculations, or septations on CT and MRI that indicate injuries of various ages. In addition, DWI has demonstrated increased sensitivity in the early detection of infarct in children with non-accidental head trauma [25]. Doppler US or MRI may distinguish external hydrocephalus (dilated subarachnoid spaces) from chronic subdural hematomas (e.g., in child abuse) when the CT demonstrates nonspecific extracerebral collections.

After initial evaluation of spine trauma with plain films and CT, radiological abnormality or changing clinical signs may indicate the need for additional imaging, i.e., MRI. Neurologic symptoms and signs out of proportion to the history of trauma should suggest an existing spinal anomaly (e.g., craniocervical anomaly) or tumor (e.g., pathologic fracture). MRI is used in acute trauma patients with progressive myelopathy or radiculopathy (e.g., intraspinal hemorrhage, cord contusion, ligamentous injury). It is also the procedure of choice for evaluating the sequelae of spinal cord trauma (e.g., syrinx, myelomalacia). SPECT imaging of the spinal column is particularly effective in delineating traumatic lesions (e.g., spondylolysis) that have not been previously identified with radiography.

Phakomatoses

The phakomatoses are malformations affecting structures of ectodermal origin [1]. These include neurofibromatosis, tuberous sclerosis, Sturge-Weber syndrome, von Hippel-Lindau disease, ataxia-telangiectasia, incontinentia pigmenti, neurocutaneous melanosis, epidermal nevus syndrome, hypomelanosis of Ito, basal cell nevus syndrome, and many others. Neurofibromatosis type 1 and 2, tuberous sclerosis, Sturge-Weber, and von Hippel-Lindau disease are discussed below.

Neurofibromatosis Type 1

Neurofibromatosis 1 (NF-1) is the most common of the phakomatoses. NF-1 is inherited as an autosomal dominant disorder with variable penetrance; it is caused by defects in the NF1 gene, located on chromosome 17, which is responsible for encoding the protein neurofibromin. This protein is a tumor suppressor that acts as a negative regulator of the Ras family GTPases. Patients with NF-1 typically present during the first decade of life. Cranial and intracranial manifestations inherent in NF-1 include white matter abnormalities, plexiform neurofibromas, and optic pathway gliomas as well as other astrocytomas, vascular dysplasias (e.g., stenoses, occlusions, moyamoya, aneurysms internal carotid dolichoectasia, AVM, and fistula), calvarial and orbital abnormalities (i.e., defects along the sphenoid wing and lambdoid suture), and neurofibromas and plexiform neurofibromas. NF1 spine patients may have scoliosis (i.e., nondystrophic vs. dystrophic) with or without kyphosis, dural ectasia, meningoceles (lateral), neurofibromas, and intramedullary tumors such as astrocytomas.

MRI studies have revealed a distinctive finding in children with NF-1 consisting of foci of hyperintense T2 signal intensity. These foci are not space-occupying and are typically located in the basal ganglia, internal capsule, brainstem, and cerebellum; they appear by 3 years of age, increasing in number and size until about 10-12 years of age, followed by a decrease during adolescence [26]. These lesions are thought to represent transient spongiotic intramyelinic vacuolization and may occur in myelin that is dysplastic [1, 27].

Neurofibromatosis Type 2

According to the NIH/NINDS, NF-2 is a rare disorder, affecting 1 in 40,000 people. NF-2 results from defects in the NF2 gene, located on chromosome 22q11. Patients with this disorder present with bilateral vestibular schwannomas, multiple cranial nerve schwannomas, meningiomas, and ependymomas. The mnemonic term MISME is used widely to refer to the disease, and is the acronym for the following anomalies: multiple inherited schwannomas, meningiomas, and ependymomas [28].

Vestibular schwannomas occur in the internal auditory canal or the porus acousticus. These tumors arise from Schwann cells, which form the myelin sheaths around the nerve root axons and are composed of Antoni A and Antoni B tissue, the composition of which is, respectively, dense and loose Vestibular schwannomas occur in 95% of adult patients with NF-2, at a mean age of 26 years [29]. On CT, these lesions are hypodense to isodense and may calcify. MRI evaluation of these patients requires thin sectioning through the posterior fossa. These tumors are hypointense on T1 images and hyperintense on T2 images. Homogeneous enhancement is present after administration of contrast material. When the lesion is large, the signal characteristics may be more heterogeneous, with necrosis or hemorrhage. Other schwannomas can involve the Vth and IXth-XIIth cranial nerves. The tumors vary in appearance from fusiform thickening of the nerve to a nodular mass; in addition, schwannomas can enlarge bony foramina.

Meningiomas can be multiple in patients with NF-2. These dural-based lesions are hyperdense on CT and avidly enhance after contrast. On MRI, they are isointense with gray matter on both T1- and T2-weighted images, but may cause displacement of the brain with associated hyperostosis or erosion of the skull. After gadolinium injection, they homogeneously enhance.

Tuberous Sclerosis

Tuberous sclerosis complex (TSC) is a multi-system genetic disease affecting 1-2 million individuals worldwide, according to the National Institutes of Health (NIH/NINDS). This complex is linked to mutations in TSC1 and TSC2, two genes located on chromosomes 9 and 16 that encode for hamartin and tuberin proteins, respectively. Neuroimaging findings in the brain include subependymal and cortical tubers, white matter lesions, subependymal giant cell astrocytoma, retinal hamartomas, and vascular dysplasias. The brain imaging findings in TSC result from a defect in the radial glial neuronal unit and may occur at any point, from a subependymal location to the cortex. The MRI intensities of subependymal nodules vary with age. During infancy, the lesions are typically T1 hyperintense and T2 hypointense. As the child ages, the lesions become isointense to white matter and are identifiable as calcified masses of variable size projecting into the ventricles. Contrast enhancement is usually mild. T2 or FLAIR hyperintense white matter lesions are also found in TSC and consist of either clusters of abnormal glial and neuronal cells or linear bands of unmyelinated fibers radiating outward from the ventricles [30]. Calcification may occur although enhancement is rare. Subependymal giant cell tumors occur in up to 10% of TSC patients. Imaging often shows an enhancing mass at the foramen of Monro with hydrocephalus. Cortical tubers consist of giant cells, disordered myelin, and gliosis. In early infancy, the lesions are CT hypodense, slightly T1 hyperintense, and T2 hypointense. With increasing age, the lesions tend to become CT isodense, T1 isointense, and T2 hyperintense. Calcification does occur but enhancement is rare.

Sturge-Weber Syndrome

Sturge-Weber syndrome, or encephalotrigeminal angiomatosis, is a neurocutaneous disorder characterized by low-flow vascular malformations of the face, globe, and leptomeninges. Most cases are sporadic although familial cases have been reported. A stereotypical "port-wine" facial nevus is almost always present and is usually unilateral, most often involving the ophthalmic division (V1) of the trigeminal nerve. Low-flow vascular malformations of the choroid of the globe are also present and may be associated with glaucoma or buphthalmos. The leptomeningeal capillary-venous malformation typically involves the parieto-occipital or temporal region and represents persistent primordial sinusoids with dysgenesis and/or thrombosis of the superficial venous system. Neurologic manifestations of the disease include seizures in up to 90% of patients, often presenting in infancy as infantile spasms or intractable epilepsy. The association of visceral, truncal, or extremity low-flow vascular malformations may be associated with the typical findings of Sturge-Weber syndrome and Klippel-Trenaunay-Weber syndrome.

Neuroimaging in Sturge-Weber syndrome is directed toward documenting the presence and extent of the pial malformation and its sequelae. Gadolinium-enhanced MRI provides the best demonstration of the extent of the pial vascular malformation. Enlarged medullary and subependymal veins are frequently present and the ipsilateral choroid plexus is often enlarged. Calcifications of the cortex underlying the pial anomaly are likely ischemic in origin, are frequently absent during infancy, and increase in frequency and extent with age. Gyriform calcific deposits, although best shown by CT, are also adequately depicted with T2 * gradient echo MRI. Atrophy of the involved hemisphere is usually evident with time. While angiography is rarely needed, it does demonstrate the absence of superficial cortical veins in the region of the capillary-venous malformation, with enlarged medullary and subependymal veins.

Von-Hippel Lindau Syndrome

Von Hippel-Lindau syndrome is an autosomal dominant disorder associated with retinal, cerebellar and spinal hemangioblastomas, pancreatic cysts, pheochromocytomas, renal cysts, endolymphatic cell tumors, and renal cell carcinoma. It is caused by a defect in the tumor suppressor gene on chromosome 3p25-p26. This is a rare disorder, seen in 1 of 30,000 live births according to the NIH/NINDS. Hemangioblastoma typically presents in the second decade of life.

Conclusions

With the introduction of ever more powerful and sophisticated imaging tools, particularly over the past decade, neuroimaging has evolved into a discrete radiological discipline that effectively detects, diagnoses, and evaluates numerous CNS diseases and disorders of childhood, both congenital and acquired. Increasingly, neuroimaging plays an important role in treatment planning, in evaluating disease progression, and in assessing treatment effects. Indeed, neuroradiologists are equipped, as never before, to assess CNS pathology with great acuity; understand underlying pathology; identify the characteristic imaging features of the various CNS diseases; and thus contribute to the clinical therapeutic options customized to the unique disease profile of each patient. With the spectacular advances in the way pediatric CNS disease is explored and examined, the neuroradiology community has growing confidence in the ability of these highly specialized imaging tools and techniques to diagnose and evaluate disease.

References

1. Barkovich AJ (2005) Pediatric neuroimaging. Lippincott Williams & Wilkins, Philadelphia
2. Veyrac C, Couture A, Saguintaah M, Baud C (2006) Brain ultrasonography in the premature infant. Pediatr Radiol 36:626-635
3. Daneman A, Epelman M, Blaser S, Jarrin JR (2006) Imaging of the brain in full-term neonates: does sonography still play a role? Pediatr Radiol 36:636-646
4. Bammer R (2003) Basic principles of diffusion-weighted imaging. Eur J Radiol 45:169-184
5. Roberts TP, Schwartz ES (2007) Principles and implementation of diffusion-weighted and diffusion tensor imaging. Pediatr Radiol 37:739-748
6. Mukherjee P, McKinstry RC (2006) Diffusion tensor imaging and tractography of human brain development. Neuroimaging Clin N Am 16:19-43, vii
7. Robertson RL, Glasier CM (2007) Diffusion-weighted imaging of the brain in infants and children. Pediatr Radiol 37:749-768
8. Rollins NK (2007) Clinical applications of diffusion tensor imaging and tractography in children. Pediatr Radiol 37:769-780
9. Medina LS, Bernal B, Dunoyer C et al (2005) Seizure disorders: functional MR imaging for diagnostic evaluation and surgical treatment – prospective study. Radiology 236:247-253
10. Zarifi MK, Astrakas LG, Poussaint TY et al (2002) Prediction of adverse outcome with cerebral lactate level and apparent diffusion coefficient in infants with perinatal asphyxia. Radiology 225:859-870
11. Tong KA, Ashwal S, Obenaus A et al (2007)Susceptibility-weighted MR imaging: a review of clinical applications in children. AJNR Am J Neuroradiol 29:9-17
12. Frieden IJ, Reese V, Cohen D (1996) PHACE syndrome. The association of posterior fossa brain malformations, hemangiomas, arterial anomalies, coarctation of the aorta and cardiac defects, and eye abnormalities. Arch Dermatol 132:307-311
13. Belman AL (1992) Acquired immunodeficiency syndrome and the child's central nervous system. Pediatr Clin N Am 39:691-714
14. Rodriguez DP, Poussaint TY (2007) Neuroimaging of the child with developmental delay. Top Magn Reson Imaging 18:75-92
15. Desprechins B, Stadnik T, Koerts G et al (1999) Use of diffusion-weighted MR imaging in differential diagnosis between intracerebral necrotic tumors and cerebral abscesses. AJNR Am J Neuroradiol 20:1252-1257
16. Poussaint TY (2001) Magnetic resonance imaging of pediatric brain tumors: state of the art. Top Magn Reson Imaging 12:411-433
17. Morris EB, Laningham FH, Sandlund JT, Khan RB (2007) Posterior reversible encephalopathy syndrome in children with cancer. Pediatr Blood Cancer 48:152-159
18. McKinney AM, Short J, Truwit CL et al (2007) Posterior reversible encephalopathy syndrome: incidence of atypical regions of involvement and imaging findings. AJR Am J Roentgenol 189:904-912
19. Barnes PD, Brody JD, Jaramillo D et al (1993) Atypical idiopathic scoliosis: MR imaging evaluation. Radiology 186:247-253
20. Poussaint TY, Moeller KK (2002) Imaging of pediatric head trauma. Neuroimaging Clin N Am 12:271-294, ix
21. Schaefer PW, Huisman TA, Sorensen AG et al (2004) Diffusion-weighted MR imaging in closed head injury: high correlation with initial Glasgow coma scale score and score on modified Rankin scale at discharge. Radiology 233:58-66
22. Ashwal S, Babikian T, Gardner-Nichols J et al (2006) Susceptibility-weighted imaging and proton magnetic resonance spectroscopy in assessment of outcome after pediatric traumatic brain injury. Arch Phys Med Rehabil 87:S50-S58
23. Ersahin Y, Gulmen V, Palali I, Mutluer S (2000) Growing skull fractures (craniocerebral erosion). Neurosurg Rev 23:139-144
24. Kleinman PK, Barnes PD (1998) Head trauma. In: Kleinman PK (ed) Diagnostic imaging of child abuse. Mosby, St. Louis, pp 285-342
25. Suh DY, Davis PC, Hopkins KL et al (2001) Nonaccidental pediatric head injury: diffusion-weighted imaging findings. Neurosurgery 49:309-318
26. Sevick RJ, Barkovich AJ, Edwards MS et al (1992) Evolution of white matter lesions in neurofibromatosis type 1: MR findings. AJR Am J Roentgenol 159:171-175
27. Di Paolo DP, Zimmerman RA, Rorke LB et al (1995) Neurofibromatosis type 1: pathologic substrate of high-signal-intensity foci in the brain. Radiology 195:721-724
28. Smirniotopoulos JG, Murphy FM (1992) The phakomatoses. AJNR Am J Neuroradiol 13:725-746
29. Parry DM, Eldridge R, Kaiser-Kupfer MI et al (1994) Neurofibromatosis 2 (NF2): clinical characteristics of 63 affected individuals and clinical evidence for heterogeneity. Am J Med Genet 52:450-461
30. Braffman B, Naidich TP (1994) The phakomatoses: Part I. Neurofibromatosis and tuberous sclerosis. Neuroimaging Clin N Am 4:299-324

Diseases of the Sella and Parasellar Region

Jean-François Bonneville[1], Walter Kucharczyk[2]

[1] Hôpital J. Minjoz, CHU Besançon, France
[2] University of Toronto, Toronto, Canada

Introduction

Pituitary adenomas are by far the most common pathology in the region of the sella turcica. Accordingly, a large part of this synopsis is devoted to them, while the remainder discusses other common lesions in this area. The emphasis is on imaging diagnosis and differential diagnosis.

Pituitary Adenomas

Magnetic resonance imaging (MRI) is usually the only imaging method needed for the morphological investigation of pituitary adenomas. Computed tomography (CT) is occasionally helpful to complement MRI examinations, as it better delineates the bony skull base, anatomic variants, calcification, and osseous malformations. Clinically, patients with microadenomas usually present with endocrine dysfunction. Rarely, the presence of these tumors may be a serendipitous discovery. On T1-weighted images, pituitary microadenomas are usually hypointense compared to the unaffected anterior pituitary gland, and round or oval in shape. In approximately 25% of cases, however, the adenoma is isointense on T1-weighted images. Pituitary microadenomas can also cause high signal intensity on T1-weighted images, probably due to internal hemorrhagic transformation of all or parts of the adenoma, a rather frequent phenomenon in prolactinomas. On T2-weighted images, the signal intensity of microadenomas typically resembles that of the temporal lobe cortex, i.e., slightly hyperintense compared to normal adenohypophysis, the intensity of which is close to that of white matter. The signal intensity on T2-weighted images varies, in particular, with the type of endocrine activity. The diagnosis of microadenomas is simple when they demonstrate high intensity on T2-weighted images, although this signal may only represent a part of the adenoma. Increased intensity on T2-weighted images is found in over 80% of microprolactinomas. Conversely, iso- or hypointensity on T2-weighted images occurs in two-thirds of all growth-hormone-secreting microadenomas. T2-weighted images are particularly helpful when looking for picoadenomas, for which T1-weighted images and even gadolinium-enhanced sequences are negative. When both the T1- and the T2-weighted images corroborate the diagnosis, which is the usual case with prolactinomas, gadolinium enhancement is unnecessary. When the diagnosis has not been established, enhanced imaging is mandatory. A half-dose of gadolinium-chelate (0.05 mmol/kg) is usually adequate. Contrast-enhanced images typically show a hypointense lesion surrounded by the intense enhancement of the normal pituitary gland, but even the contrast-enhanced images may be negative if the tumor is extremely small, the dose of gadolinium too high, or the visualization window too large. Delayed images taken 30-40 min after the injection of contrast medium may show late enhancement of the adenoma. Dynamic images are useful in the diagnosis of adenomas secreting adrenocorticotrophic hormone (ACTH), or they are used as a complementary investigation when clinical signs are strongly evocative of a pituitary adenoma, but conventional MRI results not convincing. Pituitary macroadenomas are intrasellar masses with extrasellar extension, which is usually upwards into the suprasellar cistern or laterally into the cavernous sinus. It is important to delineate this extension in relation to the various surrounding anatomical structures and to determine whether the tumor is likely to be firm, cystic, necrotic, or hemorrhagic, based on signal intensity and enhancement. Macroadenomas with suprasellar extension are often bi- or lobed in shape, with one or two extensions into the suprasellar cistern. Macroadenoma signal intensity is often inhomogeneous, particularly on T2-weighted images, with disseminated areas of hyperintensity reflecting cystic or necrotic portions of the adenoma. The adenomatous tissue usually enhances slightly after contrast-medium injection, but the object of enhanced imaging is to visualize normal pituitary tissue. It usually forms a strongly enhancing pseudocapsule around the adenoma: above it, behind it, rarely below or in front of it, and usually unilaterally. The coronal section of the enhanced T1-weighted image generally reveals a unilateral layer of normal pituitary tissue located between the adenoma and the elements of the cavernous sinus, of crucial importance to neurosurgeons. The hyperintense posterior lobe is modified: it appears either flattened or displaced and is well seen on the axial sections. Alternatively, an ectopic hyperintensity is located within the pituitary stalk, which is compressed by the superior pole of the macroadenoma. The pituitary stalk is tipped laterally. When the suprasellar extension is large, the chiasm itself may be difficult to identify. In such cases, T2-weighted coronal sections help because the optic chiasm is clearly hypointense. After gadolinium injection, discrete meningeal enhancement is usually noticeable near the area where the meninges are in contact with the adenoma, and particularly so in the anterior part of the posterior cranial fossa, along with a possible dural tail, which has previously been described with meningiomas. In our experience, the enhanced dura has no specificity whatsoever. Involvement of the cavernous sinus can modify the prognosis, but compression and invasion remain difficult to differentiate. The best sign of invasion is complete encircling of the intracavernous carotid by the tumor. Invasion can practically be eliminated if it can be demonstrated that a strip of normal pituitary tissue lies between the tumor and the cavernous sinus. Large pituitary adenomas can apply pressure onto the cavernous sinus and cause convex deformation of its external wall without necessarily involving it.

Other Considerations: Gender, Age, Hormone Secretion, Pregnancy

Prolactin-secreting microadenomas are common in young women. Some may spontaneously remain dormant over long periods. They do not develop after menopause. When prolactin-secreting adenomas are discovered in male patients, the tumors have usually reached the stage of macroadenomas. This is probably due to the fact that clinical signs are less obvious in men than in women, and to the fact that tumor development is probably different. Cavernous sinus involvement is far from exceptional. Pediatric pituitary adenomas are not only exceptional but also potentially active. Prolactin-secreting adenomas can be responsible for late puberty. Prolactinomas are usually discovered at the stage of microadenomas owing to the distinctive clinical signs occurring in young women, including amenorrhea, galactorrhea, and hyperprolactinemia (over 30-40 μg/l). Most of the time, the prolactinoma is hypointense on T1-weighted images, while it is hyperintense on T2-weighted images in four out of five cases. This high signal may only be exhibited by a portion of the adenoma. Correlation between prolactin levels and adenoma size is usually good. However, given two prolactinomas of equal size, the hypointense tumor on T2-weighted images secretes more than its counterpart. Medical treatment based on bromocriptine decreases adenoma volume drastically. As a result, diagnosis becomes difficult. We strongly recommend MRI documentation before instituting medical treatment. In some cases, when prolactinomas are imaged long after medical treatment with bromocriptine is started, peculiar scarred tissue is seen, which is evocative of a former pituitary adenoma. This is due to local remodeling of the pituitary gland, which forms a "V" on its superior aspect. While prolactinomas and growth hormone (GH)-secreting adenomas are usually located laterally in the sella turcica, ACTH-secreting adenomas in Cushing's disease, usually smaller in size, are more often located in the midline. Because of their severe prognosis and the surgical possibilities, ACTH-secreting lesions require the most detailed and exhaustive imaging. GH-secreting adenomas have the unique characteristic of exhibiting hypointensity on T2-weighted images in two-thirds of cases and are usually of the densely granulated subtype. Spontaneous infarction or necrosis of GH-secreting adenomas is far from exceptional. Some patients with acromegaly that was detected late in the course of the disease exhibited an enlarged, partially empty sella turcica, lined with adenomatous tissue that proved difficult to analyze. Medical treatment based on octreotride analogs (somatostatin) decreases the size of the adenoma by an average of 35% and brings the level of somatomedin C back to normal in 50% of patients. This therapeutic approach is useful before surgery. Macroadenomas can be nonfunctioning, but they can also be prolactin-secreting adenomas, gonadotrope adenomas, and growth hormone-secreting adenomas. The greater their size, the more heterogeneous they are, as areas of cystic necrosis are caused by poor tumoral blood supply. Gonadotrope adenomas are often massive and have a strong tendency to recur. Hemorrhage occurs in all or parts of 20% of all pituitary adenomas, but it is usually occult. Pituitary apoplexy, with the usual headache, pseudomeningeal syndrome, cranial nerve paralysis, and severe hypopituitarism, is generally caused by massive hemorrhage within a pituitary macroadenoma. Smaller-scale hemorrhage occurs much more often and can be seen within pituitary adenomas. Bromocriptine is held responsible, to a certain degree, for intratumoral hemorrhages in prolactinomas, although the phenomenon is sometimes revealed on MRI before treatment has been instituted. Recurrent hemorrhage is possible and can cause repeated headaches. Intratumoral hemorrhages are revealed by hyperintensity on the T1-weighted image, sometimes with a blood-fluid level in the mass. Normal pituitary tissue has a longer T1 in women during pregnancy. Normal pituitary tissue increases in height during pregnancy (0.08 mm per week, i.e. almost 3 mm during the course of pregnancy). Pituitary adenomas also increase in volume, especially prolactinomas. The increased volume of the prolactinoma is especially visible when medical treatment has been interrupted. Vision and tumor size should be closely monitored during this period.

Postoperative Sella Turcica and the Pituitary Gland

The surgical cavity is often filled with packing material after transphenoidal resection of a pituitary adenoma. Surgicel is frequently used and is impregnated with blood and secretions. The presence of packing material, secretions, and periadenomatous adhesions usually keeps the cavity from collapsing in the days and weeks that follow surgery. Blood, secretions, and packing material slowly involute over the following 2-3 months. Even after a few months, fragments of blood-impregnated Surgicel can still be found in the surgical cavity. If the diaphragm of the sella turcica is torn in the course of surgery, fat or muscle implants are inserted by the surgeon to prevent the occurrence of a cerebrospinal fluid fistula. Resorption of such implants takes much longer. Implanted fat involutes slowly and may exhibit hyperintensity on the T1-weighted image up to 2-3 years after surgery. Postoperative MRI 2-3 months after surgery is useful to monitor further development of a resected adenoma. An earlier MRI examination performed 48 h after surgery should be obtained to check for potential complications and to visualize any residual tumor, i.e., a mass of intensity identical to that of the adenoma before surgery that commonly occupies a peripheral portion of the adenoma. This early investigation is extremely helpful to interpret the follow-up MR images. At this stage, the remaining normal pituitary tissue can be characterized: it is usually asymmetrical, with a hyperintense area frequently observed at the base of the deviated hypophyseal stalk due to an ectopic collection of neurohypophyseal secretory vesicles. The 2-month follow-up MRI examination is essential to check for residual tumor. Late follow-up MRI, after 1-2 years or more, usually demonstrates adenoma recurrence as a rounded or convex mass that is isointense with the initial tumor.

3T MRI and Diffusion-Weighted Imaging of the Pituitary

The improved signal-to-noise (SNR) of 3T relative to 1.5T scanners can be traded-off for thinner image slices and smaller voxels, thereby offering improved spatial resolution at comparable SNR. Hence, some microadenomas may be detected at 3T that are invisible at 1.5T. Also, the cavernous sinus wall can be depicted more consistently. These facts have led us to preferentially schedule our pituitary exams on our 3T MRI. Fast spin-echo (FSE) T2-weighted images are especially useful. On the negative side of 3T imaging there are the issues of worse T1-weighting at 3T due to the lengthening of T1, greater motion artifacts, and exaggerated susceptibility effects. Diffusion-weighted imaging (DWI) and apparent diffusion coefficient (ADC) images have been employed in pituitary imaging as aids in determining tumor consistency, thereby aiding surgical planning. Early evidence suggests that soft adenomas with high cellularity and scant fibrous stroma have low ADCs, whereas firm adenomas with low cellularity and abundant fibrous stroma have high ADCs.

Craniopharyngioma

Craniopharyngiomas are epithelial-derived neoplasms that occur exclusively in the region of the sella turcica and suprasellar cistern or in the third ventricle. Craniopharyngiomas account for approximately 3% of all intracranial tumors and show no gender predominance. The tumors are hormonally inactive lesions. They have a bimodal age distribution; more than half occur in childhood or adolescence, with a peak incidence between 5 and 10 years of age, followed by a second, smaller peak in adults in the sixth decade. The tumors vary greatly in size, from a few millimeters to several centimeters in diameter. The epicenter of most is in the suprasellar cistern. Infrequently, the lesions are entirely within the sella or in the third ventricle. The majority of the discussions of craniopharyngiomas in the literature are confined to the most frequent form, the classic *adamantinomatous* type, but a distinct squamous or *papillary* type is becoming recognized with increasing frequency. Typically, the tumors are identified as suprasellar masses that occur in patients during the first two decades of life. These children most often present with symptoms and signs of increased intracranial pressure: headache, nausea, vomiting, and papilledema. Visual disturbances due to compression of the optic apparatus are also frequent but difficult to detect in young children. Other patients present with pituitary hypofunction because of compression of the pituitary gland, pituitary stalk, or hypothalamus. Occasionally, the lesions rupture into the subarachnoid space and evoke a chemical meningitis. Rarely, adamantinomatous craniopharyngiomas are found outside the suprasellar cistern, including in the posterior fossa, pineal region, third ventricle, and nasal cavity. Adamantinomatous tumors are almost always grossly cystic and usually have both solid and cystic components. Calcification is seen in the vast majority of these tumors. Extensive fibrosis and signs of inflammation are often found with the lesions, particularly when they are recurrent, so that they adhere to adjacent structures, including the vasculature at the base of the brain. Optic-tract edema on T2-weighted images is a common associated finding that is not usually seen with other suprasellar masses. The inflammatory and fibrotic nature of the lesions makes recurrence a not uncommon event, typically occurring within the first 5 years after surgery. The most characteristic MRI finding is a suprasellar mass that is itself heterogeneous but contains a cystic component that is well-defined, internally uniform, and hyperintense on both T1- and T2-weighted images. The lesions often encase the nearby cerebral vasculature. The solid portion, which is frequently partially calcified, is represented as the heterogeneous region. On rare occasions, the cyst is absent and the solid component is completely calcified. These calcified types of tumors can be entirely overlooked on MRI unless close scrutiny is paid to subtle distortion of the normal suprasellar anatomy. Contrast-medium administration causes a moderate degree of enhancement of the solid portion of the tumor, which otherwise may be difficult to see. Papillary craniopharyngiomas are typically found in the adult patient. These lesions are solid, without calcification, and often located within the third ventricle. Although surgery remains the definitive mode of therapy for all craniopharyngiomas, papillary variants are encapsulated and are readily separable from nearby structures and adjacent brain, so they are generally thought to recur much less frequently than the adamantinomatous type. On pathologic examination, papillary lesions do not show the features characteristic of the adamantinomatous variant. In papillary lesions, there is extensive squamous differentiation. Unlike their adamantinomatous counterpart, MRI shows papillary craniopharyngiomas as solid lesions. As noted previously, they are often situated within the third ventricle. These lesions demonstrate a non-specific signal intensity pattern, without the characteristic hyperintensity on T1-weighted images of the cystic component of adamantinomatous tumors. Like all craniopharyngiomas, papillary lesions typically enhance.

Rathke's Cleft Cyst

Symptomatic cysts of Rathke's cleft are less frequent than craniopharyngiomas, although they are a common incidental finding at autopsy. In a recent evaluation of 1000 non-selected autopsy specimens, 113 pituitary glands (11.3%) harbored incidental Rathke's cleft cysts. These cysts are predominantly intrasellar in location. Of the incidental Rathke's cysts > 2 mm in a large autopsy series, 89% were localized to the center of the gland, whereas the remaining 11% extended to show predominant lateral lesions. In that series, of all incidental pituitary lesions localized to the central part of the gland, 87% were Rathke's cysts. Others may be centered in the suprasellar cistern, usually midline and anterior to the stalk. Rathke's cysts are found in all age groups. They share a common origin with some craniopharyngiomas in that they are thought to originate from remnants of squamous epithelium from Rathke's cleft. The cyst wall is composed of a single cell layer of columnar, cuboidal, or squamous epithelium on a basement membrane. The epithelium is often ciliated and may contain goblet cells. The cyst contents are typically mucoid; less commonly, they are filled with serous fluid or desquamated cellular debris. Calcification in the cyst wall is rare. Most Rathke's cleft cysts are small, asymptomatic, and, as noted above, discovered only at autopsy. Symptoms occur if the cyst enlarges sufficiently to compress the pituitary gland or optic chiasm and, rarely, secondary to hemorrhage. The cysts with mucoid fluid are indistinguishable on MRI from cystic craniopharyngiomas: both are hyperintense on T1- and T2-weighted images. The serous cysts match the signal intensity of cerebrospinal fluid (CSF) and is the only subtype that has the typical imaging features of benign cysts. Those containing cellular debris pose the greatest difficulty in differential diagnosis, as they resemble solid nodules. The surgical approaches to Rathke's cleft cyst and craniopharyngioma differ. Because of infrequent postoperative recurrences, partial removal or aspiration is sufficient. Rathke's cleft cysts do not typically enhance. However, occasionally, there may be thin marginal enhancement of the cyst wall. This feature can be used to advantage to separate these cysts from craniopharyngiomas in difficult cases. CT may reveal calcification, frequently found in craniopharyngiomas, helping to distinguish the mass from a Rathke's cleft cyst.

Meningioma

Approximately 10% of meningiomas occur in the parasellar region. These tumors arise from a variety of locations around the sella, including the tuberculum sellae, clinoid processes, medial sphenoid wing, and cavernous sinus. Meningiomas are usually slow-growing lesions, with patients presenting because of symptoms related to compression of vital structures. Patients may suffer visual loss because of ophthalmoplegia due to cranial nerve involvement, proptosis due to venous congestion at the orbital apex, or compression of the optic nerves, chiasm, or optic tracts. Accurate differentiation between meningioma and pituitary adenoma is important because meningioma requires craniotomy, whereas a trans-sphenoidal route is preferred for removing most pituitary macroadenomas. Meningiomas are most frequently isointense relative to gray matter on unenhanced T1-weighted sequences, and less commonly hypointense. Approximately 50% remain isointense on the T2-weighted sequence, whereas 40% are hyperintense. Since there is little image contrast to distinguish meningiomas from brain parenchyma, indirect signs, such as a mass effect, thickening of the dura, buckling of adjacent white matter, white matter edema, and hyperostosis, are important diagnostic features. Other diagnostic signs include visualization of a cleft of CSF separating the tumor from the brain (thus denoting that the tumor has an extra-axial location) and a clear separation of the tumor from the pituitary gland (thus indicating that the tumor is not of pituitary-gland origin). The latter sign is particularly well-assessed on sagittal views of planum sphenoidale meningiomas. A peripheral black rim has been described on the edges of these meningiomas and is thought to be related to the surrounding veins. Hyperostosis and calcification are features that may be apparent on MRI but are better assessed with CT. Vascular encasement is not uncommon, particularly with meningiomas in the cavernous sinus. The pattern of encasement is of diagnostic value. Meningiomas commonly constrict the lumen of the encased vessel. This is rare with other tumors. As on CT, the intravenous administration of contrast medium markedly improves the visualization of basal meningiomas. They enhance intensely and homogeneously, often with a trailing edge of thick surrounding dura (the "dural tail sign").

Chiasmatic and Hypothalamic Gliomas

The distinction between chiasmatic and hypothalamic gliomas often depends on the predominant position of the lesion. In many cases, the origin of large gliomas cannot be definitively determined as the hypothalamus and chiasm are inseparable; therefore, hypothalamic and chiasmatic gliomas are discussed as a single entity. These tumors are for the most part tumors of childhood: 75% occur in the first decade of life. There is an equal prevalence in males and females. A definite association of optic nerve and chiasmatic gliomas with neurofibromatosis has been noted, more so for tumors that arise from the optic nerve rather than from the chiasm or hypothalamus. Tumors of chiasmal origin are also more aggressive than those originating from the optic nerves and tend to invade the hypothalamus and floor of the third ventricle and cause hydrocephalus. Patients suffer from monocular or binocular visual disturbances, hydrocephalus, or hypothalamic dysfunction. The appearance of the tumor depends on its position and direction of growth. It can be confined to either the chiasm or the hypothalamus; however, because of its slow growth, the tumor has usually attained a considerable size by the time of presentation and the site of origin is frequently conjectural. Smaller nerve and chiasmal tumors are visually distinct from the hypothalamus and their site of origin is more clear-cut. From the point of view of differential diagnosis, these smaller tumors can be difficult to distinguish from optic neuritis, which can also cause enlargement of the optic nerve. The clinical history is important in these patients (neuritis is painful, tumor is not) ; if necessary, interval follow- up of neuritis will demonstrate resolution of optic-nerve swelling. On T1-weighted images, the tumors are most often isointense while on T2-weighted images they are moderately hyperintense. Calcification and hemorrhage are not features of these gliomas but cysts are seen, particularly in the larger hypothalamic tumors. Contrast enhancement occurs in about half of all cases. Because of the tumor's known propensity to invade the brain along the optic radiations, T2-weighted images of the entire brain are necessary. This pattern of tumor extension is readily evident as hyperintensity on the T2- weighted image; however, patients with neurofibromatosis (NF) present a problem in differential diagnosis. This relates to a high incidence of benign cerebral hamartomas and atypical glial cell rests in NF that can exactly mimic glioma. Both appear as areas of high signal intensity on T2-weighted images within the optic radiations. Lack of interval growth and possibly the absence of contrast enhancement are more supportive of a diagnosis of hamartoma while enhancement suggests glioma.

Metastases

Symptomatic metastases to the pituitary gland are found in 1-5% of cancer patients. These are primarily patients with advanced disseminated malignancy, particularly breast and bronchogenic carcinoma. The vast majority die of their underlying disease before becoming symptomatic of pituitary disease. Autopsy series have demonstrated a much higher incidence of pituitary metastases, but these by and large are small and asymptomatic lesions. Intrasellar and juxtasellar metastases arise via hematogenous seeding to the pituitary gland and stalk, by CSF seeding, and by direct extension from head and neck neoplasms. There are no distinctive MRI characteristics of metastases, although bone destruction is a prominent feature of lesions that involve the base of the skull.

Infections

Infection in the suprasellar cistern and cavernous sinuses is usually part of a disseminated process, or occurs by means of intracranial extension of an extracranial infection. The basal meninges in and around the suprasellar cistern are susceptible to tuberculous and other forms of granulomatous meningitis. The cistern may also be the site of parasitic cysts, in particular cysticercosis. In infections of the cavernous sinus, many of which are accompanied by thrombophlebitis, the imaging findings on CT and MRI consist of a convex lateral contour to the affected cavernous sinus with evidence of a filling defect after contrast administration. The intracavernous portion of the internal carotid artery may also be narrowed secondary to surrounding inflammatory change. Infections of the actual pituitary gland are uncommon. Direct viral infection of the hypophysis has never been established and bacterial infections are unusual. There has been speculation that cases of acquired diabetes insipidus may be the result of a select viral infection of the hypothalamic supraoptic and paraventricular nuclei. Tuberculosis and syphilis, previously encountered in this anatomic region because of the higher general prevalence of these diseases in the population, are now rare. Gram-positive cocci are the most frequently identified organisms in pituitary abscesses. Pituitary abscesses usually occur in the presence of other sellar masses, such as pituitary adenomas, Rathke's cleft cysts, and craniopharyngiomas, indicating that these mass lesions function as predisposing factors to infection. The few reports on CT of pituitary abscesses indicate that the lesion is similar in appearance to an adenoma. As a result of the frequent coincidental occurrence of abscesses with adenomas, and because of their common clinical presentations, the correct preoperative diagnosis of abscess is difficult and rarely made. Non-contrast MRI demonstrates a sellar mass indistinguishable from an adenoma. With intravenous administration of contrast medium, there is rim enhancement of the mass with persistence of low intensity in the center.

Noninfectious Inflammatory Lesions

Lymphocytic hypophysitis is a rare, noninfectious inflammatory disorder of the pituitary gland. It occurs almost exclusively in women and particularly during late pregnancy or in the post-partum period. The diagnosis should be considered in a female patient who is in the peripartum period and has a pituitary mass, particularly when the degree of hypopituitarism is greater than that expected from the size of the mass. It is believed that, if untreated, the disease results in panhypopituitarism. Clinically, the patient complains of headache, visual loss, failure to resume menses, inability to lactate, or some combination thereof. Pituitary hormone levels are depressed. CT and MRI demonstrate diffuse enlargement of the anterior lobe without evidence of any focal abnormality or change in the internal characteristics of the gland. The distinction between simple pituitary hyperplasia and lymphocytic hypophysitis may be difficult by MRI alone, so clinical correlation is required in this setting. Sarcoid afflicting the hypothalamic-pituitary axis usually manifests itself clinically as diabetes insipidus or, occasionally, as a deficiency of one or more anterior lobe hormones. Low signal intensity on T2-weighted images is one finding that occurs in sarcoid with some frequency, but rarely in other diseases, with few exceptions (other granulomatous inflammatory diseases, lymphoma, some meningiomas). This low signal finding may aid in the differential diagnosis. Also, the presence of multiple, scattered intraparenchymal brain lesions should raise the possibility of the diagnosis, as should diffuse or multifocal lesions of the basal meninges. The latter are best defined on coronal contrast-enhanced T1-weighted images. Tolosa-Hunt syndrome (THS) refers to a painful ophthalmoplegia caused by an inflammatory lesion of the cavernous sinus; it is responsive to steroid therapy. Pathologically, the process is similar to orbital pseudotumor. Imaging in this disorder often shows normal findings, or they may be subtle, such as asymmetric enlargement of the cavernous sinus, enhancement of the prepontine cistern, or abnormal soft-tissue density in the orbital apex. The lesion resolves promptly with steroid therapy. Hypointensity on T2-weighted images may be observed; since this observation is uncommon in all but a few other diseases (e.g., meningioma, lymphoma, and sarcoid), it may be helpful in diagnosis. The clinical history allows further precision in establishing the differential diagnosis: meningioma does not respond to steroids while lymphoma and sarcoid have evidence of a primary disease elsewhere in almost all patients.

Vascular Lesions

Saccular aneurysms in the sella turcica and parasellar area arise from either the cavernous sinus portion of the carotid artery or its supraclinoid segment. These are extremely important lesions to identify correctly. Confusion with a solid tumor can lead to surgical catastrophes. Fortunately, their MRI appearance is distinctive and easily appreciated. Aneurysms are well-defined and lack any internal signal on spin-echo (SE) images, the so-called signal void created by rapidly flowing blood. This blood flow may also cause substantial artifacts on the image; these usually manifest as multiple ghosts in the phase-encoding direction, which in itself is a useful diagnostic sign. Thrombus in the aneurysm lumen fundamentally alters these characteristics, the clot usually appearing as multi-lamellated high signal on T1-weighted SE images, partially or completely filling the lumen. Hemosiderin may be visible in the adjacent brain, evident as a rim of low signal intensity on T2-weighted SE images, or on gradient echo (GE) images. If confusion exists as to the vascular nature of these lesions, MR angiography is used to confirm the diagnosis, define the neck of the aneurysm, and establish the relationship of the aneurysm to the major vessels. Carotid cavernous fistulas are abnormal communications between the carotid artery and cavernous sinus. Most cases are due to trauma; less frequently they are "spontaneous". These spontaneous cases are actually due to a variety of abnormalities, including atherosclerotic degeneration of the arterial wall, congenital defects in the media, or rupture of an internal carotid aneurysm within the cavernous sinus. Dural arteriovenous malformations of the cavernous sinus are another form of abnormal arteriovenous communication in this region. On MRI, dilatation of the venous structures, in particular the ophthalmic vein and cavernous sinus, is usually clearly visible. The intercavernous venous channels dilate in carotid cavernous fistulas and may also be seen on MRI. Furthermore, the internal character of the cavernous sinus is altered; definite flow channels become evident secondary to the arterial rates of flow within the sinus. The fistulous communication itself is most often occult on MRI. The pituitary gland has been noted to be prominent in cases of dural arteriovenous fistula without evidence of endocrine dysfunction. The exact mechanism of pituitary enlargement is not known, but venous congestion is a postulated cause. Cavernous hemangiomas are acquired lesions and not true malformations. However, there have been a few reports of extra-axial cavernous hemangiomas occurring in the suprasellar cistern. Of importance is that one of these hemangiomas did not have the features usually associated with, and so highly characteristic of, cavernous hemangiomas in the brain. The atypical appearance of extra-axial cavernous hemangiomas indicates that some caution must be exercised in the differential diagnosis of parasellar masses, because even though cavernous hemangiomas in this location are rare, failure of the surgeon to appreciate their vascular nature can lead to unanticipated hemorrhage. Cavernous hemangiomas should at least be considered in the differential diagnosis of solid suprasellar masses that do not have the classic features of more common lesions, in particular craniopharyngiomas or meningiomas. Furthermore, T2-weighted images should be a routine part of the MRI protocol for suprasellar masses because visualization of a peripheral dark rim may be the only sign of the nature of the lesion.

Other Conditions

Many other lesions may involve the sella turcica and parasellar region. These include mass lesions such as germinoma, epidermoid, dermoid, teratoma, schwannoma, chordoma, ecchordosis, choristoma, arachnoid cyst, hamartoma, and Langerhans cell histiocytosis. Also, there are several important metabolic conditions that may cause pituitary dysfunction or MRI-observable abnormalities in and around the sella; for example, diabetes insipidus, growth hormone deficiency, hemochromatosis, hypermagnesemia, and hypothyroidism.

Suggested Reading

Bonneville JF, Cattin F, Gorczyca W, Hardy J (1993) Pituitary micro-adenomas: early enhancement with dynamic CT-implications of arterial blood supply and potential importance. Radiology 187:857-861

Dietemann JL, Portha C, Cattin F et al (1983) CT follow-up of microprolactinomas during bromocriptine-induced pregnancy. Neuroradiology 25:133

Kucharczyk W, Peck WW, Kelly WM et al (1987) Rathke cleft cysts: CT, MR imaging and pathologic features. Radiology 165:491-495

Lum C, Kucharczyk W, MontaneraWJ (2002) The sella turcica and parasellar region. In: Atlas SW (ed) MRI of the brain and spine, 3rd ed. Lippincott Williams & Wilkins, Philadelphia, pp 625-667

Lundin P, Bergström K, Nyman R et al (1992) Macroprolactinomas: serial MR imaging in long term bromocriptine therapy. AJNR Am J Neuroradiol 13:1279-1291

Nagahata M, Hosoya T, Kayama T, Yamaguchi K (1998) Edema along the optic tract: a useful MR finding for the diagnosis of craniopharyngiomas. AJNR Am J Neuroradiol 19:1753-1757

Naylor MF, Scheithauer BW, Forbes GS et al (1995) Rathke cleft cyst: CT, MR, and pathology of 23 cases. J Comput Assist Tomogr 19(6):853-859

Oka H, Kawano N, Suwa T et al (1994) Radiological study of symptomatic Rathke's cleft cysts. Neurosurgery 35(4):632-636

Steiner E, Knosp E, Herold CJ et al (1992) Pituitary adenomas: findings of postoperative MR imaging. Radiology 185:521-527

Teramoto A, Hirakawa K, Sanno N, Osamura Y (1994) Incidental pituitary lesions in 1,000 unselected autopsy specimens. Radiology 193:161-164

Voelker J, Campbell R, Muller J (1991) Clinical, radiographic, and pathological features of symptomatic Rathke's cleft cysts. J Neurosurgery 74:535-544

Orbit and Visual Pathways

Bidyut K. Pramanik[1], David M. Yousem[2]

[1] New York University School of Medicine, New York, NY, USA
[2] Johns Hopkins Medical Institute, Baltimore, MD, USA

Computed tomography (CT) and magnetic resonance imaging (MRI) are excellent imaging modalities that have significantly enhanced orbital imaging in the diagnosis of ocular and orbital lesions. CT is excellent in the evaluation of the bony orbit and is the imaging modality of choice for most trauma situations. One of the most important roles played by CT is in the detection of calcification, which is crucial in the diagnosis of retinoblastoma. It is also the first choice in suspected orbital infection, especially from sinus disease. Also, orbital metallic foreign bodies are a contraindication to MRI. Rapid scanning allows for motion-free imaging and avoids the need for sedation in pediatric patients. However, it is also important to remember that CT imaging results in a radiation dose of 50 mGy to the lens. Most orbital lesions can be evaluated by CT; however, the increased spatial resolution of MRI allows better depiction of the globe, optic nerve, and orbital apex, and improved evaluation of the intracranial extension of disease. MRI differentiates among the various tissues based on signal characteristics and thus aids in differential diagnosis. Hence, it is the first choice in the diagnosis of most orbital pathologies.

Basic Orbital Anatomy

The orbit is a conical structure composed of seven bones. The major foramina of the orbit are the optic canal (OC), superior orbital fissure (SOF), and the inferior orbital fissure (IOF). The optic nerve (II) enters the orbit via the optic canal. The occulomotor (III), trochlear (IV), ophthalmic (V1), and abducens (VI) nerves exit the cavernous sinuses and enter the orbital apex via the SOF. The maxillary branch of the trigeminal nerve (V2) enters the orbit through the IOF. The orbital septum is a fibrous band that extends from the anterior orbital margin to the tarsal plates of the eyelids and serves as a limiting barrier to the spread of infectious or neoplastic processes from the subcutaneous tissues anterior to the septum and those located posteriorly.

The globe is spherical in shape and is composed of three layers: the sclera, choroid, and retina. The cornea is contiguous with the sclera and covers the anterior portion of the globe. The anterior segment lies between the cornea and the lens and is separated into an anterior and posterior chamber by the iris. Posterior to the lens is the posterior segment of the globe, which is filled with vitreous humor. The globe should not normally extend more than 21 mm anterior to the interzygomatic line. Extension beyond this point is defined as proptosis.

There are seven extra-ocular muscles: the superior, inferior, medial, and lateral rectus muscles originate at the annulus of Zinn and the optic foramen and insert on the globe. The superior and inferior oblique muscles have separate origins but also attach to the globe. The rectus and oblique muscles are responsible for positioning the eyes in all directions of gaze. The levator palpebrae muscle arises superior to the superior rectus muscle and inserts on the eyelid, which it elevates. The extra-ocular muscles avidly enhance secondary to their increased vascularity and necessity of rapid movement.

A fascial sheath encompasses the four rectus muscles and for radiographic purposes serves as a useful landmark in categorizing and formulating a differential diagnosis. Hence, lesions are classified as conal, intraconal, or extraconal.

The major vascular structures to identify in the orbit are the ophthalmic artery and the superior ophthalmic vein. The ophthalmic artery enters the orbit via the optic canal just beneath the optic nerve and may cross over to run over the nerve. The superior ophthalmic vein has a tortuous course, running anteromedial to posterolateral. Along its midpoint it becomes intraconal and runs under the superior rectus muscle. Posteriorly, it enters the superior orbital fissure and then drains into the cavernous sinus.

The optic nerve is an extension of the central nervous system (CNS). The optic nerves extend from the optic chiasm through the optic canal to the posterior globe. The optic nerve is surrounded by cerebrospinal fluid (CSF) which is contiguous with the subarachnoid space. A dural membrane surrounds the optic nerve and CSF. The nerve is approximately 50 mm long and tends to run in a sinusoidal configuration within the intraconal space. The nerve is divided into four segments: intraocular, intraorbital, intracanicular, and intracranial. The optic tracts extend from the optic chiasm to the anterior portion of the midbrain before terminating at the lateral geniculate body of the thalamus.

Orbital Pathology

Ocular Lesions

Retinoblastoma is the most common intraocular tumor of childhood. It typically presents by 5 years of age with equal frequency in males and females. Patients present with leukocoria (white reflex) on fundoscopic exam. The major diagnostic considerations in patients with leukocoria are retinoblastoma, persistent hyperplastic primary vitreous, retinopathy of prematurity, Coats disease, and toxocariasis. Retinoblastoma may present in a sporadic or familial form. The familial form is autosomal dominant. Retinoblastoma occurs as a result of a mutation in the tumor suppressor oncogene (Rb1) located on chromosome 13q14. Hereditary retinoblastoma presents as bilateral disease in 85% and as unilateral disease in 15% of patients. Those with the hereditary form are also at a lifelong risk of developing a second malignancy. In the majority of cases, the disease is sporadic and unilateral. Pineal gland tumors, typically pineoblastomas, associated with bilateral retinoblastomas are termed "trilateral" retinoblasotomas.

CT is best for demonstrating the characteristic calcifications on the posterior segment of the globe with extension into the vitreous, which maybe seen in up to 95% of patients. Calcifications maybe be punctuate or diffuse. MRI is better in assessing extra-ocular and intracranial spread of disease. On MRI, retinoblastoma demonstrates intermediate to mildly hyperintensity on T1, hypointensity on T2, and moderate enhancement.

Early diagnosis is the key. The prognosis for intraocular retinoblastoma is excellent, with a 90% cure rate. When the disease extends beyond the eye, mortality approaches 100%. Recent advances have limited the need for radiation therapy. Currently, chemotherapy is the first-line therapy.

Ocular melanoma is the most common primary intraocular malignancy in adults. Choroidal melanoma (85%) accounts for the vast majority of cases while ciliary-body and iris melanomas account for 10 and 5%, respectively. Patients typically present with painless visual disturbance and the tumor is often discovered on routine eye exam. Ocular melanomas are rare in individuals of African descent and uncommon in Asians. Congenital melanosis, ocular melanocytosis, ocudermal melanocytosis, and uveal nevi are conditions that may predispose to uveal melanoma.

On non-contrast CT, uveal melanomas are well-circumscribed hyperdense masses that avidly enhance with contrast administration. Calcifications are rare. The MRI characteristics of melanotic melanomas are related to the paramagnetic properties of melanin. Most uveal melanomas appear as areas of hyperintense signal on T1-weighted images and hypointense on T2-weighted images. Uveal melanomas demonstrate moderate enhancement. Exudative or hemorrhagic retinal detachment may be present, in which case the enhancement separates the tumor from the retinal detachment.

Ocular metastases in adults, like ocular melanomas, also primarily involve the uveal tract; thus, clinically and radiographically they can be confused with ocular melanomas. Uveal metastases, unlike melanomas, which form a protrubent mass, typically are diffuse and cause little increase in uveal thickness. They typically occur in the posterior half of the globe. The most common source is lung and breast cancer. The MRI signal characteristics of uveal metastases are similar to those of melanoma.

Retrobulbar Lesions

Optic nerve lesions encompass a wide spectrum of disease entities, including inflammatory/infectious processes as well as primary and secondary neoplastic lesions.

Optic neuritis is an inflammatory disorder of the optic nerve that typically afflicts young adults, who may present with pain, decreased visual acuity, abnormal color vision, and/or afferent papillary defect (APD). The disease is rare in children. It is the initial manifestation in 15-20% of patients who present with multiple sclerosis (MS) and maybe seen in up to 87% of MS patients. CT may demonstrate mild optic nerve enlargement and contrast enhancement. MRI is the best imaging modality to evaluate optic neuritis. It is able to evaluate the optic nerve, chiasm, and white matter. MRI findings include mild nerve enlargement, increased T2-weighted signal abnormality, and enhancement with gadolinium. The increased T2-weighted signal is the result of perivenous inflammation, which may be seen in approximately 50% of patients. Plaques can occur at the optic nerve head, intraorbital segment, intracanalicularly, or in the intracranial portions of the optic nerve.

Optic neuritis can also result from ischemia, sarcoid, systemic lupus erythematosus, syphilis, viral infection, toxoplasmosis, tuberculosis, and radiation therapy. Sarcoid involves the CNS in 5% of cases. Isolated involvement of the optic nerve is uncommon. Sarcoid granulomas cause enlargement of the optic nerve or chiasm and are associated with avid enhancement. Radiation-induced optic neuritis is suggested if a patient suffers from visual loss after radiation treatment. The average time for acute radiation-induced optic neuropathy ranges from 6 to 18 months after treatment with a total radiation dose >50 Gy. MRI demonstrates swelling and enhancement of the optic nerve or chiasm as well as occasional necrosis.

The most common optic nerve tumor is the *optic nerve glioma*, which is classified as a juvenile pilocytic astrocytoma. Optic nerve gliomas occur predominately within children and have a mean age of presentation of 8.5 years. The tumors tend to grow slowly during childhood and then stabilize. Malignant transformation is rare. Up to

70% of optic nerve gliomas are associated with neurofibromatosis (NF) I. Optic nerve gliomas most commonly affect the orbital segment of the optic nerve; in approximately 25% of patients both the orbital and intracranial segments of the optic nerve are affected. Optic nerve gliomas may have an associated cyst, resulting from ischemia, radiation therapy, or mucin deposition, which may cause nerve kinking. Typically, patients present with strabismus, visual loss, and APD followed by proptosis. CT demonstrates an enlarged optic nerve with variable enhancement. Calcification is rare. MRI is the imaging modality of choice and demonstrates hypointense T1- and hyperintense T2-weighted signal. The enhancement patterns vary from no enhancement to avid enhancement. Patients who have NF-1 may demonstrate dilation of the subarachnoid space around the optic nerve, which is termed arachnoidal gliomatosis. Optic nerve gliomas may extend posteriorly to involve the chiasm and optic tracts but less likely involve the optic radiations.

A rare form of malignant optic nerve glioma exists in adults and is distinct from the benign optic glioma of childhood. This adult form has a peak incidence between the ages of 40 and 50 and is more prevalent in males. Histologically, these tumors are anaplastic astrocytomas or glioblastoma multiforme. The adult optic nerve glioma tends to be associated with rapid loss of vision. It is usually bilateral and predominately involves the intracranial optic nerves and chiasm, with secondary extension to the hypothalamus, optic radiations, and third ventricle. The overall prognosis is poor, with death within one year.

Optic nerve meningiomas are the second most common primary optic nerve tumor. They may originate primarily from the meninges along the orbital segment of the optic nerve or may extend secondarily into the orbit from the intracranial meninges. Optic nerve meningiomas most commonly occur in middle-aged women but can occur at any age. Patients present with gradual progressive loss of vision, axial proptosis, disc edema, and pallor.

Approximately 12% of optic nerve meningiomas will contain calcifications; meningiomas near the bony apex may induce adjacent hyperostosis. Contrast enhancement of meningioma of the optic nerve sheath is intense and the tubular pattern of enhancement together with the central non-enhancing optic nerve is referred to as the "tram-track" sign.

Graves disease is a term that is best replaced with thyroid orbitopathy or thyroid eye disease (TED), to indicate that the patient may be of any hormonal state, be it hyperthyroid, hypothyroid, or euthyroid, at the time or orbital manifestations. The most common clinical manifestations of the disease are proptosis and an exposed cornea, leading to keratopathy. On imaging the findings include an increase in total orbital fat, proptosis, and enlargement of the bellies of the extraocular muscles. In the latter, the medial and inferior rectus muscles are most commonly involved, but any muscle may be affected. The retrobulbar fat may be edematous and there may be orbital apex compression of arteries and/or veins, leading to ischemic optic neuropathy syndromes or dilatation of venous structures due to outflow obstruction.

Classically, TED is not associated with pain or chemosis and therefore should not be difficulty to distinguish from *pseudotumor of the orbit*, also referred to as idiopathic granulomatous inflammation of the orbit. From an imaging standpoint, the tendons of the muscles are usually spared with TED whereas they may be involved with pseudotumor.

Pseudotumor is unique in that it can affect nearly every portion of the orbit, from the sclera to the eyelids, lacrymal apparatus muscles, optic nerves and/or sheath, and fat. Because of the associated redness and irritation, pseudotumor may be hard to distinguish clinically from orbital or periorbital cellulitis. However, the distinction is critical since pseudotumor is treated with steroids whereas cellulitis is exacerbated by steroids and is treated with antibiotics. Since sinusitis or skin infections or trauma are the most common precipitants of orbital infections, their presence may lead to the preferential diagnosis of cellulitis. Also, pseudotumor does not lead to abscess collections.

Vascular Lesions

Just as the vascular lesions elsewhere in the neck have become confusing because of the blurring of distinctions between hemangiomas (a true proliferating and involuting neoplasm) and slow-flow vascular malformations, so too are the vascular lesions of the orbit. The classic *orbital hemangioma (cavernous hemangiomas)* likely is a venous vascular malformation that may be associated with phleboliths and will not regress with age. These usually present in middle-aged women as a retrobulbar intraconal mass. This is unlike the classic capillary hemangiomas, which are childhood and adolescent phenomena that usually become smaller into adulthood. Venous vascular malformations, like venous varices, will enlarge with Valsalva maneuvers or any procedure that increases venous outflow pressure. Even cavernous carotid fistulae (vida infra) may enlarge with such maneuvers.

Orbital hemangiomas are the most common "tumors" of the orbit and are rarely seen outside the intraconal compartment. That said, the combination of lymphangiomas with venous vascular malformations is distinguished by the possibility of extraconal growth and presentation. The lymphatic vascular malformations often have fluid-fluid levels and may be bright on T1-weighted scans due to their high protein or blood content. Lymphangiomas are associated with Turner syndrome, Noonan syndrome, and fetal alcohol syndrome.

Hemangiopericytomas are more aggressive lesions that can infiltrate the orbit in a multi-compartmental fashion. They must be treated more aggressively.

Cavernous carotid fistulae (CCF) are most commonly due to traumatic injury to the orbits. Type I CCF are the most common forms and are associated with a single-hole direct communication between the cavernous carotid artery and the cavernous sinus. Arterial pressure is transmitted to the sinus and then to the draining veins, accounting for the classic enlargement of the superior (and inferior) ophthalmic veins of the orbit, with pulsating proptosis, an orbital bruit, glaucoma, and congestion. Treatment may be either via an arterial or a venous approach and may be accomplished via direct punctures or endovascular means. Plugging a single-hole CCF with balloons and/or coils is usually successful. Because of the risk of ischemic or compressive optic neuropathy, single-hole CCF are usually treated rather than watched. Carotid massage at home to induce "spontaneous" closure may also be an option.

More complicated treatments are required when there are multiple direct connections between the arteries of the internal and/or external carotid artery to the cavernous sinus or if there is a true nidus and dural arteriovenous malformation, which may be supplied by external and internal carotid feeders. These are usually congenital rather than post-traumatic. CCF may also occur when a cavernous carotid aneurysm ruptures into the cavernous sinus.

Trauma

All parts of the orbit may be subjected to traumatic injury. Most commonly seen are fractures of the walls of the orbit, with the orbital floor and medial orbital wall most commonly affected. The significance of describing entrapment of muscles with these injuries lies in the persistence of diplopia when the muscles are prevented from normal motility and for the potential for scarring, leading to permanent malpositioning. These fractures are usually accompanied by soft-tissue swelling and/or fluid levels in the maxillary and ethmoid sinus for floor and medial wall fractures, respectively.

The globe may also be traumatized from either blunt or penetrating trauma. Hemorrhage in the anterior chamber of the globe is called an anterior hyphema and is considered a type of globe rupture. This is seen as increased density to the space anterior to the lens of the eye. Radiology rarely diagnoses posterior chamber hemorrhage (posterior hyphema), which is different than vitreous hemorrhage in which the large chamber behind the lens is ruptured and may be hyperattenuated. Even less commonly seen is a detachment of either the retina or choroids, findings that may be present with neoplastic, inflammatory, or degenerative conditions.

Globe hypotony is the term used when the shape of the globe is flattened due to rupture. Other traumatic events include traumatic cataract or lens dislocation, which may be noted acutely as an abnormal density of the lens, which itself may be dislodged into an abnormal location.

The mnemonic "Vitamin C and D" provides the differential.

- Vascular (varix and hemangioma)
- Infectious (subperiosteal abscess and orbital cellulitis)
- Traumatic (hyphema, detachments)
- Acquired (thyroid eye disease, sphenoid wing dysplasia)
- Metabolic (thyroid eye disease)
- Idiopathic (sarcoidosis, Devic syndrome)
- Neoplastic (retinoblastoma, melanoma, perineural spread, optic nerve meningioma)
- Congenital (coloboma, septo-optic dysplasia, retinoblastoma, NFBT)
- Drugs

Suggested Reading

Ansari SA, Mafee MF (2005) Orbital cavernous hemangioma: role of imaging. Neuroimaging Clin N Am 15(1):137-158

Chung EM, Specht CS, Schroeder JW (2007) From the archives of the AFIP: pediatric orbit tumors and tumor-like lesions: neuroepithelial lesions of the ocular globe and optic nerve. Radiographics (4):1159-1186

Kapur R, Mafee MF, Lamba R, Edward DP (2005) Orbital schwannoma and neurofibroma: role of imaging. Neuroimaging Clin N Am 15(1):159-174

Mafee MF, Ainbinder D, Afshani E, Mafee RF (1996) The eye. Neuroimaging Clin N Am 6(1):29-59

Mafee MF, Dorodi S, Pai E (1999) Sarcoidosis of the eye, orbit, and central nervous system. Role of MR imaging. Radiol Clin North Am 37(1):73-87

Mafee MF, Inoue Y, Mafee RF (1996) Ocular and orbital imaging. Neuroimaging Clin N Am 6(2):291-318

Tan WS, Wilbur AC, Mafee MF (1987) The role of the neuroradiologist in vascular disorders involving the orbit. Radiol Clin North Am 25(4):849-861

Wenig BM, Mafee MF, Ghosh L (1998) Fibro-osseous, osseous, and cartilaginous lesions of the orbit and paraorbital region. Correlative clinicopathologic and radiographic features, including the diagnostic role of CT and MR imaging. Radiol Clin North Am 36(6):1241-1259

Temporal Bone and Auditory Pathways

Jan W. Casselman

Department of Radiology, AZ Sint-Jan AV, Brugge, Belgium

Anatomy

Today, the anatomy of the temporal bone can be evaluated in detail. Computed tomography (CT) is the method of choice to examine the external ear and middle ear. New CT devices that include helical scanning and multi-detector technology enable scanning of the temporal bone in detail. Once the images are obtained, they can be recalculated at slice thicknesses as low as 0.1 mm. On these very thin images, partial volume effects are no longer a problem and hence even very tiny structures can be seen. Moreover, excellent multi-planar reconstructions are also possible. Structures such as the branches and footplate of the stapes and the chorda tympani can now be reliably evaluated. Magnetic resonance (MR), especially T2-weighted gradient-echo (CISS) or turbo spin-echo (DRIVE, FSE, FIESTA), is used to study the inner ear. These approaches reveal the intra-labyrinthine fluid as well as the scala tympani and vestibuli separately inside the cochlea. Another advantage is that the facial nerve and the cochlear as well as the inferior and superior vestibular branches of the VIIIth cranial nerve can all be distinguished on these images. Even the posterior ampullar nerve and the ganglion of Scarpa can be identified on 0.7-mm-thick images made every 0.35 mm using a 1024 matrix (Fig. 1).

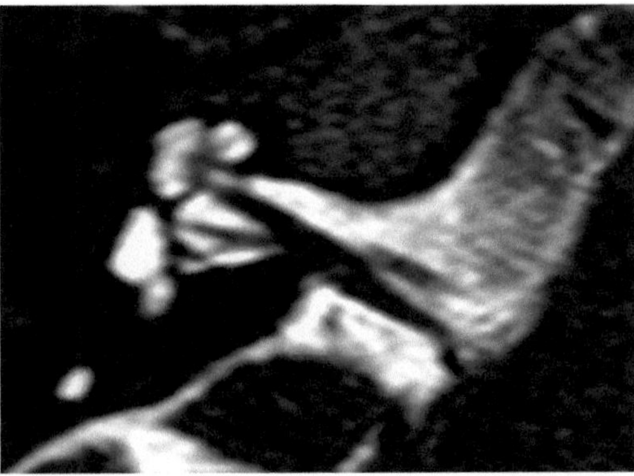

Fig. 1. This 1024 matrix 0.7-mm-thick DRIVE image shows the posterior ampullar nerve, originating from the posterior wall of the inferior vestibular nerve, and separation of the scala vestibuli and tympani inside the cochlea

MR is also the only technique that allows the visualization of lesions along the auditory pathway. Selective images through the cochlear nuclei, trapezoid body, lateral lemniscus, inferior colliculus, medial geniculate body, and auditory cortex often permit detection of the cause of deafness when selective CT and MR studies of the temporal bone are negative.

When To Use CT vs. MR

As a general rule, patients with conductive hearing loss (CHL) should be examined with CT, while those presenting with sensorineural hearing loss (SNHL), vertigo, or tinnitus should immediately be studied by MR imaging. There are, of course, exceptions and in many cases both CT and MR evaluations can contribute to making the proper diagnosis. In the following, the most frequent indications, including the choice between CT and MR, for imaging of the temporal bone are discussed.

Pathology

Otosclerosis

In otosclerosis, the dense layer of ivory-like endochondral bone that surrounds the labyrinthine capsule is replaced by foci of spongy, vascular, irregular new bone. The cause of this replacement is still under discussion. Although patients with otosclerosis present with mixed hearing loss, the conductive component is most often predominant and the lesions are often only visible on CT, making this imaging modality the method of choice. Otosclerosis/otospongiosis can be fenestral and retrofenestral. In fenestral otosclerosis, the promontory, facial nerve canal, and oval and round windows are involved. The most frequent lesion is seen as a hypodensity or even hypodense mass at the fissula antefenestrum. Similar lesions can also occur on the promontory or at the round window. At the level of the oval window, otospongiosis can block the anterior branch of the stapes, so that it can no longer move freely, thus causing CHL. Thickening of the footplate can also occur and has the same

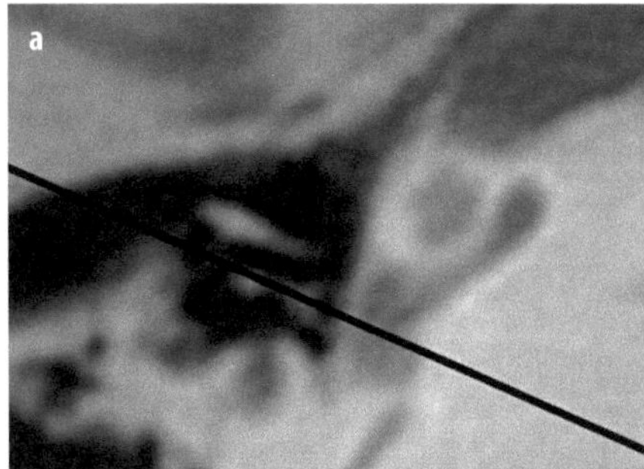

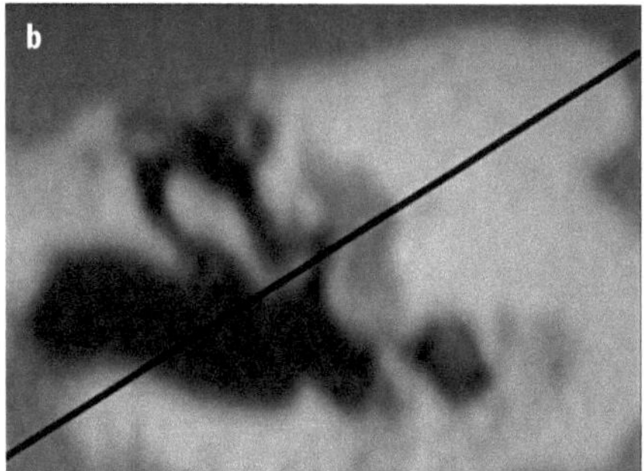

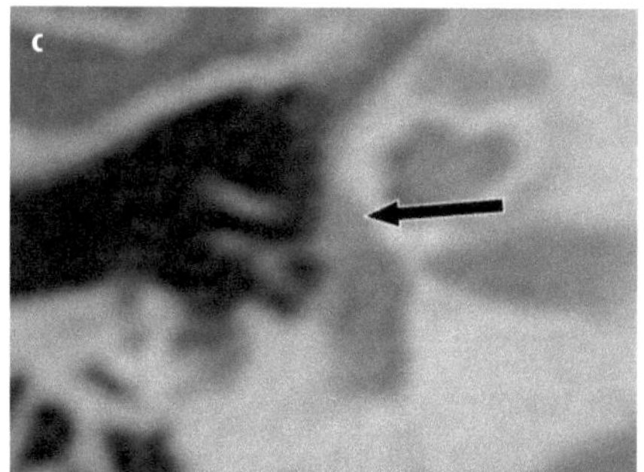

Fig. 2 a-c. **a** The only reliable way to evaluate fenestral otosclerosis is the double-oblique technique. **b** Paracoronal images are made on the axial image through the stapes. Double-oblique images are obtained when a reconstruction that lies parallel to the incudostapedial junction, as seen on the paracoronal images, is made. **c** The double-oblique image clearly shows otospongiosis at the fissula antefenestrum, encasing the anterior branch of the stapes (*arrow*)

result. The lesions near the footplate are difficult to visualize such that a double-oblique technique is required to image both branches of the stapes and the footplate in one plane (Fig. 2). Accordingly, helical acquired images should be reconstructed every 0.1 mm so that double-oblique images with sufficient quality are obtained. The round window should always be checked, as some studies have shown that surgery of the stapes and oval window are less successful when the round window is obliterated.

Retrofenestral otosclerosis involves the cochlea or the bone around the membranous labyrinth (with the exception of the lateral wall of the labyrinth). A hypodense ring, the "fourth ring of Valvassori", can develop around the complete cochlea. However, the lesions can also be more subtle and frequently a small hypodense spur can be seen anterior to the antero-inferior wall of the fundus of the internal auditory canal.

Trauma

Fractures of the temporal bone can best be seen on CT. Both longitudinal and transverse fractures can be distinguished. Longitudinal fractures follow the long axis of the temporal bone, from the surface of the petrous-mastoid bone to the middle-ear cavity and geniculate ganglion area and even the petrous apex. In transverse fractures, the fracture runs perpendicular to the long axis of the petrous bone and petrous apex and hence nearly always involves the inner ear! Post-traumatic CHL is most often explained by the CT findings and post-traumatic obliteration of the middle-ear cavity and/or fractures or luxation of the ossicles can easily be recognized on CT. However, CT cannot always explain post-traumatic SNHL and/or facial nerve palsy. In these cases, MR of the temporal bone often provides the answer, but CT is and remains the most important and first study in case of trauma.

Un-enhanced T1-weighted images must be used to recognize post-traumatic intralabyrinthine hemorrhage, which represents a concussion of the inner ear. Cloth or fibrosis formation in the labyrinth can be excluded using thin T2-weighted images (DRIVE, CISS, FIESTA). The normally high signal intensity of the fluid will disappear if fibrosis or cloth formation is present but remains when the fluid is mixed with fresh blood. Post-traumatic intralabyrinthine enhancement may also be seen. When the trauma causes a leak of intralabyrinthine fluid towards the middle ear, then the inner ear will react with higher fluid production to compensate the loss. This results in hyperemia of the labyrinth, which during the acute phase is sometimes seen as enhancement.

Fractures through the tegmen can result in meningocele or encephalocele formation. Blood or inflammation in the middle ear can only be distinguished reliably from meningo- or encephalocele formation by MR imaging.

Finally, the cause of the hearing loss may be located along the auditory pathways. The structures most frequently involved in trauma are the inferior colliculi (concussion when they are hit by the free edge of the tentorium during trauma) and the auditory cortex (hit by overlying bone or concussion/bleeding caused by the contrecoup). Again, these lesions, or their full extent, are often only visible on MR images.

Facial nerve palsy is not always caused by a fracture running through the facial nerve canal (e.g., tympanic segment); therefore, CT may remain normal in patients with post-traumatic facial nerve palsy. The labyrinthine segment of the nerve is very vulnerable because it occupies 95% of the available space of the canal. Hence, retrograde edema can easily cause compression and secondary necrosis of this facial nerve segment. This can be seen as enhancement of both the labyrinthine segment and near the fundus of the internal auditory canal – a finding that is always abnormal. In such cases, decompression of the nerve should be considered in order to save the facial nerve.

Chronic Inflammation of the Middle Ear

In chronic inflammation of the middle ear, aeration is often disturbed and hence the ear drum is frequently retracted and thickened. Moreover, mucosal thickening or even opacification of the middle-ear cavity by fluid and or glue-like thickened material can be present. Chronic infection may cause demineralization of the ossicles, and traction on the ossicles can even cause their luxation; however, their clear destruction or displacement is not seen. Middle-ear inflammation often follows the paths of pre-existing structures, such as the plicae and ligaments forming the tympanic diaphragm. Therefore, when middle-ear obliteration suddenly stops at these sites, forming a straight barrier with the aerated part of the rest of the middle ear, then the diagnosis is almost always inflammation. If the complete middle ear and mastoid are opacified, then the diagnosis is more difficult. In this case, a small cholesteatoma may be hidden somewhere in the inflamed structure(s). In these patients one should carefully check whether the bony septae between the mastoid and antral aerated cells are intact. If they are, then inflammation can be strongly suspected; if they are not, then cholesteatoma is the likely diagnosis. Comparison of the bony septae of the two ears helps in the detection of an underlying cholesteatoma. If the thickened drum or inflammatory tissue in the middle ear has calcified, then one is dealing with tympanosclerosis. Clearly, CT is the best method to depict middle-ear changes.

Cholesteatoma

Cholesteatoma is a sac lined by keratinizing stratified squamous epithelium trapped in the middle ear and growing in the middle ear or mastoid. This lesion, when large enough, will displace the ossicles, eventually destroying them and the walls of the middle-ear cavity. Typically, the lateral wall of the middle-ear cavity is eroded and the scutum is amputated. In the antrum and mastoid, the septae between the aerated cells are destroyed by the lesion. As cholesteatomas grow and become masses they have convex borders; this is, however, only visible when the surrounding part of the middle ear or mastoid is aerated. Thus, when a mass has two convex borders, it is very likely to be a cholesteatoma; when one border is convex a cholesteatoma should be suspected. If only straight or concave borders are seen, then inflammation is instead likely. Again, CT is the method of choice to evaluate the walls of the middle ear and the ossicles. The technique is also suited to determine whether residual/recurrent cholesteatoma is present and to help the surgeon decide whether a second look operation or re-intervention is necessary.

When the middle ear is completely opacified on CT, then it is often impossible to distinguish between post-surgical changes, inflammation, and (residual/recurrent) cholesteatoma. Moreover, if surgery was performed previously, landmarks such as the integrity of the ossicles and walls of the middle-ear cavity can often not be used as they have been damaged by the previous lesion and/or surgery. In these patients, CT offers no clue whether cholesteatoma is present; instead, only MR can provide the answer.

A cholesteatoma has specific signal intensities on MR: High signal intensity on T2, low on unenhanced T1, low on Gd-enhanced T1 but with a thin rim of enhancement around the lesion, and a very high signal intensity on non-echo-planar imaging (EPI) diffusion-weighted images (b = 1000). Non-EPI images are preferred as they do not suffer from susceptibility artifacts at the level of the tegmen; such artifacts often make the diagnosis of cholesteatoma impossible based on EPI images. Hence, MR results can, in most of the primary cases, inform the surgeon as to the nature of the expected lesion, obviating the need for surgery in many patients. The same goes for patients who have already undergone surgery and in whom a second-look operation is tentatively scheduled, since MR can be used to exclude residual and recurrent cholesteatoma. Problem with partial volume effects nonetheless remain, as it is difficult to acquire diffusion-weighted MR images thinner than 3 mm. Hence, very small recurrences can still be overlooked, although lesions that are 2-3 mm in diameter can currently be detected. Importantly, there are no false-positives on diffusion-weighted MR images. This means that when a high signal is present on the b-1000 images, a cholesteatoma will be found (Fig. 3).

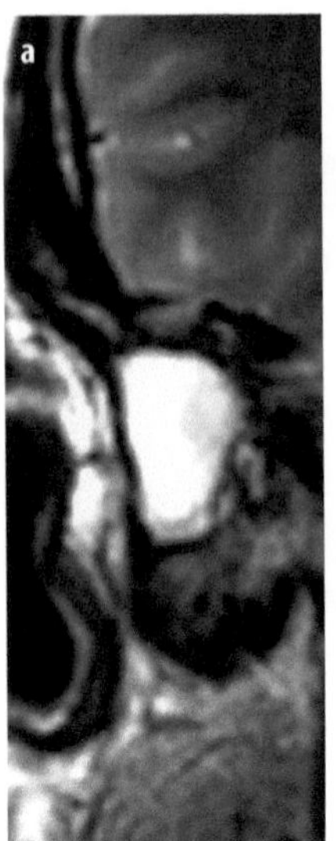

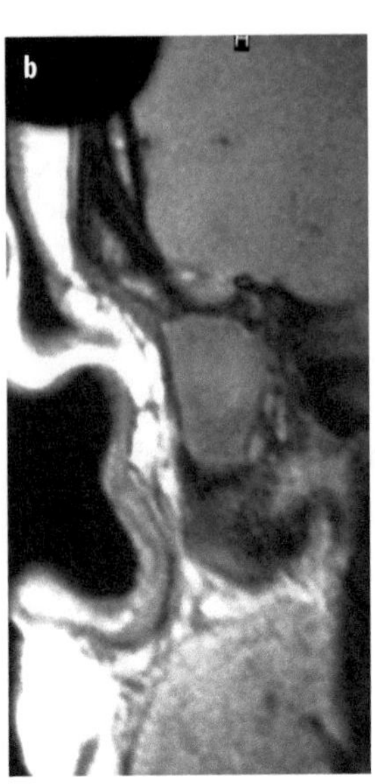

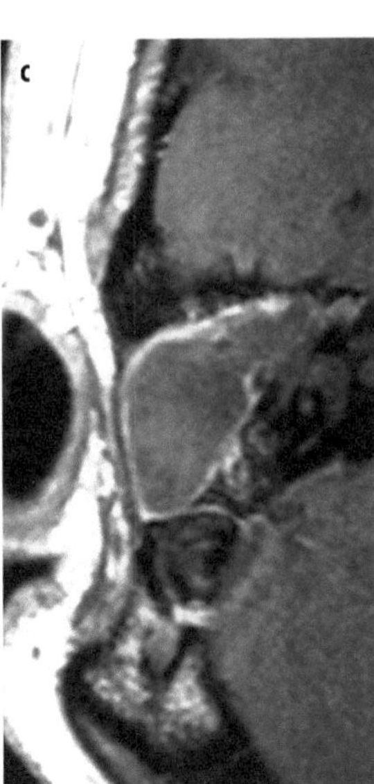

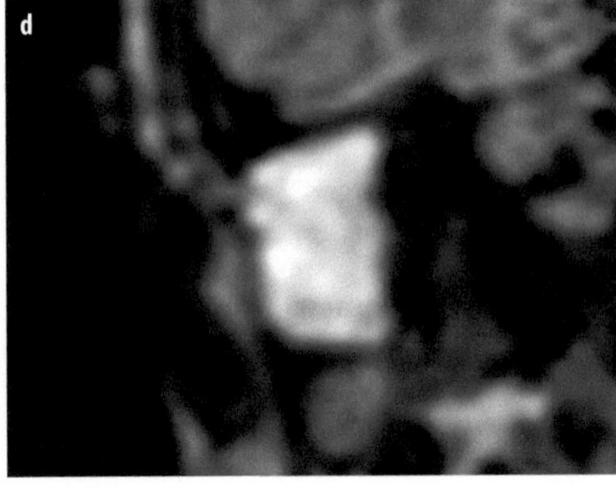

Fig. 3 a-d. Cholesteatoma in the right middle ear and mastoid. Signal intensity is high on T2 (**a**), low on T1 (**b**), low on Gd-enhanced T1 but with rim enhancement (**c**), and very high signal on b-1000 diffusion weighting (**d**)

Other lesions such as a cholesterol granuloma have very specific signal intensities as well (high on both T1 and T2, low on diffusion). Middle-ear inflammation will typically become hyperintense on contrast-enhanced T1 images. If doubt persists, "late-phase" images will often better show the enhancement and then confirm the presence of inflammation as cholesteatomas will not enhance at all.

Congenital Middle-Ear Malformations

Congenital malformations of the middle and external ear are linked embryologically and therefore often present in the same patient. CT is the preferred method to identify these congenital malformations as it most clearly reveals air and bone. In the middle ear, the status of the ossicles must be evaluated and described in detail as the surgeon must know whether hearing loss is due to a malformation of the ossicles. If they are malformed, then it is important to determine whether enough ossicles are present to reconstruct a functioning ossicular chain. Moreover the presence of a normal open round and oval window has to be confirmed. All of this information can only be provided by detailed imaging consisting of thin (0.1 mm thick) reconstructions, which will demonstrate these often subtle malformations. When the external and middle ear are malformed, then the position of the facial nerve must be checked. The nerve will often shift anteriorly and run through the middle-ear cavity (Fig. 4); it may even split into two or more mastoid branches. Since the nerve is at risk, it becomes the radiologist's responsibility to warn the surgeon if the nerve has an abnormal course. The middle ear can, of course, not be evaluated when the external auditory canal is absent or when an atresia plate is present. In these cases, the surgeon is completely dependent on the imaging findings, which will indicate whether the external ear and/or ossicular chain can be reconstructed.

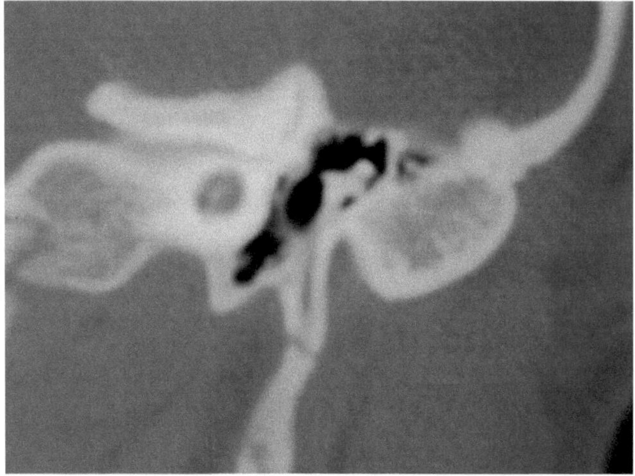

Fig. 4. Coronal CT image showing aplasia of the external auditory canal and a bony atresia plate with fixation of the fused ossicles. The facial nerve descends in the middle of the middle ear cavity

Acoustic Schwannoma

Acoustic schwannomas are the most frequent lesions found inside the internal auditory canal (IAC) and may cause SNHL, vertigo, and tinnitus. The lesions can be detected on Gd-enhanced T1-weighted images; however differentiation from neuritis can be difficult. Gradient-echo (GE) T2-weighted images are used to distinguish among the entities. Schwannoma is characterized by a nodular hypointensity along the course of the involved nerve whereas a normal or fusiform thickened nerve is present in neuritis. This applies especially to facial nerve neuritis, as enhancement of the vestibulocochlear nerve (VIIIth nerve neuritis) is rarely seen.

When the schwannoma is small, the affected branch (cochlear, inferior vestibular or superior vestibular) of the VIIIth nerve can be located. Imaging studies have shown that vertigo is more frequently correlated with very small and strictly intracanalicular schwannomas. Clinical studies have also demonstrated that purely intracanalicular acoustic schwannomas result in an earlier onset of vestibular symptoms.

Once the diagnosis of a schwannoma is made, the "growth potential" of the lesion must be assessed. This is best achieved using 1-mm-thick T1-weighted GE images (e.g., 3DFT-MPRAGE) on which volume measurements have been performed. During the first year, follow-up studies should be acquired every 6 months and then annually if the schwannoma does not grow rapidly.

If the schwannoma must be removed, then the possibility of carrying out hearing preservation surgery must be determined. Here, imaging plays a key role. First the presence of fluid between the schwannoma and the fundus of the IAC must be assessed. If fluid is still present, then the surgeon can avoid surgery close to the base of the cochlea and can choose a suboccipital or middle cranial fossa approach, thereby preserving hearing function. If no fluid is left, the surgeon has to drill in the cochlear canal and the patient will become deaf; therefore, in these patients, the less invasive translabyrinthine approach is chosen.

Another important sign is the signal intensity of the CSF between the schwannoma and fundus of the IAC and/or the intralabyrinthine fluid. Normal signal intensity of these fluid spaces seems to correlate very well with good results after hearing preservation surgery. However, when the signal intensity of the fluid is decreased, the outcome of hearing preservation surgery is significantly worse (Fig. 5).

Labyrinthitis

Only "end-phase" ossifying labyrinthitis is visible on CT. On MR acute labyrinthitis is detected by Gd-enhancement, while subacute labyrinthitis in which there is fibrosis is seen on turbo spin-echo (TSE) sequences or GE T2-weighted images. Therefore MR is the method of choice to examine patients in whom labyrinthitis is suspected. Moreover, these patients present with sensorineural hear-

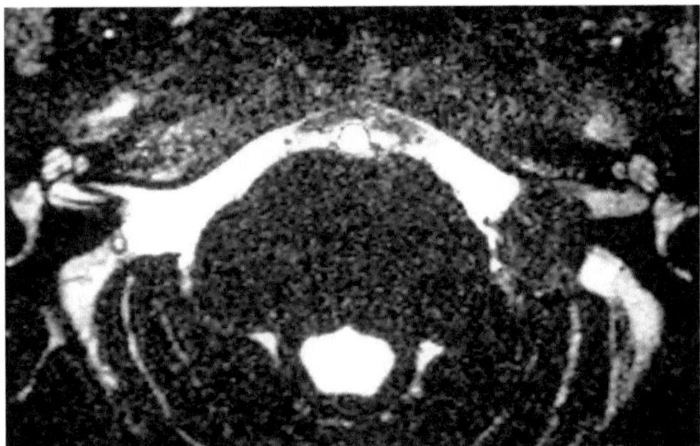

Fig. 5. Axial 0.7-mm-thick gradient-echo T2-weighted image. The signal intensity inside the left labyrinth is decreased, which is a predictor of poor outcome following attempts at hearing preservation surgery

ing loss, which also directs them towards MR examination. However, when the high signal intensity of fluid is lost on T2-weighted TSE or GE images, it is no longer possible to differentiate between fibrosis and ossification. As a rule, both MR and CT are needed to get a complete idea of the nature and extent of the labyrinthitis.

Labyrinthitis is most often viral in origin. In these cases, Gd-enhancement is seen but fibrosis and/or ossification are most often absent. Meningococcus or pneumococcus infection (meningitis) assumes a different clinical picture in that fibrosis develops very quickly and calcification can appear as early as 3-4 weeks after infection. Meningitis occurs most frequently in children, and when both ears are affected complete deafness can be the consequence. The only solution for these children is to install a cochlear implant as quickly as possible, before labyrinthine fibrosis and/or ossification occur. Since these pathological processes can set in very rapidly, CT and MR imaging have to be performed at once, as this indication must be considered as an emergency. Scheduling such a patient 1 or 2 weeks later can result in permanent deafness for the patient. Most of these children are examined under anesthesia, so it is wise to perform CT and MR at the same time in order to avoid the need for a second round of anesthesia, with its associated risks, if MR or CT alone does not provide all the answers.

Congenital Inner-Ear Malformations

Patients with inner-ear malformations present with congenital SNHL. Malformations of the bony inner ear can be seen on CT. Only MR can detect the presence of fluid inside the malformed labyrinth; it can also reliably distinguish the scala tympani and vestibuli. Moreover, MR can also be used to check whether a normal cochlear nerve is present (Fig. 6). If either the vestibulocochlear nerve or the cochlear branch of this nerve is absent, then cochlear implant surgery will no longer solve the problem and an unnecessary expensive intervention can thus be avoided.

The most frequent inner-ear malformations are an enlarged endolymphatic duct and sac (enlarged vestibular aqueduct) and a saccular lateral semicircular canal. The latter usually has no clinical consequences, whereas an enlarged endolymphatic duct and sac are linked with SNHL and frequently accompanied by intracochlear changes.

The danger of a "gusher ear", in which the CSF pressure is transmitted to the intralabyrinthine fluid, is always present when inner-ear malformations are detected. The absence of a normal bone barrier between the fundus of the IAC and the base of the cochlea (very likely) and the presence of a large vestibular aqueduct (less likely) warn the surgeon that the patient is likely to have a gusher ear. Surgery on the oval window and footplate in a patient with gusher ear may cause CSF to gush out of the oval window, leaving the patient completely deaf on that side.

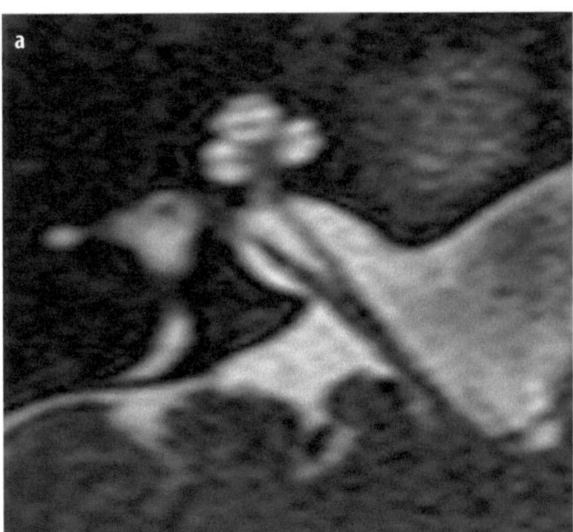

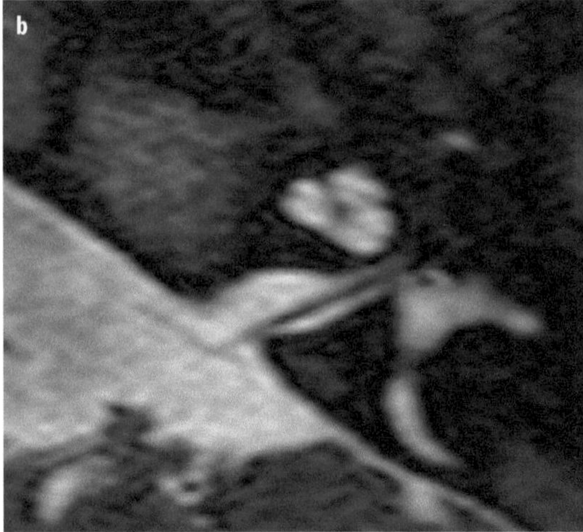

Fig. 6 a-b. a Congenital deafness on the left side due to the absence of the cochlear branch of the 8th nerve in an otherwise normal left inner ear. **b** Normal cochlear and inferior vestibular branch of the 8th nerve on the right side

Hence, the surgeon must be adequately warned if suspicious signs are noted. Unfortunately, gusher ears can also occur in radiologically completely normal inner ears.

Pathology Involving the Central Auditory Pathways

In SNHL, the pathology is frequently located along the auditory pathways. In these patients, the results of selective CT or MR studies will be normal. MR is the method of choice in these patients and selective MR of the inner ear should always be completed by a brain study. The cochlear nuclei, the trapezoid body, the lateral lemniscus, the inferior colliculus, the medial geniculate body, and the auditory cortex can all be affected. Infarctions (older patients), multiple sclerosis (younger patients), trauma, tumor, and inflammation can involve these structures and cause SNHL. Congenital malformation (pachygyria or polymicrogyria) may even be present in the auditory cortex and should be checked in all cochlear implant candidates.

Tinnitus

Patients with pulsatile tinnitus can be noninvasively examined by MR. Patients with subjective and non-pulsatile tinnitus can be examined using MR angiography but the diagnostic yield is much lower. Neurovascular conflicts near the root entry zone of the facial and vestibulocochlear nerves can best be recognized on GE T2-weighted images. These images can also be used to provide the surgeon with virtual images of the conflict in the cerebellopontine angle. Vascular time of flight images can be used to identify the vessel causing the conflict or to differentiate between arteries and veins (nonenhanced and Gd-enhanced images).

However a neurovascular conflict is not the most frequent cause of pulsatile tinnitus; rather, the condition is most often due to paragangliomas, dural arteriovenous fistulas, idiopathic venous tinnitus and benign intracranial hypertension. However, only the first two can be shown on MR.

Dural fistulas (Fig. 7), reflected as early venous drainage on nonenhanced images, can be detected by MR imaging. Glomus tumors, arteriovenous malformations, aberrant vessels running through the middle ear, high or dehiscent jugular bulbs, tortuous carotid arteries near the skull base, fibromuscular dysplasia, carotid dissection, etc., can be detected on unenhanced as well as Gd-enhanced MR angiography images. Vascularized tumors such as meningiomas have a higher arterial and venous flow in their surroundings and therefore can cause tinnitus. This is the reason why tumors near the temporal bone must be excluded in these patients. Finally, CT is sometimes necessary to find the cause of the tinnitus, e.g., in a patient with Paget's disease. However, MR angiography is the method of choice as it is able to detect many more causes of tinnitus than CT. Angiography is only used either to treat patients (embolization) or diagnostically, when pulsatile tinnitus renders a normal life impossible and MR and CT findings remain negative.

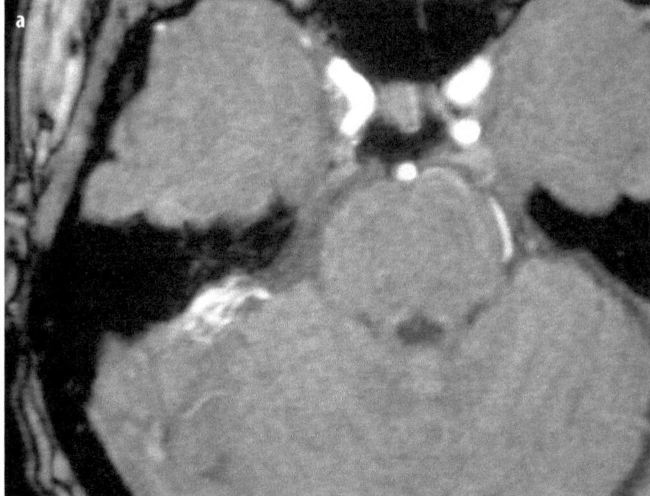

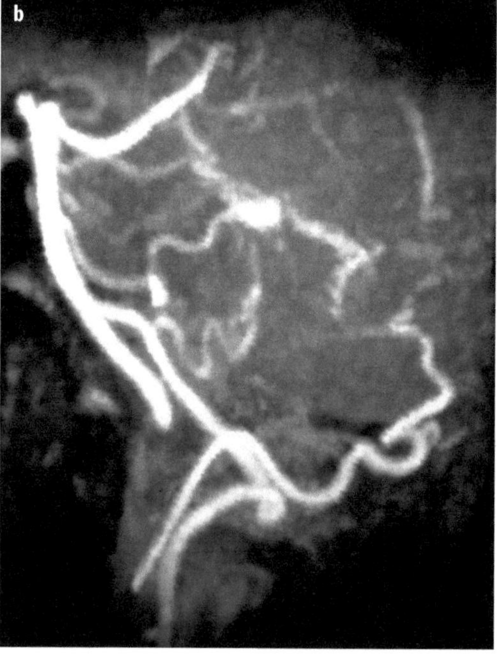

Fig. 7 a-b. Dural fistula. **a** Unenhanced time-of-flight (TOF)-MRA shows increased flow velocity in the area of the superior petrosal sinus. **b** Selective reconstructed maximum intensity projection (MIP) shows that the fistula is fed by a branch of the occipital artery as well as by branches of the posterior inferior and anterior inferior cerebellar arteries and of the superior cerebellar and posterior cerebral arteries

Suggested Reading

Alexander AE, Caldemeyer KS, Rigby P (1998) Clinical and surgical application of reformatted high-resolution CT of the temporal bone. Neuroimaging Clin N Am 8:31-50

Bradley WG (1991) MR of the brain stem: a practical approach. Radiology 179:319-332

Casselman JW (2002) Diagnostic imaging in clinical neuro-otology. Curr Opin Neurol 15:23-30

Casselman JW, Kuhweide R, Ampe W et al (1996) Inner ear malformations in patients with sensorineural hearing loss: detection with gradient-echo (3DFT-CISS) MR imaging. Neuroradiology 38:278-286

Casselman JW (1996) Temporal bone imaging. Neuroimaging Clin North Am 6:265-289

Casselman JW, Offeciers EF, De Foer B, et al (2001) CT and MR imaging of congenital abnormalities of the inner ear and internal auditory canal. Eur J Radiol (The Netherlands) 40:94-104

Casselman JW, Offeciers FE, Govaerts PJ, Kuhweide R, Geldof H, Somers Th, D'Hont G (1997) Aplasia and hypoplasia of the vestibulocochlear nerve: diagnosis with MR imaging. Radiology 202:773-781

Dietz RR, Davis WL, Harnsberger HR, Jacobs JM, Blatter DD (1994) MR imaging and MR angiography in the evaluation of pulsatile tinnitus. AJNR Am J Neuroradiol 15:890-892

De Foer B, Vercruysse J-P, Bernaerts A, Maes J, Deckers F, Michiels J, Somers T, Pouillon M, Offeciers E, Casselman JW (2007) The valueof single-shot turbo spin-echo diffusion-weighted MR imaging in the detection of middle ear cholesteatoma. Neuroradiology 49:841-848

Deplanque D, Godefroy O, Guerouaou D, Laureau E, Desaulty A (1998) Sudden bilateral deafness: lateral inferior pontine infarction. J Neurol Neurosurg Psychiatry 64:817-818

Lo WWM, Solti-Bohman LG (1996) Vascular tinnitus. In: Som PM, Curtin HD (eds) Head and neck imaging. Mosby Yearbook, St. Louis, pp. 1535-1549

Lo WW, Solti-Bohman LG (1996) Tumors of the temporal bone and the cerebellopontine angle. In: Som PM, Bergeron RT (eds) Head and neck imaging. Mosby Yearbook, St. Louis, pp 1449-1531

Maheshwari S, Mukherji SK (2002) Diffusion-weighted imaging for differentiating recurrent cholesteatoma tissue after mastoidectomy: case report. Am J Neuroradiol 23:847-849

Mark AS, Casselman JW (2002) Anatomy and diseases of the temporal bone. In: Atlas SW (ed) Magnetic resonance imaging of the brain and spine. 3rd edn. Lippincott Williams & Wilkins, Philadelphia , pp. 1363-1432

Mark AS (1994) Contrast-enhanced magnetic resonance imaging of the temporal bone. Neuroimaging Clin North Am 4:561-578

Nayak S (2001) Segmental anatomy of the temporal bone. Semin Ultrasound CT MR 22:184-218.

Nair SB, Abou-Elhamd KA, Hawtorne M (2000) A retrospective analysis of high resolution computed tomography in the assessment of cochlear implant patients. Clin Otolaryngol 25:55-61

Phelps PD, Reardon W, Pembrey M (1991) X-linked deafness, stapes gushers and a distinctive defect of the inner ear. Neuroradiology 33:326-330

Sartoretti-Schefer S, Kollias S, Wichmann W, Valavanis AS (1998) T2-weighted three-dimensional fast spin-echo MR in inflammatory peripheral facial nerve palsy. AJNR Am J Neuroradiol, 19:491-495

Sartoretti-Schefer S Wichmann W et al (1997) Contrast enhanced MRI of the facial nerve in patients with posttraumatic peripheral facial nerve palsy. AJNR Am J Neuroradiol 18:1115-1125

Sasaki O, Ootsuka K, Taguchi K, Kikukawa M (1994) Multiple sclerosis presented acute hearing loss and vertigo. ORL J Otorhinolaryngol Relat Spec 56:55-59

Somers T, Casselman J, de Ceulaer G et al (2001) Prognostic value of MRI findings in hearing preservation surgery for vestibular schwannoma. Am J Otology 22:87-94

Swartz JD, Harnsberger HR (1998) Temporal bone vascular anatomy, anomalies, and diseases, emphasizing the clinical-radiological problem of pulsatile tinnitus. In: Swartz JD, Harnsberger HR (eds) Imaging of the temporal bone. Thieme, New York, pp 170-239

Swartz JD, Harnsberger HR (1998) The otic capsule and otodystrophies. In: Swartz JD, Harnsberger HR (Eds) Imaging of the temporal bone. Thieme, New York, pp 240-317

Van den Brink JS, Watanabe Y, Kuhl CK et al (2003) Implications of SENSE MR in routine clinical practice. Eur J Radiol 46:3-27

Veillon F, Riehm S, Emachescu B et al (2001) Imaging of the windows of the temporal bone. Semin Ultrasound CT MR 22:271-280

Veillon F, Baur P, Dasch JC et al (1991) Traumatismes de l'os temporal. In: Veillon F (ed) Imagerie de l'oreille. Médecine-Sciences Flammarion, Paris, pp 243-281

Vercruysse JP, De Foer B, Pouillon M et al (2006) The value of diffusion-weighted MR imaging in the diagnosis of primary acquired and residual cholesteatoma: a surgical verified study of 100 patients. Eur Radiol 16:1461-1467

Williams MT, Ayache D, Alberti C et al (2003) Detection of residual cholesteatoma with delayed contrast-enhanced MR imaging: initial findings. Eur Radiol 13:169-174

Imaging of Temporal Bone Pathology

Francis Veillon, Sophie Riehm, Maher Abu Eid, Luciana Ramos Taboada

Service de Radiologie I, Hopital de Hautepierre, 67098 Strasbourg, France

Anatomy

The temporal bone is made up of three bones: the *tympanic*, *squamous*, and *petrous* bones. It contains three cavities: the external auditory meatus, the middle ear or tympanic cavity, the inner ear or labyrinth, and, more medially, the internal auditory meatus. The facial nerve is located within the temporal bone: first in the internal auditory meatus, between the anterior and posterior labyrinth, and then between the inner and middle ear. The VIIIth and VIIth cranial nerves are located in the internal auditory meatus. The VIth cranial nerve runs close to the anterior part of the petrous apex. The mixed nerves (IX-XI) are located in the anterior part of the jugular foramen.

The tympanic bone is cylinder-shaped (Fig. 1), open at its upper end, and closed by the squamous bone. The parotid gland is located below.

The squamous bone consists of a vertical and a horizontal part. The vertical part, at its external face, is in close contact with the temporal muscle. On the inner face, lie the meninges and the temporal lobe. The horizontal part is made up anterior (superior to the mandibular condyle), middle (superior to the external auditory meatus), and posterior (lateral to the antrum, the biggest posterior cell of the middle ear) components.

The petrous bone is pyramid-shaped and located in the axial plane, oriented anteriorly and medially (Fig. 2). It contents the middle ear (and all its walls except the lateral one) and the inner ear (or labyrinth). Medially, the brainstem (pons), cerebellum, meninges, cerebrospinal fluid, temporal lobe are found; inferiorly lie the vascular space with the internal carotid artery, the jugular vein (Fig. 3), and two important nerves: the inferior tympanic nerve (Jacobson) entering the petrous bone between the internal carotid artery and the jugular vein, and the facial nerve which leaves the petrous bone in the stylomastoid foramen. The nasopharynx is another important relationship of the inferior part of the petrous apex.

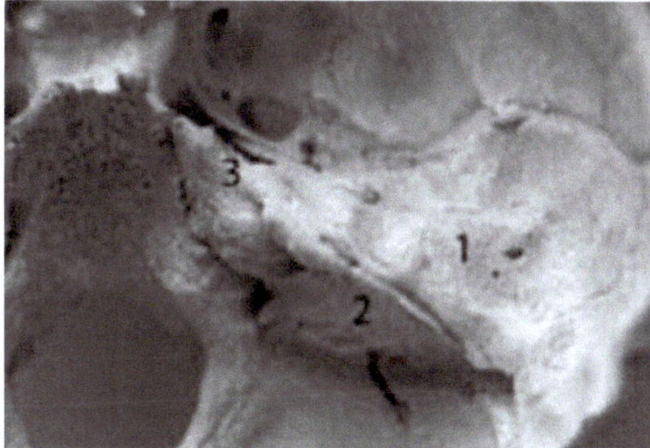

Fig. 2. Superior view of a dry temporal bone. *1*, External wall of the petrous bone; *2*, inner wall of the petrous bone; *3*, petrous apex

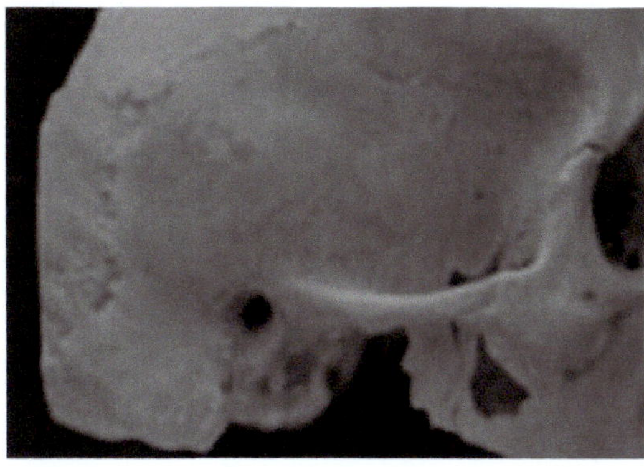

Fig. 1. Lateral view of a dry temporal bone with the external auditory meatus

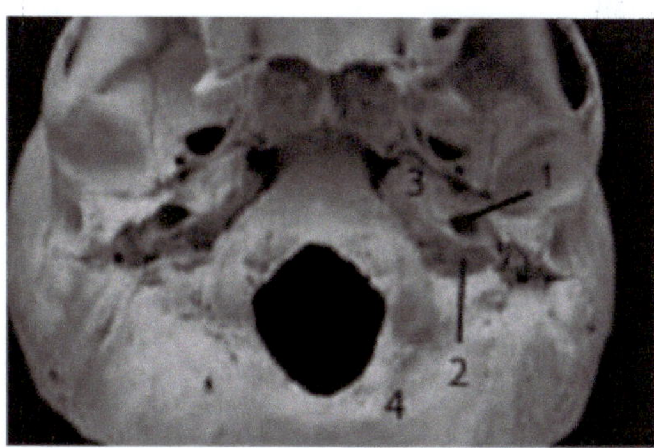

Fig. 3. Inferior view of a left temporal bone. *1*, Inferior foramen of the internal carotid artery; *2*, jugular foramen; *3*, petrous apex; *4*, occipital bone

Imaging Techniques

Computed Tomography of the External, Middle, and Inner Ear

The following CT imaging parameters are recommended:
- Thickness: 0.4-0.7 mm
- Increment: 0.1-0.2
- Filter: high-resolution
- Plane: Axial (Fig. 4) (parallel to the lateral semicircular canal)
  Coronal
  Sagittal
  Oblique (stapes incus)
- Reconstructions: 0.4-0.5 mm

Magnetic Resonance Imaging of the Adult External, Middle Ear

- T1 spin-echo (SE) fat sat axial parallel to the roof of the orbit 1-1.5 or 2 mm without and with intravenous gadolinium injection
- Diffusion (SE): 2 mm axial, coronal
- High-resolution axial 3D T2 0.4-0.7 mm (parallel to the lateral semicircular canal)

Magnetic Resonance Imaging of the Middle Ear in a Young Child

- Diffusion (SE) 2 mm axial, coronal
- T1 SE fat sat axial

Magnetic Resonance Imaging of the Inner Ear and Internal Auditory Meatus

- T1 SE fat sat axial parallel to the roof of the orbit 1-1.5 or 2 mm without and with intravenous gadolinium injection

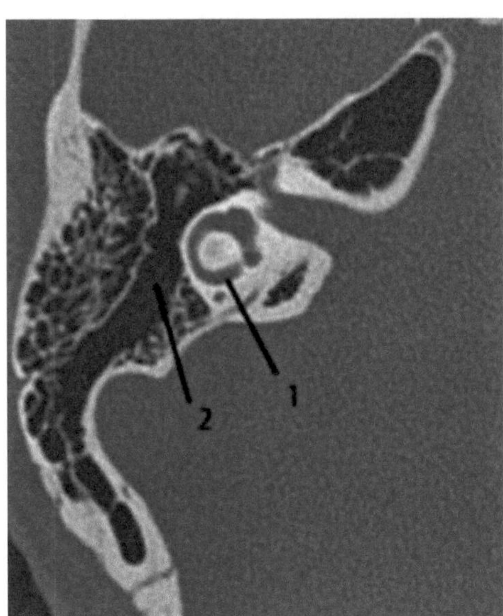

Fig. 4. CT axial view in the plane of the lateral semicircular canal (CISS sequence). *1*, Lateral semicircular canal; *2*, middle ear

- High-resolution axial 3D T2 0.4-0.7 mm (Figs. 5, 6) (parallel to the lateral semicircular canal)
- Sagittal high-resolution T2 (from the 3D) centred in the internal auditory meatus

Examination of the Different Cavities

The lumen of the external auditory meatus is easily analyzed by the otologist during the clinical examination. The tympanic bone is studied with CT. The adjacent temporomandibular joint, located anteriorly, is studied with CT and MRI; the inferiorly located parotid gland is studied with MRI. The mastoid part of the facial nerve, lo-

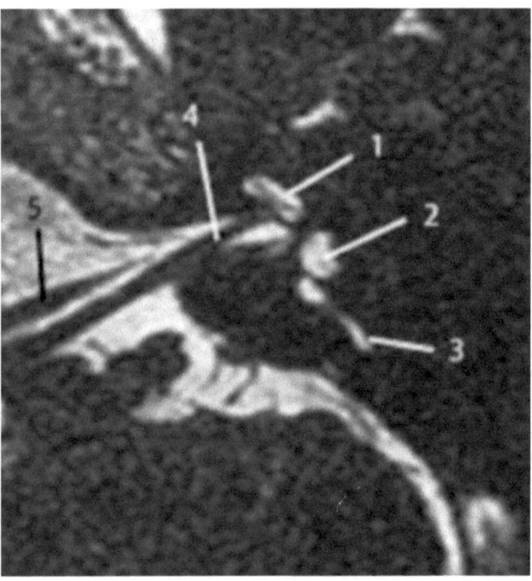

Fig. 5. MRI. The axial high-resolution T2-weighted image shows the cochlea (*1*), the vestibule (*2*), the posterior semicircular canal (*3*), the vestibulocochlear nerve (*4*), and the facial nerve (*5*)

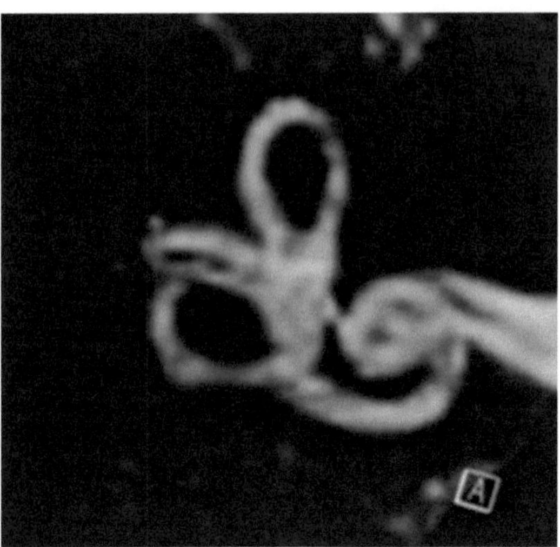

Fig. 6. High-resolution 3D T2-weighted image of a normal labyrinth

cated in the posterior wall of the middle ear not far from the external cavity, is studied with CT and MRI.

The walls of the middle ear (superior, inferior, external, anterior, posterior, inner walls) are studied with CT. MRI in the coronal plane is used to study the superior wall and the relationship (particularly in T2) with the meninges, CSF, and temporal lobe. The three ossicles, malleus, incus, and stapes, are well-studied with CT in the axial, coronal, sagittal, and oblique planes. Normally, the middle ear is filled with air. CT may provide useful information about pathological soft-tissue content, particularly the presence of skin (or cholesteatoma). When difficulties are encountered in analyzing the origin of the pathological tissue in the middle ear, MRI can distinguish between fibrosis, hyperplasia of the mucosa, serous fluid, abscess, and cholesteatoma.

The inner ear is made up of very dense bone, which constitutes the walls of the anterior labyrinth, integrated in the auditory system, and the posterior labyrinth, which forms part of the vestibular system. These cavities contain the membranous labyrinth, which is filled with endolymphatic fluid and is surrounded by the perilymphatic fluid.

CT provides information about the shape of the bony labyrinth, its dense structure, and the lumen which does not contain any calcification. MRI is very useful for analyzing the perilymphatic fluid within the anterior and posterior labyrinths (in T1 and T2), the shapes of these labyrinths, and the absence of any abnormal uptake of gadolinium in T1 in the bone and the lumen. The origin of the vestibular nerve within the posterior labyrinth is also visible in MRI.

The oval and round windows must also be analyzed. The oval window is closed by the footplate of the stapes, the round window by a small membrane. CT is the best way to studying these windows, with images obtained in the axial and coronal planes.

Pathology

There are five main pathologies that affect the temporal bone: inflammation, trauma, malformations, pseudotumors or tumors, and otosclerosis.

Here, the cavities of the temporal bone and their pathologies will be discussed separately.

The External Auditory Meatus

Trauma

Trauma to the temporal bone, particularly in the external auditory meatus, is a frequent occurrence. Usually the anterior wall of the tympanic bone is fractured, resulting in the presence of blood in its lumen. The roof (horizontal squamous bone) of the external auditory meatus is also frequently involved by trauma. CT usually demonstrates the course of the fracture. A small part of the anterior tympanic wall may be displaced within the lumen, a finding that can be detected by CT.

Benign Bony Lesions

Exostoses are a very frequent pathology. The increased thickness of the bony walls of the tympanic bone makes the clinical examination difficult. CT in the axial and sagittal planes measures the importance of the increased bony thickness. Usually, the middle and inner ears are normal. This benign pathology is frequent in individuals who frequently swim in cold water (Fig. 7).

Fibrous dysplasia is a rare pathology in which the lumen of the external auditory meatus is reduced due to the increased thickness of the tympanic bone. The increase in thickness is the result of swelling, which is more or less heterogeneous and involves the tympanic, squamous, and posterior part of the petrous bone.

Osteomas are rare in the temporal bone and are more or less pedicled.

Malformations

Malformations are frequent in the external auditory meatus. The tympanic bone may be small or absent, and the external lumen narrow or absent without any drum. The middle ear is often the site of abnormalities, including fixed and deformed ossicles. The inner ear is usually normal. CT demonstrates the presence or absence of the external lumen and ear drum. The deformed malleus and incus are often fixed to the external wall of the middle ear.

Inflammation of the External Auditory Meatus

Infections in diabetic patients are very common, especially external osteitis and abscess in the adjacent tempo-

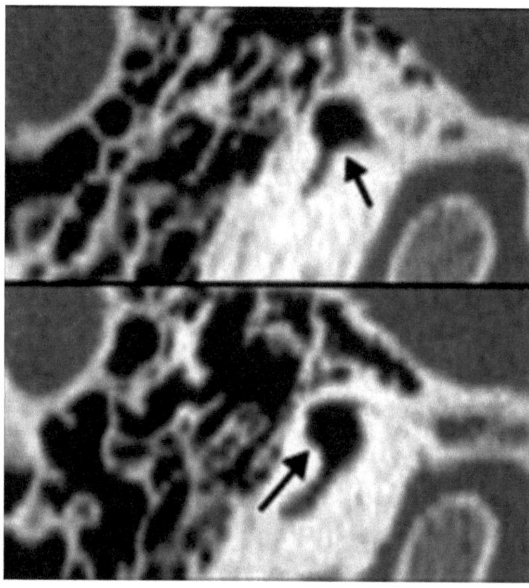

Fig. 7. CT sagittal section showing exostoses of the external auditory meatus (*arrows*)

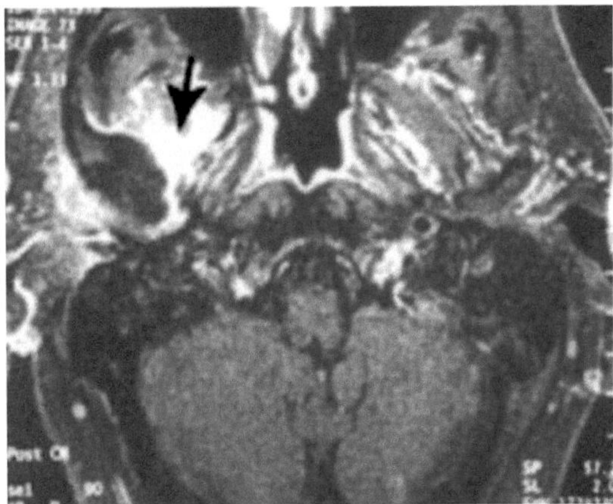

Fig. 8. Malignant external otitis. MRI, axial T1 spin-echo, intravenous gadolinium injection. High enhancement is present in the region of the right temporomandibular joint and the parapharyngeal space

ral tissues, temporomandibular joint, the mastoid bone, and parapharyngeal space. CT reveals the bony defects, and MRI the soft-tissue inflammation. The best sequence to obtain in elderly patients is the axial T1 with fat saturation and intravenous gadolinium injection. Contrast uptake in the pathological region is usually very high. MRI is also a very good way to follow up patients after medical treatment. A biopsy is often needed to find the etiology of infection (usually, *Pseudomonas aeruginosa*) and may suffice to eliminate a cancer (Fig. 8).

Secondary cholesteatoma is rare in the external ear; when clinically diagnosed, CT and MRI are used to evaluate the extension of the lesions. CT analyzes possible bony destruction, while in MRI cholesteatoma is of low signal intensity in T1 without any uptake of gadolinium. The signal is high in diffusion-weighted imaging.

A carcinoma may develop in the mucosa of the external auditory meatus or originate in the parotid gland, with extension to the tympanic bone. CT and MRI show the extension of the lesion, particularly in the vicinity of the facial nerve canal (the mastoid part). There is usually more or less important uptake in T1 after intravenous gadolinium injection.

The Middle Ear

Otitis

In infectious otitis without any complications, there is no need for CT, neither are CT studies required in cases of serous otitis media in children.

In mastoiditis, imaging is required to demonstrate osteitis of the inner wall of the petrous bone (CT) and thrombosis of the lateral sinus, or the presence/absence of an abscess in the posterior or middle cranial fossa (MRI).

In serous otitis media in an adult without any history of chronic inflammation, CT and/or MRI are needed to eliminate the possibility of a tumor, particularly a nasopharyngeal cancer, a meningioma of the middle or posterior cranial fossa, or any process in the deep regions of the face that compresses the Eustachian tube.

Tympanosclerosis

A consequence of chronic otitis media is tympanosclerosis, which is characterized by hyalinization and calcification of the mucosa. This pathology includes many findings: a small calcification of the drum, calcified tendons and ligaments, and an ossified mass in the epitympanum and/or antrum. The stapes may be very dense, particularly the footplate. CT is very useful to demonstrate the various calcified anatomical areas.

The Ossicles and Chronic Otitis Media

Prior to surgery, CT can be used to evaluate the ossicles, which may be partially or totally destroyed even without cholesteatoma. Special attention must be paid to a bony fixation of the head of the malleus or lysis of the long process of the incus and/or stapes. CT easily analyzes these destructions in the different planes of the ossicles and in 3D.

Cholesteatoma

Clinical diagnosis of cholesteatoma is usually made by the otologist. In certain circumstances, the diagnosis of cholesteatoma is not easy, particularly when the drum is not open, the lesion is small, or is situated very high in the attic. In postoperative patients it may be clinically difficult to demonstrate the recurrence of a cholesteatoma in a surgical cavity. CT shows the cholesteatoma as a bowl-shaped mass in the external epitympanum. The scutum is often destroyed; the cholesteatoma may extend in the internal epitympanum, mesotympanum (Fig. 9), and or antrum. The superior wall of the tympanic cavity may be open. In 10% of the cases, there is a fistula of the lateral semicircular canal. A fistula of the superior semicircular

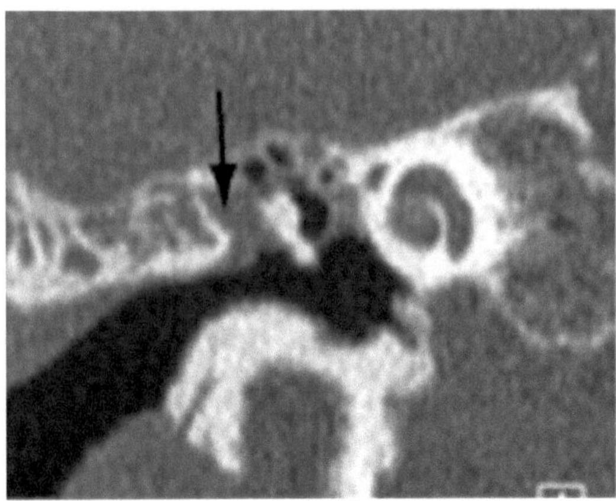

Fig. 9. Cholesteatoma of the lateral epitympanic recess. CT coronal view (*arrow*)

canal is rare, as is an opening of the posterior semicircular canal. In some cases, CT diagnosis of the cholesteatoma is also difficult particularly in postoperative cavities in which the soft tissues fill up the entire surgical area. In these cases, MRI is very useful for diagnosing the recurrent cholesteatoma. T1-weighted imaging shows a nodule of intermediate signal without any enhancement after intravenous gadolinium injection (Fig. 10). In diffusion-weighted imaging, the signal is high (Fig. 11). In high-resolution T2-weighted images, the signal is intermediate or low. If a fistula of the lateral semicircular canal has been diagnosed in CT, the MRI shows the usual conservation of the endosteal layer without any invasion of the perilymphatic space. In rare cases, the keratoma invades the lumen of the lateral semicircular canal.

In unusual cases, a secondary cholesteatoma may be very large, with significant destruction of the inner wall of the petrous bone but without any opening of the dura.

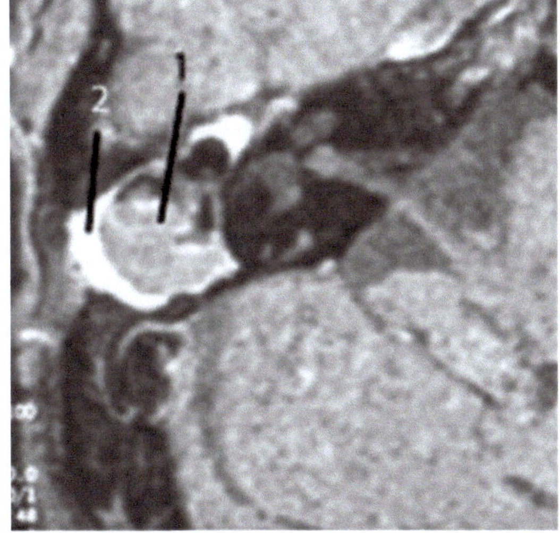

Fig. 10. Postoperative recurrent cholesteatoma. Axial T1 (spin-echo, intravenous gadolinim injection). *1*, Cholesteatoma; *2*, hyperplasia of the mucosa

Malformations

Malformations of the tympanic cavity and ossicles are very frequent findings. CT well-delineates fixation, deformity, fusion, and partial or total absence of the ossicles. CT, with the possibility of reconstruction in the direction of each ossicle and 3D presentation, is the best procedure to obtain the diagnosis.

The abnormalities may be associated or not with a small cavity. The superior wall may be lowered or open, the jugular bulb protruding or not into the inferior part of the middle ear. There is no need for MRI when investigating a malformation of the middle ear associated with a conductive hearing loss.

Trauma

Fractures of the middle ear are very frequent. Usually the trauma follows the axis of the tympanic cavity, from the posterolateral part to the anteromedial area. The fracture may enter the different portions of the horizontal squamous bone. The anterior and superior walls of the middle ear are often involved by the traumatic process. In most cases, there is a longitudinal extra-labyrinthine fracture of the temporal bone. Disjunction of the incudo-stapedial joint is frequent as is a fracture of the long process of the incus. Disjunction between the malleus and incus and fracture of the stapes are other possible findings.

Tumors

In adult most of the lesions are benign: tympanic paragangliomas, adenomas, meningiomas, and neuromas of the VIIth and VIIIth nerves.

Malignant tumors may extend into the middle ear: carcinomas (external auditory meatus, parotid gland, minor salivary glands, pharynx), lymphomas, or metastasis. In all of these lesions, CT and MRI provide the correct diagnosis and take into account the structure, margins, and location of the tumor.

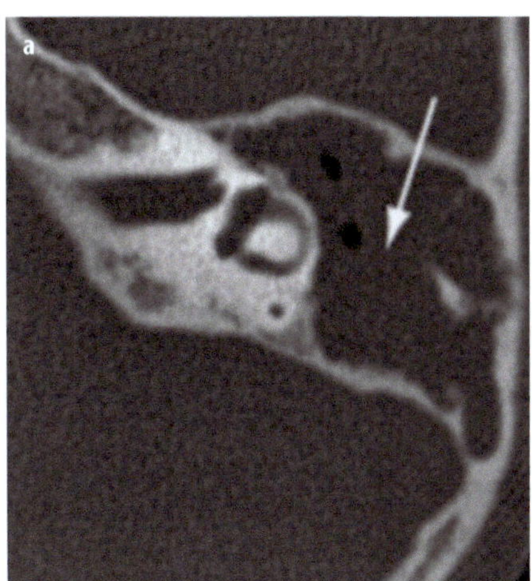

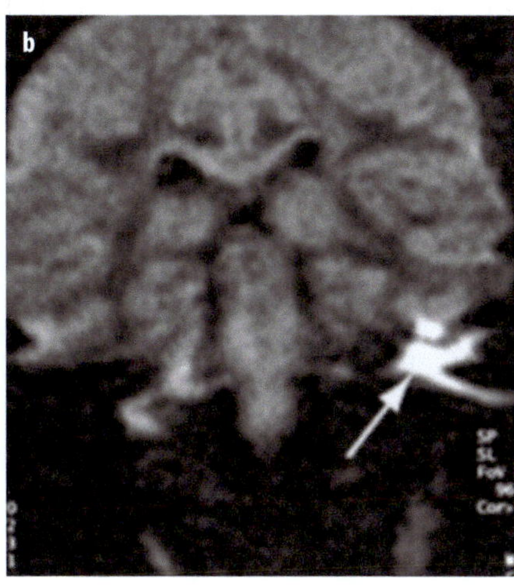

Fig. 11 a, b. a Recurrent postoperative cholesteatoma in a child (*arrow*); axial CT. **b** Same patient as in (**a**). Coronal diffusion shows high signal in the left middle ear (*arrow*)

In children, primitive cholesteatoma, associated or nor with malformations, is easily diagnosed by CT. There is a mesotympanic round mass with or without destruction of the long process of the incus. This congenital lesion is associated with good aeration of the middle ear.

Histiocytosis is an aggressive process in which histiocytic cellular sheets are responsible for the destruction of the mastoid, with or without inner ear extension. In CT, bony destruction of the posterior petrous bone is very well-delineated. In T1-weighted imaging after intravenous gadolinium injection, there is strong enhancement of the soft-tissue content in the middle ear. Optical microscopy shows Langerhans cells, which are large, with abundant pink cytoplasm and reniform nuclei. Immunohistochemical techniques specific for CD1a (Langerhans cellular specific cytoplasmic membranous tracer) are positive. The presence of destruction of the posterior petrous and squamous bones, with strong enhancement in T1 after gadolinium injection, together with the immunohistochemical results lead to the correct diagnosis.

Sarcomas are rare tumors diagnosed on the basis of biopsy findings. Metastasis (often from a neuroblastoma) is detected by ultrasound examination of the abdomen.

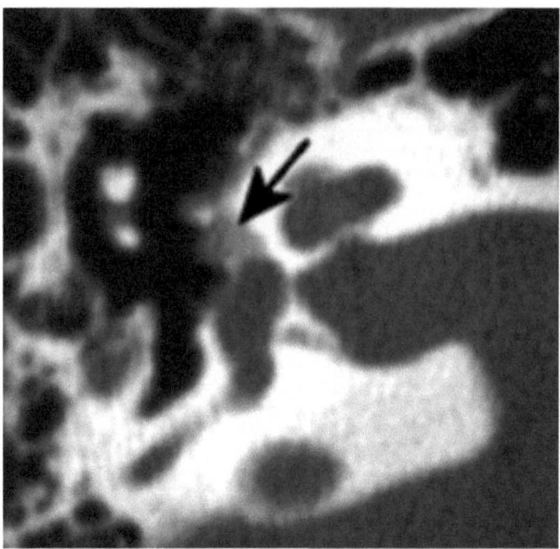

Fig. 12. Otosclerosis. Axial CT (high resolution). Hypodensity close to the vestibule (*arrow*)

The Inner Ear

The labyrinthic cavities are involved by five pathologies: otosclerosis, malformation, inflammation, trauma, and tumors.

Otosclerosis

This disease consists of dystrophy of the labyrinthic bone, with ossification of cartilaginous remnants. In more than half of the patients there is a genetic history. Otosclerosis occurs preferentially in women, particularly after two pregnancies.

The labyrinthic bone anterior to the oval window is most often affected, with the process originating in a cartilaginous remnant, the fissula ante fenestram. The main clinical sign is conductive hearing loss due to limited vibrations of the stapes. The stapedial reflex is absent. CT is the best way to confirm the clinical diagnosis and provides anatomical and prognostic information. In CT, the otosclerotic focus appears as a hypodensity anterior to the oval window (Fig. 12), usually with an increased thickness of the adjacent footplate. Hypodensities may also involve other parts of the middle layer of the labyrinthine capsule. Locations in the posterior labyrinth are rare. In 7% of the cases there is a focus in the margins (lateral and/or medial) of the round window. In rare cases, there is an extension from the pathological labyrinthine bone to the tympanic cavity, with possible encroachment of the ossicles. Associations with inner-ear malformations or chronic otitis media are possible.

CT also yields information about the long process of the incus (for fixation of the prosthesis) and the position of the facial nerve (surgical approach to the footplate). CT and MRI are also useful in follow-up of patients with postoperative complications: lateral luxation of the prosthesis (CT), too long prosthesis (CT and MRI), granuloma within the vestibule (MRI), and perilymphatic fistula through the oval window (MRI).

CT allows also diagnosis of other etiologies of conductive hearing loss: malformations of the ossicles, gusher syndrome, calcified stapes, primitive cholesteatoma, neuroma of the VIIth nerve.

Malformations

Malformations of the inner ear are very common abnormalities. Usually, the most important sign is dilatation of the posterior structures, particularly the lateral semicircular canal. In the majority of cases, these abnormalities are discovered by chance. In other cases, the vestibule is dilated, with or without abnormal segmentation of the anterior labyrinth.

Dilatation of the vestibular aqueduct is very common and is usually associated with abnormal segmentation of the anterior labyrinth.

The posterior labyrinth may be absent in the CHARGE syndrome, whereas the absence of the anterior labyrinth is very rare. In very exceptional cases all of the inner ear is absent.

The absence of the modiolus can be diagnosed with CT and may be associated with an abnormally shaped anterior or posterior labyrinth and dilatation of the vestibular aqueduct. In this syndrome the CSF of the internal auditory meatus is located in the perilymphatic spaces of the inner ear, associated with an abnormal footplate. In such case, any surgical procedure on the stapes, particularly the footplate, is dangerous and carries a risk of postsurgical total deafness.

CT is very useful for analyzing malformations of the inner ear, which are often associated with congenital abnormalities of the windows and middle ear.

In MRI, the segmentation of the anterior labyrinth is better demonstrated than with CT. The fluid content is also easily analyzed with T1- and T2-weighted sequences. The presence or absence of the VIIIth nerve as well as the course of the facial nerve in the internal auditory meatus and adjacent to the cochlea is nicely demonstrated with MRI.

Infectious complications of inner ear malformations are very well-analyzed by MRI. Granulation tissue in the middle ear, with extension to the perilymphatic spaces shows strong enhancement in T1 after intravenous gadolinium injection.

Inflammation

Labyrinthitis is a common pathology of the inner ear. It may be due to viral or bacterial infections or autoimmune pathology. The T1-weighted images may be normal or slightly hyperintense, depending on the infection. Usually, there is a contrast enhancement in the perilymphatic spaces after intravenous gadolinium injection. High-resolution T2-weighted images may be normal or show slight filling with a more or less solid material.

In rare cases, there is a bony infection with slight hypodensities of the anterior and or posterior labyrinth, as seen on CT studies; MRI shows contrast enhancement of the pathological bone in T1 after intravenous gadolinium injection.

To summarize, in viral labyrinthitis there is a diffusion of gadolinium in the perilabyrinthine spaces with a strong signal in T1. High-resolution T2 is often normal. In bacterial infections there is also a diffusion of gadolinium within the inner ear but the signal in high-resolution T2 is decreased.

Secondary cholesteatomas extend to the labyrinth, usually the lateral semicircular canal, in about 10% of cases. In the majority of cases, however, the endostum is normal and the lumen of the lateral semicircular canal is not affected. In rare cases, there is an opening of the endosteum.

Trauma

Traumas of the inner ear account for only 7% of all temporal bone traumas. Usually, the fractures run from the occipital bone to the inner wall of the petrous bone. The otic capsule is crossed by the shock wave. All the cavities of the inner ear may be involved: the semicircular canals, the vestibule, the cochlea. In some cases, the lesion is very thin and magnified CT sections are needed. If CT is negative, MRI may be useful, revealing possible hemorrhage within the lumen of the labyrinthine bone.

In 5% of cases, the fracture runs in the internal and middle ear with an opening of the windows (round and/or oval window with or without lesions of the footplate). CT is the best way to diagnose these lesions.

Tumors

Intralabyrinthine schwannomas originate at the beginning of the VIIIth nerve and develop in the scala tympani. Extension in the vestibule and semicircular canals is possible. In rare cases, the lesion extends to all compartments of the inner ear and invades the round window recess and the middle ear. High-resolution T2 shows solid material in the cochlea and/or the posterior labyrinth. After gadolinium injection in T1, there is contrast enhancement of the entire mass with sharp margins.

Papillary tumors of the endolymphatic sac occur particularly in patients with Von Hippel Lindau disease; 7% of these patients will develop a tumor of the endolymphatic sac. In some cases the tumor is bilateral. The clinical signs are hearing loss, vertigo, deafness. CT shows a heterogeneous legion with hazy margins and destruction of the bone surrounding the endolymphatic canal. On MRI, T1-weighted images part of the content of the mass is of high signal intensity. Other solid areas are also visible with, a high enhancement in T1 after intravenous gadolinium injection. In T2, the signal is bright.

Other pseudotumoral or tumoral lesions erode the otic capsule: primitive cholesteatomas; paragangliomas; neuromas of the Vth, VIIth, and mixed nerves; carcinomas of the pharynx, minor salivary glands, and sphenoid sinus; and malignant bony lesions or metastases.

The Windows of the Temporal Bone

The oval and round windows may be affected by all the pathologies of the temporal bone: otosclerosis, trauma, inflammation, malformations, and even tumors.

Otosclerosis

This is the most frequent pathology of the stapes and oval windows, with an increased thickness of the anterior part of the footplate. It is usually associated with a hypodensity of the prevestibular area. Otosclerosis of an isolated round window is extremely rare; instead, the condition is usually associated with a lesion of the oval window.

Trauma

Trauma affecting the windows is very common. For example, the footplate may be displaced medially in the vestibule by a foreign body, with leakage of perilymphatic fluid from the vestibule to the middle ear.

Fractures of the footplate are also possible, with or without leakage of fluid. This is a common occurrence in trauma to the middle and inner ear.

Perilymphatic fistulae without any fracture may be encountered after cranial trauma, diving, flying, slaps, and sound trauma. In such cases, fluid material is diagnosed by CT and high-resolution T2-weighted MRI.

Inflammation

Tympanosclerosis is very common in the oval window. The increased thickness of a calcified footplate is well-delineated with CT. The new spiral machines ably demonstrate the calcified stapes. The round window recess is usually filled with serous fluid or there are signs of hyperplasia. In some circumstances, cholesteatoma may invade this recess.

Malformations

These are also frequent in narrow oval and/or round windows. In rare cases, the windows are absent, with a lowering of the tympanic facial nerve canal. In gusher syndrome there is a congenital abnormality of the oval window, which is sometimes visible in CT studies.

Tumors

The extension of tumors from the tympanic cavity to the inner ear, or from the labyrinthine lumen to the middle ear is rare. An intralabyrinthine Schwannoma of the VIIIth nerve may run from the scala tympani to the round window recess and the tympanic cavity.

Internal Auditory Meatus

Schwannoma of the VIIIth nerve is the most frequent tumor in this region. It appears as a nodule centred in the vestibular and/or cochlear nerves and is particularly visible in the sagittal 3D high-resolution T2. There is a high enhancement in T1 after intravenous gadolinium injection. The margins of the nodule are very well-delimited. In high-resolution T2, the nodule is solid and well-delimited while the signal of the perilymphatic spaces is often decreased.

Neuromas of the VIIth nerve are very rare compared to those of the VIIIth nerve. The diagnosis is usually easy in the internal auditory meatus when the lesion is centered in the facial nerve but may be more difficult when the lesion is centered in the cerebellopontine angle.

Meningomas present as an increased thickness of the dura. They may occur in the internal auditory meatus, with nodule enhancement after gadolinium injection. Usually, the dura is thickened in the posterior wall of the petrous bone and in the region surrounding the inner part of the internal auditory meatus.

Lipomas are diagnosed in MRI on T1-weighted images because of a high spontaneous signal, without the need for contrast medial injection.

Vascular hamartomas appear in association with fatty tissues and vascular abnormalities.

Meningitis is a benign increased thickness of the meninges and sometimes is present after an infection. It may disappear after medical treatment.

Metastasis in the internal auditory meatus is very common in cases of diffuse metastasis to the meninges. The metastases are seen on T1 with contrast as small nodules in the internal auditory meatus, with an increased thickness of the adjacent meninges. In rare cases some are found in the labyrinth.

Conclusions

The temporal bone and adjacent regions can be evaluated in detail by CT and MRI, which not only provide important diagnostic information but also insight into pathological procedures and their extension within these structures. To benefit from these technologies, the radiologist and clinician knowledge of the anatomy of this region is absolutely necessary.

Suggested Reading

Harnsberger HR (2004) Diagnostic Imaging of the Head and Neck. Amirsys, Salt Lake City

Schuknecht JF (1993) Pathology of the ear. Lea & Febiger, Philadelphia

Swartz JD, Harnsberger HR (1998) Imaging of the temporal bone, 3rd edn. Thieme, New York

Veillon F (1991) Imagerie de l'oreille. Flammarion, Paris

Veillon F, Riehm S, Enachescu B et al (2001) Imaging of the windows of the temporal bone. Semin Ultrasound CT MR 2:271-280

Imaging Diseases of the Pharynx and Oral Cavity

Bernard Schuknecht[1], Wendy Smoker[2]

[1] Division of Neuroradiology, MRI Medizinisch Radiologisches Institut, Zurich, Switzerland
[2] Division of Neuroradiology, University of Iowa Hospitals & Clinics, Iowa City, IA, USA

Imaging the Nasopharynx

Anatomy

The pharynx is subdivided into the nasopharynx, oropharynx, and hypopharynx. The nasopharynx joins the oropharynx at the level of the hard and soft palates, while the hypopharynx is the continuation of the oropharynx into the piriform sinus below the level of the pharyngo- and aryepiglottic folds. The pharynx is formed by the superior, middle, and inferior constrictor muscles. The nasopharynx is attached to the skull base by the pharyngobasilar fascia, a musculo-aponeurotic continuation of the middle layer of the deep cervical fascia (ML-DCF) that invests the pharyngeal muscles [1]. The ML-DCF represents the anterior wall layer of the retropharyngeal space. The suprahyoid retropharyngeal space houses fat and medial and lateral (Rouviere) lymph nodes. It is separated by a transversely oriented duplication of the deep layer of the deep cervical fascia (DL-DCF) from the danger space and the perivertebral space. The ML-DCF and the constrictor pharyngeal muscles house the pharyngeal mucosal space and Waldeyer's lymphatic ring with adenoid tissue in the roof of the nasopharynx and the faucial and lingual tonsils within the oropharynx.

The posterosuperior wall of the nasopharynx abuts the floor of the sphenoid sinus and foramen lacerum, and is lined by the lateral and posterosuperior walls of the soft palate. The nasopharynx extends laterally into the pharyngeal recess or fossa of Rosenmüller, which is bordered anteriorly by the torus tubarius. The Eustachian tube and levator veli palatini muscle perforate the lateral pharyngobasilar facia through the hiatus of Morgagni. Extension of malignancy may occur via the foramen lacerum and hiatus of Morgagni to reach the skull base, internal carotid artery, trigeminal nerve, and cavernous sinus.

The oropharynx is located posterior to the oral cavity and includes the soft palate with the faucil tonsils, the oropharyngeal wall, and the posterior third of the tongue dorsal to the circumvallate papillae. It further includes the vallecula and lingual surface of the epiglottis. Adjacent spaces, such as the parapharyngeal, masticator, buccal, and perivertebral spaces, are only exceptionally involved by lesions arising from the naso- or oropharynx.

The hypopharynx consists of three regions: the piriform sinus, posterior hypopharyngeal wall, and postcricoid region. The hypopharynx abuts the laryngeal vestibule and larynx posteriorly and is continuous with the cervical esophagus.

Imaging Issues

Imaging of the pharynx and oral cavity is important in determining the precise origin and location of a lesion and for delineating involvement of adjacent fascia, muscles, vessels, cranial nerves, and bone. Recognition of infiltration of the skull base, jaws, spine, and laryngeal and cricoid cartilages is of particular diagnostic and therapeutic relevance. Malignancy and infection may involve regional and distal lymph nodes as well as extralymphatic sites, such as the lung and the bone marrow.

Magnetic resonance (MR) and computed tomography (CT) are the imaging modalities most frequently applied to assess location, extent, and potential lymph node involvement by tumors arising from the naso- and oropharynx. MR imaging is best to assess intraspatial, trans-spatial, and perineural extension of malignancy and for identification of fascial plane violations. Involvement of the periosteum, perichondrium, cartilage, and cancellous bone by neoplasm or infection is significantly better delineated by MR than by CT. The internal morphology of congenital lesions, vascular malformations, hemangiomas, and salivary-gland and neural-tissue tumors is best defined by MRI. Magnetic resonance angiography (MRA) at higher field strength [2] or time-resolved MRA with improved time resolution [3] renders visible the vascular supply, angioarchitecture of vascular tumors, and the degree of vascularization. Advances in contrast media, such as the first blood-pool agent available for clinical use (Gadofosveset, Vasovist) rely on prolonged retention time within the circulation to enhance macrovascular and intralesional microvascular signal [4]. Furthermore, ultra-small iron oxide particles (USPIO) provide an opportunity to improve sensitivity and specificity for the detection of lymph node metastases [5]. Reactive adenopathy takes up USPIO and displays susceptibility-induced signal loss on T2*-weighted images, while nodal metastases do not show a change in signal.

CT, however, is best to assess cortical bone involvement (e.g., skull base, jaws,), suspected calcification, calculus-related glandular duct obstruction, or the status of cervical lymph nodes. CT-guided biopsies enable tissue from deeply located lesions to be obtained, thus allowing histologic diagnosis. For superficial lesions, sonography is ideal to assist in performing fine needle biopsies (lymph nodes, localized tumors) and in the follow-up evaluation of cervical lymph nodes in patients after treatment of head and neck cancers. Positron-emission tomography (PET)-CT has evolved as an important diagnostic technique to search for primary-tumor location in patients with metastatic lymph node manifestations, and in the staging of advanced cancer [6].

The choice of imaging modality depends on the specific diagnostic strength of the technique and the suspected disease. The decision to use a particular technique requires that patient age (e.g., small children), clinical status (dyspnea, swallowing disorders), and the presence of dental amalgams, be taken into account as these may severely compromise the results of the examination. Additional factors to be considered include iodine allergy, hyperthyroidism, iodine-131 treatment for thyroid cancer, implanted pacemakers, and ferromagnetic osteosynthetic materials in the area of interest.

The key to interpreting pathology of the aerodigestive tract relies on differences in signal intensity on T2-, T1-, and Gd-enhanced T1-weighted images. T1-weighted images outline the musculofascial anatomy best and provide a notion of fat and fascial infiltration and cancellous bone involvement by neoplasm or infection. T2-weighted images readily distinguish between mucosa and superficial adenoidal tissues, display increased signal as a correlate of fluid within cysts and dilated ducts, and optimally demonstrate the higher fluid content within the matrix of benign tumors or areas of necrosis in neoplasms. Tumors with high cellularity, such as lymphoma, or fibrous-rich tissue, such as seen in aggressive fibromatosis, exhibit markedly decreased signal on T2-weighted images. Fat-suppressed T1-weighted images are helpful to depict soft-tissue extension, bone marrow infiltration, and metastatic lymph node involvement. CT examination requires sufficient time for the contrast medium to accumulate within tumors, sites of infection, and lymph nodes. A typical protocol for multi-detector CT thus requires 40 s (flow rate 2 ml/s) for the contrast medium to enter the vasculature and parenchyma before CT scanning of the neck can be performed.

Benign Lesions of the Pharynx

Benign lesions of the pharynx may be epithelial (e.g., papilloma, adenoma) or mesenchymal (e.g., hemangioma, angiofibroma, chondroma, chordoma) in origin, or may originate from specialized tissues (e.g., teratoma, paraganglioma).

Chordoma

Chordomas, arising from notochordal remnants, most commonly arise in the sacrum but the second most common site of occurrence is the clivus, where they typically destroy the adjacent skull base. Large tumors show extensive bony inclusions or calcifications within the soft-tissue mass. So-called inferoclival chordomas may protrude anteriorly into the nasopharynx. These tumors may occur at any age but most commonly affect men in the third and fourth decades. Chordomas are predominantly hyperintense on T2-weighted images. A heterogeneous pattern on MRI and CT is due to the presence of residual bone, calcification, or hemorrhage. Most chordomas display marked heterogeneous contrast enhancement. MRI delineates relationships to the prevertebral fascia anteriorly, the dura posteriorly, adjacent neural foramina, and internal carotid arteries. A characteristic pattern on CT may support the diagnosis. CT is frequently obtained preoperatively to delineate the extent of osseous infiltration and to obtain data for CT-guided intraoperative navigation.

Juvenile Nasopharyngeal Angiofibroma

Angiofibromas are benign, locally infiltrative, nonencapsulated vascular tumors that arise in adolescent males, most commonly in or near the sphenopalatine foramen. The tumors expand the pterygopalatine fossa and extend into the sino-nasal cavities, nasopharynx, orbital apex, and cavernous sinus. Presenting symptoms include recurrent spontaneous epistaxis and nasal obstruction. More advanced cases may cause proptosis or cranial nerve deficits. Angiofibromas consist of fibrous tissue with many thin-walled vessels that lack contractile tissue. Preoperative embolization is advocated via the feeding arterial pedicles in order to reduce intraoperative blood loss. The strong vascularity of these tumors is evidenced by intratumoral flow voids on T2-weighted images and by time-resolved MRA. There is typically prominent enhancement on both CT and post-contrast T1-weighted images. CT shows a permeative type of bone erosion. Image fusion of CT with MRI and navigation CT may increase the likelihood of radical resection of tumors confined to the nasal cavity, paranasal sinuses, and skull base.

Neoplasms of the Pharynx

Nasopharyngeal Carcinomas

Nasopharyngeal carcinomas account for 70% of nasopharyngeal malignancies and represent 0.25% of all malignancies in Caucasian patients. There is an incidence of 1 per 100,000 men and 0.4 per 100,000 women. These neoplasms are much more common in patients of southern Chinese origin, with an incidence of 18 per 100,000. There is a strong indication of viral origin, as elevated titers of Epstein-Barr virus antibodies are found in almost all patients with advanced nasopharyngeal carcinoma.

Nasopharyngeal carcinoma affects men more often than women, typically in the sixth decade of life [7]. The most common presenting symptom is unilateral or bilateral conductive hearing loss, primarily due to obstruction of the Eustachian tube and the resultant serous otitis media. The second most common symptom is a cervical mass resulting from metastatic lymphadenopathy. Approximately one-third of patients present with nasal obstruction, congestion, rhinorrhea, or epistasis. The World Health Organization classifies epithelial nasopharyngeal carcinomas into two subtypes depending on whether the squamous cell carcinoma is keratinizing (type 1) or non-keratinizing (type 2). The latter type is further subdivided into differentiated (2a) and undifferentiated (undifferentiated carcinoma of nasopharyngeal type) (2b) forms. Because nasopharyngeal squamous cell carcinoma is often heavily infiltrated with lymphocytes, subtypes 2a and 2b are often termed lymphoepitheliomas.

The nonkeratinizing undifferentiated carcinoma is the most common histologic type, while keratinizing variety, unlike squamous cell carcinomas encountered in other head and neck locations, is the most uncommon type. The majority of tumors arise in the lateral recess of the nasopharynx (Fig. 1).

Lymphomas account for about 20% of nasopharyngeal malignancies. The remaining 10% of nasopharyngeal tumors comprise a diverse group that includes tumors of minor salivary gland origin, melanomas, rhabdomyosarcomas, and extramedullary plasmacytomas. MRI is particularly superior to CT in assessing tumor extension in this location. Tumors can spread directly (exophytically) into the airway and/or extend in a submucosal manner to invade the tonsillar pillars inferiorly, the soft palate anteriorly, or the skull base posterosuperiorly. MRI depicts disruption of the buccopharyngeal fascia along the tensor and levator veli palatini muscles, skull-base invasion, and spread along the deep musculofascial planes or neural pathways. Extension toward the foramen caroticum via the hiatus of Morgagni and along the petrous and cavernous segments of the internal carotid artery via the foramen lacerum is common. Deep infiltrating carcinomas may extend to involve both the pre-and post-styloid compartments of the parapharyngeal space [8]. CT is superior in detecting erosion of the cortical skull base and sphenoid sinus floor, as well as enlargement of the foramen rotundum, vidian canal, and foramen ovale. Bone marrow infiltration is delineated to better advantage by MRI. With any malignant lesion of the nasopharynx, evaluation of cervical lymph nodes, either by MRI or CT, is mandatory. In addition to involvement of nodes in levels II-IV, retropharyngeal lymph node involvement is common.

The most effective treatment for epithelial nasopharyngeal carcinomas is radiation therapy, either with or without adjunct chemotherapy. Radiation therapy results in a 5-year survival rate of approximately 40-60%. Follow-up MRI requires inclusion of the cavernous sinus and cervical lymph nodes in the examination because recurrence is most likely to occur at the borders of the radiation field. PET-CT should be performed when MRI is ambiguous with respect to small recurrent tumor or lymph node metastases.

Lymphoma

Malignant lymphoid neoplasms of the nasopharynx are usually non-Hodgkin lymphomas or lymphosarcomas [9]. Hodgkin lymphoma rarely presents as extranodal disease (1-4%) while non-Hodgkin lymphoma occurs in extranodal sites in 25-30% of cases. Lymphomas constitute approximately 20% of malignant neoplasms of the nasopharynx, the second-most common site after the faucial tonsils. Patients typically present in the fourth through eighth decades. In young adults and children, there is a higher incidence of Hodgkin lymphoma and Burkitt lymphoma. The Epstein-Barr virus is strongly associated with the development of lymphoproliferative disorders in post-transplant patients.

On MRI and CT, a large bulky bilateral mass that presents with little or no bony erosion strongly suggests the diagnosis of lymphoma. Lymphomas typically have intermediate signal intensity on T1-weighted images, moderate contrast enhancement, and low, homogeneous signal intensity on T2-weighted images. Lymphoid hyper-

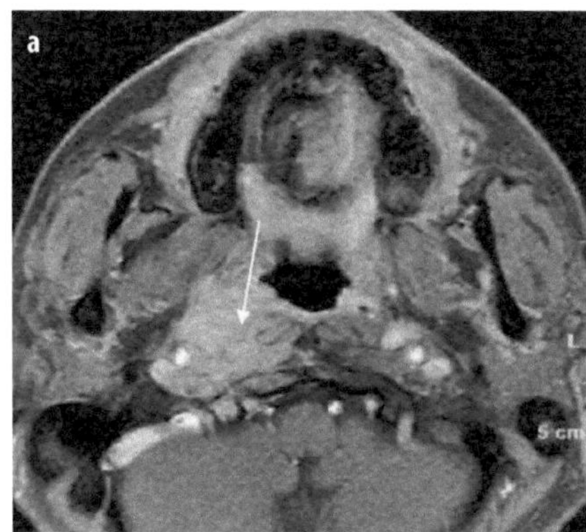

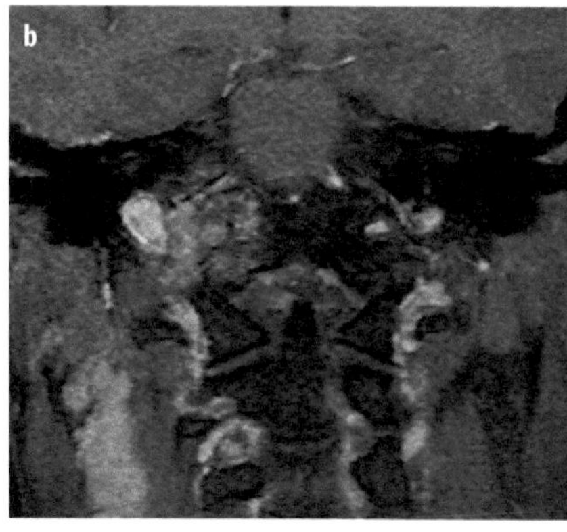

Fig. 1 a, b. Axial (**a**) and coronal (**b**) T1-weighted fat-suppressed contrast-enhanced images depict nasopharyngeal carcinoma with infiltration of the right perivertebral space, clivus, hypoglossal canal, and parapharyngeal (post-styloid carotid) space

plasia in Waldeyer's ring also enhances, but typically demonstrates internal septations and a more heterogeneous signal on T2-weighted images. These features may help distinguish reactive lymphoid hypertrophy from neoplasm. On CT, Waldeyer's ring lymphomas are characterized by homogenous submucosal masses, isodense to muscle, associated with enlarged lymph nodes. Necrosis and extranodal extension are not encountered. Treatment for lymphoma consists of chemotherapy.

Rhabdomyosarcoma

Rhabdomyosarcoma is the second most common soft-tissue sarcoma and the second most frequent head and neck malignancy in children. Nearly one-third of head and neck rhabdomyosarcomas involve the pharynx. The peak incidence is between 2 and 5 years of age, with 70% of all cases observed in subjects <10 years of age. Rhabdomyosarcoma is a malignant mesenchymal tumor believed to arise from cells related to the skeletal muscle lineage. Among the three main histopathologic types, the embryonal type is most common (75%), followed by alveolar (20%) and pleomorphic tumors (5%) [10]. The incidence of metastatic cervical lymph node involvement at the time of initial manifestation is 3-25%.

Imaging findings in rhabdomyosarcomas are similar to those of malignant epithelial carcinomas. Since these neoplasms arise from muscle, they may not necessarily involve the pharyngeal mucosal space. The most typical finding is a bulky nasopharyngeal mass producing heterogeneous signal intensities on both T1- and T2-weighted images. These features are caused by areas of necrosis. Following administration of contrast medium, variable heterogeneous enhancement is observed of both the primary neoplasm as well as associated metastatic lymph nodes. CT provides complimentary information regarding skull-base destruction and the occasional associated remodeling of bone.

Malignant Melanoma

Primary nasopharyngeal melanomas are rare, accounting for <1% of all malignant melanomas. Melanomas rarely metastasize to the nasopharynx from other sites. The melanocytes in the nasal cavity are located primarily in the nasal septum or the turbinates. The nasopharynx is involved by direct extension. Melanomas have relatively homogeneous signal intensity, typically exhibit high signal due to melanin or hemorrhage on T1-weighted images, and are isointense or hyperintense on T2-weighted images. Melanomas show moderate contrast enhancement. Post-contrast T1-weighted fat-suppressed scans are useful to assess for evidence of parapharyngeal, skull-base, and intracranial involvement.

Extramedullary Plasmocytoma

This tumor is composed almost exclusively of plasma cells, without intervening stroma. Extramedullary plasmocytoma occurs in the head and neck in 80% of affected patients, with the nasopharynx as the most common location. A polypoid appearance with submucosal extension and pure osteolysis is indicative of a plasmocytoma.

Squamous Cell Carcinoma of the Oropharynx

Oropharyngeal squamous cell carcinomas are usually poorly differentiated [11, 12]. These tumors are characterized by extensive primary disease, with a 50-70% incidence of cervical lymph node metastasis at the time of presentation (Table 1) and a 10-20% incidence of bilateral lymph node disease if midline structures are affected. Early disease is rarely recognized since patients usually are asymptomatic. Some lesions may be detected on discovery of a neck mass (lymphadenopathy). Persistent unilateral sore throat, referred otalgia, and difficulty with speech or swallowing are symptoms of advanced disease. Squamous cell carcinomas of the oropharynx have a propensity to spread extensively along the mucosal surfaces of the soft palate, lateral pharyngeal wall, and base of the tongue.

Carcinoma of the tonsil tends to spread posteriorly to the lateral pharyngeal wall, inferiorly to the base of the tongue via the glossotonsillar sulcus (Fig. 2) and superiorly to the soft palate. This tumor can also grow directly into the soft tissues of the neck and posterolaterally to invade the adventitia of the carotid artery. Lymph node metastases are present in 60-70% of patients with T3 and T4 tumors at the time of diagnosis. Bilateral nodal involvement is seen in 15-20% of patients in whom a large portion of the base of the tongue or soft palate is involved. Tonsillar carcinomas primarily drain to lymph nodes in levels I-V. Small carcinomas are difficult to detect by imaging studies, CT in particular. Infection, lymphoid hyperplasia, and postoperative asymmetry may all simulate the presence of a tonsillar mass on CT or MRI. PET-CT has proven extremely useful in the evaluation of the patient with an "unknown primary". More often than not, the tumor is located in the tonsil. Occasionally, tonsillectomy is performed for both diagnosis and treatment.

Table 1. Incidence and location of cervical lymph node metastases according to the site of the primary tumor

Site of primary tumor	Incidence of lymph node metastasis at presentation (%)	Nodal level involved
Nasopharynx	86-90	II, III, IV
Tongue (base)	50-83	II, III, IV
Tonsillar fossa	58-76	I, II, III, IV
Hypopharynx	52-75	II, III, IV
Oropharynx	50-71	II, III
Tongue (oral portion)	34-65	I, II, III
Floor of mouth	30-59	I, II
Retromolar trigone	39-56	I, II, III
Soft palate	37-56	II
Supraglottic larynx	31-54	II, III, IV

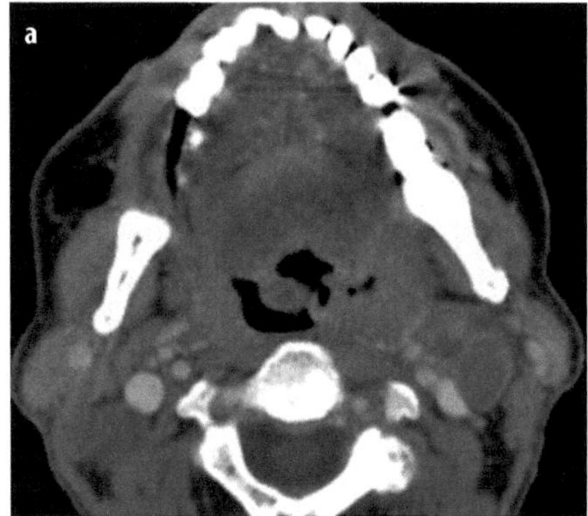

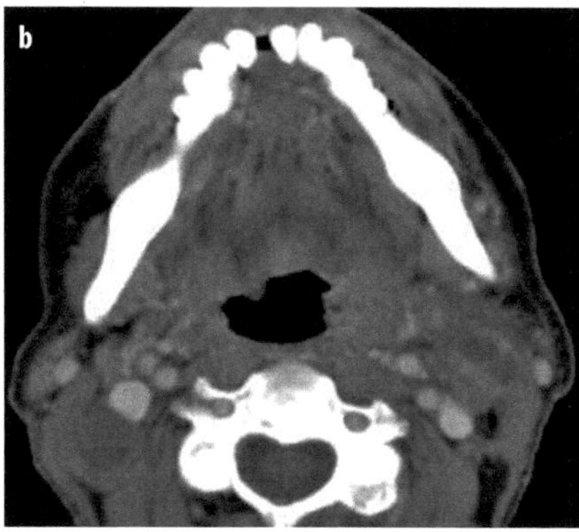

Fig. 2 a, b. Axial contrast-enhanced CT images show left tonsillar carcinoma with ulceration (**a**) extending down the glossotonsillar sulcus (**b**); bilateral lymph node metastases to right level IA and left level IIB are visible

Squamous cell carcinomas of the base of the tongue are aggressive, deeply infiltrative, moderately or poorly differentiated neoplasms. There is a 75% incidence of lymph node metastases (33-50% of which are bilateral) at the time of presentation due to a rich lymphatic network. The most commonly involved lymph nodes are those of the internal jugular chain (levels II-V). As many as 10-20% of clinically normal lymph nodes harbor occult metastatic disease. Early disease is radiosensitive and curable by radiation alone, with results comparable to those of surgery without mutilation. Late disease requires combined radiation and surgical treatment or chemotherapy.

Sagittal images obtained with MRI permit excellent appreciation of the volume of tumor in the tongue base and infiltration of the vallecula. Such carcinomas are usually hyperintense on T2-weighted images, may form ulcerative bulky masses, or may present as deeply infiltrative processes along the muscle planes. Carcinoma of the base of the tongue is distinguished from hyperplasia of the lingual tonsil by invasion and disruption of the muscle bundles of the tongue. The administration of contrast results in intense enhancement on CT or MRI.

The lateral and posterior portions of the oropharynx and the posterior tonsillar fossa form the oropharyngeal wall. Squamous cell carcinomas of this region are often ulcerated and may infiltrate inferiorly into the hypopharynx. Such tumors are usually moderately or poorly differentiated. Because of the lack of early symptoms, 75% of patients present with extensive primary disease and lymph node metastases, frequently bilateral. The most commonly involved lymph nodes are those of levels II and III and the lateral retropharyngeal lymph nodes [13].

Minor salivary gland tumors commonly occur in the oropharynx and oral cavity. Adeno-, adenoid cystic, and mucoepidermoid carcinomas, along with malignant mixed tumors, constitute the principle histologic subtypes.

Squamous Cell Carcinoma of the Hypopharynx

Squamous cell carcinomas of the hypopharynx are predominantly moderately or poorly differentiated tumors [14]. These neoplasms spread with ease from one anatomic site to another, as well as from the hypopharynx to the larynx, since there are no fascial boundaries between these structures. Common sites are the piriform sinus (65%), followed by the post-cricoid area (20%) and the posterior pharyngeal wall (15%). The incidence of lymph node metastases is 50-70%, with 10-20% bilateral involvement owing to the rich lymphatic pathways in the hypopharynx.

Early symptoms of hypopharyngeal carcinoma include sore throat, intolerance to hot and cold liquids, dysphasia, odynophagia, and ipsilateral otalgia. Whenever otalgia is present, the tumor is large and has invaded the superior laryngeal nerve with referred pain back to the vagus nerve. Involvement of the post-cricoid area leads to dysphagia, while extensive carcinomas of the piriform sinus result in hoarseness, laryngeal stridor, and hemoptysis.

Piriform sinus carcinomas are often bilateral and submucosal in location. Deep extension of disease and lymph node metastases are well-evaluated with CT and MRI. T1-weighted images maximize contrast between the intermediate signal of the tumor and the bright signal in adjacent loose areolar tissue. Tumors originating from the apex of the piriform sinus are aggressive and infiltrative and may extend into the adjacent posterior margin of the thyroid cartilage and infrahyoid muscles. Spread of disease towards the larynx and trachea is common.

Carcinoma of the post-cricoid area is usually well-differentiated. Despite aggressive surgery, 5-year survival is only 10-20%, owing to extensive spread of disease at the time of initial presentation. This site has the worst prognosis of all three sites of hypopharyngeal carcinoma.

Carcinoma of the posterior pharyngeal wall is the least common location for carcinomas of the hypopharynx. Such lesions are large and exophytic at the time of presentation and may extend to the lateral pharyngeal wall or the cervical esophagus below. The perivertebral muscles and vertebral bodies may not be involved until late in the disease, due to the presence of the prevertebral fascia. About 50% of afflicted patients have cervical lymph node metastases, often bilateral, at the time of diagnosis.

CT frequently is sufficient to delineate the origin and extent of tumor, to recognize cartilage invasion in post-cricoid locations, and to identify infiltration of the paraglottic space anteriorly. Differentiation of anterior from posterior wall location may be difficult unless a supplementary scan is performed with Valsalva maneuver. Assessment of craniocaudal tumor extension, delineation of the relationship to the prevertebral fascia, and evaluation of cervical lymph nodes requires coronal and sagittal multiplanar CT reconstructions and/or coronal and sagittal MRI sequences.

Imaging the Oral Cavity

Anatomy

The oral cavity includes the floor of the mouth, the anterior two-thirds of the tongue, the lips, and gingivobuccal (oral vestibule) and buccomasseteric regions. The oral cavity is separated from the oropharynx at the level of the circumvallate papillae. The tongue is composed of the intrinsic musculature (superior and inferior longitudinal, transverse and vertical muscle fibers) and extrinsic muscles (genioglossus, styloglossus, hyoglossus, and palatoglossus muscles), which originate external to the tongue but insert into the tongue itself.The floor of the mouth is composed of the mylohyoid muscles, united by a median raphe, and the midline geniohyoid muscles, located below the genioglossus muscles. It is supported by the anterior bellies of the digastric muscles, which border the triangular submental space that contains fat and lymph nodes (nodal level IA). At the posterior margin of the mylohyoid muscle, the submandibular gland extends through a gap between the hyoglossus and mylohyoid muscles. Its deep portion is contained in the sublingual space together with the sublingual gland, the lingual nerves laterally, and the lingual artery and vein medially. Posteriorly, the sublingual space freely communicates with the submandibular space as no fascial boundary separates them. The submandibular space contains lymph nodes (level IB) and the submandibular gland, with the facial artery medially and the facial vein laterally.

The oral vestibule separates the lips and cheeks form the teeth and alveolar process by a reflection of buccal mucosa onto the maxilla and mandible. Adjacent to the alveolar process, the gingivobuccal and the glossoalveolar sulci are common locations for squamous cell carcinoma of the vestibule and floor of the mouth, respectively. The retromolar trigone, between the third molar and the mandibular ramus, is another frequent site of squamous cell carcinoma. The pterygomandibular raphe is a fascial band extending from the hamulus of the medial pterygoid plate to the mylohyoid ridge of the mandible and provides origin for the buccinator and superior pharyngeal constrictor muscles. Retromolar malignancies may spread along this raphe to the maxillary tuberosity superiorly and to the retroantral masticator space posteriorly and inferiorly to reach the floor of the mouth. The buccomasseteric region is composed of the buccal space, traversed by the parotid duct, the buccinator and masseter muscles, and the body of the mandible.

Benign Lesions of the Oral Cavity

Germ Cell Derivatives

Germ cell derivatives comprise epidermoid, dermoid, and teratoid cysts. These developmental lesions are formed by inclusion of ectodermal (epidermoid), ecto- and mesodermal tissue (dermoids), and components of all three germ layers (teratoid cysts) during midline closure of the first and second branchial arches.

Epidermoid cysts are composed of squamous epithelium contained within a fibrous wall. Dermoids additionally consist of hair follicles, sebaceous glands, and fat. Teratoid cysts are composed of ecto-, meso-, and entodermal tissue and bear the designation "teratoma" if recognizable organs (e.g., teeth) are found histologically and/or on imaging. Dermoids occur along the floor of the mouth. Depending on the amount of fat they contain, they display negative CT values, are less dense than epidermoids (0-15 HU), and are of higher signal intensity on T1-weighted images. T2 hyperintense signal is typical and the walls display mild contrast enhancement. Unlike epidermoids, dermoids and teratomas bear malignant potential, while teratoid cysts in the floor of the mouth or nasopharynx are usually composed of well-differentiated tissues.

Vascular Lesions

In infancy and childhood, two types of vascular lesions are encountered: *hemangiomas* and *vascular malformations* [10]. Hemangiomas are tumors characterized by endothelial cell proliferation and the formation of vascular channels within a soft-tissue stroma. They commonly become apparent within the first months of life; enlarge rapidly during a proliferative phase, and subsequently regress by adolescence. Bluish discoloration of the skin and compressibility are encountered when these tumors are subcutaneous in location. Deep lesions may affect the pharynx, oral cavity, or orbits. Hemangiomas require no treatment unless functional compromise (respiration, deglutition, vision) occurs. They are typically hyperintense on T2-weighted MRI, enhance moderately, and may contain flow voids in the proliferative stage.

Vascular malformations, or angiomas, are not tumors but inborn errors of vascular morphogenesis. Based on the predominant vascular component, vascular malformations are classified into capillary, arterial, venous, lymphatic, or mixed types. Vascular malformations are present at birth, grow commensurate with growth of the child, and do not involute. Endocrine stimuli or trauma, including surgery, may cause exacerbation. Capillary malformations (port-wine stain, nevus flammeus) are slow-flow malformations that may occur as isolated lesions or as part of a syndrome (e.g., Sturge-Weber, ataxia-telangiectasia, Rendu-Osler-Weber, Wyburn-Mason, or Cobb syndromes). Venous malformations commonly affect the oral cavity or may be entirely intramuscular, most often within the masseter muscle. T2 hyperintensity, gadolinium enhancement on MRI, muscle isodensity on CT, and phleboliths are characteristic findings. Arteriovenous malformations are high-flow lesions with abundant flow voids; they may become quite large, and affect the midface, masticator space, and oral cavity. Lymphatic malformations, or lymphangiomas, may display increased signal intensity on T1-weighted images and mild hyperdensity on CT due to their high protein content. Lymphangiomas represent a continuum of lesions that include cystic lymphangiomas, (previously termed cystic hygromas), cavernous and capillary lymphangiomas, and lymphangiomas with additional vascular elements (hemangio-lymphangiomas, venolymphatic malformations). Any of these components may be found in a single lesion. Fluid-fluid levels due to hemorrhage may be present. Capillary and cavernous malformations are preferentially located in the posterior cervical, sublingual, and submandibular spaces. The cavernous type may present with a permeative pattern within the tongue and floor of the mouth.

Benign Cystic Lesions

Ranulas are mucous retention cysts due to obstruction of a salivary gland, most commonly the sublingual gland. Simple ranulas are true epithelial-lined cysts, while the plunging (diving) ranula develops following rupture of the simple ranula cyst wall (pseudocyst) and presents as a lesion primarily centered in the submandibular space, although a small residual "tail" can usually be identified extending from the sublingual space. Therefore, a "cystic" lesion in relationship to the submandibular gland may be a ranula (medially): a second *branchial cleft cyst* (posteriorly); a third branchial cleft cyst inferiorly; or, more commonly, anteriorly a dermoid, cystic hygroma, or lipoma [15]. The suprahyoid *thyroglossal duct cyst,* the most common congenital lesion, is located in the midline between the foramen cecum and the level of the hyoid. Infrahyoid cysts (50-65%) frequently extend off-midline, encased within the infrahyoid strap muscles along the course of the embryonic thyroglossal duct (Fig. 3). Persistent thyroid tissue may occur anywhere along the duct and typically enhances markedly on post-contrast CT and MRI studies. The possibility of malignancy (usually papillary carcinoma) or infection should be taken into consideration.

Inflammatory and Infectious Lesions

Inflammation of the floor of the mouth, submental or submandibular spaces, and buccomasseteric region may arise from dental disease, ductal obstruction due to sialolithiasis, strictures, or a neoplasm obliterating the orifice of Wharton's (submandibular) duct or Stensen's (parotid) duct. Glandular inflammation (sialadenitis) may display swelling and increased contrast enhancement by the gland and its fascial lining. CT may be required to demonstrate sialotlithiasis in glandular inflammation. This holds true despite advanced techniques such as MR sialography. Frank *abscess* formation is rare and, in the absence of a predisposing condition, should initiate a search for a specific etiology (e.g., tuberculosis). Inflammation within the oral cavity may, alternatively, arise from infection in a pre-existing lesion (ranula, dermoid, thyroglossal duct cyst) or may be of odontogenic origin (Fig. 4).

Periapical or periodontal disease that gains access to the sublingual, submandibular, or masticator spaces may eventually lead to perimandibular phlegmonous or abscess formation. Extension to cancellous and cortical bone via Volkmann's canals results in mandibular osteomyelitis. An orthopantomogram, supplemented by CT with bone window algorithm, is the imaging modality of choice to demonstrate complications of odontogenic infection. Early signs are cortical bone erosion and periosteal reaction. Later signs include sequestration, pathologic fracture, and progressive bone sclerosis. MRI, however, is superior to CT for demonstration of the bone marrow involvement characteristic of the acute and chronic stages of osteomyelitis [16].

A recently detected complication of prolonged biphosphonate treatment, "biphosphonate related osteonecrosis of the jaws", evidences increased density of the periodontal ligament, cancellous bone and cortical thickening

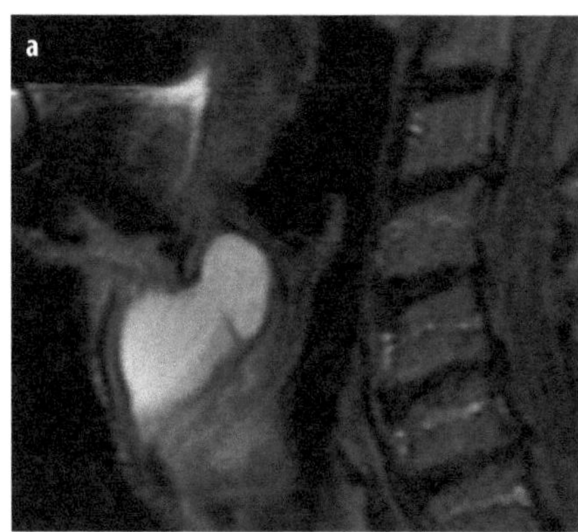

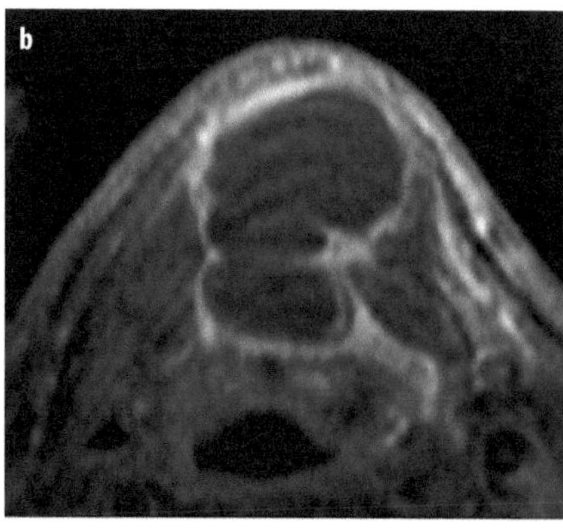

Fig. 3 a, b. Sagittal T2-weighted (**a**) and axial T1-weighted (**b**) images demonstrate an infrahyoid large thyroglossal durct cyst with mild linear thickening and contrast-enhancing walls, indicating previous infection

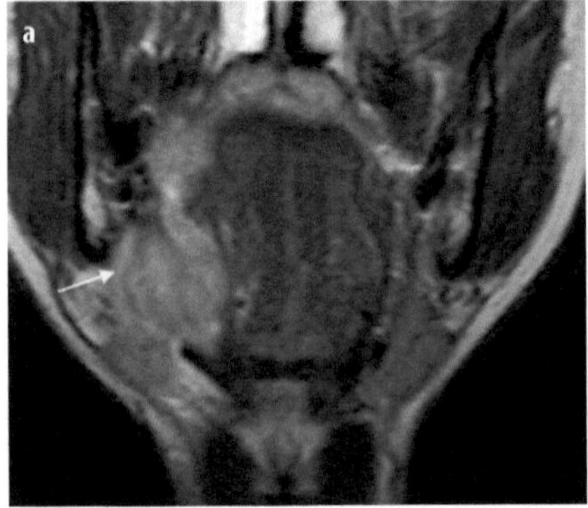

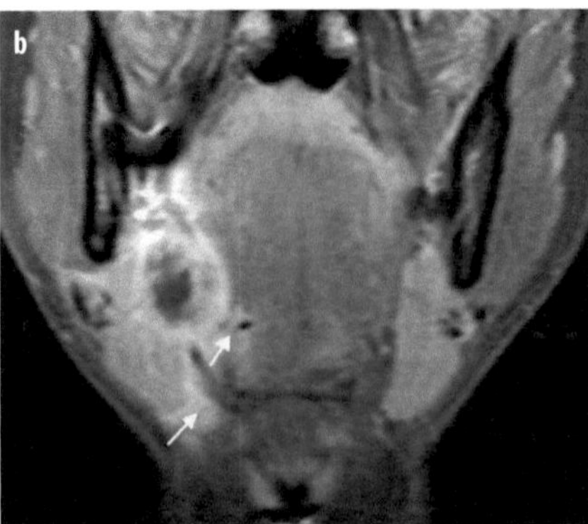

Fig. 4 a, b. Coronal T2-weighted (**a**) and T1-weighted fat-suppressed (**b**) images display an abscess of the floor of the mouth with lateral displacement of the deep lobe of the submandibular gland (*arrow* in **a**) and little involvement of the submandibular space (*short arrow* in **b**) and sublingual space (*arrowhead* in **b**) This is of odontogenic (last molar, 38) origin with signal inhomogeneity noted in the retromolar trigone and inferior soft palate

as direct effects of inhibition of osteoclast-mediated bone resorption. Superimposed infection of exposed bone is common and modifies the clinical and radiographic presentation by the presence of periosteal calcifications, sequestra and, rarely, fistulae.

Benign Tumors of the Oral Cavity

In the oral cavity and buccal space, *pleomorphic adenomas* are the most common benign glandular tumors. Such lesions may cause pressure erosion of the posterior hard plate and display cystic changes, hypodensity with little enhancement on CT, T2 hyperintensity, and inhomogeneous enhancement on MRI. *Schwannomas* and *malignant minor salivary gland tumors* are often also well-defined and therefore have a similar imaging appearance. *Rhabdomyomas* are rare, benign, frequently encapsulated tumors of striated muscle that occur in middle-aged men and preferentially affect the base of the tongue, floor of the mouth, and pharynx. *Granular cell myoblastomas* contain neurogenic and muscular elements and are most probably of primitive neuroectodermal origin. As nonencapsulated tumors, they may display a somewhat infiltrating appearance. The oral tongue, the dorsum and lateral tip in particular, is affected in 50% of cases. The lesions are of muscle density (CT) and signal intensity (MRI).

Malignant Neoplasm of the Oral Cavity

The squamous epithelium within the oral cavity originates from ectoderm and thus gives rise to better-differentiated neoplasms than the entodermally derived mucosa of the oropharynx. Squamous cell carcinomas (SCCa) account for 90% of oral cavity malignancies. Other malignant neoplasms include minor salivary gland tumors (e.g. adenocystic, adeno-, and mucoepidermoid carcinomas), sarcomas, and lymphomas [17].

Imaging must be tailored to provide specific information for the clinicians: (1) precise description of tumor location; (2) assessment of the extent of submucosal disease; (3) presence or absence of sublingual space and neurovascular pedicle involvement; (4) presence or absence of perineural tumor spread; (5) evidence of cortical bone involvement; and (6) the status of regional lymph nodes. Common sites for oral cavity SCCa are the lower lip, oral tongue, floor of the mouth, gingival/ etromolar trigone, and hard palate, in decreasing order of frequency.

SCCas of the oral tongue typically originate along the middle and posterior thirds, along the plane of occlusion, and tend to invade the intrinsic and extrinsic tongue muscles [12]. Assessment of the relationship of the tumor to the midline of the tongue and floor of the mouth/neurovascular bundles is critical, as contralateral tongue and neurovascular bundle invasion dictate total glossectomy or nonsurgical organ preservation therapy. Tumors may also extend to the base of the tongue, the anterior tonsillar pillar (via the glossotonsillar sulcus), and into the soft palate.

SCCas of the floor of the mouth are most commonly found in the anterior third and may spread medially to obstruct the submandibular duct as well as laterally and posteriorly within the glosso-alveolar sulcus along the mylohyoid muscle to affect the lingual and occlusal cortical mandibular surfaces. They may also extend along the neurovascular bundle within the sublingual space. Small tumors may be missed on axial sections, either by CT or MRI, unless the coronal images are scrutinized. Lymph node drainage affects the submental (nodal level IA), submandibular (IB) and jugulodigastric (II) lymph nodes. Carcinomas of the gingiva, gingivobuccal sulcus, and retromolar trigone are prone to cause mandibular erosion and to spread into the buccal and masticator spaces [18].

Tumors arising in the retromolar trigone may extend along the palatoglossus muscle and the pterygomandibular raphe, occasionally mimicking tonsillar SCCa. Oral tongue and retromolar trigone tumors commonly drain to lymph nodes in levels I-III.

MRI in most instances is devoid of dental artifacts and is superior to CT in recognition of tumor extension. Obliteration of fat by tumor extension along the nasopalatine nerves into the pterygopalatine fossa and widening of the descending palatine canal are signs indicating perineural tumor spread of hard-palate tumors. Early recognition of cortical bone erosion, however, requires high-resolution CT [19, 20].

Imaging Cervical Metastasis

Imaging is especially useful to detect pathologic lymph nodes in a clinically negative neck. Non-necrotic lymph node enlargement or groups of enlarged lymph nodes suggest Hodgkin or non-Hodgkin lymphoma [21]. Carcinoma of unknown primary represents 3-5 % of head and neck cancers; SCCa account for 70-90% of these lesions [22]. The main imaging criteria for assessing nodal metastases include the size and shape of the node, the presence of necrosis, and the presence of a localized group of nodes in an expected nodal-draining area for a specific primary tumor (Table 1).

Lymph nodes are considered abnormal if they are >10 mm in diameter. Exceptions include the larger level II nodes and the smaller retropharyngeal nodes, which are considered abnormal if their diameters exceed 15 mm and 8 mm, respectively. Imaging cannot yet identify microscopic tumor foci. Normal lymph nodes are oval or oblong, while metastatic lymph nodes are round or spherical. Central nodal necrosis is the most specific sign of metastasis but has to be differentiated from hilar fat.

Transcapsular extranodal tumor spread decreases survival by 50% compared to confined tumors. Extranodal extension is seen on CT and MRI as a poorly defined nodal border with variable enhancement [22]. In addition, there may be obliterated fat planes adjacent to the node. Any lymph node with ill-defined margins is abnormal. Nodal capsular penetration and the presence of a nodal mass surrounding at least 75% of an adjacent structure are highly suggestive of fixation to the adjacent structure.

SCCa of the nasopharynx, tonsil, and base of the tongue are the primary neoplasms of the head and neck that commonly metastasize to cervical lymph nodes. These areas must be carefully examined in the search for an unknown primary tumor.

Staging of Cancer of the Pharynx and Oral Cavity

Accurate staging is the most important factor in the assessment, treatment planning, and prognosis of patients with head and neck cancer. The staging system of the American Joint Cancer Committee (AJCC) [20] incorporates three aspects of tumor assessment: the extent of primary tumor (T), involvement of regional lymph nodes (N), and distant metastases (M).

The primary tumor (T) is scored as:

- TX: Primary tumour cannot be assessed
- T0: No evidence of primary tumour
- Tis: Carcinoma in situ
- T1-T4 Increasing size or local extent of the primary tumor

Table 2. Definitions of T1-T4 for tumors of the pharynx and oral cavity. (Adapted from [20])

Primary tumor	Definition
Nasopharynx	
T1	Tumor confined to one site of nasopharynx or no tumor visible (positive biopsy only)
T2	Tumor involving two sites (both posterosuperior and lateral walls)
T3	Extension of tumor into nasal cavity or oropharynx
T4	Tumor invasion of skull base or cranial nerve involvement, or both
Oropharynx and oral cavity	
T1	Tumor ≤2 cm in the greatest diameter
T2	Tumor >2 cm but not >4 cm in the greatest diameter
T3	Tumor >4 cm in greatest diameter
T4	Massive tumor >4 cm in diameter, with invasion of contiguous structures
Hypopharynx	
T1	Tumor confined to site of origin
T2	Extension of tumor to adjacent region or site without fixation of hemilarynx
T3	Extension of tumor to adjacent region or site with fixation of hemilarynx
T4	Massive tumor invading bone or soft tissues of the neck

The exact definitions of T1-T4 depend on the actual site of the primary tumor (Table 2). T4 lesions are further subdivided into: T4A (resectable), T4B (unresectable), and T4C (advanced distant metastases).

Nodal involvement (N) is scored as:

- NX: Regional lymph nodes cannot be assessed
- N0: No regional lymph node metastases
- N1: Metastasis in a single ipsilateral lymph node, ≤3 cm in the greatest dimension
- N2a: Metastasis in a single ipsilateral lymph node, >3 cm but not >6 cm in the greatest dimension
- N2b: Metastases in multiple ipsilateral lymph nodes, not >6 cm in the greatest dimension
- N2c: Bilateral or contralateral metastatic lymph nodes, none >6 cm in the greatest dimension
- N3: Metastasis in a lymph node, >6 cm in the greatest dimension

Distant metastases (M) are scored as:

- Mx: Distant metastases cannot be assessed
- M0: No known distant metastases
- M1: Distant metastasis present (specify area or structure)

The resulting tumor stages are then defined by the combination of tumor (T), node (N), and metastasis (M) scores:

- Stage I: T1, N0, M0
- Stage II: T2, N0, M0
- Stage III: T3, N0, M0
T1 or T2 or T3, N1, M0
- Stage IV: T4, N0 or N1, M0
Any T, N2 or N3, M0
Any T, Any N, M1

References

1. Harnsberger HR (2004) Pharyngeal mucosal space. Introduction and overview III-1-2. In: Harnberger HR (ed) Diagnostic Imaging: Head and Neck. Amirsys, Salt Lake City, pp 2-5
2. DeLano MC, DeMarco JK (2006) 3.0 T versus 1.5 T MR angiography of the head and neck. Neuroimag Clin N Am 16:321-341
3. Krings T, Hans F (2004) New developments in MRA: time resolved MRA. Neuroradiology 46:(Suppl 2)s214-s222
4. Fink C, Goyen M, Lotz J (2007) Magnetic resonance angiography with blood-pool contrast agents: future applications. Eur Radiol 17(Suppl 2):B38-B44
5. Baghi M, Mack MG, Hambek M et al (2005) The efficacy of MRI with ultrasmall superparamagnetic iron oxide particles (USPIO) in head and neck cancers. Anticancer Res 25:3665-3667
6. Paul SA, Stoeckli SJ, von Schulthess GK, Goerres GW, (2007) FDG PET and PET/CT for the detection of the primary tumour in patients with cervical non-squamous cell carcinoma metastasis of an unknown primary. Eur Arch Otorhinolaryngol 264:189-195
7. Weber AL, Al Areyedh S, Rashid A (2003) Nasopharynx: clinical, pathologic and radiologic assessment. Neuroimag Clin N Am 13:465-483
8. Dubrulle F, Souillard, Hermans R (2007) Extension pattern of nasopharyngeal carcinoma. Eur Radiol 17:2622-2630
9. Sakai O, Curtin HD, Romo LV, Som PM (2000) Lymph node pathology: benign proliferative, lymphoma, ands metastatic disease. Radiol Clin North Am 22:631-636
10. Robson CD (2003) Cyst and tumours of the oral cavity, oropharynx and nasopharynx in children. In: Weber AL (ed) Imaging of the mandible, maxilla and pharynx. Neuroimag Clin N Am 13:427-442
11. Laine FJ, Smoker WR (1995) Oral cavity: anatomy and pathology. Semin Ultrasound CT MR 16:527-545
12. Smoker WRK (2003) The oral cavity. In: Som PM, Curtin HD (eds) Head and neck imaging. 5th edn. Mosby Year Book, St Louis, pp 1377-1464
13. MacDonald AJ, Harnsberger HR (2004) Oral cavity and imaging issues III-4-2. In: Harnsberger HR (ed) Diagnostic imaging: head and neck. Amirsys, Salt Lake City
14. Schmalfuss IM (2002) Imaging of the hypopharynx and cervical esophagus. Mag Reson Imaging Clin N Am10: 495-509
15. Som PM, Smoker WRK, Curtin HD et al (2003) Congenital lesions. In: Som PM, Curtin HD (eds) Head and neck imaging. 5th edn. Mosby year Book, St Louis pp 1828-1864
16. Schuknecht B, Valavanis A (2003) Osteomyelitis of the mandible. Neuroimaging Clin N Am 13:605-618
17. Hoang TA, Hasso AN (1994) Magnetic resonance imaging of the oral cavity and tongue. Magn Reson Imaging 6(4):241-253
18. Kurabayashi T, Ida M, Ohbayashi N et al (2002) MR Imaging of benign and malignant lesions in the buccal space. Dentomaxillofacial Radiol 31:344-349
19. Kimura Y, Sumi M, Yoshiko A et al (2002) Deep extension from carcinoma arising from the gingiva: CT and MR imaging features. AJNR Am J Neuroradiol 23:468-472
20. American Joint Committee on Cancer (2002) AJCC cancer staging manual, 6th edn. Lippincott-Raven, New York
21. Urquhart A, Berg R (2001) Hodgkin's and non-Hodgkin's lymphoma of the head and neck. Laryngoscope 111:1565-1569
22. Donta TS, Smoker WR (2007) Head and neck cancer: carcinoma of unknown primary. Top Magn Reson Imaging 18:281-292

Imaging of the Larynx and Hypopharynx

Minerva Becker

Division of Diagnostic and Interventional Radiology, Geneva University Hospital, Geneva, Switzerland

Imaging Techniques

The larynx and hypopharynx are imaged with either computed tomography (CT) or magnetic resonance (MR). A standard CT examination is done with the patient in the supine position; the patient is also instructed to resist swallowing or coughing. Axial slices are obtained from the base of the skull to the trachea with a scan orientation parallel to the true vocal cords. Iodinated contrast material (total dose: 35-40 g iodine) is given intravenously with an automated power injector. Images are obtained during quiet breathing rather than during apnea because the abducted position of the true vocal cords facilitates evaluation of the anterior and posterior commissures. Acquisitions with 3-mm collimation at pitch 1 and overlapping reconstruction intervals of 2 mm are the minimum settings necessary to evaluate the larynx. With multi-slice CT scanners, a slice thickness of 1.3 and overlapping reconstructions every 0.6 mm are used routinely by many investigators, including ourselves, as these settings yield high-quality 2D-reconstructions in the coronal or sagittal plane.

To date, MR imaging of the larynx and hypopharynx is done using dedicated surface neck coils in phased array (multi-coil) configuration. Two basic pulse sequences are currently used by most investigators, namely T1-weighted sequences and T2-weighted sequences. Axial T2-weighted fast spin-echo (FSE) and T1-weighted SE or T1-weighted FSE images are obtained with a scan orientation parallel to the true vocal cords. Typical image parameters for a standard examination include a slice thickness of 3 or 4 mm with a 0- to 1-mm intersection gap and a field of view of 18 × 18 cm or less. The acquisition matrix should be 256 × 512 or 512 × 512. Additional axial T1-weighted images after intravenous administration of gadolinium chelates are obtained routinely. Fat-saturated T1-weighted images with or without contrast-material enhancement and fat-saturated T2-weighted images are optional. Images in the coronal or sagittal plane may be obtained in order to evaluate certain anatomic spaces, such as the pre-epiglottic space in the sagittal plane, or the paraglottic space and the ventricle in the coronal plane.

Pathologic Conditions of the Larynx and Hypopharynx

The most common indications to perform cross-sectional imaging of the larynx include: (1) squamous cell carcinoma, (2) nonsquamous cell tumors, (3) cysts and laryngoceles, (4) vocal-cord paralysis, (5) inflammatory lesions, and (6) traumatic lesions.

Squamous Cell Carcinoma

Over 90% of laryngeal and hypopharyngeal tumors are squamous cell carcinomas. With very few exceptions, squamous cell tumors are located at the mucosal surface, and the clinical diagnosis is readily confirmed by endoscopic biopsy. However, submucosal tumor extension cannot be assessed reliably with endoscopy alone. Since the degree of infiltration into the surrounding deep anatomic structures has implications for treatment and prognosis, cross-sectional imaging – either CT or MR – is required for the diagnostic workup of laryngeal and hypopharyngeal tumors. Unusual malignant neoplasms of the laryngo-hypopharyngeal region, such as chondrosarcomas, lymphomas, or lipomas, are often entirely located submucosally. The origin and extension of these tumors are difficult to diagnose with endoscopy, such that biopsy and treatment planning usually depend on the imaging findings.

Patterns of Tumor Spread

Carcinoma of the larynx arises in the supraglottic region (30%), glottis (65%), or subglottic region (5%).

Supraglottic tumors originating from the epiglottis primarily invade the pre-epiglottic space. The MR imaging diagnosis of tumor spread to the pre-epiglottic space is made when the high signal intensity of fat normally seen on the T1-weighted image is replaced by a mass with low signal intensity and when enhancement of the pre-epiglottic mass is observed (Fig. 1). Although sagittal images are best-suited to delineate the extent of tumor spread within the pre-epiglottic space (Fig. 2), standard axial images are sufficient to establish the diagnosis. Similarly, on CT, the diagnosis of pre-epiglottic space in-

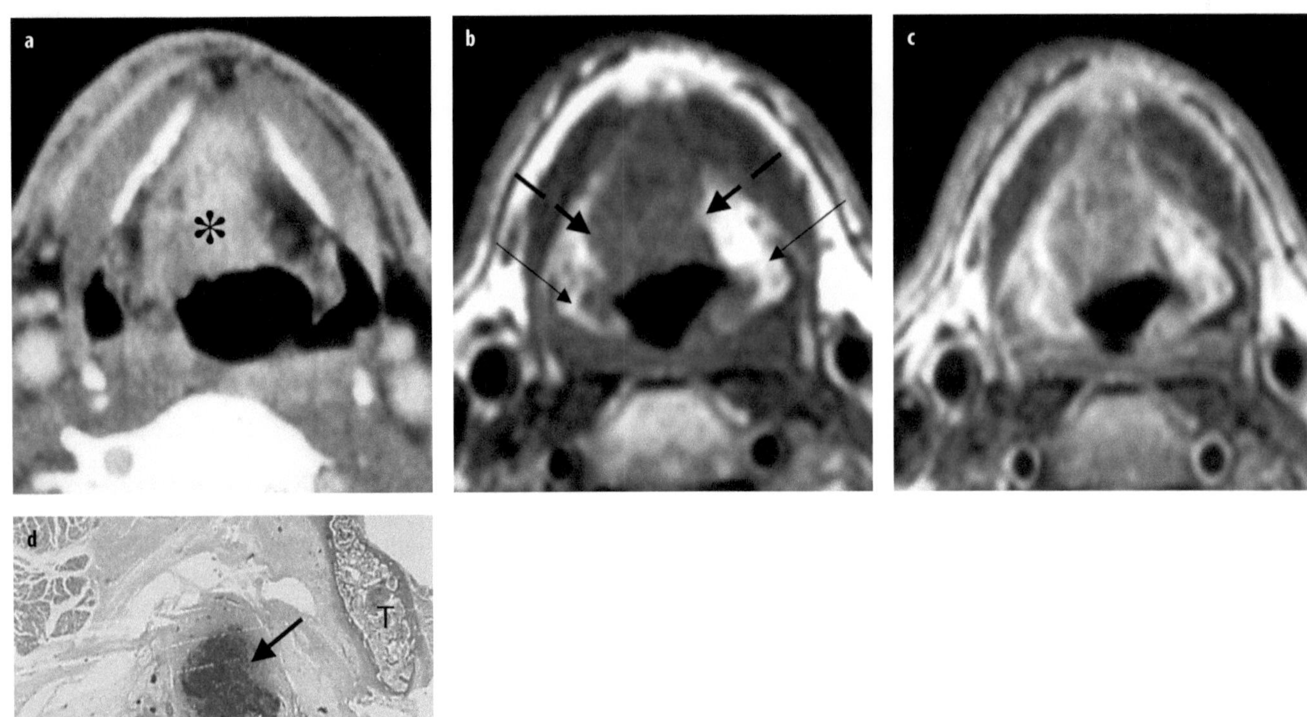

Fig. 1 a-d. Neoplastic invasion of the pre-epiglottic space due to supraglottic cancer. **a** Axial, contrast-enhanced CT image at the supraglottic level shows an enhancing mass invading the preepiglottic space (*asterisk*). **b** Axial, unenhanced T1-weighted image at the supraglottic level shows a tumor mass with intermediate signal intensity as it extends into the pre-epiglottic space (*dashed arrows*). Note the high signal intensity of the noninvaded paraglottic space due to the high content of fatty tissue (*thin arrows*). **c** Axial gadolinium-enhanced T1-weighted image at the same level shows enhancement of the tumor mass invading the pre-epiglottic space. **d** Whole-organ, axial histologic slice from a supraglottic horizontal laryngectomy specimen confirms tumor invasion of the pre-epiglottic space (*arrows*). *E*, Epiglottis; *T*, thyroid cartilage. From Becker (2001), with permission

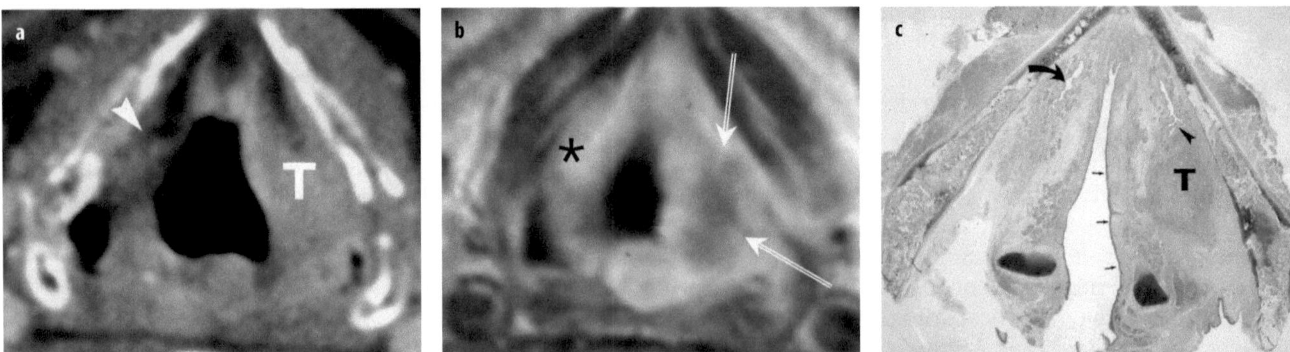

Fig. 2 a-c. Neoplastic invasion of the left paraglottic space due to ventricular cancer. Endoscopically, only a very small mucosal lesion was present within the left laryngeal ventricle. **a** Axial contrast-enhanced CT image at the supraglottic level shows a tumor mass (*T*) invading the left paraglottic space. Note the normal appearance of the contralateral paraglottic space (*arrowhead*). **b** Axial contrast-enhanced T1-weighted image shows an enhancing tumor mass (*arrows*) invading the left paraglottic fat; normal right paraglottic fat space (*asterisk*). **c** Whole-organ axial slice from the specimen confirms extensive paraglottic space invasion by a predominantely submucosal tumor mass (*T*). The tumor mass originates from the left laryngeal ventricle (*arrowhead*). The *curved arrow* points to the right laryngeal ventricle. Note the normal aspect of the laryngeal mucosa overlying the tumor mass (*thin arrows*)

vasion is made when an enhancing mass is seen within the pre-epiglottic fat (Fig. 1). Supraglottic tumors originating from the false cord, laryngeal ventricle, or aryepiglottic fold primarily infiltrate the paraglottic space. The primary sign of tumor spread to the paraglottic space on MR imaging or CT is replacement of fatty tissue by tumor tissue (Fig. 2). Although the sensitivity of MRI and CT for the detection of neoplastic spread to the pre-epiglottic and paraglottic space is high, the corresponding specificity is limited. This is due to the fact that peritumoral inflammatory changes may lead to overestimation of tumor spread with either method and thus to false-positive assessments. The primary lymphatic spread of supraglottic carcinomas is directed toward the superior jugular lymph nodes. Lymph node metastases are common and often bilateral.

Glottic carcinoma typically arises from the anterior half of the vocal cord and primarily spreads into the anterior commissure. Invasion of the anterior commissure is seen on CT and MR imaging as a soft-tissue thickening of >1-2 mm. Once the tumor has reached the anterior commissure, it may easily spread into the thyroarytenoid muscle, contralateral cord, paraglottic space, supraglottis, or subglottis. On axial CT or MR images, neoplastic invasion occurring at the subglottic level below the anterior commissure appears as an irregular thickening of the cricothyroid membrane. Further spread occurs mainly in a cephalad or caudad direction or, via the cricothyroid membrane, into the perilaryngeal tissue. Paraglottic tumor spread in glottic cancer may be entirely occult clinically and detectable only by means of CT or MR imaging. Subglottic spread is relatively common in glottic cancer and may either occur superficial or deep to the elastic cone. Deep subglottic spread is very difficult to detect endoscopically, the extent of the tumor may be underestimated unless CT or MR imaging is performed. The degree of subglottic spread is best displayed on axial images (Fig. 3); coronal images are of limited help in the assessment of subglottic spread because they are difficult to interpret except in the midcoronal plane. Lymphatic metastases from glottic carcinoma are uncommon as long as the tumor is confined to the endolarynx. However, once the tumor has spread into the soft tissues of the neck, the frequency of lymph node metastases increases significantly.

Primary subglottic carcinoma is uncommon and tends to spread to the trachea or invade the thyroid gland and the cervical esophagus. Lymph node metastases are much more common than in glottic carcinoma and they involve the paratracheal and pretracheal nodes. These nodes drain to the lower jugular or upper mediastinal nodes. Cross-sectional imaging performed in patients with primary subglottic tumors should therefore include the upper mediastinum.

Carcinoma of the hypopharynx may arise in the piriform sinus (65%), postcricoid area (20%), and posterior

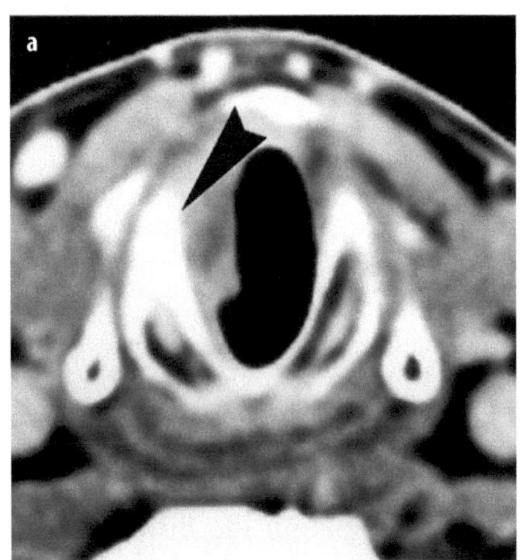

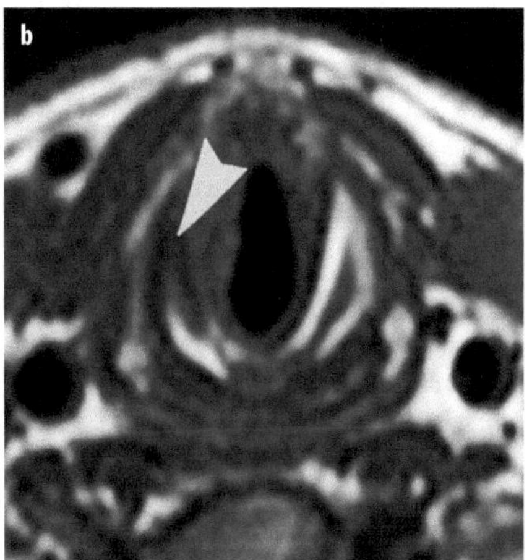

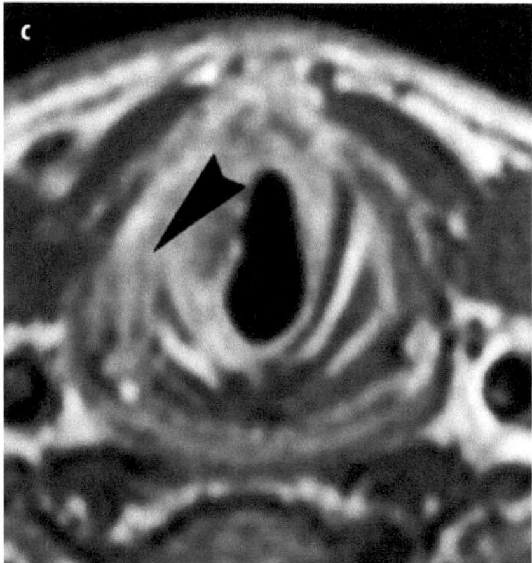

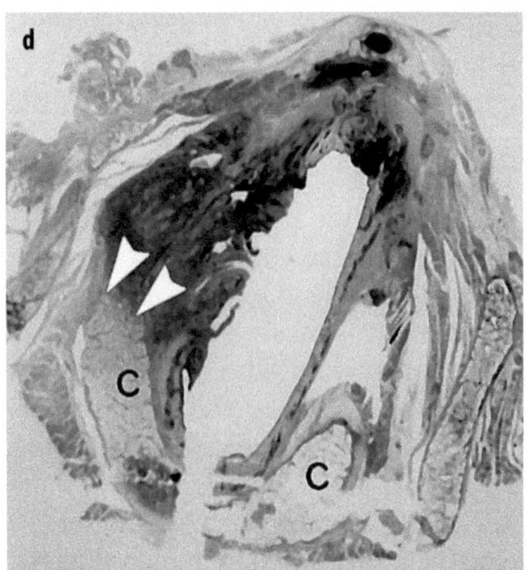

Fig. 3 a-d. Neoplastic invasion of the cricoid cartilage. Glotto-subglottic carcinoma of the larynx in a 46-year-old male patient. **a** Contrast-enhanced CT at the subglottic level shows a right-sided tumor mass adjacent to a sclerotic cricoid cartilage. Sclerosis suggests invasion of the adjacent cricoid cartilage. **b** Axial T1-weighted image: a mass with intermediate signal intensity infiltrates the right subglottic region. The signal intensity of the right cricoid cartilage is decreased (*arrowhead*). **c** Contrast-enhanced axial T1-weighted image shows extensive contrast enhancement of the right subglottic tumor mass as well as of the adjacent cricoid cartilage. The extensive enhancement of the right cricoid cartilage (*arrowhead*) suggests tumor invasion. **d** Axial slice from specimen at the same level shows a large subglottic tumor mass invading the right cricoid cartilage (*arrowheads*). *C*, Cricoid cartilage. From Becker et al. (1995), with permission

pharyngeal wall (15%). Carcinoma of the piriform sinus is readily detected with endoscopy while very early superficially spreading tumors that are limited to the mucosa may be invisible at cross-sectional imaging. In most cases, however, patients with piriform sinus tumors initially present with advanced lesions and diagnosis at CT or MR imaging is straightforward. Since the piriform sinus is usually collapsed during quiet respiration, the exact tumor location (medial wall vs. lateral wall) may be difficult to determine radiologically; thus, very close cooperation with the head and neck surgeon is essential. Tumors originating from the lateral wall of the piriform sinus have a tendency to infiltrate very early the soft tissues of the neck. Tumors originating from the medial wall or the angle of the piriform sinus may infiltrate the larynx by growing anteriorly into the paraglottic space. Piriform sinus carcinoma frequently invades the paraglottic space and the laryngeal cartilages (see below).

Postcricoid carcinoma is uncommon but observed in certain groups at risk (patients with Plummer-Vinson syndrome). These tumors spread submucosally, most often toward the cervical esophagus. Tumor growth is mainly submucosal such that the true extent only becomes apparent with axial or sagittal MR images.

Carcinoma of the posterior pharyngeal wall commonly involves both the oropharynx and hypopharynx. On axial MR images, these tumors appear as asymmetrical thickening of the posterior pharyngeal wall. Invasion of the prevertebral muscles is unusual at initial presentation.

Squamous cell carcinoma of the hypopharynx has a relatively poor prognosis, with up to 75% of patients having metastases to cervical lymph nodes at initial presentation.

Neoplastic Cartilage Invasion

Invasion of the hyaline laryngeal cartilage by squamous cell carcinoma alters staging, prognosis, and, in most centers, the therapeutic approach. Most investigators feel that radiation therapy cannot eradicate tumor within cartilage but may result in perichondritis and chondronecrosis, although others believe that radiation therapy can sterilize the tumor even in cases in which the cartilage is invaded. Invasion of the thyroid, cricoid, and both arytenoid cartilages precludes classical voice-sparing partial laryngectomy; instead, total laryngectomy, an extremely invasive procedure, is required. Recent direct comparison studies with histologic correlation have shown that CT has a high sensitivity and a high negative predictive value for the detection of cartilage invasion provided that the following criteria are used: sclerosis, erosion, lysis and extralaryngeal spread. Sclerosis is a sensitive sign for the detection of neoplastic cartilage invasion and enables diagnosis of early or microscopic intracartilaginous tumor spread (Fig. 3). It corresponds to bone remodeling and new bone formation induced by the presence of tumor cells in the immediate vicinity. The specificity of this sign varies considerably from one cartilage to another, being lowest in the thyroid cartilage (40%) and higher in the cricoid and arytenoid cartilages (76 and 79%, respectively). Therefore, if a tumor mass is seen adjacent to a sclerotic cartilage, this does not automatically imply that tumor cells are found within the remodeled marrow cavity (Fig. 4). Conversely, failure at surgery to remove a cartilage that exhibits sclerosis on CT carries a 50-60% risk of leaving tumor behind. As the process of cartilage invasion progresses, minor and major osteolysis is seen within the areas of new bone formation. Minor areas of osteolysis correspond to the CT criteria of erosion, while major areas of osteolysis correspond to the CT criteria of lysis. Histologically, erosion and lysis correspond to destruction of bone due to osteoclastic activity. Consequently, erosion and lysis can be considered specific criteria for the detection of neoplastic invasion in all cartilages. The overall specificity of erosion and lysis is 93%. However, neither criterion is very sensitive as each is affected by the presence of more advanced invasion of laryngeal cartilage. Extralaryngeal spread is the result of tumor invasion through a cartilage into the extralaryngeal soft tissues. This CT sign is highly specific (overall specificity: 95%) but, because it is only seen very late in the disease process, its sensitivity is as low as 44%. A combination of the criteria of extralaryngeal tumor, sclerosis, and erosion/lysis with respect to all cartilages increases the overall sensitivity to as high as 91%. As the negative predictive value of this combination is 95%, CT may be considered as an excellent test to exclude cartilage invasion prior to treatment.

The sensitivity for the detection of cartilage invasion based on MR criteria is very high. The reported sensitivity of MR imaging for the detection of neoplastic cartilage invasion is 89-94%, the specificity 74-88%, and the negative predictive value 94-96%. Extensive tumor invasion involving both inner and outer aspects of the cartilage can be diagnosed with a high degree of accuracy with MR imaging. In addition, MR imaging enables detection of intracartilaginous tumor spread. If tumor is present only adjacent to the inner aspect of a cartilage, the radiologist can differentiate between tumor and nonossified cartilage by comparing the different MR pulse sequences. Cartilage invaded by tumor displays an intermediate to low signal intensity on T1-weighted images, a higher signal intensity on proton-density and T2-weighted images, and areas of enhancement within the cartilage adjacent to the tumor after injection of gadolinium chelates (Fig. 3). If these signs are absent, cartilage infiltration can be ruled out with a high level of confidence, since the negative predictive value of MR imaging is very high (Fig. 5). Unfortunately, the MR findings suggesting neoplastic cartilage invasion are not as specific as was expected initially, but may yield false-positive results in a considerable number of instances; the positive predictive value is only 71%. This is because reactive inflammation, edema, fibrosis, and ectopic red bone marrow in the vicinity of the tumor may display similar diagnostic features as cartilage infiltrated by tumor (Fig. 4).

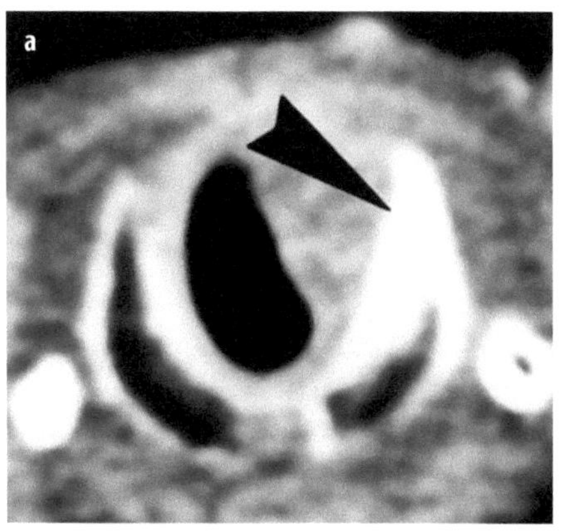

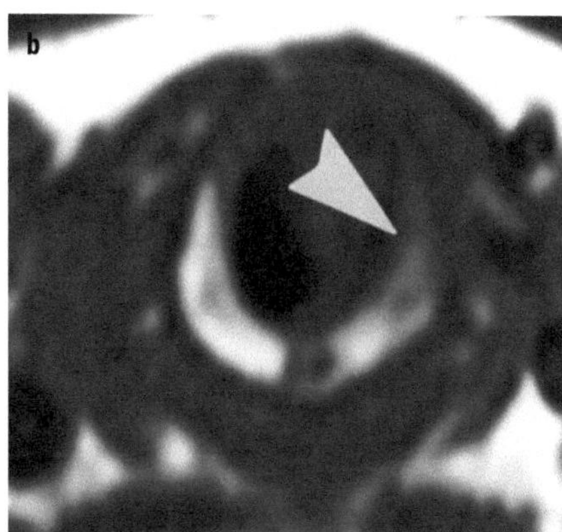

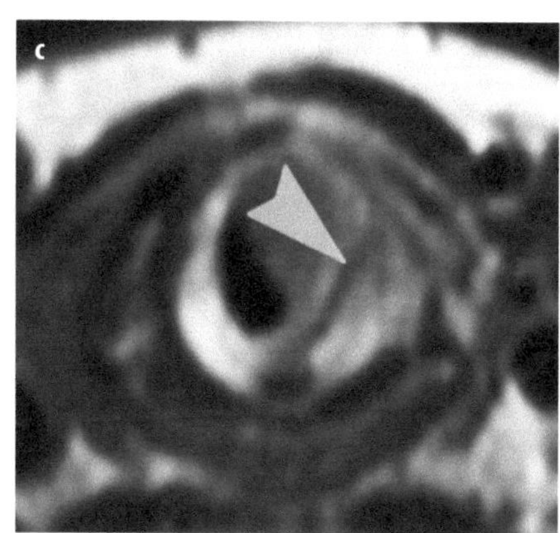

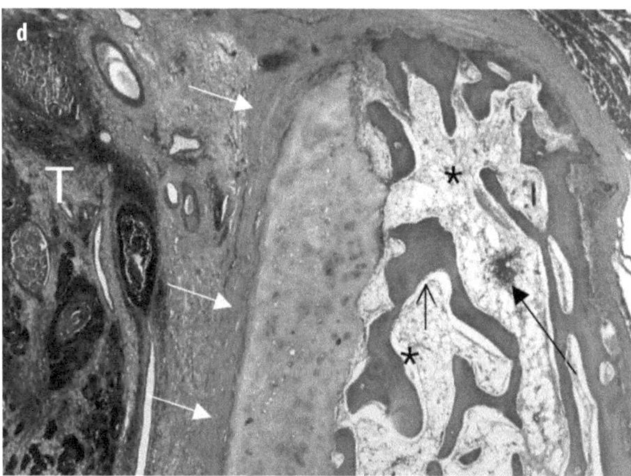

Fig. 4 a-d. CT and MR imaging false positive results for neoplastic cartilage invasion due to inflammatory changes. Glotto-subglottic carcinoma of the larynx in a 71-year-old female patient. **a** Contrast-enhanced CT shows sclerosis of the left cricoid cartilage, suggesting invasion by the adjacent tumor. **b** T1-weighted axial image: a mass with low signal intensity infiltrates the left subglottic region. The signal intensity of the adjacent left cricoid cartilage is decreased (*arrowhead*). **c** Contrast-enhanced T1-weighted image: contrast enhancement is seen within the left cricoid cartilage (*arrowhead*) as well as within the subglottic tumor mass, suggesting invasion. **d** Axial slice from specimen shows a large, left-sided subglottic tumor mass (*T*) but no evidence of cartilage invasion. The cricoid cartilage shows extensive inflammatory changes with lymph follicles (*black arrow*), fibrosis (*asterisks*), and bone resorption (*open arrows*) but with an intact perichondrium (*white arrows*). From Becker et al. (1998), with permission

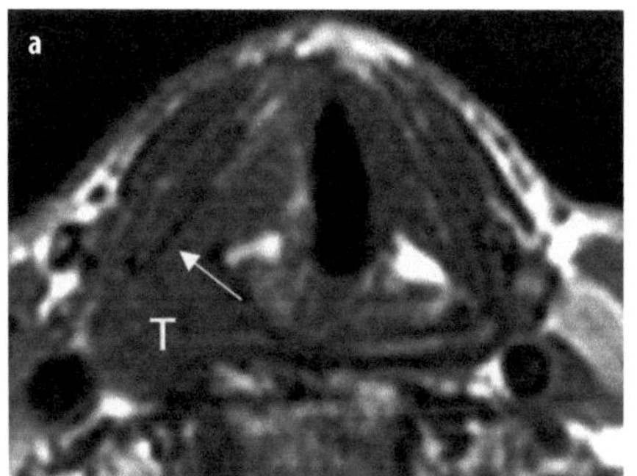

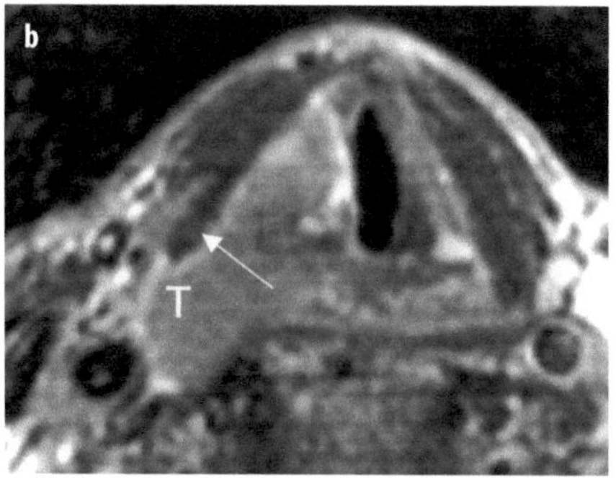

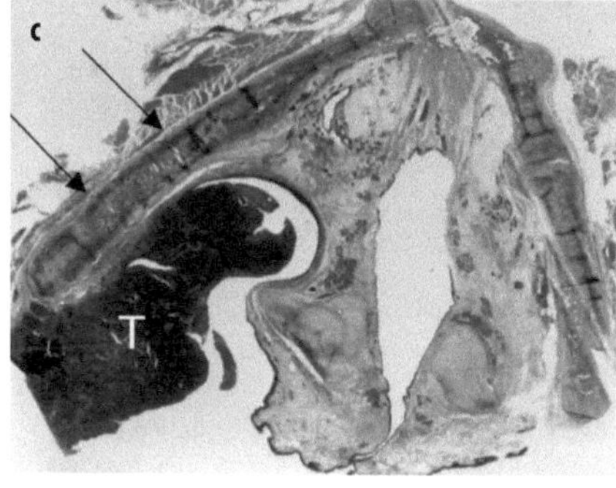

Fig. 5 a-c. True negative MR imaging findings for neoplastic invasion of the thyroid cartilage. **a** T1-weighted image obtained at the supraglottic level shows a right-sided piriform sinus tumor with intermediate to low signal intensity (*T*). The signal intensity of the adjacent right thyroid lamina is also intermediate (*arrow*). **b** T1-weighted spin-echo (SE) image obtained after intravenous administration of contrast material shows contrast enhancement of the tumor mass (*T*) but no enhancement of the adjacent thyroid lamina (*arrow*). This suggests that the thyroid cartilage is composed of nonossified hyaline cartilage and that no intracartilaginous tumor spread is present. **c** Corresponding axial slice from surgical specimen at the same level confirms that the right thyroid lamina is composed of nonossified hyaline cartilage (*arrows*). No cartilage invasion was found at histology. The tumor (*T*) arises from the lateral wall of the right piriform sinus. From Becker (1998), with permission

Since inflammatory changes are most common in the thyroid cartilage, the specificity of MR imaging to detect neoplastic invasion of the thyroid cartilage is only 56%, as opposed to 87 and 95% in the cricoid and arytenoid cartilage, respectively. The positive diagnosis of neoplastic invasion of the thyroid cartilage should, therefore, be made with extreme caution at MR imaging.

TNM Classification of Laryngeal and Hypopharyngeal Carcinoma

Laryngeal and hypopharyngeal carcinomas are staged according to the criteria recommended by the International Union Against Cancer (UICC) or according to the criteria recommended by the American Joint Cancer Committee (AJCC). The guidelines of both the UICC and the AJCC, which are now almost identical, recommend the use of cross-sectional imaging. Several studies as well as the experience at our institution have shown that the use of CT or MR imaging greatly improves the accuracy of the pre-therapeutic T-classification of laryngeal and hypopharyngeal tumors. In our own experience, the overall pretherapeutic staging accuracy of CT and MRI is 80 and 85%, respectively.

Nonsquamous Cell Laryngeal Neoplasms

Carcinomas of histologies other than the squamous cell type occur only very occasionally in the laryngo-hypopharyngeal region. Adenocarcinoma and adenosquamous carcinoma typically originate and extend beneath the mucosal surface. Therefore, these carcinomas are more difficult to detect with endoscopy than squamous cell carcinoma. Although none of the unusual types of carcinoma has any signal characteristics allowing its distinction from squamous cell carcinoma on CT or MR imaging, the discrepancy between the presence of a tumoral soft-tissue mass on MR imaging and an intact mucosa at endoscopy should always raise the suspicion of a neoplasm of nonsquamous cell origin. In such cases, CT and MR imaging serve not only to assess the degree of tumor spread, but also to direct the endoscopist to the appropriate site where the deep aggressive biopsies necessary to establish the correct histologic diagnosis must be performed.

Laryngeal chondrosarcoma predominantly affects males in their sixth or seventh decade of life and more commonly originates from the cricoid than from the thyroid cartilage. As in chondrogenic tumors of other locations, the tumor matrix is of high signal intensity on T2-weighted images, corresponding to hyaline cartilage with its low cellularity and high water content (Fig. 6). Small areas of low signal intensity correspond to stippled calcifications; these changes are, however, not as well-demonstrated as with CT, where characteristic "pop-corn" calcifications may be seen. Although the injection of gadolinium chelates may lead to a diffuse central or peripheral enhancement on T1-weighted images, these findings are nonspecific and do not help in differentiating low-grade chondrosarcomas from benign chondroma. While the diagnosis of laryngeal chondrosarcoma can be strongly suspected based on CT or MR imaging findings, it must be confirmed with deep biopsy. Surgery is regarded as the treatment of choice and is increasingly done in the form of function-preserving laryngeal resection. Imaging studies are important for follow-up after treatment, since chondrosarcoma has a tendency to recur locally.

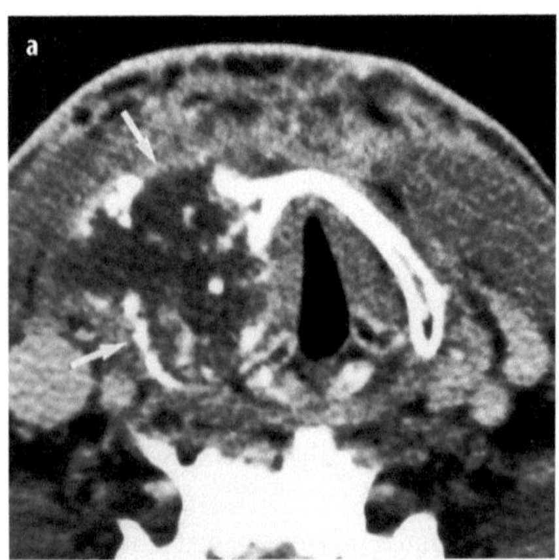

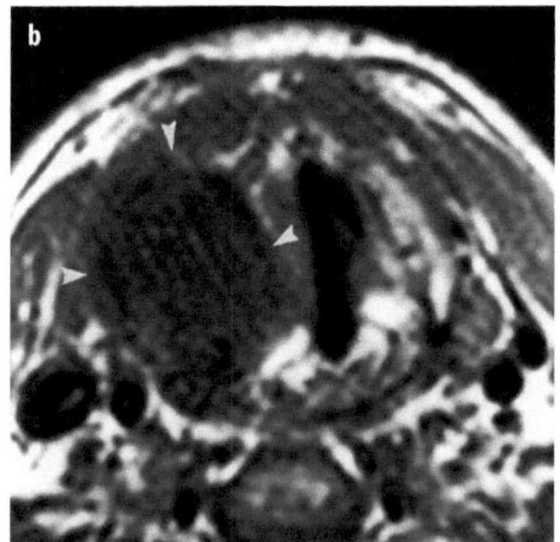

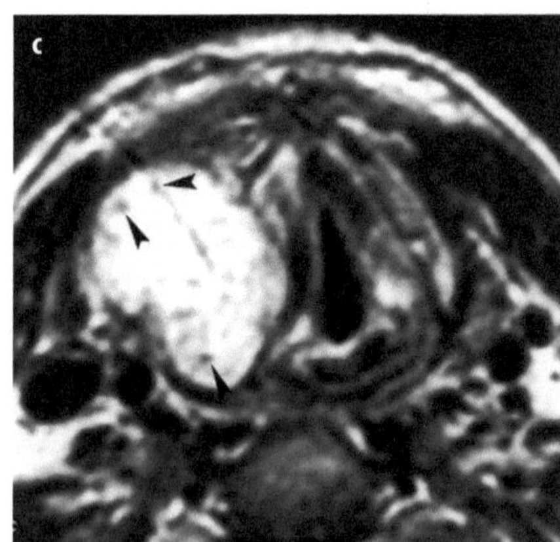

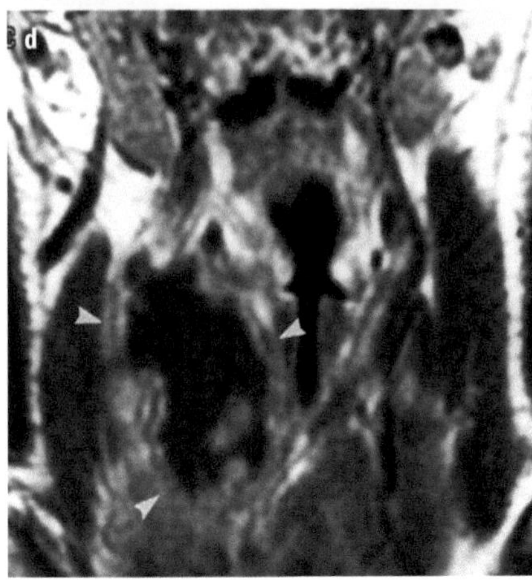

Fig. 6 a-d. Chondrosarcoma of the thyroid cartilage: CT and MR imaging appearance. A 47-year-old male patient presenting with a hard lump in the neck. **a** Axial contrast-enhanced CT scan shows a large, lobulated mass with coarse and stippled calcifications characteristic of chondrosarcoma (*arrows*). **b** T1-weighted, axial MR image shows a lobulated mass with low signal intensity that arises from the right thyroid lamina (*arrowheads*). Note the normal aspect of the left thyroid lamina. (**c**) T2-weighted fast spin-echo (FSE) image. The tumor mass has a very high signal intensity due to its high water content. The hypointense areas within the tumor correspond to intratumoral calcifications (*arrowheads*). **d** T1-weighted, contrast-enhanced, coronal image. Note the moderate peripheral enhancement (*arrowheads*) and the extramucosal location of the tumor. The patient underwent voice-preserving laryngeal resection and was free of recurrence 5 years later. From Becker (1998) (Fig. 6a), and Becker et al. (1998b) (Figs. 6b-d), with permission

Cysts and Laryngoceles

Laryngeal cysts arise from the mucosa and are related to minor salivary glands, whereas laryngoceles (also called saccular cysts) are dilatations of the saccule of the laryngeal ventricle. A laryngocele occurs when there is obstruction of the ventricle, sometimes by a small cancer located near the neck of the saccule. Laryngoceles may contain air or fluid. An internal laryngocele extends superiorly in the paralaryngeal space; it may present as a submucosal supraglottic mass at endoscopic evaluation. If the laryngocele extends through the thyrohyoid membrane into the soft tissues of the neck, it is called an external laryngocele. On CT or MR imaging, a laryngocele presents as a well-circumscribed, air- or fluid-filled structure extending from the laryngeal ventricle into the paralaryngeal space or through the thyrohyoid membrane into the soft tissues of the neck.

Vocal-Cord Paralysis

Paralysis of the recurrent laryngeal nerve is the most common type of vocal-cord paralysis. The CT and MR imaging features of recurrent laryngeal-nerve paralysis are explained by atrophy of the thyroarytenoid muscle and include an enlarged ventricle, ipsilateral enlargement of the piriform sinus, and decreased size or fatty infiltration seen at the level of the true vocal cord. A patient with recurrent laryngeal-nerve paralysis of unknown origin should undergo imaging of the entire pathway of the vagus and recurrent laryngeal nerve to exclude a tumor mass.

Inflammatory Lesions

Epiglottitis and croup are diagnosed clinically and do not require imaging. In the Western hemisphere, the larynx is rarely affected by granulomatous diseases. Tuberculosis, numerous mycotic infections, leprosy and syphilis appear to be more common in Asia and Africa and may affect the larynx and pharynx. Relapsing polychondritis affects laryngeal cartilages, and rheumatoid arthritis affects the cricoarythenoid and the cricothyroid joints. Necrotizing fasciitis of the head and neck is a severe, acute, and potentially life-threatening bacterial soft-tissue infection with a very rapid clinical evolution. It affects both immunocompetent and immunocompromised patients and, unless immediate surgical treatment is provided, leads invariably to mediastinitis and fatal sepsis. CT or MR imaging findings include cellulitis, multiple fluid collections with or without gas in various neck compartments, diffuse enhancement of neck fasciae, and myositis. The larynx is often involved by the inflammatory, edematous process, necessitating intubation; myositis with or without abscess formation or myonecrosis is seen in the pharyngeal constrictor muscles. In the acute and subacute phase, CT and MR imaging may demonstrate contrast enhancement of the pharyngeal constrictor muscles or frank disruption of the pharyngeal wall.

Trauma

Trauma to the larynx can cause mucosal tears, submucosal hematomas, avulsion of the epiglottis, fractures of the laryngeal cartilages, and joint dislocation. Both fractures and hematomas may lead to severe airway compromise. Fractures of the thyroid cartilage may be vertical, horizontal, or the entire thyroid cartilage may be shattered (Fig. 7). Fractures of the cricoid cartilage tend to occur bilaterally. Cricothyroid dislocations tend to occur with severe trauma, while cricoarytenoid dislocations are frequently the result of minor trauma. Most patients with laryngeal trauma undergo CT, which allows excellent delineation of most traumatic lesions. However, MR imaging may provide significant additional information in young patients, in whom the laryngeal cartilages are not ossified and therefore not well-visualized on CT.

Stenosis of the larynx or cervical trachea can be a sequel of trauma or prolonged intubation. MR imaging (axial, coronal, and sagittal images) and CT with 2D reconstructions are very useful in exactly defining the vertical extent of a stenosis.

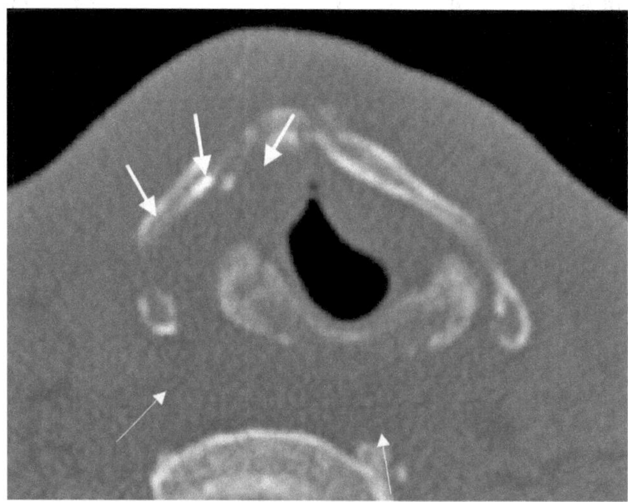

Fig. 7. Laryngeal trauma following a motor-vehicle accident: comminuted fracture of the thyroid cartilage (*arrows*) and bilateral fracture of the cricoid cartilage (*thin arrows*)

Suggested Reading

Becker M (1998) Larynx and hypopharynx. Radiologic Clinics North Am 36:891-920

Becker M (2001) Malignant lesions of the larynx and hypopharynx. In: Baert AL, Sartor K, Hermans R (eds) Imaging of the larynx. Springer, Berlin-Heidelberg-New York, pp 55-84

Becker M (2004) The larynx. In: Valvassouri G, Mafee M, Becker M (eds) Imaging of the head and neck. Thieme, New York-Stuttgart, pp 731-777

Becker M, Zbären P, Laeng H et al (1995) Neoplastic invasion of the laryngeal cartilage: Comparison of MR imaging and CT with histopathologic correlation. Radiology 194:661-669

Becker M, Zbären P, Delavelle J et al (1997a) Neoplastic invasion of the laryngeal cartilage: reassessment of criteria for diagnosis at CT. Radiology 203:521-532

Becker M, Zbären P, Hermans R et al (1997b) Necrotizing fasciitis of the head and neck: role of CT in diagnosis and management. Radiology 202:471-476

Becker M, Moulin G, Kurt AM et al (1998a) Atypical squamous cell carcinoma of the larynx and hypopharynx: radiologic features and pathologic correlation. Eur Radiol 8:1541-1551

Becker M, Moulin G, Kurt AM et al (1998b) Non-squamous cell neoplasms of the larynx: radiologic-pathologic correlation. Radiographics 18(5):1189-1209

Castelijns JA, Gerritsen GJ, Kaiser MC et al (1988) Invasion of laryngeal cartilage by cancer: comparison of CT and MR imaging. Radiology 167:199-206

Castelijns JA, Becker M, Hermans R (1996a) The impact of cartilage invasion on treatment and prognosis of laryngeal cancer. Eur Radiol 6:156-169

Castelijns JA, van den Brekel MW, Tobi H et al (1996b) Laryngeal carcinoma after radiation therapy: correlation of abnormal MR imaging signal patterns in laryngeal cartilage with the risk of recurrence. Radiology 198:151-155

Curtin HD (1996) The larynx. In: Som PM, Curtin HD (eds) Head and neck imaging, 3rd edn. Mosby, St. Louis, pp 612-707

Loevner LA, Yousem DM, Montone KT et al (1997) Can radiologists accurately predict preepiglottic space invasion with MR imaging? AJR Am J Roentgenol 169:1681-1687

Mancuso AA (1991) Evaluation and staging of laryngeal and hypopharyngeal cancer by computed tomography and magnetic resonance imaging. In: Silver CE (ed) Laryngeal cancer. Thieme, New York-Stuttgart, pp 46-94

Sobin LH, Wittekind C (2002) TNM classification of malignant tumors, 6th edn. UICC, Wiley-Liss

Stiglbauer R, Steurer M, Schimmerl S et al (1992) MRI of cartilaginous tumors of the larynx. Clin Radiol 46:23-27

Zbären P, Becker M, Laeng H (1996) Pretherapeutic staging of laryngeal cancer: clinical findings. Computed tomography and magnetic resonance imaging versus histopathology. Cancer 77(7):1263-1273

Imaging of the Larynx

Hugh D. Curtin

Harvard Medical School, and Massachusetts Eye and Ear Infirmary Hospital, Boston, MA, USA

Imaging of the larynx must be coordinated with the clinical examination [1, 2]. The information acquired at imaging usually emphasizes the deeper tissues, as superficial assessment is done by direct visualization. A description of the anatomy is key to the description of any lesion.

Anatomy

Important Mucosal Landmarks

Several anatomic structures are important to the radiologist seeking to evaluate the larynx. Perhaps the most important relationship in the larynx is that of the false vocal fold, true vocal fold, and ventricle complex. The ventricle is a crucial reference point. Much imaging of tumors is aimed at defining the position of a lesion relative to this region. Another important landmark is the upper margin of the cricoid cartilage. This cartilage is the only complete ring of the cartilage framework and is essential to the integrity of the airway.

The true vocal folds (cords) play a major role in speech. The cords stretch across the lower larynx and lie in the horizontal or axial plane. There is a small crease just above the true vocal fold called the ventricle. Immediately above the ventricle and again parallel to both the ventricle and the true fold is a second pair of folds, called the false vocal folds. Above the false folds, the mucosa curves out laterally to the upper edges of the larynx, at the aryepiglottic folds, which, in turn, curve around and extend up to the margins of the epiglottis.

These structures are the basis for anatomic localization within the larynx. The glottic larynx refers to the true vocal folds. The glottis has been defined as extending from the ventricle to a plane approximately 1 cm below the ventricle. Here, the glottis merges with the subglottis (the lower part of the larynx). The subglottis extends from the lower margin of the glottis to the inferior margin of the cricoid cartilage. Everything above the ventricle of the larynx is referred to as the supraglottis.

Another important anatomic term is the anterior commissure. This is the point where the true folds converge anteriorly and insert into the thyroid cartilage.

Cartilage Framework

The cartilages make up the framework of the larynx and gives it structure (Fig. 1). The cricoid cartilage is the foundation of the larynx and the only complete ring. Above the cricoid and attached to the lateral margins of the cricoid cartilage is the thyroid cartilage. This shield-like cartilage provides protection to the inner workings of the larynx. The arytenoid cartilages perch upon the posterior edge of the cricoid. The epiglottis is made up of fibrocartilage and extends behind the thyroid cartilage in the supraglottic larynx.

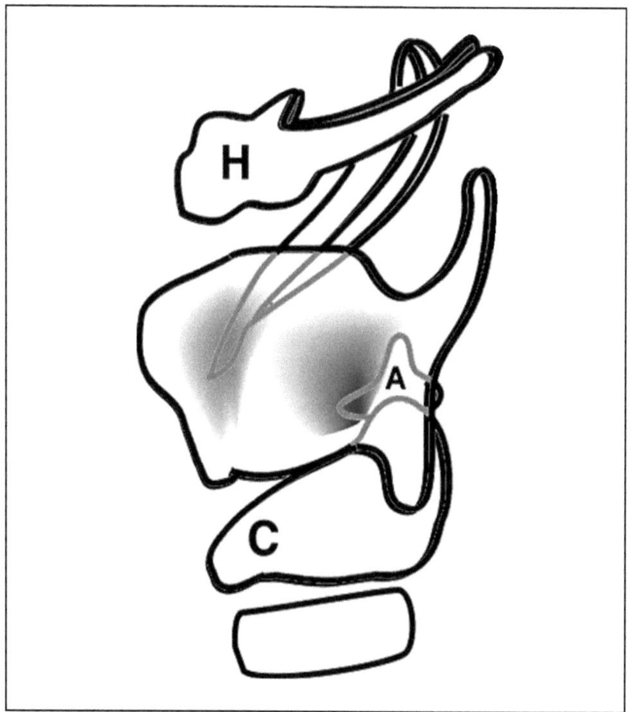

Fig. 1. Line diagram showing the relationships of the laryngeal cartilages. The thyroid cartilage attaches to the signet-ring-shaped cricoid cartilage (*C*). The arytenoid cartilages (*A*) perch on the posterior aspect of the cricoid cartilage. The epiglottis is protected by the hyoid bone (*H*) and the thyroid cartilage

In axial imaging, the cartilages can help the radiologist in orienting the mucosal levels in the larynx (Fig. 2). The cricoid is at the level of the glottis and subglottis. The upper posterior edge of the cricoid cartilage is actually at the level of the true folds or ventricle. The lower edge of the cricoid cartilage represents the lower boundary of the larynx and, therefore, the lower edge of the subglottis.

The arytenoid cartilage spans the ventricle. The upper arytenoid is at the level of the false fold, whereas the vocal process defines the position of the vocal ligament and, therefore, the true fold. The epiglottis is totally within the supraglottic larynx.

Deep Soft Tissues

There are many *muscles* within the larynx. The key muscle for the radiologist is the thyroarytenoid muscle. This forms the bulk of the true fold or cord and extends from the arytenoid to the anterior part of the thyroid cartilage at the anterior commissure. The radiologist should be familiar with this muscle because identifying it is very helpful in attempting to identify the true fold and ventricle.

The *paraglottic space* refers to the major part of the soft tissue between the mucosa and the cartilaginous framework of the larynx. At the level of the supraglottis or false fold, this space predominantly contains fat, whereas at the level of the true fold, the paraglottic region is filled by the thyroarytenoid muscle (Fig. 3). Again, this concept is helpful in orienting one to the level within the larynx. The level of the ventricle is identified as the transition between fat and muscle. At the level of the subglottis, the paraglottic space essentially disappears.

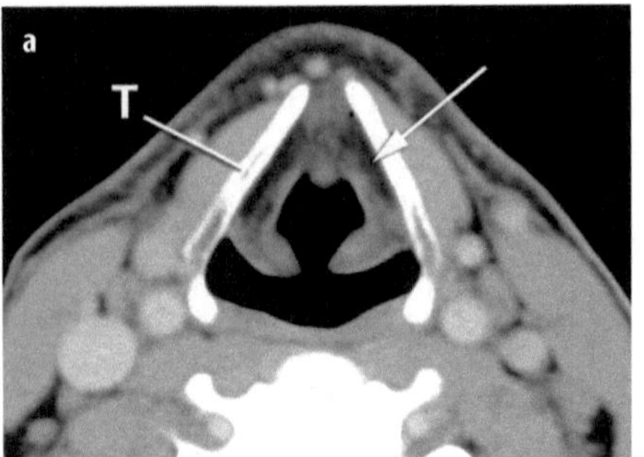

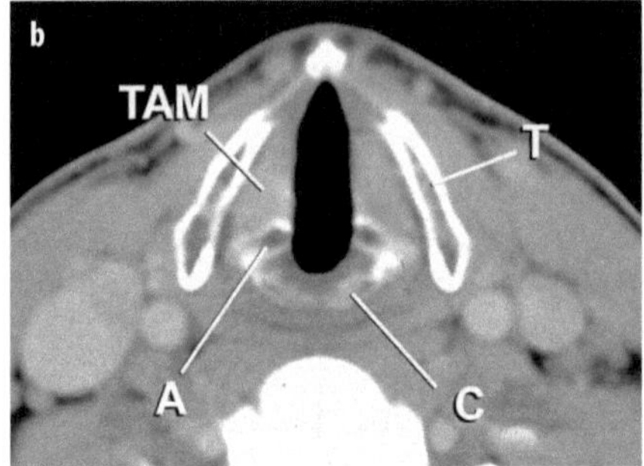

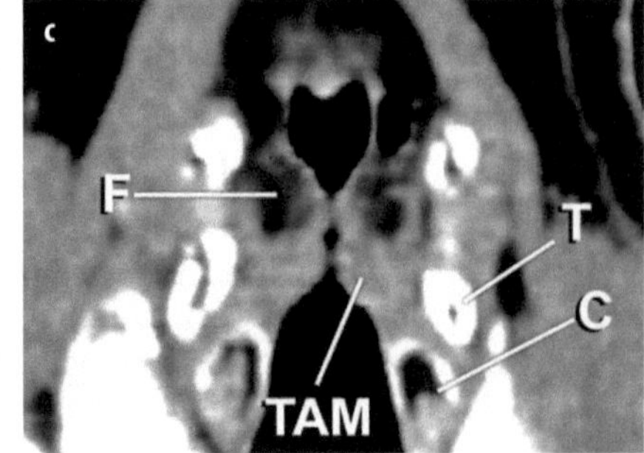

Fig. 2 a-c. Computed tomography image of the normal larynx. **a** Axial image through the supraglottis. Notice the fat (*arrow*) in the paraglottic space of the lateral larynx. *T*, thyroid cartilage. **b** Axial image through the level of the true cord. The thyroarytenoid muscle (*TAM*) makes up the bulk of the true cord. Other structures seen at this level include the thyroid cartilage (*T*), the upper edge of the posterior cricoid cartilage (*C*), and the arytenoid cartilage (*A*). The vocal ligament attaches to the anterior margin or vocal process of the arytenoid cartilage. **c** Coronal image through the larynx. The TAM makes up the bulk of the true cord or fold. Note the fat (*F*) in the paraglottic space of the supraglottis. The ventricle is not seen but can be predicted to be at the level of the transition of fat to muscle. *C*, Cricoid cartilage; *T*, thyroid cartilage

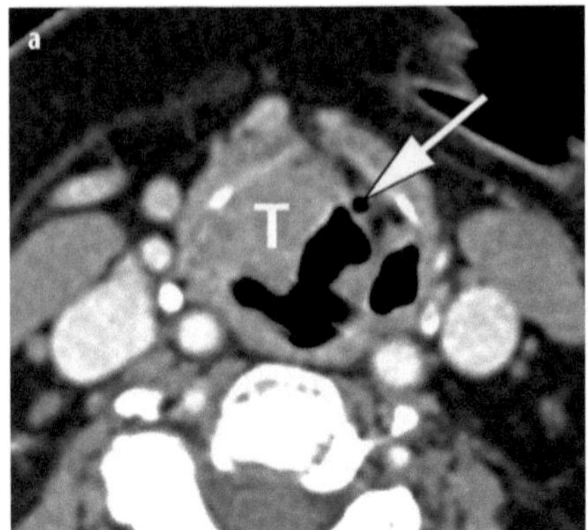

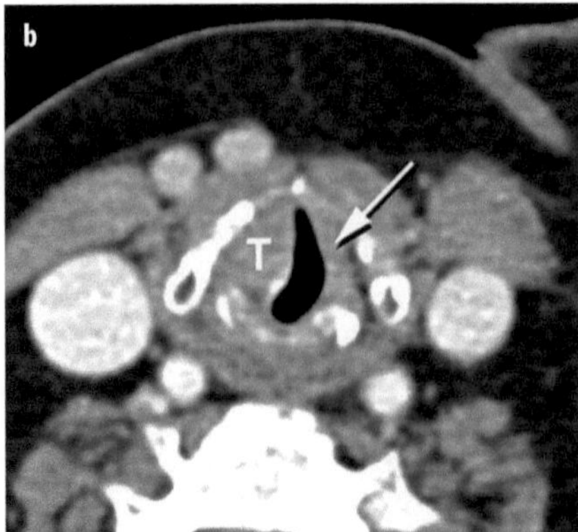

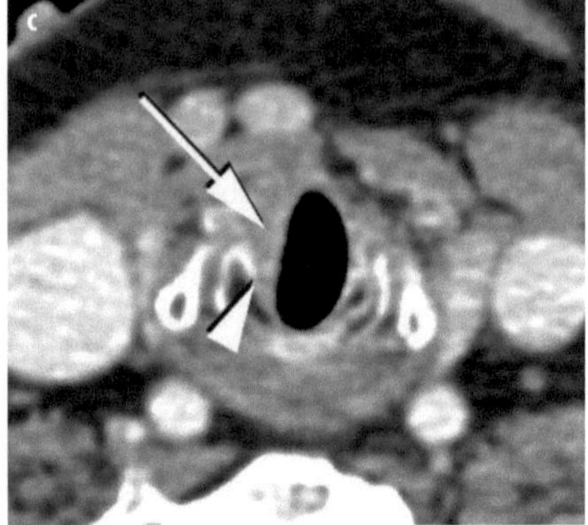

Fig. 3 a-c. Carcinoma of the larynx crossing the laryngeal ventricle (transglottic). **a** Axial image; supraglottic level. Tumor (*T*) is seen obliterating the right supraglottic fat in the paraglottic and pre-epiglottic areas. Note the small amount of air in the ventricular appendix (*arrow*) in the normal paraglottic fat on the left. **b** Axial image; true cord (glottic) level. Tumor (*T*) enlarges the cord on the right side. Note the typical appearance of the thyroarytenoid muscle (*arrow*) on the left, indicating that the image is at the level of the cord. **c** Axial image; subglottic level. The tumor (*arrow*) spreads along the inner cortex of the cricoid cartilage (*arrowhead*)

Pathology and Imaging

Imaging of the larynx and upper airway is required in many situations. At our institution, most laryngeal imaging studies relate to tumor evaluation or to trauma.

Tumors of the Larynx

Tumors of the larynx can be separated into two categories. Most tumors of the larynx are squamous cell carcinomas and arise from the mucosa [3]. A few tumors arise from the cartilaginous skeleton or from the other submucosal tissues [4].

The endoscopist almost always detects and diagnoses mucosal lesions. Indeed, imaging should not be used in an attempt to "exclude" squamous cell carcinoma of the larynx. In such cases, the role of the radiologist is almost always determination of the depth of spread and the inferior limit of spread. Submucosal tumors are, however, somewhat different. They can usually be visualized by the endoscopist; however, since they are covered by mucosa there may be considerable difficulty in making the diagnosis. In these cases the clinician may rely on the radiologist to determine the identity of the lesion.

Squamous Cell Carcinoma

Imaging is most often used to determine the depth of extension. The presence of submucosal disease can make a difference in the choice of therapy. It is therefore important for radiologists to be aware of the indications and contraindications of various alternatives to total laryngectomy. The following descriptions refer to standard classic partial laryngectomies [5, 6]. In many institutions, similar surgeries are now done via endoscopic approaches. If the information needed for these procedures is gathered through imaging, then there is more than enough information for radiotherapists as well as other clinical specialists.

Supraglottic laryngectomy: In this procedure, everything above the level of the ventricle is removed. It is used for tumors arising above the ventricle in the epiglottis area, false fold, or aryepiglottic folds. Tumor may obstruct the endoscopist's view of the lower margin of the tumor or tumor can cross the ventricle by "tunneling" beneath the mucosal surface. This type of submucosal spread can travel along the paraglottic pathway around the ventricle. Such extension is a contraindication to supraglottic laryngectomy and, since it can be missed by direct visualization, the radiologist must try to detect it (Figs. 3, 4).

Cartilage involvement is another contraindication, but this is extremely rare in supraglottic cancers unless the lesion has actually crossed the ventricle to become transglottic. Other contraindications include significant extension into the tongue or significant pulmonary problems. These mostly relate to patient difficulty in learning how to swallow once the key part of the laryngeal protective mechanism has been removed.

Vertical hemilaryngectomy: A vertical hemilaryngectomy is done for lesions of the true fold. The aim is to remove the tumor but to retain enough of one true fold so that the patient can still create speech using the usual mechanism. Actually, even if the lesion extends onto the anterior part of the opposite fold satisfactory removal is still possible. In these areas, the radiologist looks most closely at the inferior extension. Does the tumor reach the upper margin of the cricoid cartilage (Fig. 3c)? In most institutions, such extension would mean that the patient is not a candidate for vertical hemilaryngectomy but rather should have a total laryngectomy or alternative therapies.

Lesions of the anterior commissure may extend anteriorly into either the thyroid cartilage or through the cricothyroid membrane into the soft tissues of the neck. This may be invisible to the examining clinician and is again a key point to evaluate. Involvement of both the arytenoid cartilages is another contraindication to vertical hemilaryngectomy but this is usually evaluated by direct visualization.

Radiotherapy or combination radiation/chemotherapy: Radiation, with or without chemotherapy, is another speech-conservation treatment. Here, the therapist needs to know the extent of the lesion, according to the same landmarks used for surgical planning. Cartilage invasion and the volume of the tumor are also important [7].

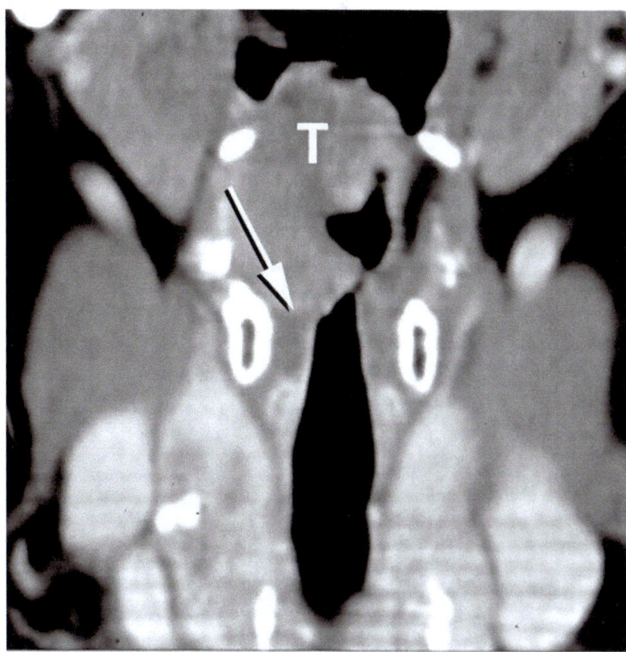

Fig. 4. Carcinoma of the supraglottis extending to the level of the ventricle. The tumor (*T*) was visible by mirror. Coronal CT shows the tumor extending down to the level of the ventricle (*arrow*). The tumor enhances slightly more than the thyroarytenoid muscle

Imaging Laryngeal Squamous Cell Carcinoma

At our institution we begin with computed tomography (CT). The new multi-detector CT (MDCT) scanners give excellent resolution as well as good coronal and sagittal plane image reformats. The study can be done in a very short time interval, with newer scanners performing the entire study during a single breath-hold. Magnetic resonance (MR) is reserved for the evaluation of lesions close to the cartilage or ventricle. A limited study may be done to clarify a particular margin and to evaluate the cartilage.

Imaging of cartilage involvement is controversial [8-10]. Some investigators favor CT and some MR imaging. At CT, sclerosis of the cartilage and obliteration of the low-density fat in the medullary space can indicate involvement. The negative finding, intact fat in the medullary space, with a normal cortex is considered reliable. On MR imaging, the T1-weighted image is acquired first. If there is high signal intensity (fat) in the medullary space, the cartilage is considered normal. If the area is dark, then the T2-weighted image is examined. Non-ossified cartilage remains dark whereas tumor is usually brighter. High signal intensity on T2-weighted images can mean tumor or edema related to tumor. At our institution, high signal intensity is presumed to represent tumor. More research is needed to determine the significance of signal changes with respect to prognosis.

Submucosal Lesions

These may arise from the cartilages, the minor salivary glands, or from other soft-tissue structures [4].

CT with intravenous contrast can be very helpful in visualizing submucosal lesions. Chondromatous lesions can arise from any cartilage, often have demonstrable cartilage matrix [11], and tend to expand the parent cartilage (Fig. 5). Hemangiomas enhance intensely as do the very rare glomus (paraganglioma) tumors. There are other lesions that arise in the submucosal region but they do not enhance as avidly nor do they involve the cartilage. Such lesions cannot be identified precisely but it is very helpful to the clinician if a very vascular lesion or a chondroid lesion can be excluded.

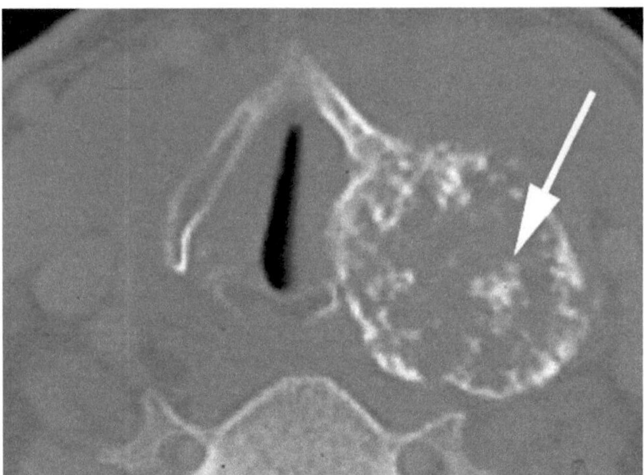

Fig. 5. Chondrosarcoma of the larynx. The tumor expands the cricoid cartilage. Note the small bits of cartilage matrix (*arrow*) within the tumor

Another submucosal lesion that is very important is the laryngocele, or saccular cyst. This lesion can present as a submucosal swelling but it is actually totally benign, representing an obstructive dilatation of the small saccule (appendix) of the ventricle. Thus, the lesion can be thought of as a supraglottic, paraglottic cyst. Although benign, it may be associated with a malignancy at the level of the ventricle. It is very important to carefully evaluate this level. Radiologically, small lesions of the mucosa cannot be totally excluded; this must be done endoscopically.

Trauma

Trauma to the airway can obviously be life-threatening. Most patients who have a demonstrable fracture of the larynx undergo endoscopy to rule out mucosal tears. If a fragment of cartilage is exposed to the airway, then chondritis and eventual chondronecrosis can be expected. The integrity of the thyroid cartilage and the cricoid ring should be carefully evaluated. Laryngeal fractures are associated with edema or hemorrhage of the endolarynx. These findings are very helpful especially when, as in a young patient, the cartilages are not completely calcified.

Fractures

Fractures of the cricoid usually involve "collapse" of the ring. The anterior arch of the cricoid is pushed posteriorly into the airway. There is usually swelling, as indicated by fluid/soft-tissue density within the cricoid ring. The thyroid can fracture vertically or horizontally. Hemorrhage in the adjacent pre-epiglottic fat may be a clue to this type of fracture. The arytenoid does not commonly fracture but can be dislocated.

Dislocations

Dislocations can occur at the cricothyroid articulation or the cricoarytenoid joint. Cricothyroid dislocation is usually associated with significant trauma. There is usually a fracture of the inferior horn of the thyroid cartilage rather than a true dislocation. Cricoarytenoid dislocation may occur with minor trauma. The status of these joints can be difficult to determine at imaging but the radiologist should indicate whether the cartilages appear to be normally aligned.

Conclusions

At our institution, CT is the first step in the evaluation of cancer of the larynx. MR imaging is used for additional evaluation of the cartilage. The ventricle and the upper margin of the cricoid are the two most important landmarks.

For submucosal lesions, an enhanced CT scan can detect chondroid lesions or laryngoceles. If these are excluded, the vascularity of a lesion should be determined.

In trauma patients, CT is used to identify fractures or dislocations.

References

1. Becker M (1998) Larynx and hypopharynx. Radiol Clin North Am 36:891-920
2. Curtin HD (2003) Larynx. In: Som PM, Curtin HD (eds) Head and neck imaging. 4th ed. Mosby, St Louis, pp 1595-1699
3. Pilch BZ (2001) Larynx and hypopharynx. In: Pilch BZ (ed) Head and neck surgical pathology. Lippincott Williams & Wilkins, Philadelphia, pp 230-283
4. Becker M, Moulin G, Kurt AM et al (1998) Non-squamous cell neoplasms of the larynx: radiologic-pathologic correlation. Radiographics 18:1189-1209
5. Bailey BJ (2006) Early glottic and supraglottic carcinoma: vertical partial laryngectomy and laryngoplasty. In: Bailey BJ, Johnson JT, Newlands SD (eds) Head & neck surgery – otolaryngology. 4th ed. Lippincott Williams & Wilkins, Philadelphia, pp 1727-1741
6. Zeitels SM (2006) Early glottic and supraglottic carcinoma: endoscopic techniques. In: Bailey BJ, Johnson JT, Newlands SD (eds) Head & neck surgery – otolaryngology. 4th ed. Lippincott Williams & Wilkins, Philadelphia, pp 1721-1726
7. Mancuso AA, Mukherji SK, Schmalfuss I et al (1999) Preradiotherapy computed tomography as a predictor of local control in supraglottic carcinoma. J Clin Oncol 17:631-637
8. Becker M, Zbaren P, Delavelle J et al (1997) Neoplastic invasion of the laryngeal cartilage: reassessment of criteria for diagnosis at CT. Radiology 203:521-532
9. Becker M (2000) Neoplastic invasion of laryngeal cartilage: radiologic diagnosis and therapeutic implications. Eur J Radiol 33:216-229
10. Castelijns JA, van den Brekel MW, Smit EM et al (1995) Predictive value of MR imaging-dependent and non-MR imaging-dependent parameters for recurrence of laryngeal cancer after radiation therapy. Radiology 196:735-739
11. Franco RA Jr, Singh B, Har-El G (2002) Laryngeal chondroma. J Voice 16:92-95

Sinonasal Imaging: Normal Anatomy and Pathologic Processes

Laurie A. Loevner

Department of Radiology, Hospital of the University of Pennsylvania, Philadelphia, PA, USA

Development

The maxillary sinuses are the first of the paranasal sinuses to develop, beginning in the first trimester of gestation and usually completed by adolescence. The ethmoid air cells arise from numerous evaginations from the nasal cavity, starting with the anterior air cells and progressing to the posterior air cells. The ethmoid air cells develop between the end of the first trimester and the mid-second trimester of gestation, although their final adult proportions are usually attained during puberty. The sphenoid sinus is present by the second trimester of pregnancy, and usually finishes its growth by the time a child reaches 10 years of age. The frontal sinuses are the only sinuses that are consistently absent at birth. Their development is variable, beginning during the first few years of life, and completed in early adolescence.

Anatomy

In order to understand the disease processes that may affect the paranasal sinuses and the nasal cavity, it is important to understand the normal anatomy as well as the normal drainage patterns of these structures. The paranasal sinuses and nasal cavity are lined by ciliated columnar epithelium that contains both mucinous and serous glands. The common drainage pathway for the frontal sinuses, maxillary sinuses, and anterior ethmoid air cells is through the ostiomeatal complex. The ostiomeatal unit is made up of a drainage pathway that consists of the maxillary sinus ostium, the infundibulum, the hiatus semilunaris, and the middle meatus. This drainage conduit is centered around the uncinate process (an osseous extension of the lateral nasal wall). Secretions that accumulate within the maxillary sinuses circulate towards the maxillary sinus ostium propelled by cilia within this sinus. From the maxillary ostium, mucus circulates through the infundibulum, located lateral to the uncinate process. From the infundibulum, secretions progress through the hiatus semilunaris, an air-filled channel anterior and inferior to the ethmoidal bulla (the largest ethmoid air cell), and then pass into the middle meatus, into the nasal cavity, and ultimately into the nasopharynx.

The frontal sinuses drain inferiorly via the frontal ethmoidal recess/nasofrontal duct into the middle meatus. This the common drainage site also for the anterior ethmoid air cells, whose ostia contact the infundibulum of the ostiomeatal complex. The nasofrontal duct is the channel between the inferomedial frontal sinus and the anterior part of the middle meatus. The anterior-most ethmoid air cells, the agger nasi cells, are located in front of the middle turbinates. The latter are positioned anterior, lateral, and inferior to the frontal ethmoidal recess. Inconstant ethmoid air cells located along the anterosuperior maxillary surface just inferior to the orbital floor are called maxilloethmoidal or Haller cells; they are present in less than one-half of imaged patients.

The posterior ethmoid air cells are located behind the middle turbinate and secretions drain through the superior meatus, the supreme meatus, and/or other tiny ostia under the superior turbinate into the sphenoethmoidal recess, the nasal cavity, and finally into the nasopharynx. Cilia are necessary for the drainage of the sphenoid sinus, as secretions must be propelled to the ostia of this sinus which is located above the sinus floor.

The three sets of turbinates in the nasal cavity include the superior, middle, and inferior turbinates. Occasionally, there may be a supreme turbinate located above the superior turbinate. When the middle turbinate is aerated, it is termed a concha bullosa, present in 30-50% of patients. Large or opacified concha bullosa may obstruct the ostiomeatal complex, the common drainage passageway of the frontal sinus, maxillary sinus, and anterior ethmoid air cells.

The nasal septum separates the right and left nasal turbinates, dividing the nasal cavity in half. The anterior and inferior nasal septum is made up of cartilage. The posterior portion of the nasal septum is osseous. Specifically, the supero-posterior osseous portion is the perpendicular plate of the ethmoid bone, while the infero-posterior osseous portion is the vomer. The septum within the nasal cavity is lined by squamous epithelium while the remainder of the nasal cavity and the paranasal sinuses are lined by columnar epithelium.

The nasolacrimal duct courses from the lacrimal sac at the medial canthus, then along the anterior and lateral nasal wall, before draining into the inferior meatus. There is normal cyclical passive congestion and decongestion of each side of the nasal cavity and ethmoid air cells, including temporary mucosal thickening in these structures.

The blood supply to the sinonasal structures comes from both the internal and external carotid arteries. The arterial supply to the frontal sinuses is from supraorbital and supratrochlear branches of the ophthalmic artery, while venous drainage is through the superior ophthalmic vein. The ethmoid air cells and sphenoid sinus also receive their blood supply from branches of the sphenopalatine artery (arising from the external carotid circulation) as well as ethmoidal branches of the ophthalmic artery (arising from the internal carotid circulation). Venous drainage is via nasal veins into the nasal cavity, and/or ethmoidal veins which drain into the ophthalmic veins, which then subsequently drain into the cavernous sinus. The maxillary sinuses are supplied predominantly by the external carotid circulation, namely, by numerous branches of the maxillary artery. These sinuses drain through facial as well as maxillary veins, the latter communicating with the pterygoid venous plexus. It is the venous drainage pattern of the paranasal sinuses (ultimately communicating with the cavernous sinus and pterygoid venous plexus) that is responsible for the potential intracranial complications of sinusitis, including meningitis, subdural empyema, and cavernous sinus thrombosis.

Pathology and Disease Processes of the Paranasal Sinuses

Congenital Lesions

Many congenital or developmental abnormalities that occur within the nasal cavity are related to aberrant invagination of the neural plate. During neural plate retraction in embryogenesis, the dura contacts the dermis. Normally, this dermal connection regresses. When it does not, congenital abnormalities may develop, including sinus tracts, dermoid cysts, encephaloceles, and nasal gliomas. The term nasal glioma is in fact a misnomer as it is not a true neoplasm. With nasal gliomas, there is a fibrous connection with the intracranial compartment.

Inflammatory Disease/Sinusitis

Most cases of acute sinusitis are related to an antecedent viral upper respiratory tract infection. There is resultant swelling that causes apposition of the mucosal surfaces within the paranasal sinuses, leading to obstruction of the normal drainage pathways. Inadequate drainage of secretions results in bacterial overgrowth.

In patients with sinusitis who are therefore candidates for fundoscopic sinus surgery (FESS), it is important to evaluate certain anatomic landmarks on high-quality, thin-section unenhanced computed tomography (CT) images of the sinonasal cavity. Either direct coronal images or direct thin-section axial images with subsequent coronal reformations should be obtained. Specifically, the medial orbital walls, cribiform plate, and roof and lateral walls of the sphenoid sinus should be examined for defects or deficiencies in these osseous structures. A defect in the lamina papyracea may result in orbital penetration and subsequent hematoma formation, whereas a dehiscence in the cribiform plate or sphenoid sinus could result in a cerebrospinal fluid (CSF) leak, intracranial (meningitis, encephalocele), or carotid artery complications (perforation with acute subarachnoid hemorrhage; pseudoaneurysm formation).

Evaluations of the paranasal sinuses should include comments on mucosal apposition or inflammatory changes in the region of the ostiomeatal unit and the sphenoethmoidal recess. Obscuration of the infundibulum best predicts which patients will be at risk for sinusitis. The presence of air-fluid levels should be noted. Hyperdense secretions on CT can suggest the presence of inspissated secretions, fungal disease/elements, or hemorrhage in the setting of trauma. Sinonasal secretions have variable signal intensity patterns on magnetic resonance (MR) imaging. MR signal-intensity characteristics are related to the protein concentration and mobile water protons within the secretions. As the protein concentration in secretions increases, the signal intensity on T1-weighted imaging changes from hypointense to hyperintense, to hypointense again. On T2-weighted images, low-protein secretions are initially bright; however, as the protein content and viscosity increase, the signal intensity decreases.

The complications of sinusitis include periorbital cellulitis, meningitis, thrombophlebitis (including cavernous sinus thrombosis), subdural empyema, intraparenchymal brain abscesses, and perineural and perivascular spread of infection (particularly in invasive fungal disease). Mucoceles may also be a complication of sinusitis and are most common in the frontal sinuses and ethmoid air cells, but least common in the sphenoid sinus. Mucoceles may show a spectrum of signal characteristics on MR imaging, depending on their protein content, and usually demonstrate rim enhancement (compared to tumors, which typically show more solid enhancement).

Neoplasms

Computed tomography and MR imaging play complementary roles in the evaluation of tumors of the sinonasal cavity; frequently, both are employed in the assessment of patients with newly diagnosed sinonasal masses. CT provides bone detail, while MR provides superior soft-tissue resolution as well as multi-planar capabilities. MR is also better in evaluating the intraorbital and intracranial extension of neoplastic processes.

Typically, benign neoplasms, when large enough, expand the affected paranasal sinus and secondarily remodel the adjacent bone; however, osseous destruction from benign lesions is less common than with malignancies. Nonetheless, it should be noted that in the paranasal sinuses it is not unusual for contained malignant tumors to have benign features. The contrary is also true; that is, benign tumors may have a relatively aggressive appearance. Caution is always required when evaluating masses within the sinuses. Fibro-osseous lesions that may involve the paranasal sinuses include osteomas, fibrous dysplasia, ossifying or non-ossifying fibromas, and chondromas or other chondroid lesions. These lesions frequently have radiologically characteristic appearances.

Papillomas

Papillomas arise from the columnar epithelium and are classified in three subtypes: inverted, cylindric, and fungiform. In general, papillomas tend to occur unilaterally in the sinonasal cavity. The most common papilloma affecting the paranasal sinuses is the inverted papilloma. These are more common in men in the fourth through sixth decades of life. While this is a benign neoplasm, squamous cell carcinoma is present in up to 15% of cases. Inverted papillomas may show a rather aggressive appearance, with bony destruction. They typically arise from the lateral nasal wall at the level of the middle turbinate, or less commonly, within the maxillary sinus itself. While there are no imaging features that characteristically suggest the diagnosis of an inverted papilloma, the location is usually a tip-off to the diagnosis. Inverted papillomas may occasionally erode the skull base (as may benign polyps), simulating an aggressive cancer.

Malignant Neoplasms

It is essential that patients with sinonasal malignancies undergo MR imaging to distinguish sinus opacification related to tumor from opacification related to inspissated secretions. Most neoplasms can be distinguished from inflammatory conditions based on their imaging characteristics as well as their more solid enhancement pattern following intravenous contrast administration (compared to rim enhancement in benign inflammatory disease). In addition, T2-weighted imaging may be helpful, as most malignancies are heterogeneous and intermediate in signal compared to inflammatory secretions, which tend to be hyperintense and more homogeneous in character. Sinonasal secretions are complex and have variable signal-intensity patterns on MR imaging; this is related to the protein concentration and mobile water protons within the secretions, as described above. Fungus is frequently black on T2-weighted images, mimicking an "aerated sinus". Imaging of sinonasal malignancies must also include high-resolution views of the orbit, skull base, and the intracranial compartment. Direct tumor extension or perineural spread outside the sinonasal cavity and into these important adjacent anatomic locations may occur. Such findings significantly impact upon the patient's operability, the type of resection that is required, and the necessity for radiation therapy. An especially important anatomic location for detection of tumor spread is the pterygopalatine fossa. If tumor from the sinonasal cavity spreads to this site, then extension into the adjacent orbit, infratemporal fossa, skull base, and intracranial compartment may subsequently occur.

Squamous cell carcinoma is the most common malignancy of the paranasal sinuses and nasal cavity, representing two-thirds of all cancers in this region. Occupational exposures, including radium, Thorotrast, and, especially, nickel, are causative factors. The majority of squamous cell carcinomas originate in the maxillary sinus anthrum, with the next most common site the nasal cavity septum. Adenocarcinomas, lymphoma, undifferentiated carcinomas, esthesioneuroblastomas, and sarcomas may also occur in the sinonasal structures. Following squamous cell carcinoma, minor salivary gland tumors and melanomas (which arise from melanocyte rests in the sinonasal mucosa) are the next most common malignancies to affect the nasal cavity. Minor salivary gland tumors represent a wide spectrum of histologic subtypes including adenoid cystic carcinoma, mucoepidermoid carcinoma, and acinic cell carcinomas. Of these, adenoid cystic carcinoma is the most frequently reported. Metastatic disease to the paranasal sinuses is unusual, with renal cell carcinoma the most commonly reported.

Suggested Reading

Babbel RW, Harnsberger HR, Sonkens J et al (1992) Recurring patterns of inflammatory sinonasal disease demonstrated on screening sinus CT. Amer J Neuroradiol 13:903-912

Barkovich AJ, Vandermarch P, Edwards MSB et al (1991) Congenital nasal masses: CT and MR imaging features in 16 cases. Am J Neuroradiol 12:105-116

Dillon KB, Som PM, Fullerton GD (1990) Hypointense MR signal in chronically inspissated sinonasal secretions. Radiology 174:73-78

Eisen MD, Yousem DM, Loevner LA et al (2000) Preoperative imaging to predict orbital invasion by tumor. Head Neck Surg 22:456-462

Kallman JE, Loevner LA, Yousem DM et al (1996) Heterotopic brain in the pterygopalatine fossa. Am J Neuroradiol 18:176-179

Lanzieri CF, Shah M, Krauss D et al (1991) Use of gadolinium-enhanced MR imaging for differentiating mucoceles from neoplasms in the paranasal sinuses. Radiology 178:425-428

Lasser A, Rothfeld PR, Shapiro RS (1976) Epithelial papilloma and squamous cell carcinoma of the nasal cavity and paranasal sinuses: a clinicopathologic study. Cancer 38:2503-2510

Loevner LA, Sonners AI (2004) Imaging of neoplasms of the paranasal sinuses. Neuroimag Clin North Am 14(4):625-646

Loevner LA, Yousem DM, Lanza DC et al (1995) MR evaluation of frontal osteoplastic flaps using autogenous fat grafts to obliterate the sinus. Am J Neuroradiol 16:1721-1726

Schaeffer JP (1920) The embryology, development and anatomy of the nose, paranasal sinuses, nasolacrimal passageways and olfactory organs in man. Blakiston, Philadelphia, PA

Sigal R, Monnet O, de Baere T et al (1992) Adenoid cystic carcinoma of the head and neck: evaluation with MR imaging and clinical-pathologic correlation in 27 patients. Radiology 184:95-101

Som PM, Lidov M, Brandwein M et al (1994) Sinonasal esthesioneuroblastoma with intracranial extension: marginal tumor cysts as a diagnostic MR finding. Am J Neuroradiol 15:1259-1262

Som PM, Lawson W, Lidov MW (1991) Simulated aggressive skull base erosion in response to benign sinonasal disease. Radiology 180:755-759

Som PM, Shapiro MD, Biller HF et al (1988) Sinonasal tumors and inflammatory tissues: differentiation with MR. Radiology 167:803-808

St Pierre S, Baker SR (1983) Squamous cell carcinoma of the maxillary sinus: analysis of 66 cases. Head Neck Surg 5:508-513

Woodruff WW, Vrabec DP (1994) Inverted papilloma of the nasal vault and paranasal sinuses: spectrum of CT findings. AJR Am J Roentgenol 162:419-423

Yousem DM, Li C, Montone KT et al (1996) Primary malignant melanoma of the sinonasal cavity: MR evaluation. Radiographics 16:1101-1110

Zinreich SJ, Kennedy DW, Kuman AJ et al (1988) MR imaging of normal nasal cycle: comparison with sinus pathology. J Comput Assist Tomogr 12:1014-1019

CT and MRI of the Nose, Paranasal Sinuses, and Adjacent Spaces

Roberto Maroldi, Davide Farina, Andrea Borghesi, Marco Ravanelli

Department of Radiology, University of Brescia, Brescia, Italy

Introduction

The impressive development of endonasal surgical techniques during the last two decades has been made possible by the detailed pre-operative information provided by computed tomography (CT) and magnetic resonance imaging (MRI). For each imaging technique, specific fields of clinical application have been described in the medical literature [1]. As CT supplies excellent details about the thin bony sinonasal walls, it reveals the precise individual anatomy of the nose and paranasal sinuses. It is on the basis of this *internal map* that endonasal surgery for rhinosinusitis is planned. Therefore, inflammatory diseases belong to the domain of CT, whereas benign and malignant neoplasms are covered by the MRI. The main advantages of MRI are that it more precisely distinguishes tumor signal from adjacent structures, more accurately demonstrates two critical periosteal linings (periorbita, dura mater), and allows the early detection of perineural spread of disease. In addition, as endonasal surgeons are confronted with new challenges, such as endoscopic craniofacial resection, radiologists must be able to provide answers to questions regarding the precise grading of the intracranial neoplastic extent [2].

Whereas MRI reliably identifies pre-treatment tumor extent, early submucosal local recurrences are still difficult to demonstrate because of post-treatment changes in the anatomy and signal of treated tissues. Although diffusion-weighted imaging and dynamic contrast-enhanced techniques are promising developments, positron emission tomography (PET)-CT is the imaging technique expected to overcome the limits of morphological MRI.

Essential Anatomy of the Sinonasal Area

Three anatomic areas, corresponding to the narrowest tracts of drainage pathways, are crucial for endoscopic surgery planning: the ostiomeatal complex, the frontal recess, and the spheno-ethmoid recess.

The ostiomeatal complex is located at the crossroads of anterior ethmoid, frontal sinus, and maxillary sinus mucus drainage. It includes the maxillary sinus ostium, the ethmoid infundibulum, the ethmoid bulla, and the uncinate process. The ethmoid infundibulum is the air passage connecting the maxillary sinus ostium to the middle meatus. It is bordered superiorly by the ethmoid bulla, the most posterior cell within the anterior ethmoid, protruding in the middle meatus. The vertical portion of the uncinate process is a key component of the ostiomeatal complex. Depending on the nature of its superior attachment, the *frontal recess* (i.e., the mucus drainage path of the frontal sinus) may open into the middle meatus medially or laterally to the uncinate process [3]. Correct assessment of the frontal recess opening is essential in planning the proper endonasal approach to the frontal recess and adequate exposure of the frontal sinus (Fig. 1). Medially, the middle turbinate borders the ostiomeatal complex, its vertical lamina is anchored on the cribriform plate while its ground lamella inserts laterally onto the posterior part of the lamina papyracea.

The *spheno-ethmoid recess* is outlined by the anterior sphenoid sinus wall and by the posterior wall of posterior ethmoid cells. It conveys sphenoid sinus secretions in the superior meatus and is more clearly shown on axial CT images.

There are several variants of sinonasal anatomic structures. Most of them are due to the variable extent of ethmoid sinus pneumatization into adjacent sinuses, i.e., infraorbital ethmoid cells (maxillary sinus), frontal cells, Onodi cells (sphenoid sinus); bones, i.e., agger nasi (lacrimal bone), supraorbital ethmoid cells (frontal bone); or laminae belonging to the ethmoid bone (concha bullosa). Extensive pneumatization of the sphenoid sinus may result in dehiscence of its bony boundary with the internal carotid artery or optic nerve. Similarly, dehiscences of the lamina papyracea increase the risk of complications due to damage of intraorbital structures.

The pterygopalatine fossa is a narrow fat space located between the pterygoid process/plates and the vertical process of the palatine bone (merged with the wall of the posterior maxillary sinus). Both CT and MRI demonstrate the foramina and canals through which the pterygopalatine fossa directly communicates with the middle cranial fossa (vidian canal and foramen rotundum), the orbit (inferior orbital fissure), the masticatory space

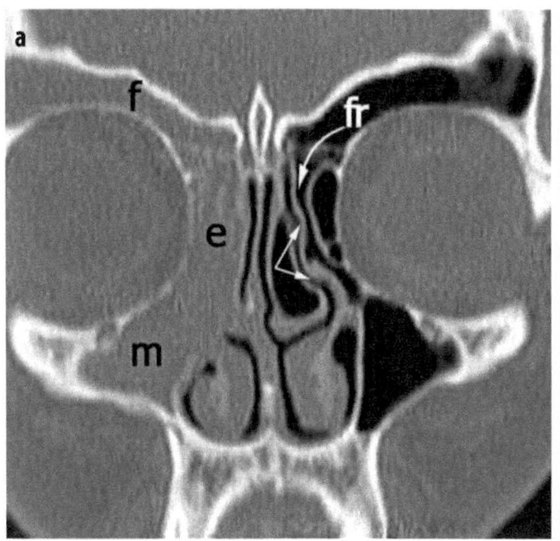

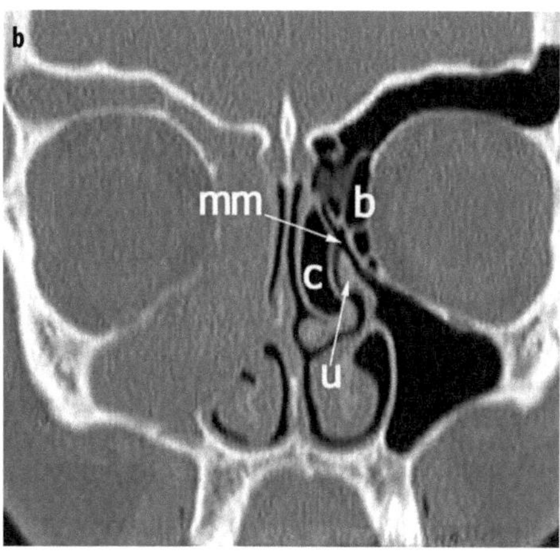

Fig. 1 a, b. Chronic rhinosinusitis. Computed tomography (CT) in the coronal plane. **a** On the right side, the maxillary (*m*), anterior ethmoid (*e*), and frontal sinuses (*f*) are filled by fluid, suggesting blockage at the level of the middle meatus with rhinosinusitis involving all the three sinuses. On the left normal side, the path of the frontal recess (*fr*, *curved arrow*) runs medial to the superior attachment of the vertical portion of the uncinate process (*arrows*). **b** On the left side, the coronal plane shows the narrow space of the middle meatus (*mm*), located between the ethmoid bulla (*b*), the middle pneumatized turbinate ("concha bullosa", *c*), and the horizontal part of the uncinate process (*u*)

(pterygomaxillary fissure), the choana (sphenopalatine foramen), and the oral cavity (greater and lesser palatine canals). Within the pterygopalatine fossa are the pterygopalatine ganglion, part of the maxillary nerve, terminal branches of the internal maxillary artery (the sphenopalatine artery), and fat.

Imaging the Patient with Acute or Chronic Rhinosinusitis

Patients with acute rhinosinusitis do not require radiological studies of the paranasal sinuses because the symptoms noted in association with the endoscopic examination are the only steps required for making a correct diagnosis [4]. Contrast-enhanced CT is indicated if an orbital complication, generally secondary to acute ethmoiditis, and/or intracranial complication are suspected. CT can discriminate between preseptal cellulitis, subperiosteal inflammation, and intraorbital (extra- or intraconal) spread. [5].

Overall, CT allows correct diagnosis of orbital complication in up to 91% of cases and is significantly more accurate than clinical examination alone (81%) [6].

Intracranial complications are generally secondary to frontal sinusitis. They are observed even in the absence of sinus wall defects as they may be secondary to thrombophlebitis of the valveless diploic veins [7]. Imaging is mandatory in order to correctly assess the degree of involvement of intracranial structures. In this setting, MRI is the technique of choice, with an accuracy superior to that of CT, in particular in differentiating dural reaction from epidural/subdural or intracerebral abscess and in demonstrating thrombosis of the sagittal or cavernous sinus [6, 8].

CT evaluation of patients complaining of chronic rhinosinusitis and nasal polyposis is essentially focused on the accurate delineation of those elements – inflammatory mucosal changes and/or predisposing anatomic factors – that may impair mucociliary drainage and on the extent of the lesion.

Patients affected by chronic rhinosinusitis should receive adequate medical treatment before CT examination of the paranasal sinuses, in order to treat acute infection and resolve mucosal edema. Courses of oral antibiotics and the use of nasal steroids and antihistamines, prescribed at least 3 weeks before the CT examination, decrease the risk of overestimating chronic inflammation and polypoid reaction of the mucosa.

Because of the high contrast between air, mucosa, and bone, low-dose protocols should be adopted by decreasing tube current down to 30-50 mAs [9]. This results in a considerable decrease of the eye-lens dose [10] without a significant loss of diagnostic information.

The volume acquired by CT should be reconstructed in the coronal, axial, and sagittal planes. Coronal images are the mainstay of imaging in chronic rhinosinusitis. These images, which are oriented perpendicular to the hard palate, demonstrate the patency, width, and morphology of the middle and superior meatus, which are hidden by the turbinates and are thus difficult to access at clinical examination. Moreover, coronal imaging clearly shows both the superior and the lateral insertion of the middle turbinate, as well as the cribriform plate. Thin slices (1-2 mm) minimize partial volume artifacts that may mimic mucosal thickenings along small-caliber drainage pathways. Axial images better demonstrate the anterior and posterior walls of the frontal, maxillary, and sphenoid sinuses. Sagittal reconstructions are essential in assessing the anatomy of the recesses of the frontal sinuses.

According to Sonkens et al. [11], five different patterns of chronic rhinosinusitis may be described at CT, all but one are based on the obstruction of different mucus-drainage pathways:

- The infundibular pattern is mainly due to the presence of mucosal thickenings or isolated polyps along the ethmoid infundibulum with blockage of maxillary sinus drainage alone.
- The ostiomeatal unit pattern reflects obstruction of all drainage systems in the middle meatus, leading to maxillary, frontal, and anterior ethmoid sinusitis. The most frequent causes are nonspecific mucosal thickenings or nasal polyps (Fig. 1). This pattern may also be observed in the presence of benign or malignant neo-

plasms arising from the lateral nasal wall.

- The spheno-ethmoid recess pattern is rather rare, consisting of sphenoid sinusitis and/or posterior ethmoiditis secondary to spheno-ethmoid recess obstruction.
- The pattern of nasal polyposis is usually characterized by bilateral involvement of the middle meati as well as the ethmoid infundibular and paranasal cavities by inflammatory polyps. At CT, solid lobulated lesions filling the ethmoid, the nasal fossae, and the sinusal cavities are seen. Bone remodeling is triggered by mechanical pressure exerted by the polyps but also by the local release of inflammatory mediators and by bacterial invasion of bone and periosteum [12]. Widening of the ethmoid infundibulum (or infundibula) and truncation of the middle turbinate(s) is observed bilaterally in up to 80% of patients indicate nasal polyposis. A peculiar variant of sinonasal polyp is the antrochoanal polyp, which arises from the maxillary sinus and bulges into the middle meatus, where it extends between the middle turbinate and the lateral nasal wall to reach the choana. Antrochoanal polyp is of low density (fluid-like) on CT, while on MRI it resembles inflammatory polyps. Since the waist of the polyp may be strangled as it passes through constrictive ostia, dilation and stasis of the feeding vessels combined with the presence of edema causes the lesion to show non-homogenous enhancement, i.e., an angiomatous polyp [13].
- The sporadic pattern includes a wide list of different conditions (such as isolated sinusitis, retention cyst, mucocele, post-surgical changes) unrelated to the impairment of mucociliary drainage. CT findings consist of partial or complete obliteration of a sinusal cavity by means of a thickened mucosa with a smooth, occasionally lobulated, surface and homogeneously low density [14].

Imaging the Patient with Fungal Rhinosinusitis or Aggressive Inflammatory Lesions

Fungal rhinosinusitis can be defined as an infection of the paranasal sinuses in which fungi are the primary pathogens or an inflammation that is due to their presence. According to the presence or absence of invasion of the sinonasal mucosa [15], fungal rhinosinusitis is classified into non-invasive and invasive forms. The former includes fungus ball and eosinophilic fungal rhinosinusitis [16]; acute fulminant rhinosinusitis, chronic invasive fungal rhinosinusitis, and granulomatous invasive fungal rhinosinusitis make up the latter.

In non-invasive fungal rhinosinusitis, the lesion is usually confined for a long time by the sinusal walls. Eventually, there is remodeling and destruction of the walls due to the fungus ball, a mass-like accumulation of fungal debris and mucus within the sinus, usually appearing as an isolated lesion, or to the mechanical pressure exerted by the diffuse accumulation of mucin. The latter is referred to as eosinophilic fungal rhinosinusitis and is frequently associated with sinonasal polyposis. CT and MRI findings in non-invasive forms reflect the high calcium, iron, and manganese content within fungal hyphae. On CT, spontaneous hyperdensities and scattered calcifications may be observed. Both iron and manganese cause relevant shortening of T1 and T2. Therefore, on MRI, both fungus ball and eosinophilic fungal rhinosinusitis will appear as hypointense/signal-void lesions filling the naso-sinusal cavity. A hyperintense signal on T1 has been shown in bipolaris infection [17]. In eosinophilic rhinosinusitis the mucosa is undamaged; this thickened non-invaded mucosa bordering the sinonasal cavities has high signal intensity on T2-weighted images and enhances on post-contrast T1-weighted images [8]. Expansion of the sinusal walls and bone thinning are more commonly observed in eosinophilic fungal rhinosinusitis [18] (Fig. 2), whereas sclerosis of the sinusal walls is more typical of a fungus ball (Fig. 3).

Invasion of mucosa, bone, and vessels is the hallmark of invasive fungal rhinosinusitis. These forms are generally encountered in immunocompromised patients. Acute fulminant and chronic invasive fungal rhinosinusitis share common imaging features; the differential diagnosis is therefore based on the severity and rapidity of the clinical course, which in the acute fulminant form is often lethal.

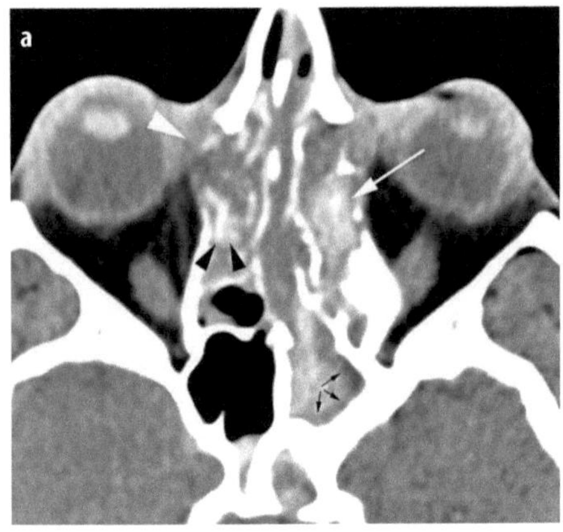

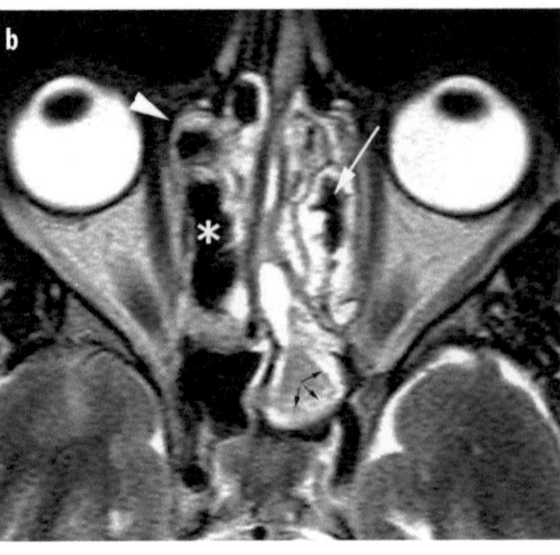

Fig. 2 a, b. Eosinophilic fungal rhinosinusitis. **a** On CT, the content of the sinuses ranges from calcifications (*black arrowheads*) in the right ethmoid cells to high densities in the left ethmoid cells (*white arrow*) and left sphenoid sinus. In both sinuses, the high density filling the cavity is separated by thickened mucosa (*black arrows* in the left sphenoid sinus). **b** On MRI, the mycotic content appears as hypointense signal in the right (*asterisk*) and left (*white arrow*) ethmoid sinuses. Remodeling of the lacrimal bone is demonstrated on CT and by magnetic resonance imaging (MRI) (*white arrowheads*)

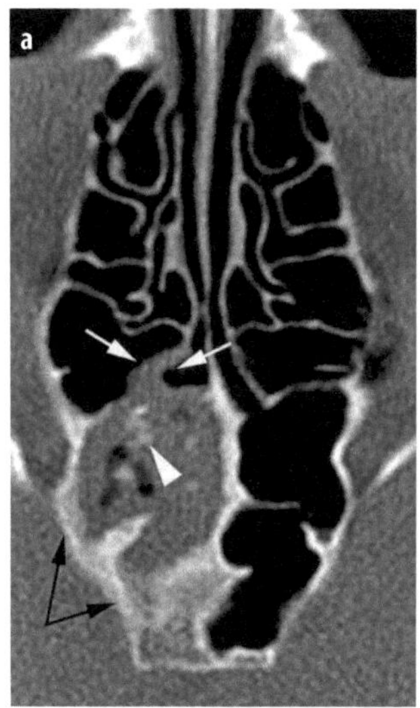

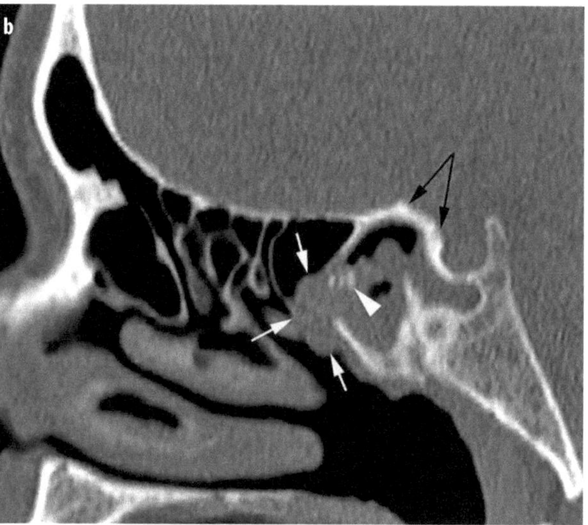

Fig. 3 a, b. Fungus ball. **a** The right sphenoid sinus is filled by non-homogeneous signal and calcifications (*arrowhead*). Increased thickness and sclerosis of the sinusal wall are present (*black arrows*). The fungus ball extends through the spheno-ethmoidal recess (*white arrows*). **b** In the sagittal plane, the lesion abuts the superior meatus

On MRI, due to vascular invasion, the necrotic mucosa does not enhance. It may show variable signal intensity on T2-weighted images, perhaps reflecting different stages of tissue ischemia. Frequently, the infected devascularized tissue extends beyond the sinusal walls, with involvement of the dura, dural sinuses, and the brain. Early extension into the orbital apex and invasion of the skull base (with cavernous sinus involvement) can be observed, particularly in acute fulminant disease [19].

Wegener's granulomatosis is a chronic, granulomatous necrotizing vasculitis affecting the upper and lower respiratory tract and the kidneys. At imaging, sinonasal mucosal changes in the early stage of the disease are nonspecific and very similar to chronic inflammatory changes. Only in the late stage of the disease does the signal intensity of the mucosa and submucosa switch to hypointensity on both T2-and T1-weighted sequences, with variable degrees of contrast enhancement [20]. This is mostly due to submucosal granuloma formation. In advanced disease stages, the inflammatory infiltrate and granulomatous lesions within small vessels walls lead to obliteration of the lumen and avascular necrobiosis. This is the pathologic basis of bone destruction, often involving midline structures such as the nasal septum. A similar pattern of bone destruction can be observed in advanced cocaine abusers (midline destructive syndrome). Imaging may be useful for the differential diagnosis. In cocaine abusers, not only the septum but also the adjacent turbinates may be destroyed, roughly in a centrifugal pattern [21]. In addition, unlike in Wegener's granulomatosis, the hard and soft palates are eventually destroyed. Wegener's granulomatosis may involve the deep spaces of the face and spread to the central skull base. MRI is decisive in identifying the cause of nerve impairment:

- Direct granuloma extension into the fissures or foramina of the skull base, such as the pterygopalatine fossa, the orbital fissure or the vidian canal. On MRI, the granulomatous lesions show hypointense signal on both T2-weighted and plain T1-weighted sequences. Contrast enhancement ranging from mildly inhomogeneous to hyperintense is usually observed [22].
- Perineural granulomatous spread along trigeminal/parasympathetic nerve branches. MRI findings include asymmetric nerve thickening, enlargement, and late destruction of the related foramina and fissures [23].
- Localization of the disease to the central nervous system.

However, involvement of deep spaces of the face and/or perineural spread is indistinguishable on MRI from malignant neoplasms, such as non-Hodgkin lymphoma.

Imaging the Patient with a Sinonasal Mass: CT and MRI Techniques

The first step in the diagnostic work-up of benign and malignant sinus neoplasms consists of fiberoptic examination. Endoscopy allows adequate demonstration of the superficial spread of the lesion and may guide biopsy. The discrimination between benign and malignant tumors and the precise characterization of the lesion are, in most cases, far beyond the capabilities of CT [17]. The main goals of imaging are therefore to provide a precise map of deep tumor extension in all those areas not visible at fiberoptic examination, especially the anterior cranial fossa, orbit, and pterygopalatine fossa.

In this setting, MRI is the technique of choice because it clearly differentiates tumor from retained secretions; allows early detection of perivascular/perineural spread; and provides higher contrast resolution. Nonetheless, the strengths of CT consist of its superior definition of bone structures, even in the case of subtle erosions; faster and easier use; superior accessibility; and lower cost.

Despite the relevant improvements provided by multislice technology, i.e., fast coverage of the volume of interest, thin collimation, and acquisition of nearly isotropic voxels, CT indications are nowadays restricted to imaging patients who were not preliminarily examined by the otolaryngologist (to rule out non-neoplastic lesions) or of patients with contraindications to MRI.

A key aspect of the MRI protocol is the spatial resolution. The nasal cavity and paranasal sinuses are a complex framework of airspaces bordered by thin bony boundaries. A thin osteo-periosteal layer separates the sinonasal region from the anterior cranial fossa (cribriform plate and dura) and the orbit (lamina papyracea and periorbita). Adequate depiction of these structures mandates high field equipment and a dedicated circular coil (head coil). In addition, a high-resolution matrix should be applied along with the smallest field-of-view (FOV) achievable. It is also recommended that the slice thickness not exceed 3-3.5 mm, with an interslice gap of 1.5-2.4 mm (50-70%). The parameters listed above, applied to TSE T2 and SE T1 sequences, are an acceptable compromise between the need to attain small pixel size and the risk of significantly decreasing the signal-to-noise ratio.

Inverted Papilloma and Juvenile Angiofibroma: CT and MRI Findings

Inverted papilloma (IP) is an epithelial benign neoplasm characterized by infolding of the mucosa in the underlying stroma without crossing of the basement membrane. It is one of the most common benign neoplasms of the sinonasal tract [18, 19], and its association with sinonasal malignancies, in particular squamous cell carcinoma, is well-established. IP may be suspected whenever an isolated, unilateral polypoid lesion is detected by imaging studies. At CT, IP appears as a soft-tissue density mass with non-homogeneous contrast enhancement; calcifications represent residues of involved bone [20]. Turbo spin-echo (TSE) T2 and enhanced T1 may reveal IP's "septate striated appearance" [21], "convoluted cerebriform pattern" [22], or "columnar pattern", depending on the macro-architecture of the lesion (Fig. 4). Juxtaposition of several epithelial and stromal layers – the first being hypointense on TSE T2 because of the papilloma's high cellularity and mildly enhancing on post-contrast SE T1; the second being hyperintense on TSE T2 due to edematous changes and highly enhancing on post-contrast SE T1 – results in a quite regular columnar pattern on MRI. Thin SE T1 sections and slice acquisition in three spatial planes improve identification of the particular pattern.

Juvenile angiofibromas (JAs) are composed of vascular and fibrous elements, and typically occur in adolescent males. It was recently suggested that JA is a vascular malformation [23] (or hamartoma) rather than a tumor. The specific findings of JA are the tendency of the lesion to grow in the submucosal plane and early invasion of the cancellous bone of the pterygoid root; the lesion may then grow laterally into the greater wing of the sphenoid bone. From its site of origin in the pterygopalatine fossa, the JA extends: (a) medially into the nasal cavity (and nasopharynx) via enlargement and erosion of the sphenopalatine foramen; (b) anteriorly with bowing of the maxillary sinus wall [24]; (c) laterally, via the pterygomaxillary fissure; (d) superiorly into the apex of the orbit through the inferior orbital fissure, and into the middle cranial fossa via the superior orbital fissure.

Enhanced CT or MRI precisely maps the extent into these spaces by detecting the enhancing finger-like projections of JA and the lesion's sharp and lobulated mar-

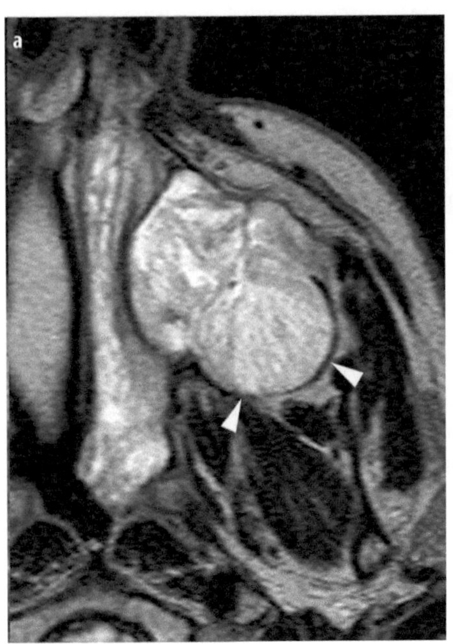

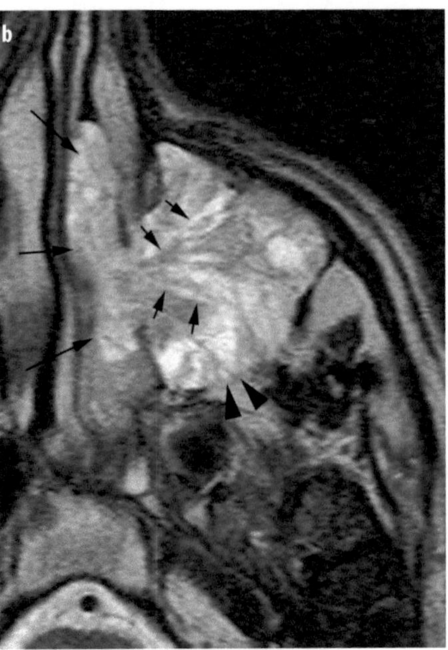

Fig. 4 a, b. Inverted papilloma. T2-weighted sequence. **a** The mass totally fills the left maxillary sinus, displacing and remodeling the posterolateral wall. A hypointense interface between the tumor and the infratemporal fat tissue (*arrowheads*) indicates the periosteal covering. **b** The characteristic parallel columnar pattern of the inverted papilloma is clearly demonstrated (*short arrows*). The mass exits the sinus and expands into the nasal cavity (*long arrows*). Extreme thinning of the bony periosteal covering of the posterolateral maxillary sinus is seen (*arrowheads*)

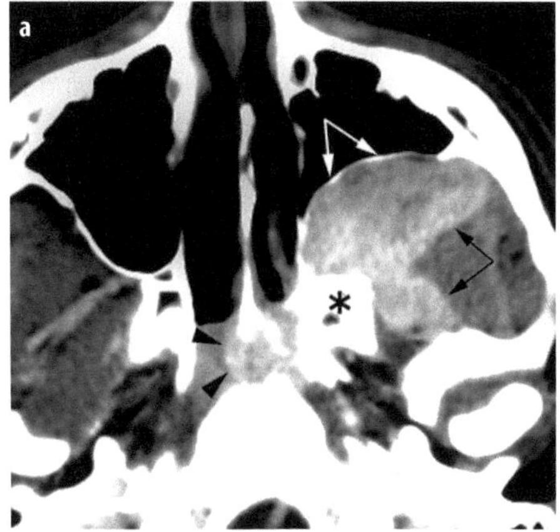

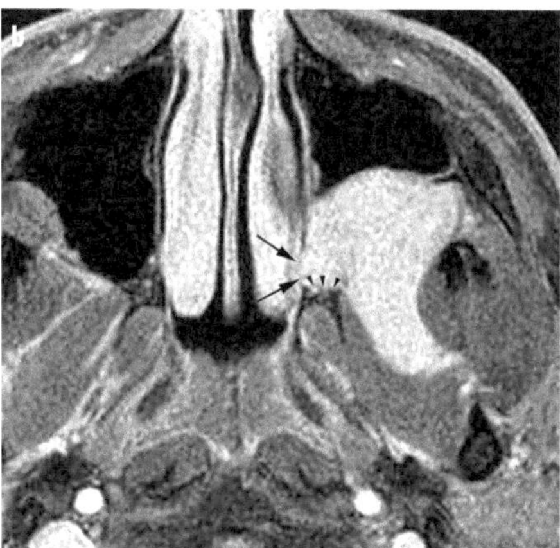

Fig. 5 a, b. Juvenile angiofibroma. **a** On enhanced CT, the lesion anteriorly displaces the posterolateral maxillary sinus wall (*white arrows*). Involvement of the spongiotic bone of the pterygoid process (*asterisk*) is suspected. There is submucosal spread deep to the nasopharyngeal roof (*black arrowheads*). **b** On MRI, the post-contrast GET1 fat-sat (VIBE) sequence shows extension of the tumor towards the sphenopalatine foramen (*arrows*) and erosion of the pterygoid process (*arrowheads*)

gins (Fig. 5). At CT, intradiploic spread may be demonstrated by differentiating normal medullary content from the strongly enhancing JA. On MRI, this discrimination is achieved by combining a plain T1 with a post-contrast T1 without or with fat saturation. The latter permits the hyperintense enhanced JA to be easily distinguished from the suppressed signal of the surrounding bone marrow. Intracranial extent is mainly due to the finger-like projections running along canals or through foramina; extension through destruction of the inner table of the greater wing or the lateral sphenoid sinus walls is rare.

Essential Information in Managing Naso-sinusal Neoplasms

Although infrequent, sinonasal neoplasms are characterized by numerous different histotypes, a distinctive feature that reflects the peculiar densities of the diverse anatomic structures present in this area. About 80% of these neoplasms arise from the maxillary sinus, with up to 73% being squamous cell carcinoma [25]; most of the remaining tumors arise from the ethmoid sinus [26]. Among these malignancies, adenocarcinoma, squamous cell carcinoma, and olfactory neuroblastoma are the most common. As a result, patterns of tumor spread may be generalized into two different models according to their site of origin: maxillary vs. naso-ethmoidal.

Mapping Malignancies of the Maxillary Sinus

The critical areas of neoplasms arising from the maxillary area include the posterior wall of the maxillary sinus, the infratemporal and pterygopalatine fossa, and the orbital floor. The main goal of imaging is to assess the integrity of the bony-periosteal barrier. It is well-known that MRI is less accurate than CT in the assessment of focal bone erosions, since the calcium content cannot be adequately detected by magnetic resonance techniques [27, 28]. Nevertheless, it is also known that the most effective barrier to spread of aggressive lesions beyond the sinusal walls is the periosteum, rather than the mineralized bony walls [29]. Therefore, in such cases, neoplastic spread beyond the periosteum is, in effect, the critical information needed for therapeutic planning because this pattern indicates extrasinusal infiltration (Fig. 6).

The thin sinusal walls appear hypointense in every MRI sequence because of the reduced water content of the cortical bone and periosteum. The entire thickness of the wall can be appreciated when invested by thickened mucosa or when the air on one/both side(s) has been replaced by mucous secretions or neoplastic tissue [30].

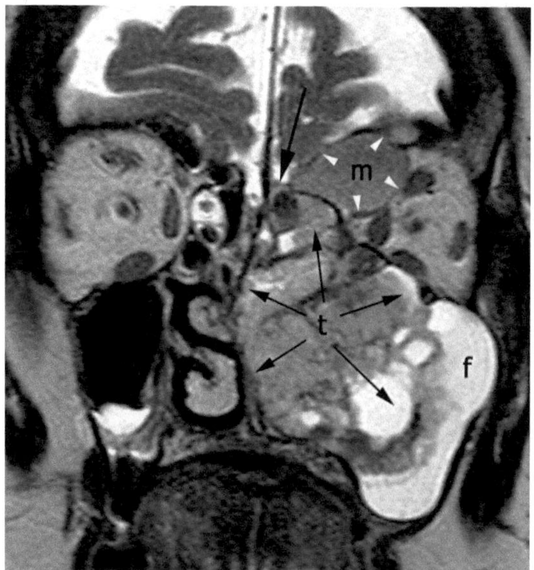

Fig. 6. Squamous cell carcinoma of left maxillary sinus. On MRI, the T2-weighted coronal sequence shows a solid mass (*t*) extending into the nasal fossa and the ethmoid. The inferior and medial orbital walls are remarkably displaced. A hypointense interface between tumor and intraorbital fat suggests that the periorbita still separates the two structures. A fronto-ethmoidal mucocele, secondary to the tumor, remodels and displaces the left orbital roof (*white arrowheads*). A second, small ethmoidal mucocele displaces the left cribriform plate (*long black arrow*). Fluid retention (*f*) within the maxillary sinus

The proper frequency encoding direction has to be selected in order to avoid the asymmetric appearance of cortical bone due to chemical shift artifacts [31].

Mapping Naso-ethmoidal Malignancies

In managing naso-ethmoidal neoplasm, the most critical areas include the orbit (particularly the roof and the posterior lamina papyracea, where most postoperative recurrences occur), the floor of the anterior cranial fossa (ACF), and the sphenoid sinus. It is a widely accepted notion that the orbit can be preserved at surgery, even when its bony walls are completely eroded, as long as the periorbita is not (or minimally) invaded. In fact, it has been demonstrated that a more aggressive approach does not improve survival [24].

Displacement and distortion of the orbital walls by ethmoid neoplasms occur frequently. The mineral content of the wall may be partially or completely eroded, leading to a questionable CT evaluation. On MRI, when a thin and regular hypointensity between neoplasm and orbital fat is still detectable on T2 images, the periorbita should be considered intact [25, 26] (Fig. 7). Although definitive assessment of the integrity of the periorbita is obtained in most cases intraoperatively, the information provided by MRI may be crucial for surgical planning. Furthermore, if imaging suggests orbital infiltration, the patient should be informed that an exenteratio orbitae may be required.

An assessment of the anterior cranial fossa floor invasion is also relevant for treatment planning.

Similar to invasion of the orbital wall, bone destruction at the skull base is better demonstrated by CT. However, at this level the imaging findings differ from those observed in other bone interfaces of the paranasal sinuses. This is due to the fact that when the skull base is invaded, the dura mater usually shows abnormal thickening and enhancement related either to neoplastic invasion or to an inflammatory, non-neoplastic reaction.

Since dural invasion implies a worse prognosis and a wider surgical resection, imaging should focus on precisely identifying the depth of skull base invasion [27, 28]. Here, MRI has been reported to be more accurate than CT. The key aspect is analysis of the MRI signal intensity of the structures located at the interface between the ethmoid roof (below) and brain (above): the cribriform plate and its double periosteal covering (lower layer), the dura mater (middle layer), the subarachnoid space (superior layer).

On enhanced sagittal and coronal SE T1 or 3D GE fat sat T1 (VIBE) sequences, the three layers constitute a "sandwich" of different signals (bone-periosteum complex, dura mater, CSF) [29]. When a sinonasal neoplasm abuts the cribrifom plate interface, without interrupting its hypointense signal, the lesion should be considered extracranial. Effacement of the hypointense signal of the lower layer by tumor implies bone-periosteum penetration. In this case, if an uninterrupted thickened and enhancing dura mater (middle layer) is seen, the neoplasm is graded as intracranial-extradural. Conversely, focal or more extensive replacement of enhanced thickened dura mater by tumor signal indicates intracranial-intradural invasion. Brain invasion is suspected in the presence of edema. Patients with limited brain invasion treated by craniofacial resection were reported to have a non-significant decrease in survival compared to those with dural invasion only.

Imaging of the Perineural Spread

Although the term "perineural spread" should be limited to tumor spreading along the perineurium that envelopes the nerve bundles, the term actually encompasses either

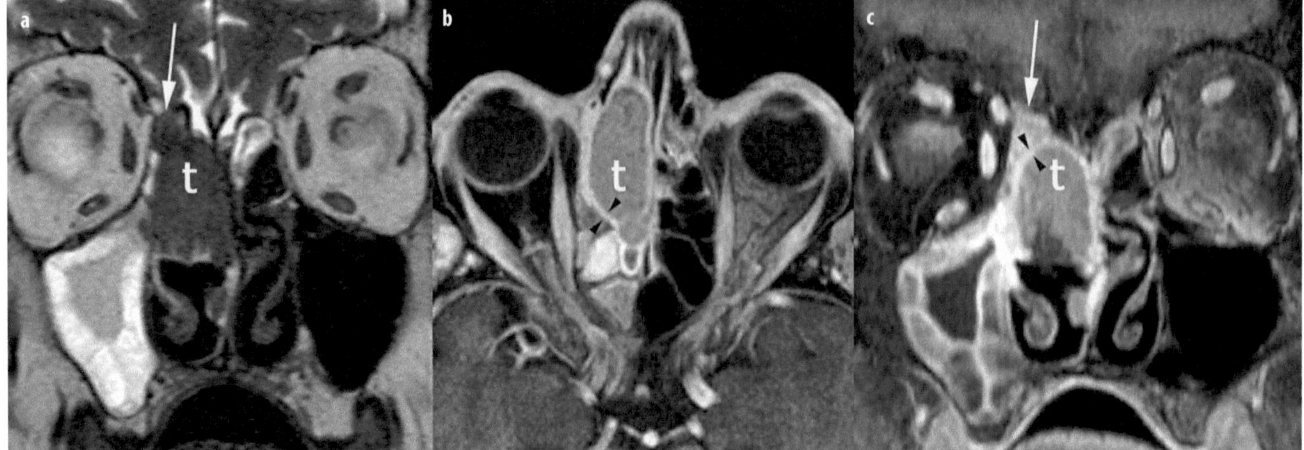

Fig. 7 a-c. Adenocarcinoma of right ethmoidal sinus. **a** In the T2-weighted coronal plane, the mass (*t*) occupies the right anterior ethmoid, abuts the cribriform plate, and possibly reaches the fovea ethmoidalis (*white arrow*). On the post-contrast GET1 fat-sat (VIBE) sequences in the axial (**b**) and coronal (**c**) planes, an enhancing peripheral rim (*arrowheads*) clearly separates the tumor (*t*) from the medial orbital wall. Note that the lesion is not in contact with the fovea ethmoidalis (*white arrow*)

neoplasms invading all compartments and their neural sheaths or tumor involving single compartments, such as the space between the epineurium and the nerve bundles, or single sheaths (mainly the perineurium). Nerve enhancement and nerve enlargement are more predictive of perineural spread.

Tumor growth induces an increased permeability of the endoneurial capillaries and, eventually, disruption of the perineurium. Rupture of the blood-nerve barrier allows leakage and accumulation of iodinated or paramagnetic contrast agents, resulting in segmental nerve enhancement on MRI. Accordingly, the detection of segmental nerve enhancement by MRI is more sensitive than by CT [30-33]. Several MRI techniques have been proposed, with or without fat-saturation. The use of high spatial resolution, post-contrast fat saturation VIBE (with isotropic voxels ranging from 0.5 to 0.7 mm) permits a detailed evaluation of the skull base foramina that is free of artifacts. The spatial resolution of this approach allows the normal nerve and the surrounding vascular plexus to be clearly imaged [1, 34].

Segmental nerve enhancement, however, is not unique to perineural spread. It may be present in several non-neoplastic lesions that result in blood-nerve barrier disruption, such as inflammation, ischemia, infarct, trauma, demyelination, and axonal degeneration. These conditions may account for false-positive results on MRI.

Moreover, for segments such as the V2, V3, XIIth, and inferior alveolar nerves crossing foramina/canals, the "target" or "tram-track-like" enhancement patterns are normally present and do not represent abnormal findings [35]. Conversely, if these enhancement patterns are demonstrated in the labyrinthine and/or mastoid segments of the facial nerve, disruption of the blood-nerve barrier should be suspected [36]. Abnormal enhancement of the central nerve on "target" or "tram-track-like" patterns without nerve enlargement has been correlated with minimal burden of perineural spread [37,38]. Further growth of tumor cells along the nerve gives rise to an increased nerve diameter (Fig. 8), which can be directly demonstrated on MRI, with or without abnormal nerve enhancement. Direct detection of an enlarged nerve is possible on CT, as long as the nerve is mainly surrounded by fat (i.e., the infraorbital nerve). Indirect signs at CT are widening and, eventually, erosion of bony fissures and foramina. The enlarged nerve may, however, recover its normal diameter as it runs along a bony canal, instead of remodeling or eroding the inner surface of the bone while skipping the tract. Once the nerve exits on the opposite side, perineural spread is once again macroscopic. This "resurfacing phenomenon" is a mechanism of perineural extension, which deserves particular attention on CT and MRI. It can be observed with tumors of the hard or soft palate that "resurface" into the pterygopalatine fossa.

Retrograde (central) spread may lead the tumor to Meckel's cave (through V2 or V3) and to the cavernous sinus. Replacement of fluid signal in Meckel's cave by solid enhancing tissue and bulging and enlargement of the cavernous sinus indicate neoplastic invasion. If an intravascular paramagnetic contrast agent is used and high-definition post-contrast GE sequences (VIBE) are acquired with a delay of about 2 min, the tumor can be better separated from the venous signal within the cavernous sinus. Furthermore, when perineural spread leads to damage of a motor branch of a cranial nerve, MRI can detect the changes in the denervated muscles during both the acute phase (hyperintensity in T2 images and abnormal enhancement) and the chronic phase (atrophy and fat replacement).

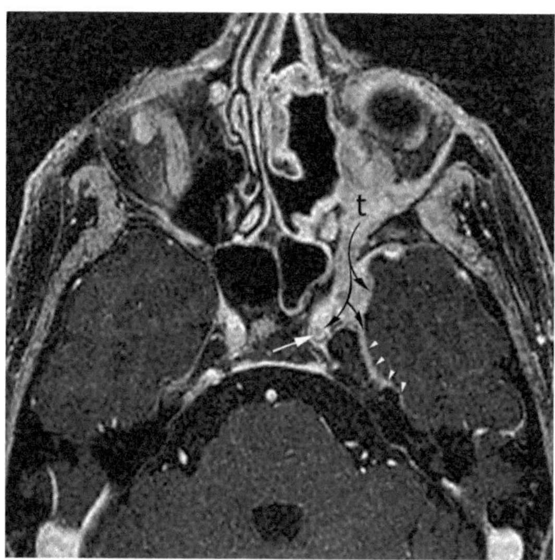

Fig. 8. Squamous cell carcinoma of the ethmoid invading the pterygopalatine fossa and orbital apex. Contrast-enhanced 3D GE T1 VIBE sequence, axial reconstruction (1-mm slice thickness). The tumor (*t*) grows along V2 (*curved arrows*) to reach posteriorly the internal carotid artery (*white arrow*). Subtle linear enhancement along the lateral surface of Meckel's cave and the anterior aspect of the petrous apex (*arrowheads*) confirms perineural tumor spread along the greater superficial petrosal nerve

Follow-up

During follow-up, the role of MRI is to detect asymptomatic extramucosal disease. The interpretation of post-treatment imaging studies may be quite challenging because of the anatomical and functional changes induced by treatment(s). These changes greatly reduce the morphological and signal differences between persistent/recurrent disease and the adjacent tissues. Tissue changes secondary to resection can be predicted based on the surgical report. As craniofacial resection is the surgical treatment of choice, thorough knowledge of the normal appearance after open or endoscopic or combined craniofacial resection is necessary. Since these surgical approaches are indicated because a portion of the skull base floor is invaded, recurrences are more frequently expected at the boundaries of the resection and reconstruction. Hence, the meningo-galeal complex, which replaces the anterior skull base floor, must be evaluated in detail. Both coronal and sagittal T2 and post-contrast non-fat-suppressed T1 images are indicated. Focal thickness changes and lost of the "multiple-layer aspect" of the meningo-galeal complex during follow-up are clues suggesting neoplastic recurrence. When a local or revascularized flap is used after orbital or maxillary resection, the regularity of the interface between the flap and the adjacent tissues must be assessed. Reactive mucosal changes resulting from radiation therapy or bone resection and subperiosteal dissection may be present and are difficult to separate from recurrent disease, especially during the early post-treatment phase [39]. In the late phase, progression towards a mature scar is suggested by hypointensity on T2 and the absence of enhancement [40, 41].

The difficulty in discriminating between post-treatment changes and residual/recurrent disease accounts for the growing interest in more sophisticated ways to examine tissues. Dynamic contrast-enhanced MRI exploits the vascularization and permeability of the endothelium of neoplastic microvessels [42, 43]. Diffusion-weighted imaging studies the diffusion motion of water protons in the tissues. With this technique, signal is related to the freedom of water molecules to move within intercellular spaces. This movement can be taken advantage of to distinguish highly cellular tissues (tumor), in which the movement of water molecules is restricted, from inflammatory changes [44-46]. PET/CT may demonstrate the increased glucidic metabolism of neoplastic tissues.

While all of the above-mentioned techniques are promising, none of them are currently used routinely as part of standardized follow-up protocols.

References

1. Maroldi R, Nicolai P (2005) Imaging in treatment planning for sinonasal diseases, Springer, Berlin-New York
2. Nicolai P, Castelnuovo P, Lombardi D et al (2007) Role of endoscopic surgery in the management of selected malignant epithelial neoplasms of the naso-ethmoidal complex. Head Neck 29:1075-1082
3. Landsberg R, Friedman M (2001) A computer-assisted anatomical study of the nasofrontal region. Laryngoscope 111:2125-2130
4. Phillips CD (1997) Current status and new developments in techniques for imaging the nose and sinuses. Otolaryngol Clin North Am 30:371-387
5. Hahnel S, Ertl-Wagner B, Tasman AJ et al (1999) Relative value of MR imaging as compared with CT in the diagnosis of inflammatory paranasal sinus disease. Radiology 210:171-176
6. Younis RT, Lazar RH, Bustillo A, Anand VK (2002) Orbital infection as a complication of sinusitis: are diagnostic and treatment trends changing? Ear Nose Throat J 81:771-775
7. Lerner DN, Choi SS, Zalzal GH, Johnson DL (1995) Intracranial complications of sinusitis in childhood. Ann Otol Rhinol Laryngol 104:288-293
8. Rao VM, Sharma D, Madan A (2001) Imaging of frontal sinus disease: concepts, interpretation, and technology. Otolaryngol Clin North Am 34:23-39
9. Hagtvedt T, Aalokken TM, Notthellen J, Kolbenstvedt A (2003) A new low-dose CT examination compared with standard-dose CT in the diagnosis of acute sinusitis. Eur Radiol 13:976-980
10. Sohaib SA, Peppercorn PD, Horrocks JA et al (2001) The effect of decreasing mAs on image quality and patient dose in sinus CT. Br J Radiol 74:157-161
11. Sonkens JW, Harnsberger HR, Blanch GM et al (1991) The impact of screening sinus CT on the planning of functional endoscopic sinus surgery. Otolaryngol Head Neck Surg 105:802-813
12. Giacchi RJ, Lebowitz RA, Yee HT et al (2001) Histopathologic evaluation of the ethmoid bone in chronic sinusitis. Am J Rhinol 15:193-197
13. De Vuysere S, Hermans R, Marchal G (2001) Sinochoanal polyp and its variant, the angiomatous polyp: MRI findings. Eur Radiol 11:55-58
14. Scuderi AJ, Babbel RW, Harnsberger HR, Sonkens JW (1991) The sporadic pattern of inflammatory sinonasal disease including postsurgical changes. Semin Ultrasound CT MR 12:575-591
15. deShazo RD, O'Brien M, Chapin K et al (1997) A new classification and diagnostic criteria for invasive fungal sinusitis. Arch Otolaryngol Head Neck Surg 123:1181-1188
16. Ponikau JU, Sherris DA, Kern EB et al (1999) The diagnosis and incidence of allergic fungal sinusitis. Mayo Clin Proc 74:877-884
17. Aribandi M, Bazan C 3rd (2007) CT and MRI features in Bipolaris fungal sinusitis. Australas Radiol 51:127-132
18. Mukherji SK, Figueroa RE, Ginsberg LE et al (1998) Allergic fungal sinusitis: CT findings. Radiology 207:417-422
19. Howells RC, Ramadan HH (2001) Usefulness of computed tomography and magnetic resonance in fulminant invasive fungal rhinosinusitis. Am J Rhinol 15:255-261
20. Muhle C, Reinhold-Keller E, Richter C et al (1997) MRI of the nasal cavity, the paranasal sinuses and orbits in Wegener's granulomatosis. Eur Radiol 7:566-570
21. Trimarchi M, Gregorini G, Facchetti F et al (2001) Cocaine-induced midline destructive lesions: clinical, radiographic, histopathologic, and serologic features and their differentiation from Wegener granulomatosis. Medicine (Baltimore) 80:391-404
22. Keni SP, Wiley EL, Dutra JC et al (2005) Skull base Wegener's granulomatosis resulting in multiple cranial neuropathies. Am J Otolaryngol 26:146-149
23. Marsot-Dupuch K, De Givry SC, Ouayoun M (2002) Wegener granulomatosis involving the pterygopalatine fossa: an unusual case of trigeminal neuropathy. AJNR Am J Neuroradiol 23:312-315
24. Perry C, Levine PA, Williamson BR, Cantrell RW (1988) Preservation of the eye in paranasal sinus cancer surgery. Arch Otolaryngol Head Neck Surg 114:632-634
25. Kim HJ, Lee TH, Lee HS et al (2006) Periorbita: computed tomography and magnetic resonance imaging findings. Am J Rhinol 20:371-374
26. Curtin HD, Rabinov JD (1998) Extension to the orbit from paraorbital disease. The sinuses. Radiol Clin North Am 36:1201-1213
27. Kraus DH, Lanzieri CF, Wanamaker JR et al (1992) Complementary use of computed tomography and magnetic resonance imaging in assessing skull base lesions. Laryngoscope 102:623-629
28. Shah JP, Kraus DH, Bilsky MH et al (1997) Craniofacial resection for malignant tumors involving the anterior skull base. Arch Otolaryngol Head Neck Surg 123:1312-1317
29. Ishida H, Mohri M, Amatsu M (2002) Invasion of the skull base by carcinomas: histopathologically evidenced findings with CT and MRI. Eur Arch Otorhinolaryngol 259:535-539
30. Hanna E, Vural E, Prokopakis E et al (2007) The sensitivity and specificity of high-resolution imaging in evaluating perineural spread of adenoid cystic carcinoma to the skull base. Arch Otolaryngol Head Neck Surg 133:541-545

31. Chang PC, Fischbein NJ, McCalmont TH et al (2004) Perineural spread of malignant melanoma of the head and neck: clinical and imaging features. AJNR Am J Neuroradiol 25:5-11
32. Caldemeyer KS, Mathews VP, Righi PD, Smith RR (1998) Imaging features and clinical significance of perineural spread or extension of head and neck tumors. Radiographics 18:97-110
33. Ginsberg LE, DeMonte F (1998) Imaging of perineural tumor spread from palatal carcinoma. AJNR Am J Neuroradiol 19:1417-1422
34. Maroldi R, Ambrosi C, Farina D (2005) Metastatic disease of the brain: extra-axial metastases (skull, dura, leptomeningeal) and tumour spread. Eur Radiol 15:617-626
35. Williams LS, Schmalfuss IM, Sistrom CL et al (2003) MR imaging of the trigeminal ganglion, nerve, and the perineural vascular plexus: normal appearance and variants with correlation to cadaver specimens. AJNR Am J Neuroradiol 24:1317-1323
36. Martin-Duverneuil N, Sola-Martinez MT, Miaux Y et al (1997) Contrast enhancement of the facial nerve on MRI: normal or pathological? Neuroradiology 39:207-212
37. Williams LS (1999) Advanced concepts in the imaging of perineural spread of tumor to the trigeminal nerve. Top Magn Reson Imaging 10:376-383
38. Williams LS, Mancuso AA, Mendenhall WM (2001) Perineural spread of cutaneous squamous and basal cell carcinoma: CT and MR detection and its impact on patient management and prognosis. Int J Radiat Oncol Biol Phys 49:1061-1069
39. Loevner LA, Sonners AI (2002) Imaging of neoplasms of the paranasal sinuses. Magn Reson Imaging Clin N Am 10:467-493
40. Gong QY, Zheng GL, Zhu HY (1991) MRI differentiation of recurrent nasopharyngeal carcinoma from postradiation fibrosis. Comput Med Imaging Graph 15:423-429
41. Lell M, Baum U, Greess H et al (2000) Head and neck tumors: imaging recurrent tumor and post-therapeutic changes with CT and MRI. Eur J Radiol 33:239-247
42. Fischbein NJ, Noworolski SM, Henry RG et al (2003) Assessment of metastatic cervical adenopathy using dynamic contrast-enhanced MR imaging. AJNR Am J Neuroradiol 24:301-311
43. Shah GV, Fischbein NJ, Gandhi D, Mukherji SK (2004) Dynamic contrast-enhanced MR imaging. Top Magn Reson Imaging 15:71-77
44. White ML, Zhang Y, Robinson RA (2006) Evaluating tumors and tumorlike lesions of the nasal cavity, the paranasal sinuses, and the adjacent skull base with diffusion-weighted MRI. J Comput Assist Tomogr 30:490-495
45. Hermans R, Vandecaveye V (2007) Diffusion-weighted MRI in head and neck cancer. Cancer Imaging 7:126-127
46. Vandecaveye V, De Keyzer F, Nuyts S et al (2007) Detection of head and neck squamous cell carcinoma with diffusion weighted MRI after (chemo)radiotherapy: correlation between radiologic and histopathologic findings. Int J Radiat Oncol Biol Phys 67:960-971

Lumbar Degenerative Disc Disease

Michael T. Modic[1], Sean Symons[2]

[1] Division of Radiology, Lerner College of Medicine, Cleveland, OH, USA

[2] Department of Medical Imaging, Sunnybrook Healt Sciences Centre, Toronto, ON, Canada

The sequelae of disc degeneration remain among the leading causes of functional incapacity in both men and women and are a common source of chronic disability in the working years. A significant portion of the cost of the morbidity associated with neck and back disorders is related to diagnostic testing, mostly medical imaging, the results of which may rightly or wrongly provide the basis for subsequent, more invasive treatments.

Traditionally, disc degeneration has been linked to mechanical loading, which brings about structural disruption and cell-mediated changes in disc composition – but which occurs first is not clear. Biochemical factors can increase the susceptibility to mechanical disruption and this could adversely influence disc cell metabolism. Regardless of the initiating mechanism, the contributing factors are interactive and additive, with the end result being an altered functional ability of the disc to resist applied forces. In addition to mechanical and nutritional causes, a genetic predisposition for degenerative disease has also been suggested by both animal models and human studies [1-3].

Abnormalities of collagen are most often cited to support a genetic influence in degenerative disc disease. Type II collagen is the most abundant collagen of cartilaginous tissues and is often referred to as the "major" collagen, forming heterotypic fibrils with the less abundant "minor" collagens, IX and XI. These fibrils provide the strength necessary to resist tensile forces. Disease causing mutations in types II and XI collagen have been demonstrated in a number of chondrodystrophies. In a study looking for additional disease-producing mutations, amino acid substitutions were identified that are significantly more prevalent in patients with lumbar degenerative disc disease than in normal controls [2, 4].

Several other studies suggested that not just the process of degenerative disc disease but perhaps even its sequelae, including disc herniation, low back pain and radiculopathy, are strongly influenced by genetic factors [5-8]. Clearly, there are many interactive factors – mechanical, traumatic, nutritional, and genetic – all of which may play a role in the cascade of disc degeneration, albeit to variable degrees in different individuals. Whatever the etiology, by the age of 50 years, 85-95% of adults show evidence of degenerative disc disease at autopsy [9].

Morphologic Alterations and Imaging

No less a problem than understanding the etiology of disc degeneration is agreeing on a terminology to reliably and reproducibly describe the morphologic alterations produced by the degenerative process [10-13]. For the purposes of this review, we have used the terminology proposed by Millette et al. [14]. While there is confusion in differentiating between pathological degenerative processes in the disc and those of normal aging, here the term "degenerative" includes all such changes [15-17].

The manner of degeneration of the various components of the spine is mediated and manifested by the specific structure involved. Cartilaginous, synovial, and fibrous structures each degenerate in a specific manner, which is associated with characteristic pathologic and thus imaging aberrations.

The major cartilaginous joint of the vertebral column is the intervertebral disc. Each disc consists of an inner portion, the nucleus pulposus, surrounded by a peripheral portion, the annulus fibrosus. The nucleus pulposus is eccentrically located, more closely related to the posterior surface of the intervertebral disc. With degeneration and aging, the amount of type II collagen increases outwardly in the annulus and there is greater water loss from the nucleus pulposus than from the annulus. This results in a loss of the hydrostatic properties of the disc, with an overall reduction of hydration in both areas to about 70%. In addition to water and collagen, the other important biochemical constituents of the intervertebral disc are proteoglycans. The individual chemical structures of the proteoglycans do not change with degeneration, but their relative composition does. The decrease in water-binding capacity of the nucleus pulposus is thought to be related to the decreased molecular weight of its nuclear proteoglycan complexes (aggregates). The disc becomes progressively more fibrous and disorganized, with the end stage represented by amorphous fibrocartilage and no clear distinction between nucleus and annulus [18, 19]. On T2-weighted images, the signal intensity of the central disc is usually markedly decreased and at distinct variance to that seen in unaffected discs of the same individual. Studies using T2-weighed spin-echo sequences

[20] suggested that magnetic resonance imaging (MRI) is capable of detecting changes in the nucleus pulposus and annulus fibrosus relative to degeneration and aging. This ability is based on a loss of signal presumed to be secondary to known changes of hydration that occur within the intervertebral disc. In work with cadaver spines of various ages, absolute T2 measurements correlated more closely with glycosaminoglycan (GAG) concentration than with absolute water content [21]. Thus, the signal may not be related to the total amount of water but rather to the state of the water.

Conventional theory would imply that degeneration and aging are very similar processes, albeit occurring at different rates. It has been proposed that annular disruption is the critical factor in degeneration; when a radial tear develops in the annulus, there is shrinkage, accompanied by disorganization of the fibrous cartilage of the nucleus pulposus, and replacement of the disc by dense fibrous tissue with cystic spaces [17-19, 22, 23]. The terms "tear" and "fissure" describe the spectrum of such lesions without implying that the lesion is consequent to trauma. Although it has certainly been verified that annular disruption is a sequela of degeneration, and that the two are often associated, its role as the causal agent of disc degeneration has not been proved definitively.

With loss of water and proteoglycans, the nucleus pulposus becomes desiccated and friable, with yellow-brown discoloration. Radiolucent collections representing gas, principally nitrogen, occur at sites of negative pressure produced by the abnormal spaces [24]. Progression of intervertebral (osteo)chondrosis may lead to calcification of the disc. Calcification has usually been described on MRI as a region of decreased or absent signal. There is, however, variability of signal intensity of calcium on various sequences; and the type and concentration of calcification are probably important factors Hyperintense discs on T1-weighted images may be secondary to calcification.

The relationship among the vertebral body, endplate, annulus, and disc has been studied [25-28] using degenerated and chymopapain-treated discs as models. Signal intensity changes in the vertebral body marrow adjacent to the endplates of degenerated discs are a common observation on MRI and seem to take one of three main forms. Type I changes are characterized by decreased signal intensity on T1-weighted images and increased signal on T2-weighted images. They have been identified in approximately 4% of patients scanned for lumbar disease. Histopathologic sections of discs with type I changes show disruption and fissuring of the endplate and vascularized fibrous tissues within the adjacent marrow, prolonging T1 and T2. Mild enhancement of type I changes in the vertebral body marrow is seen with Gd-DTPA and at times extends to involve the disc itself, presumably due to the vascularized fibrous tissue within adjacent marrow. Type II changes are represented by increased signal on T1-weighted images and isointense or slightly hyperintense signal on T2-weighted images. They have been identified in approximately 16% of patients studied by MRI. Discs with type II changes also show evidence of endplate disruption, with yellow (lipid) marrow replacement in the adjacent vertebral body resulting in a shorter T1. Type III changes are represented by a decreased signal intensity on both T1- and T2-weighted images that appears to correlate with extensive bony sclerosis on plain radiographs. Similar marrow changes have been noted in the pedicles. While originally described as being associated with spondylolysis, such changes have also been noted in patients with degenerative facet disease and pedicle fractures. Again, the changes are probably a reflection of abnormal stresses, be they loading or motion [29].

Like all diarthrodial synovium-lined joints, the lumbar facet joints are predisposed to arthropathies, with alterations of the articular cartilage. Disc degeneration and loss of disc space height place increased stresses on the facet joints, with craniocaudal subluxation resulting in arthrosis and osteophytosis. The superior articular facet is usually more significantly involved. It has been proposed that facet arthrosis occurs independently and is a source of symptoms on its own [30, 31].

The important ligaments of the spine include the anterior longitudinal ligament, the posterior longitudinal ligament, the paired sets of ligamenta flava (connecting the laminae of adjacent vertebrae), the intertransverse ligaments (extending between the transverse processes), and the unpaired supraspinous ligament (along the tips of the spinous processes). As these ligaments normally provide stability, any alteration in the vertebral articulations can lead to ligamentous laxity and subsequent deterioration. Loss of elastic tissue, calcification and ossification, and bone proliferation at sites of ligamentous attachment to bone are recognized manifestations of such degeneration.

Common, potential complications of degenerative disc disease include alignment abnormalities, intervertebral disc displacement, and spinal stenosis. The various types of alignment abnormalities can exist alone or in combination, but the two most frequent are segmental instability and spondylolisthesis.

Herniation refers to localized displacement of the nucleus, cartilage, fragmented apophyseal bone, or fragmented annular tissue beyond the intervertebral disc space. The disc space is defined rostrally and caudally by the vertebral body endplates and, peripherally, by the outer edges of the vertebral ring apophyses, exclusive of osteophytic formations. The term "localized" contrasts with "generalized", the latter being arbitrarily defined as >50% (180°) of the periphery of the disc [14]. Since details of the integrity of the annulus are often unknown, herniation is usually distinguished by the observation of "localized" displacement of disc material beyond the edges of the ring apophyses, meaning <50% (180°) of the circumference of the disc.

Localized displacement in the axial (horizontal) plane can be "focal", signifying <25% of the disc circumference, or "broad-based", meaning between 25 and 50% of the disc circumference. The presence of disc tissue "circumferentially" (50-100%) beyond the edges of the ring apophyses may be called "bulging" and is not considered a form of herniation. A disc may have more than one herniation. The term "herniated disc" does not imply any knowledge of etiology, relation to symptoms, prognosis, or need for treatment.

When images are sufficient to make the distinction, a herniated disc may be more specifically characterized as "protruded" or "extruded". These distinctions are based upon the shape of the displaced material. Protrusion is present if the greatest distance, in any plane, between the edges of the disc material beyond the disc space is less than the distance between the edges of the base in the same plane. Extrusion is present when, in at least one plane, any one distance between the edges of the disc material beyond the disc space is greater than the distance between the edges of the base in the same plane, or when no continuity exists between the disc material beyond the disc space and that within the disc space. Extrusion may be further specified as a sequestration. Herniated discs in the craniocaudal (vertical) direction through a break in the vertebral body endplate are referred to as intravertebral herniations.

Spinal stenosis was defined in 1975 as any type of narrowing of the spinal canal, nerve root canals, or intervertebral foramina [32]. Two broad groups have been defined, acquired (usually related to degenerative changes) and congenital or developmental. In the acquired type, there has been no association documented between the severity of pain and the degree of stenosis. The imaging changes are generally more extensive than expected from the clinical findings [33]. While there does appear to be a correlation between cross-sectional area and mid-sagittal measurements in patients with symptomatic spinal stenosis, absolute values and correlations between measurements and symptoms are lacking. Unfortunately, there does not appear to be reliable prognostic imaging findings that would correlate with surgical success or even whether patients would benefit from surgery [34].

Symptoms

The etiology of symptoms in patients with degenerative disc disease is diverse The symptom complexes are more often characterized by variability and change rather than predictability and stability. The most common symptom is pain. Anatomic areas of the spine can serve as sites of pain generation through intrinsic or acquired innervation, the latter as a product of soft-tissue repair. Mechanisms, often acting in combination, include: (1) instability with associated disc degeneration, facet hypertrophic, and arthopathy; (2) mechanical compression of nerves by bone, ligament, or disc material; and (3) biochemical mediators of inflammation/pain.

It is important to reemphasize that disc degeneration per se is not painful and, in fact, has a very high prevalence in the asymptomatic population. In addition, the finding of degenerative disc disease by imaging does not predict subsequent symptom development over time [35].

Mechanical compression/deformity of the nerve roots as a cause of pain or nerve dysfunction is the classic working concept, related to displacement and effacement of neural tissue by disc herniation; it dates to the observation of Mixter and Barr [36]. Nerve fibers have been identified in the outer third of the annulus in the normal state, but may extend into the inner annulus and nucleus pulposus, accompanied by blood vessels, in patients with chronic back pain [37].

The concept of neural compression by itself is inadequate to explain part or all of many symptom complexes.

The perplexing clinical scenario of patients who complain of incapacitating back pain but have no overt morphologic abnormality has given rise to the concept of the disc as a pain generator [38]. This was classically described by Crock [39] as "chronic internal disc disruption syndrome" (IDDS).

The concept of disc tissue producing an inflammatory response is not new, but has become more sophisticated and targeted with the application of monoclonal antibody technology and other assay techniques [40]. "Chemical radiculitis" was thought to be related to the suggestion that the nuclear material and its glycoproteins are strong irritants of nerve tissue. As a manifestation of this inflammatory response, higher systemic plasma levels of C-reactive protein have been measured in patients with sciatica vs. healthy controls [41].

Disc cells are also capable of expressing pro-inflammatory substances, such as tumor necrosis factor α (TNF-α), which can produce radicular morphologic abnormalities similar to those seen with nucleus pulposus application [42]. Olmarker [43] showed that inhibition of TNF-α prevented thrombus formation and intraneural edema, and reduced nerve conduction velocity. This set the stage for an open-label trial of anti-TNF therapy in sciatic patients [44-46]. Infliximab (Remicade, Centocor) (a chimeric monoclonal human/mouse antibody) inhibits TNF-α-induced infiltration of leukocytes to the site of injury. A single infusion of infliximab produced a rapid beneficial effect on pain, which persisted over one year following a dose of 3 mg/kg.

Sensory and motor deficits appear to be the result of a combination of mechanical deformation and the presence of inflammatory agents. Clearly, the etiology of pain in degenerative disease is much more complex than suggested by a simple mechanical explanation. Investigation of these other factors will hopefully bring a greater understanding of the relationship between morphologic alteration and clinical symptoms.

Significance of Imaging Findings

The role of an imaging is to provide accurate morphologic information that will, in turn, influence therapeutic decision making [47]. A necessary component is accurate data on the natural history of the pathology.

Disc herniations can be demonstrated in 20-28% of asymptomatic patients and the majority have evidence of additional degenerative disc disease [48-50]. Degenerative disc space narrowing, facet disease, and stenosis tend to slowly progress over time. Eventual stabilization of the three-joint discovertebral complex is thought to be part of the evolution of degenerative disease and is assumed to be accompanied by a decrease in pain. In a study of symptomatic patients, the prevalence of disc herniations in patients with low back pain and radiculopathy at presentation was similar. There was a higher prevalence of herniations (57% in the low back pain and 65% in the radiculopathy group) than the 20-28% reported in the asymptomatic series. In general, one-third of patients with disc herniations at presentation showed significant resolution or disappearance of symptoms by 6 weeks and two-thirds by 6 months [51, 52]. The type, size, and location of herniation at presentation and changes in herniation size and type over time did not correlate with outcome. In fact, the presence of a herniation on MRI was a positive prognostic finding.

Interestingly, not only do discs have a tendency to regress, but 13% of patients in a symptomatic series developed new or larger disc herniations over time. In a study of patients with low back pain or radiculopathy, MRI did not have additive value over clinical assessment. This lack of prognostic value also appears to apply to the conservative management of spinal stenosis. There are no reliable prognostic imaging findings that would correlate with surgical success or even indicate whether patients would benefit from surgery and spinal stenosis [34].

The clinical significance of marrow changes associated with degenerative disc disease remains unclear. Type I changes seem to be associated with a higher prevalence of active low back symptoms. The exact etiologic mechanism or mechanisms, while unknown, are thought to be related to some unusual stresses, micro- or macroinstabilility, or microtrauma. Surgical studies have suggested that patients with type I marrow changes who undergo fusion for low back pain do better than those without endplate changes or type II patterns [53-55]. The presumption is that type I changes are related to or are an indicator of some degree of instability. In a surgical study that examined the prognostic value of type I marrow changes related to surgical outcome, the authors demonstrated that persistence of type I marrow changes following fusion was associated with significantly worse outcome [55].

Degeneration of the intervertebral disc complex begins early in life and is a consequence of a variety of genetic, physiologic, and environmental factors as well as normal aging. Given the ubiquitous nature of the process and its high prevalence in both symptomatic and asymptomatic individuals, the leap from identifying an anatomic derangement to proposing a symptom complex must be made with caution [56]. Thus, there is a unique opportunity for imaging to further our understanding of degeneration.

What separates individuals with dramatic morphologic findings who have no symptoms from individuals with identical alterations who are symptomatic? Understanding the relationship of etiologic factors, the morphologic alterations which can be characterized by imaging, the mechanisms of pain production, and their interactions in the production of symptoms will require more accurate and reproducible stratification of patient cohorts. This may be a strong suit of imaging, i.e., the phenotyping of morphologic alterations which can be compared to results of emerging genotyping work relative to etiology and clinical manifestations. The ultimate translational goal is the integration of this information into the therapeutic decision-making process.

References

1. Hestbaek L, Iachine IA, Leboeuf-Yde C et al (2004) Heredity of low back pain in a young population: a classical twin study. Twin Res 7:16-26
2. Marini JC (2001) Genetic risk factors for lumbar disk disease. JAMA 285:1886-1888
3. Modic M (2007) Degenerative disc disease: genotyping, MR imaging and phenotyping. Skeletal Radiol 36:91-93
4. Annunen S, Paassilta P, Lohiniva J et al (1999) An allele of COL9A2 associated with intervertebral disc disease. Science 285:409-412
5. Nelson CL, Janecki CJ, Gildenberg PL, Sava G (1972) Disk protrusions in the young. Clin Orthop Relat Res 88:142-150
6. Varlotta GP, Brown MD, Kelsey JL, Golden AL (1991) Familial predisposition for herniation of a lumbar disc in patients who are less than twenty-one years old. J Bone Joint Surg Am 73:124-128
7. Matsui H, Terahata N, Tsuji H et al (1992) Familial predisposition and clustering for juvenile lumbar disc herniation. Spine 17:1323-1328
8. Scapinelli R (1993) Lumbar disc herniation in eight siblings with a positive family history for disc disease. Acta Orthop Belg 59:371-376
9. Quinet RJ, Hadler NM (1979) Diagnosis and treatment of backache. Semin Arthritis Rheum 8:261-287
10. Bonneville JF, Dietemann JL (1992) Imaging in sciatica. Rev Prat 42:554-566
11. Brant-Zawadzki MN, Jensen MC, Obuchowski N, Ross JS, Modic MT (1995) Interobserver and intraobserver variability in interpretation of lumbar disc abnormalities. A comparison of two nomenclatures. Spine 20:1257-1263
12. Breton G (1991) Is that a bulging disk, a small herniation or a moderate protrusion? Can Assoc Radiol J 42:318
13. Fardon DF, Balderston RA, Garfin SR et al (1991) Disorders of the spine, a coding system for diagnoses. Hanley and Belfus, Philadelphia, pp 20-22
14. Milette PC (2001) Reporting lumbar disk abnormalities: at last, consensus! AJNR Am J Neuroradiol 22:428-429
15. Czervionke LF (1993) Lumbar intervertebral disc disease. Neuroimaging Clin N Am 3:465-485
16. Modic MT, Herfkens RJ (1990) Intervertebral disk: normal age-related changes in MR signal intensity. Radiology 177:332-333
17. Sether LA, Yu S, Haughton VM, Fischer ME (1990) Intervertebral disk: normal age-related changes in MR signal intensity. Radiology 177:385-388
18. Yu S, Haughton VM, Sether LA et al (1989) Criteria for classifying normal and degenerated lumbar intervertebral disks. Radiology 170:523-526
19. Friberg S, Hirsch C (1949) Anatomical and clinical studies on lumbar disc degeneration. Acta Orthop Scand 19:222-242

20. Modic MT, Pavlicek W, Weinstein MA et al (1984) Magnetic resonance imaging of intervertebral disk disease. Clinical and pulse sequence considerations. Radiology 152:103-111
21. Majors AW, McDevitt CA, Silgalis I, Modic MT (1994) A correlative analysis of T2, ADC and MT radio with water, hydroxyproline and GAG content in excised human intervertebral disk. Orthopedic Research Society, New Orleans, pp 116-120
22. Hirsch C (1959) Studies on the pathology of low back pain. J Bone Joint Surg Br 41-B:237-243
23. Coventry MB (1969) Anatomy of the intervertebral disk. Clin Orthop Relat Res 67:9-15B
24. Knutsson F (1942) The vacuum phenomenon in the intervertebral discs. Acta Radiol 23:173-179
25. Bangert BA, Modic MT, Ross JS et al (1995) Hyperintense disks on T1-weighted MR images: correlation with calcification. Radiology 195:437-443
26. de Roos A, Kressel H, Spritzer C, Dalinka M (1987) MR imaging of marrow changes adjacent to end plates in degenerative lumbar disk disease. AJR Am J Roentgenol 149:531-534
27. Masaryk TJ, Boumphrey F, Modic MT et al (1986) Effects of chemonucleolysis demonstrated by MR imaging. J Comput Assist Tomogr 10:917-923
28. Modic MT, Steinberg PM, Ross JS et al (1988) Degenerative disk disease: assessment of changes in vertebral body marrow with MR imaging. Radiology 166:193-199
29. Modic MT (2007) Modic type 1 and type 2 changes (editorial). J Neurosurg Spine 6:150-151
30. Harris RI, Macnab I (1954) Structural changes in the lumbar intervertebral discs; their relationship to low back pain and sciatica. J Bone Joint Surg Br 36-B:304-322
31. Schellinger D, Wener L, Ragsdale BD, Patronas NJ (1987) Facet joint disorders and their role in the production of back pain and sciatica. Radiographics 7:923-944
32. Arnoldi CC, Brodsky AE, Cauchoix J et al (1976) Lumbar spinal stenosis and nerve root entrapment syndromes. Definition and classification. Clin Orthop Relat Res 115:4-5
33. Amundsen T, Weber H, Lilleas F et al (1995) Lumbar spinal stenosis. Clinical and radiologic features. Spine 20:1178-1186
34. ECRI (2001) Treatment of degenerative lumbar spinal stenosis. Volume 1: Evidence report. AHRQ Publication No. 01-E048 32
35. Borenstein DG, O'Mara JW Jr., Boden SD et al (2001) The value of magnetic resonance imaging of the lumbar spine to predict low-back pain in asymptomatic subjects: a seven-year follow-up study. J Bone Joint Surg Am 83-A:1306-1311
36. Mixter W, Barr JS (1934) Rupture of the intervertebral disc with involvement of the spinal canal. N Engl J Med 211:210-214
37. Freemont AJ, Peacock TE, Goupille P et al (1997) Nerve ingrowth into diseased intervertebral disc in chronic back pain. Lancet 350:178-181
38. Von Korff M, Saunders K (1996) The course of back pain in primary care. Spine 21:2833-2837
39. Crock HV (1986) The presidential address: ISSLS, internal disc disruption, a challenge to disc prolapse fifty years on. Spine 11:650-653
40. Marshall LL, Trethewie ER, Curtain CC (1977) Chemical radiculitis. A clinical, physiological and immunological study. Clin Orthop Relat Res 129:61-67
41. Lee G (2000) Systemic inflammatory response with plasma C-reactive protein elevation in disk-related lumbosciatic syndrome. Joint Bone Spine 67:452-455
42. Igarashi T, Kikuchi S, Shubayev V, Myers RR (2000) Volvo Award winner in basic science studies: exogenous tumor necrosis factor-alpha mimics nucleus pulposus-induced neuropathology. Molecular, histologic, and behavioral comparisons in rats. Spine 25:2975-2980
43. Olmarker K, Rydevik B (2001) Selective inhibition of tumor necrosis factor-alpha prevents nucleus pulposus-induced thrombus formation, intraneural edema, and reduction of nerve conduction velocity: possible implications for future pharmacologic treatment strategies of sciatica. Spine 26:863-869
44. Genevay S, Stingelin S, Gabay C (2004) Efficacy of etanercept in the treatment of acute, severe sciatica: a pilot study. Ann Rheum Dis 63:1120-1123
45. Karppinen J, Korhonen T, Malmivaara A et al (2003) Tumor necrosis factor-alpha monoclonal antibody, infliximab, used to manage severe sciatica. Spine 28:750-753
46. Korhonen T, Karppinen J, Malmivaara A et al (2004) Efficacy of infliximab for disc herniation-induced sciatica: one-year follow-up. Spine 29:2115-2119
47. Sox H, Stern S, Owens D, Abrams HL (1989) Assessment of diagnostic technology in health care. Rationale, methods, problems and directions. National Academy Press, Washington DC
48. Wiesel SW, Tsourmas N, Feffer HL et al (1984) A study of computer-assisted tomography. I. The incidence of positive CAT scans in an asymptomatic group of patients. Spine 9:549-551
49. Boden SD, Davis DO, Dina TS et al (1990) Abnormal magnetic-resonance scans of the lumbar spine in asymptomatic subjects. A prospective investigation. J Bone Joint Surg Am 72:403-408
50. Jensen MC, Brant-Zawadzki MN, Obuchowski N et al (1994) Magnetic resonance imaging of the lumbar spine in people without back pain. N Engl J Med 331:69-73
51. Modic MT, Ross JS, Obuchowski NA et al (1995) Contrast-enhanced MR imaging in acute lumbar radiculopathy: a pilot study of the natural history. Radiology 195:429-435
52. Modic MT, Obuchowski NA, Ross JS et al (2005) Acute low back pain and radiculopathy: MR imaging findings and their prognostic role and effect on outcome. Radiology. 237:597-604
53. Vital JM, Gille O, Pointillart V et al (2003) Course of Modic 1 six months after lumbar posterior osteosynthesis. Spine 28:715-720
54. Braithwaite I, White J, Saifuddin A et al (1998) Vetebral endplate (Modic) changes on lumbar spine MRI: correlation with pain reproduction at lumbar discography. Eur Spine J 7 363-368
55. Buttermann GR, Heithoff KB, Ogilvie JW et al (1997) Vertebral body MRI related to lumbar fusion results. Eur Spine J 6:115-120
56. White AA 3rd, Gordon SL (1982) Synopsis: workshop on idiopathic low-back pain. Spine 7:141-149

Acute Spinal Trauma

Pia C. Sundgren[1], Adam E. Flanders[2]

[1] Department of Radiology, University of Michigan Health Systems, Ann Arbor, MI, USA
[2] Department of Radiology, Thomas Jefferson University Hospital, Philadelphia, PA, USA

Introduction

Injuries to the spinal column and the spinal cord are a major cause of disability, affecting predominately (60%) affecting young healthy males between 15 and 35 years of age. This prevalence has important socioeconomic consequences and the costs of lifetime care and rehabilitation are extremely high.

The main cause for spinal injuries is blunt trauma, most commonly due to motor vehicle accidents (48%) followed by falls (21%), and sport injuries (14.6%). Assault and penetrating trauma account for approximately 10-20% of the cases.

The majority of spinal injuries involve the cervical spine, with over 10,000 cervical fractures, followed by over 4000 thoracolumbar fractures diagnosed per year in the USA alone. Almost half of the spinal injuries result in neurological deficits, often severe and sometimes fatal [1]. Survival is inversely related to the patient's age; mortality during the initial hospitalization is reported to be almost 10% [2].

Injury to the spinal cord occurs in 10-14% of spinal fractures and dislocations, with injuries of the cervical spine being by far the most common cause of neurological deficits (up to 40% of cases) [3, 4]. Most (85%) injuries to the spinal cord occur at the time of trauma, whereas 5-10% of cord injuries present in the immediate post-injury period [5].

The imaging of patients with acute spinal trauma has dramatically changed in the last decade due to the development of more advanced computed tomography (CT) scanners, such as the use of helical CT, to evaluate the vertebral column, and magnetic resonance imaging (MRI), which has become the method of to evaluate spinal cord, soft-tissue, and ligamentous injuries.

Imaging Modalities

Plain Film Radiography

If multi-slice CT is not available, plain-film radiographs remain the initial imaging modality. To clear the cervical spine, a minimum of three sets of views must be obtained: lateral, anteroposterior, and an open-mouth odontoid view. Often, additional views, such as oblique views and/or swimmer's view, are obtained in an attempt to clear the cervicothoracic junction.

Computed Tomography

Nowadays, multi-slice or single-slice helical CT is the initial method of choice when evaluating the cervical spine for bone injuries after blunt trauma. Either technique allows examination of the entire spine within a very short time. In addition, fast reformatting of images in multiple planes allows for better and more exact diagnosis of bone and soft-tissue abnormalities [6-11]. With the introduction of these new CT imaging techniques, most trauma centers have set up dedicated acute (multi-) trauma protocol(s) that include CT of the brain, cervical spine, thorax, and abdomen, with subsequent reformatting of images of the thoracic and lumbar spine. In addition, several institutions have completely replaced plain films by multi-slice CT, including 2D and 3D reformatting, in patients with blunt spinal trauma, especially in cases involving the cervical spine. CT not only detects fractures with higher sensitivity than obtained with plain films, it also can detect soft-tissue abnormalities, such as disc herniation as well as paravertebral soft-tissue- and epidural hematomas.

A high-resolution CT imaging protocol with reformatted 1.25-2mm thin slices in the C1-C2 region, 2- to 3-mm thin slices in the rest of the cervical spine and 3- to 4-mm thin slices in the thoracic and lumbar spine are typically chosen for axial presentation. Reformatted sagittal and coronal images of the entire spine are produced from contiguous sub-millimeter (0.3-0.75 mm) axial images, or, on the older scanners, from thicker overlapping slices. Reconstructions are always performed with both bone and soft-tissue algorithms.

Magnetic Resonance Imaging

Today, MRI is considered the method of choice for assessing soft tissue injuries, spinal cord injury (SCI), intervertebral discs and ligaments, and vascular injuries

[12-14]. The greatest impact that MRI has made in the evaluation of SCI has been in assessment of the soft-tissue component of the injury. No other imaging modality has been able to faithfully reproduce the internal architecture of the spinal cord, and it is this particular feature of MRI that promises to have the greatest impact on the management of the SCI patient. An MRI examination in the acute period is warranted in any patient who has a persistent neurological deficit after spinal trauma. MRI is the examination of choice to exclude instability, prove/exclude injury to the cord or disc in patients with focal neurological signs, and in those who need pre-operative spinal canal clearance. In addition, post-traumatic sequelae, such as syrinx formation, myelomalacia, cord atrophy, and tethering, are typically examined and evaluated with MRI.

In acute spinal trauma, the MR imaging protocol of the cervical spine includes 3-mm-thick sagittal T1-weighted (T1W) and T2-weighted (T2W) and short tau inversion recovery (STIR) sequences as well as 3-mm-thick axial T2*-gradient recalled echo (GRE) images without contrast. In the thoracic and lumbar spine, 4-mm-thick sagittal T1W, T2W, and STIR sequences and axial 4-mm-thick T1W, T2W, and T2*GRE images without contrast is recommended. Fat-saturated T2W images are valuable to evaluate ligamentous and soft-tissue injuries, while T2* GRE is used to detect small hemorrhages or foci of blood products in the spinal cord.

One of the critical decisions in the emergency setting is determining which patients require imaging of the spine and what type of imaging is called for. The appropriate selection of imaging depends upon several factors, such as availability of the different imaging modalities, the patient's clinical and neurological condition, the type of trauma (blunt, single or multi-trauma), and other associated injuries to the brain, thorax, or abdomen. Clinical factors to consider also include the quality of pain, limitations in motion, or the presence of permanent or transient neurological deficits. MRI is reserved for those patients who require clearance of the spinal cord and spinal canal prior to surgery, and for patients with symptoms that cannot be explained by findings on plain films or CT.

Injuries to the Vertebral Column

The thoracolumbar spine can be divided into three osteoligamentous columns: anterior, middle, and posterior. The anterior column includes the anterior longitudinal ligament and anterior two-thirds of the vertebral body and disc, including the annulus fibrosus. The components of the middle column are the posterior third of the vertebral body and disc, including the annulus fibrosus, and the posterior longitudinal ligament. The posterior column is composed of the pedicles, articular processes, facet capsules, laminae, ligamenta flava, spinous processes, and the interspinous ligaments. Depending on the mechanism of injury, there are several different types of traumatic injuries to the cervical as well as to the thoracic and lumbar spines, all of which may result in stable or unstable spine injuries.

The type of injury to the cervical column can simplistically be divided into three major groups based on the biomechanics of the injury: hyperflexion, hyperextension, and vertical compression. Hyperflexion injuries include anterior subluxation, bilateral interfacetal dislocation, simple wedge fracture, fracture of the spinous process, teardrop fracture, and odontoid (dens) fracture. Bilateral interfacetal dislocation and the teardrop fracture are considered unstable. The odontoid fracture can be considered stable or unstable depending on the fracture type. The remaining injuries are considered stable. Hyperextension injuries are less frequent than hyperflexion injuries and result in the following types of fractures: dislocation, avulsion fracture or fracture of the posterior arch of C1, teardrop fracture of C2, laminar fracture, and the so-called hangman's fracture. Most of these injuries with the exception of hangman's fracture are considered stable. The hyperextension injuries are often associated with central cord syndrome, especially in patients with pre-existing cervical spondylosis, and usually produce diffuse pre-vertebral soft-tissue swelling. Vertical compression results in the Jefferson fracture, which involves the atlas and is considered an unstable or burst fracture.

Fractures in the lower thoracic and lumbar spine are often complex and are due to a combination of mechanisms. The most common fracture is the simple compression, or wedge fracture (50% of all fractures), which is stable. The remaining types of fractures are considered unstable. The "seat-beat injury" can be divided into three subtypes: type I (Chance fracture) involves the posterior bony elements, type II (Smith fracture) involves the posterior ligaments, and in type III the annulus fibrosus is ruptured, allowing for subluxation [15]. Burst fractures can be divided into five subtypes and account for 64-81% of all thoracolumbar fractures. They are associated with a high incidence of injuries to the spinal cord, conus medullaris, cauda equina, and nerve roots [16]. It is important to remember that a burst fracture involving the anterior and middle column can be misdiagnosed as a mere compression fracture on plain films. Consequently, it may be erroneously treated as a stable compression or mild wedge fracture that involves only the anterior column. CT is required for accurate characterization.

Traumatic Disc Herniation and Ligamentous Injury

Traumatic disc injury should be considered when the disc exhibits high signal intensity on T2W images or when severe traumatic vertebral-body fractures and/or ligamentous injury is present [17]. Traumatic disc herniation is commonly caused by distraction and shearing in sudden extension but can also occur in flexion injuries. Extruded disc material may extend into the epidural or pre-vertebral space.

Ligamentous injury has to be suspected when there is a gap between parts of the vertebrae or by increased signal in the ligament or adjacent structures on T2W and STIR images. Ligamentous injury without underlying fracture in the cervical spine is rare [18]. Disruption of the anterior longitudinal ligament is often seen in hyperextension injuries, with associated injury to the pre-vertebral muscles and intervertebral discs, and may have a poor clinical outcome if not surgically treated to prevent instability. It can be seen as interruption of the normal linear band of hypointense signal of the ligament on T1W images. Disruption of the posterior ligamentous complex is caused by distraction and flexion forces and is manifested by an increase in the distance between interspinous processes during flexion.

Injuries to the Spinal Cord

Assessment of the spinal-cord-injured patient includes evaluation of mental status, cranial nerves, motor and sensory function, and autonomic-system coordination and gait. Nearly all SCIs damage both upper and lower motor neurons. The symptoms of complete spinal cord transection depend upon the level of injury. The etiology for mechanical spinal cord transection is often the result of penetrating trauma; however, it can also occur with severe fracture/dislocations. Incomplete SCIs are further categorized clinically into anterior cord syndrome, Brown-Sequard syndrome, central cord syndrome, conus medullaris syndrome, cauda equina syndrome, and spinal cord contusions.

Spinal Cord Hemorrhage

Post-traumatic spinal cord hemorrhage (i.e., hemorrhagic contusion) is defined as the presence of a discrete focus of hemorrhage within the substance of the spinal cord after an injury. The most common location is within the central gray matter of the spinal cord and centered at the point of mechanical impact [19-21]. Experimental and autopsy pathologic studies have shown that the underlying lesion most often consists of hemorrhagic necrosis of the spinal cord. True hematomyelia is rarely found [22]. MRI identification of hemorrhage in the spinal cord following trauma has significant clinical implications. It was originally thought that detection of intramedullary hemorrhage was predictive of a complete injury. However, the increased sensitivity and spatial resolution of current MRI techniques have shown that even small amounts of hemorrhage are identifiable in incomplete lesions. Therefore, the basic premise has been altered, such that the detection of a sizable focus of blood (> 4 mm in length on sagittal images) in the spinal cord is often indicative of a complete neurological injury [23]. The anatomic location of the hemorrhage closely corresponds to the neurological level of injury and the presence of frank hemorrhage implies a poor potential for neurological recovery [19-21, 24-26].

Spinal Cord Edema

Spinal cord edema is defined on MRI as a focus of abnormally high signal intensity on T2W images [27]. This signal abnormality presumably reflects a focal accumulation of intracellular and interstitial fluid in response to injury [20, 21, 27, 28]. Edema is usually well-defined on the mid-sagittal long TR image. Axial T2W images offer supplemental information with regard to involvement of structures, as seen in cross-section. Edema involves a variable length of spinal cord above and below the level of injury, with discrete boundaries adjacent to uninvolved parenchyma. Spinal cord edema is invariably associated with some degree of spinal cord swelling; however, it can occur without MRI evidence of intramedullary hemorrhage. The length of spinal cord affected by edema is directly proportional to the degree of initial neurological deficit [19, 29]. Cord edema alone connotes a more favorable prognosis than cord hemorrhage [21, 23, 24].

Clinical outcome

Many clinical investigations have reported that the MRI patterns of SCI correlate with the neurological deficit at presentation [19-21, 23, 24, 29, 30]. Intramedullary hemorrhage (type I injury) is equated with a severe neurological deficit and a poor prognosis. Cord edema alone (type II injury) was found in patients with mild to moderate initial neurological deficits who subsequently showed neurological improvement [19-21, 23, 24, 30]. The extent of the cord edema may also play a role in neurological outcome. For example, cord edema extending for more than the span of one vertebral segment was shown to be associated with a more severe initial deficit than smaller areas of edema. Cord hemorrhage is associated with the most severe neurological abnormalities, and portends for a poor prognosis [20, 29].

References

1. Hill MW, Dean SA (1993) Head injury and facial injury: is there an increased risk of cervical spine injury? J Trauma 34:549-554
2. Pope AM, Tarlov AR (1991) Disability in America: toward a national agenda for prevention. Washington: National Academy Press
3. Riggins RS, Kraus JF (1997) The risk of neurological damage with fractures of the vertebrae. J Trauma 17:126-130
4. Castellano V, Bocconi FL (1970) Injuries of the cervical spine with spinal cord involvement (myelic fractures): statistical considerations. Bull Hosp J Dis Orthop Inst 31:188-198
5. Rogers WA (1957) Fractures and dislocations of the cervical spine; an end-result study. J Bone Joint Surg 39:341-351
6. Diaz JJ Jr, Gillman C, Morris JA Jr et al (2003) Are five-view plain films of the cervical spine unreliable? A prospective evaluation in blunt trauma in patients with altered mental status. J Trauma 55:658-663
7. Griffen MM, Frykberg, Kerwin AJ et al (2003) Radiographic clearance of blunt cervical spine injury: plain radiograph or computed tomography scan? J Trauma 55:222-226

8. Holmes JF, Mirvis SE, Panacek et al for the NEXUS Group (2002) Variability in computed tomography and magnetic resonance imaging in patients with cervical spine injuries. J Trauma 53:524-529
9. Kligman M, Vasili C, Roffman M (2001) The role of computed tomography in cervical spine injury due to diving. Arch Orthop Trauma Surg 121:139-141
10. Schenarts PJ, Diaz J, Kaiser C et al (2001) Prospective comparison of admission computed tomographic scan and plain films of the upper cervical spine in trauma patients with altered mental status. J Trauma 51:663-668
11. Berne JD, Velmahos GC, El Tawil Q et al (1999) Value of complete cervical helical computed tomographic scanning in identifying cervical spine injury in the unevaluable blunt trauma patient with multiple injuries: a prospective study. J Trauma 47:896-902
12. Flanders AE, Schaefer DM, Doan HT et al (1990) Acute cervical spine trauma; correlation of MR imaging findings with degree of neurological deficit. Radiology 177:25-33
13. Sliker CW, Mirvis SE, Shanmuganathan K (2005) Assessing cervical spine stability in obtunded blunt trauma patients; review of medical literature. Radiology 234:733-739
14. Wilmink JT (1999) MR imaging of the spine: trauma and degenerative disease. Eur Radiol 9:1259-1266
15. Rogers LF (1971) The roentgenographic appearances of transverse or chance fractures of the spine: the seat belt fracture. Am J Roentgenol 111:844-849
16. Gertzbein SD (1992) Scoliosis Research Society: multicenter spine fracture study. Spine 17:528-540
17. Van Goethem JW, Maes M, Özsarlak Ö et al (2005) Imaging of the spinal trauma. Eur Radiol 15:582-590
18. Diaz JJ, Aulino JM, Collier B et al (2005) The early work-up for isolated ligamentous injury of the cervical spine; does computed tomography scan have a role. J Trauma 59:897-904
19. Bondurant FJ, Cotler HB, Kulkarni MV et al (1990) Acute spinal cord injury. A study using physical examination and magnetic resonance imaging. Spine 15(3): 161-168
20. Flanders AE, Schefer DM, Doan HT et al (1990) Acute cervical spine trauma: correlation of MR imaging findings with degree of neurologic deficit. Radiology 177(1):25-33
21. Kulkarni MV, McArdle CB, Kpanicky D et al (1987) Acute spinal cord injury: MR imaging at 1.5 T. Radiology 164(3):837-843
22. Schouman-Claeys e; Frija G, Cuenod CA et al (1990) MR imaging of acute spinal cord injury: results of an experimental study in dogs. AJNR Am J Neuroradiol 11(5):959-965
23. Ramon S, Dominguez R, Ramirez L et al (1997) Clinical and magnetic resonance imaging correlation in acute spinal cord injury. Spinal Cord 35(10):664-673
24. Cotler HB, Kulkarni MV, Bondurant FJ (1988) Magnetic resonance imaging of acute spinal cord trauma: preliminary report. J Orthop Trauma 2(1):1-4
25. Sato T, Kokubun S, Rijal KP et al (1994) Prognosis of cervical spinal cord injury in correlation with magnetic resonance imaging. Paraplegia 32(2):81-85
26. Marciello MA, Flanders AE, Herbison GJ et al (1993) Magnetic resonance imaging related to neurologic outcome in cervical spinal cord injury. Arch Phys Med Rehabil 74(9):940-946
27. Goldberg AL, Rothfus WE, Deeb ZL et al (1988) The impact of magnetic resonance on the diagnostic evaluation of acute cervicothoracic spinal trauma. Skeletal Radiol 17(2): 89-95
28. Wittenberg RH, Boetel U, Beyer HK (1990) Magnetic resonance imaging and computer tomography of acute spinal cord trauma. Clin Orthop Relat Res 260:176-185
29. Schaefer DM, Flanders A Northrup BE et al (1989) Magnetic resonance imaging of acute cervical spine trauma. Correlation with severity of neurologic injury. Spine 14(10):1090-1095
30. Kulkarni MV, Narayana PA, McArdle CB et al (1988) Cervical spine MR imaging using multislice gradient echo imaging: comparison with cardiac gated spin echo. Magn Reson Imaging 6(5):517-525

Spinal Cord Inflammatory and Demyelinating Diseases

Claude Manelfe[1], Jean-Luc Sarrazin[2]

[1] Department of Diagnostic and Therapeutic Neuroradiology, Hôpital Purpan, Toulouse, France
[2] Department of Radiology, American Hospital of Paris, Neuilly, France

Introduction

Clinical presentation and imaging findings of inflammatory and demyelinating diseases of the spinal cord are protean and often nonspecific. They may mimic neoplastic lesions either clinically or radiologically. Magnetic resonance imaging (MRI) is the best imaging modality to screen patients who are clinically suspected of having myelitis.

The most challenging imaging presentation is that of an enlargement (focal or more diffuse) of the spinal cord. Neither spinal cord enlargement nor gadolinium enhancement is synonymous with spinal cord tumor as both can be found in myelitis, myelopathies, or syringohydromyelia.

Since myelitis is relatively rare, the works-up is often delayed and incomplete. Among the causes of myelitis, demyelinating and viral diseases are the most frequent. MRI is very sensitive but lacks specificity and most of the lesions feature high signal intensity on T2-weighted images. The clinical presentation of the patient, anamnesis, mode of onset, underlying disease, and duration can point to the diagnosis. An acute or rapidly progressive clinical onset suggests a vascular (mainly arterial), infectious, viral or inflammatory origin; a slowly progressive onset is more likely due to compression, demyelination, vascular (mainly venous), or metabolic or toxic causes.

Clinical Presentation

The most frequent clinical picture is an *acute transverse myelitis* (ATM). This is an inflammatory or infectious process involving the entire cross-sectional area of the cord at a particular level. The most prominent findings on histopathological examination are found in the blood vessels and perivascular spaces of the gray and white matter: hyperemia, perivascular cellular exudate and edema, as well as hemorrhage. ATM can result from an autoimmune or allergic response, vasculitis, direct viral invasion, or demyelination. Clinically, ATM is characterized by acute or subacute (from 4 days to 4 weeks) paraparesis, with bilateral sensory findings and sphincters disorders, a clearly defined sensory level, a stable nonprogressive course, and no clinical or laboratory evidence of spinal cord compression. A set of uniform and diagnostic criteria and nosology for ATM has been proposed to avoid confusion.

Diagnosis of ATM requires evidence of inflammation within the spinal cord. Since spinal cord biopsy is not a practical option in routine evaluation of these patients, enhanced spinal MRI and lumbar puncture with cerebrospinal fluid (CSF) analysis are the only tools currently available to determine the presence of inflammation. Abnormal enhancement of the spinal cord or CSF pleocytosis or an elevated CSF IgG index is required for the diagnosis of ATM. Serologic and culture examinations of blood, CSF, and biopsy specimens may obviate surgical biopsy of the spinal cord. Analysis of the viral genome in CSF by the polymerase chain reaction (PCR) is a fast (<24 h) and sensitive test; its specificity is superior to viral serologies.

Differentiating idiopathic ATM from ATM attributed to an underlying disease, or disease-associated ATM (demyelinating, infectious, systemic, inflammatory and autoimmune, metabolic and nutritional diseases) is important.

Imaging Techniques

Magnetic resonance imaging is the best technique due to its multi-planar capabilities and superior tissue sensitivity:

- Sagittal and axial T1- and T2-weighted fast spin echo (FSE) are the most frequently used sequences. Spin echo (SE) sequences are superior to gradient echo (GE) sequences except when associated acute hemorrhage is suspected. The study of patients with suspected intramedullary lesions (mainly multiple sclerosis) is improved by including a separate sagittal proton-density-weighted FSE scan, which generally confirms the lesions suspected on T2-weighted sequences and frequently may detect additional cord lesions.
- FSE with longer TR/TE (3000/150) results in poorer lesion-cord contrast than obtained with more moderate TR/TE (2500/90). The slice thickness must be 3 mm or less when a spinal cord lesion is suspected.

- SE sequences with short time inversion (TI) recovery (STIR) (TR: 3000 m, TE: 40 ms, TI: 140-160 ms) are well-suited for evaluating intramedullary lesions and are particularly helpful in the detection of multiple sclerosis plaque.
- Sequence with long TI (FLAIR, TR: 10000 m, TE: 180 ms, TI: 2000 ms) have less sensitivity in the detection of intramedullary lesions, but can be useful to differentiate an intramedullary cyst from myelomalacia or edema.
- In the axial plane, T2-weighted SE sequences are more sensitive to flow artifacts, while T2-weighted* GE sequences are more efficient, mainly at the cervical level.
- Gadolinium (Gd) injection increases conspicuity and specificity, and improves the localization and detection of subtle areas of infection or inflammation. Post-Gd fat suppression T1-weighted sequences are very useful for analyzing not only the bone marrow and epidural space but also the spinal cord and nerve roots.
- Magnetic resonance angiography (MRA, black blood technique) of the spinal cord lacks sufficient spatial resolution and presently cannot replace spinal cord angiography when the medullary vessels are not dilated. Gd-enhanced MRA has increased spatial resolution, and preliminary studies with this technique have shown promising results.
- Magnetic resonance myelography (MRM), using ultrafast techniques, such as HASTE (half Fourier acquisition single-shot turbo spin echo) or CISS (constructive interference steady state) 3D sequences, is a valuable method to explore the spine and spinal cord pathology. It is, however, less useful in imaging intramedullary pathologies than in intra- or extradural lesions (tumors, degenerative disk disease, spinal stenosis).
- Diffusion-weighted imaging (DWI), in which molecular water motion is imaged, has been applied recently to the study of spinal cord diseases.
- Diffusion tensor tractography (DTI) can display vectors corresponding to the strength and direction of movement of water molecules. The first reports of DTI studies of spinal cord pathologies were recently published.

Demyelinating Diseases

Multiple Sclerosis

Multiple sclerosis (MS) is the most frequent demyelinating disease of the central nervous system (CNS) of autoimmune origin. MS affects young adults and has three main clinical forms: (a) relapsing-remitting (25%), (b) secondary progressive (40%), and (c) primary progressive (12%). Diagnostic criteria are based on clinical history, physical examination, and paraclinical tests, such as CSF analysis (oligoclonal bands and IgG index), visual evoked potentials, and MRI findings. It is worthy of note that ATM may be the first presentation in patients who are ultimately diagnosed with MS.

Spinal abnormalities are present in 83% of patients with MS; approximately 10-15% of patients with spinal cord plaques have no intracranial disease. In the new imaging criteria for diagnosing MS, a medullary plaque is equivalent to a posterior fossa plaque or to an enhancing plaque.

MS affects mainly the cervicothoracic cord: plaques are elongated, extend over one to two vertebral segments, and do not respect boundaries between tracts of gray and white matter. Cord enlargement may be noted in acute lesions and Gd enhancement may be observed. On axial sections, plaques are located at the periphery of the cord, mainly in the posterior (41%) and lateral (25%) aspects. More than half the cord plaques longer than two vertebral segments are accompanied by cord atrophy, by cord swelling. STIR sequence improves lesion detection or while DWI demonstrates increased mean diffusivity. Diffuse cord abnormalities seem to be correlated with primary or secondary progressive clinical MS subtypes. Diffuse disease is more frequently associated with cord atrophy and has a weak but significant correlation with clinical disability. The magnetization transfer ratio (MTR) in the cervical cord of MS patients may be lower than in normal controls, even in the absence of detectable cord lesions on T2-weighted sequences.

Differential diagnosis with neoplasm, granulomatous infection or viral diseases may be difficult. The disappearance of enhancing lesions on follow-up examinations and associated brain lesions suggest MS.

Acute Disseminated Encephalomyelitis

Acute disseminated encephalomyelitis (ADEM) is an acute or subacute demyelinating process of autoimmune origin mediated by antibody-antigen complexes. The disease has a monophasic course, typically following a specific viral illness, vaccination, or non-specific respiratory infection. Mortality is approximately 10-20% in the acute phase, but 60% of patients recover completely. Pathological analysis shows perivenous demyelination with variable inflammatory cell infiltration of the white matter.

MRI findings in ADEM are non-specific, showing punctuate to segmental high signal intensity on T2-weighted images in the white matter. In the brain, lesions are usually bilateral, asymmetric, and widely distributed without mass effect. ADEM can be indistinguishable from MS on a single study. The monophasic course of ADEM, the involvement of the cranial nerves, basal ganglia and thalami, and gadolinium enhancement differentiate it from MS.

Devic's Neuromyelitis Optica

Neuromyelitis optica or Devic's disease is defined as the association of myelitis with optic neuritis, which is often bilateral. It is regarded as a particular and severe form of MS. MRI shows a cord swelling with diffuse intramedullary hyperintensity on T2-weighted images. Optic nerve(s) enhancement can be present following Gd injection. Brain MRI is usually negative.

Guillain-Barré Syndrome

Guillain-Barré syndrome is an acute inflammatory demyelinating polyradiculoneuropathy. Distal paresthesias and sensory loss are common, followed by ascending paralysis, which is frequently bilateral and symmetric. Cranial nerve involvement is frequent, with bilateral facial paralysis in 50% of patients. CSF analysis shows a typical elevated protein level without pleocytosis. MRI findings are an intense enhancement of the nerve roots of the cauda equina on T1-weighted sagittal and axial images, sometimes associated with pial enhancement of the conus.

The differential diagnosis includes chronic inflammatory demyelinating polyneuropathy (CIDP), which differs from Guillain-Barré syndrome by the presence of relapsing or progressive sensorimotor deficit. MRI demonstrates enlargement and abnormal T2-weighted hyperintensity of the nerve roots of the cauda equina and proximal peripheral nerves. Gd enhancement of the nerve roots is mild to moderate.

Systemic Inflammatory Diseases

Sarcoidosis

Neurosarcoidosis is an idiopathic, multi-systemic, noncaseating granulomatous disease. Spinal cord involvement is present in 6-8% of these patients. The clinical picture is nonspecific, and clinical and laboratory tests are mandatory (Kvein skin test, serum levels of angiotensin-converting enzyme (ACE), CSF studies, chest radiograph). Histologic examination of biopsies of skin, nasal mucosa, and lymph nodes is of great value and can obviate the need for cord biopsy.

As in MS, cervical cord involvement is frequent in spinal sarcoidosis. T1- and T2-weighted images are not specific, as they show an enlarged cord and hyperintensity on T2-weighted imaging, mimicking a tumor or an MS plaque. Four patterns of enhancement correspond to different stages of the disease: (a) linear, leptomeningeal; (b) parenchymal, associated with cord swelling; (c) focal or multi-focal with abnormal cord; and (d) atrophy. Associated leptomeningeal cranial involvement is helpful for the diagnosis of sarcoidosis but may also be present in tuberculosis or non-Hodgkin's lymphoma.

Other infectious granulomatous disease includes tuberculosis. Intramedullary tuberculomas have been reported, but are extremely rare. The ratio of intracranial to intraspinal tuberculomas ranges from 20:1 to 42:1. MRI can demonstrate a fusiform swelling of the cord, with iso- or hyperintensity on T1-weighted images; hypo- or iso intensity on T2-weighted images is suggestive of tuberculoma. Because of the increase in drug-resistant tuberculosis and the AIDS epidemic, spinal tuberculosis must be considered in the differential diagnosis of patients at risk.

Systemic Lupus Erythematosus

Systemic lupus erythematosus (SLE) is a systemic disease with multi-organ involvement. Occasionally, the CNS is the main site of clinical involvement, with minimal evidence of skin or articular disease. Although much less common than cerebral, myelopathy may occur in an acute or subacute fashion. MRI may show focal areas of cord edema and hyperintensities on T2-weighted images. Serologic (anti-DNA antibodies, antiphospholipid antibodies) or clinical evidence of connective tissue disease is helpful.

Sjogren's Syndrome

The prevalence of CNS involvement in patients with Sjogren's syndrome varies from 2 to 20%. The clinical presentation and CSF studies may mimic the pattern seen in MS. In some cases, an acute onset of pain and myelopathy suggests a vascular origin. Involvement of multiple organs, such as lacrimal and salivary glands, lungs, kidneys, thyroid, muscles, and peripheral nerves suggests the diagnosis.

Infectious Diseases

This class of non-granulomatous diseases comprises viral, bacterial, parasitic, and toxic myelopathies.

Viral Infections

The clinical picture is frequently represented by ATM. It affects individuals of all ages with bimodal peaks between the ages of 10 and 19 years, and 30 and 39 years, with no sex or familial predisposition. Transverse myelitis is an inflammatory or infectious process involving the entire cross-sectional area of the cord at a particular level.

Acute paraparesis with motor, sensory, and sphincters disorders is the most common clinical presentation. In children, ATM is commonly preceded by infection (herpes, rabies, varicella, mumps, rubeola) or vaccination. In adults, the most frequent causes of ATM are acquired immune deficiency syndrome (AIDS), vasculitis (systemic lupus erythematosus) and paraneoplastic syndromes.

The MRI appearance of transverse myelitis is nonspecific: focal or extended cord enlargement is present in 40% and Gd enhancement in 60% of patients. On axial sections, the high signal intensity on T2-weighted images occupies more than two-thirds of the cross section of the cord.

AIDS

Patients infected with the human immunodeficiency virus (HIV) frequently experience vacuolar myelopathy, HIV myelitis, opportunistic infections, lymphomas, and vascular or metabolic disorders.

Vacuolar myelopathy is the most common spinal cord disease in AIDS (30-50% in autopsy studies). It is characterized by a spongy degeneration (vacuolization) of spinal white matter affecting predominantly the lateral and posterior columns of the thoracic cord. The histopathological features are similar to those of subacute combined degeneration of the spinal cord secondary to vitamin B_{12} deficiency. Vacuoles are the result of edematous swelling within myelin, with splitting of the lamellae. The axons are usually normal until severe vacuolation, secondary Wallerian degeneration, and axonal disruption occur. The exact cause of vacuolar myelopathy remains unclear; it may be secondary to a combination of immune-mediated myelin and oligodendrocyte injuries and simultaneous impairment of repair mechanisms due to a deficiency of S-adenosylmethionine.

Common clinical manifestations are progressive spastic paraparesis, incontinence, and ataxia. Dementia is observed in 70% of cases. MRI usually shows diffuse and symmetric hyperintensities on T2-weighted images of the dorsal and lateral columns in a normal or atrophic spinal cord, more often without Gd enhancement since the inflammatory component is missing.

HIV myelitis occurs in 5-8% of AIDS patients and is caused by direct HIV infection. Lesions are focal, have high signal intensity on T2-weighted images, and predominate in the central gray matter.

Opportunistic infections in AIDS patients may be caused by cytomegalovirus (CMV), fungi, herpes simplex virus (HSV), and varicella-zoster virus (VZV). Other common opportunistic infections are tuberculosis, toxoplasmosis, syphilis and progressive multi-focal leukoencephalopathy (PML).

CMV infection, the most common opportunistic infection in AIDS patients and frequently involves the conus medullaris and cauda equina. Myelitis and necrotizing polyradiculitis are the most common pathological findings. Back and radicular pain, flaccid paraparesis, urinary retention, saddle anesthesia, and an inflammatory CSF profile (polymorphonuclear pleocytosis, low sugar and high protein contents) are usual. Retinitis, pneumonia, and gastrointestinal infections are frequently associated. PCR in the CSF allows better characterization and improves the diagnosis of CMV infection. MRI shows clumping of the nerve roots of the cauda equina and leptomeningeal enhancement of the conus.

In VZV myelitis the posterior horns and dorsal roots are affected in 100 and 90%, respectively; the spinal ganglion is involved in 25% of cases. In the immunocompetent patient, VZV myelitis usually follows (2-3 weeks) cutaneous vesicular eruption; more rarely it can precede it, and exceptionally can be isolated. In the immunodepressed patient, clinical manifestations of ATM are more insidious and progressive. PCR in the CSF allows the diagnosis. On MRI, hyperintensity on T2-weighted images and enhancement of the posterior horns are demonstrated. Dorsal nerve root and spinal ganglia can be involved in some cases.

One must keep in mind that neurological symptoms during a zona are not always synonymous of VZV myelitis: zona can be secondary to a neoplastic vertebral lesion causing spinal cord compression.

Spinal cord *Toxoplasma gondii* infection occurs rarely in AIDS patients and is always associated with coexisting cerebral infection. MRI is nonspecific. When focal spinal cord enlargement with Gd enhancement is present, toxoplasmic myelitis and lymphoma should be considered; brain involvement is present in both conditions, but a positive thallium-201 single photon emission computed tomography (SPECT) scan makes a diagnosis of lymphoma more likely. When spinal cord enlargement and abnormal signal (hyperintensity on T2-weighted images) are associated with meningeal enhancement, CMV infection and tuberculosis should be considered.

Tropic Spastic Paraparesis

Human T-cell lymphotrophic virus type I (HTLV-I) is an endemic infection in the Caribbean and some parts of Africa and is called tropical spastic paraparesis (TSP). In Japan, this myelopathy was found to be associated with leukemia and was thus called HTLV-1-associated myelopathy (HAM). Neuropathology reveals demyelination in the lateral and dorsal tracts as well as axonal loss. Clinical presentation usually consists of progressive weakness of the lower limbs with paresthesias. MRI may show either diffuse atrophy and abnormal signal intensity on T2-weighted images or, at the acute stage, spinal cord swelling with peripheral Gd enhancement. Associated white matter lesions in the brain have been reported.

Bacterial Infections

Bacterial infections and abscesses of the spinal cord are extremely rare. Clinical presentation can be acute, subacute, or chronic, mimicking a tumor. Predisposing factors include cardiopulmonary infections, immunosuppression, diabetes, and drug abuse. Fever is present in 40% of patients. The most common causative agent is *Staphylococcus aureus*. Cord swelling and extensive edema are present at the initial stage (phlegmon) with or without nodular or ring enhancement. A rim-enhancing cavity is seen at the abscess stage.

Listeria monocytogenes can cause abscesses of the brain stem and upper cervical cord.

Syphilitic myelitis is a very rare manifestation of neurosyphilis. Pathology shows an endarteritis with thrombosis of the spinal cord vessels. MRI is not specific, demonstrating more or less extended hyperintensity of the cord on T2-weighted images, with leptomeningeal enhancement. Final diagnosis rests on serum and CSF tests (VDRL, Venereal Disease Research Laboratory).

Lyme disease is a multi-systemic chronic disease due to infection with *Borrelia burgdorferi*. The CNS is involved in 10-20% of cases (neuroborreliosis). Lymphocytic meningoradiculitis and acute transverse myelitis are the most common clinical presentations. Leptomeningeal enhancement of the spinal cord, nerve roots and cranial nerves is usual.

Parasitic and Fungal Infections

Parasitic infections such as schistosomal myelitis, toxocarosis, bilharziosis, and cysticercosis are suspected in patients who have been in countries where these diseases are endemic, and in patients who have hypereosinophilia (in blood or CSF). Spinal cord lesions are far less frequent than brain lesions. Pain, spastic paraplegia and sphincter disturbances comprise the most frequent presentation.

MRI shows non-specific focal mass effect, low signal intensity on T1-weighted images, and high signal intensity on T2-weighted images. Cysts in the subarachnoid spaces compressing the spinal cord and/or nerve roots are seen in neurocysticercosis; they are isointense to the CSF, and their mobility in the CSF can be helpful for the diagnosis of cysticercosis. Peripheral enhancement of the cyst(s) is present after the death of the parasite, consistent with an intense inflammatory reaction of the host.

Fungal myelitis is exceptional and occurs almost exclusively in immunocompromised patients. It manifests as abscesses, meningitis, or granuloma. The most common causes are cryptococcosis, histoplasmosis, and coccidiomycosis.

Metabolic and Nutritional Deficiency Myelitis

Subacute Combined Degeneration

Subacute combined degeneration (SCD) of the spinal cord is due to vitamin B_{12} deficiency and is often associated with megaloblastic anemia. Degenerative and demyelinating changes occur in the white matter of the dorsal and lateral columns of the spinal cord. MRI shows hyperintensity on T2-weighted images in the dorsal columns (mainly cervical and thoracic) with or without cord enlargement or Gd enhancement. Following vitamin B_{12} supplementation, improvement is seen clinically and on MRI.

Radiation Myelitis

Atrophy is the most common appearance of radiation myelitis. It can mimic, however, tumoral infiltration when transient enlargement of the cord with high signal intensity on T2-weighted images is present. Focal enhancement after Gd injection may be seen. The thoracic cord is more sensitive to radiation. A spinal lesion attributed to radiation myelitis should lie in the radiation portal and appears at least 6-12 months after radiotherapy. Associated bony changes (fatty degeneration of the vertebral bodies) in the radiation portal help in differentiating myelitis from tumor. Overall, radiation myelitis is related to tumors of the head and neck in 82% of cases.

Conclusions

Even if demyelinating and inflammatory diseases of the spinal cord are relatively rare, a rapid and accurate diagnosis will ensure not only that a spinal cord compression is ruled out, but also that idiopathic ATM is distinguished from ATM secondary to a known underlying disease.

Suggested Reading

Byrne ThN, Benzel EC, Waxman SG (2000) Diseases of the spine and spinal Cord. Oxford University Press, Oxford

Colimon R (2002) Introduction to the virological diagnosis of the most frequent infections of the central nervous system. J Clinical Virology 25:1-3

Cosnard G, Lecouvet F (2002) Imagerie du rachis, des méninges et de la moelle épinière. Masson, Paris

D'Angelo CM, Whisler W (1978) Bacterial infections of the spinal cord and its coverings. In: Vinken PJ, Bruyn (eds) Handbook of clinical neurology, vol. 33. North-Holland, Amsterdam, pp 187-194

Manelfe C (1992) Imaging of the spine and spinal cord. Raven, New York

Ross JS, Brant-Zawadzki M, Moore KR et al (2005) Spine, diagnostic imaging. Amirsys, Salt Lake City

Thurnher MM (2007) Spinal Infections. In : Van Goethem JWM, Van Den Hauwe L, Parizel PM (eds) Spinal imaging. Springer, Berlin-Heidelberg-New York, pp 521-541

Thurnher MM, Bammer R (2006) Diffusion-weighted magnetic resonance imaging of the spine and spinal cord. Semin Roentgenol 41 (4):294-311

Transverse Myelitis Consortium Working Group (2002) Proposed diagnostic criteria and nosology of acute transverse myelitis. Neurology 59:499-505

Vargas MI, Delavelle J, Jlassi H et al (2008) Clinical applications of diffusion tensor tractography of the spinal cord. Neuroradiology 50:25-29

Spine Inflammatory and Infectious Diseases

Jeffrey S. Ross

Southwest Neuro-Imaging, Neuroradiology, Barrow Neurological Institute, St. Joseph's Hospital, Phoenix, AZ, USA

Introduction

The neuroimaging evaluation of patients with myelopathy is a fundamental magnetic resonance imaging (MRI) application, although it can be one of the more challenging examinations from a technical, interpretative, and differential diagnostic standpoint. The common pathologic lesions responsible for producing myelopathic symptoms in patients include intrinsic and extrinsic compressive, neoplastic, and inflammatory processes. This article focuses on spinal inflammatory diseases, and will review the MRI interpretative and clinicopathologic features of several important disease entities that produce a spine inflection and intrinsic inflammatory myelopathy.

Extradural Infection

The sources for the bacterial seeding that cause vertebral osteomyelitis include genitourinary, dermal, and respiratory ones. In children, the bacteria find their way to the vascularized disk, where the resulting destruction causes loss of disk space height. As the infection spreads to the adjacent endplates, plain films show the characteristic irregularity. Hematogenous spread also occurs in adults, even though the disk has lost a great deal of its vascularity. The seeding is to the vascularized endplates, with the disk and opposite endplates becoming infected secondarily.

The radionuclides most commonly used for detecting inflammatory changes of the spine are technetium 99m (^{99m}Tc) phosphate complexes, gallium (^{67}Ga) citrate, and indium-111-labeled white blood cells. Although scintigraphy with ^{99m}Tc and ^{67}Ga compounds is sensitive to infection, it is also nonspecific. Healing fractures, sterile inflammatory reactions, tumors, and loosened prosthetic devices can show increased uptake [1-3].

Indium-111 has several advantages over other radionuclides, including higher target-to-background ratios, better image quality (compared to gallium), and more intense uptake by abscesses. Its main disadvantage is its accumulation within any inflammatory lesion, whether infectious or not [4]. The radionuclide study also takes time (hours to days) to perform. Computed tomography (CT) has played a minor role in cases with bony or soft-tissue components and is not considered a mainstay for the diagnosis of disk space infection (DSI) [5]. In appropriate situations, MRI appears to have a sensitivity for detecting vertebral osteomyelitis that exceeds that of plain films and CT and approaches or equals that of radionuclide studies [6, 7].

In MRI, it is imperative to obtain both T1-weighted (T1W) and T2-weighted (T2W) images in the sagittal plane for optimum disease sensitivity. The T1W spin-echo (SE) image allows detection of the increased water content or marrow fluid seen with inflammatory exudates or edema. Like most pathologic processes, DSI or vertebral osteomyelitis results in increased signal intensity on T2W images. The diagnostic specificity of MRI is provided by the signal intensity changes on T1- and T2-weighted images, as well as by the anatomic pattern of disease involvement and the appropriate clinical situation (Fig. 1).

On T2W images, the normal intervertebral disk usually shows increased signal intensity within its central portion, which is bisected by a thin horizontal line of decreased signal, termed the intranuclear cleft. In people over 30 years of age, the cleft is almost a constant feature of normal intervertebral disks.

The typical MR appearance of DSI is a confluent decreased signal intensity of the adjacent vertebral bodies and the involved intervertebral disk space on T1W images as compared to the normal vertebral body marrow. A well-defined endplate margin between the disk and adjacent vertebral bodies cannot be defined. T2W images show increased signal intensity of the vertebral bodies adjacent to the involved disk, and an abnormal morphology and increased signal intensity from the disk itself, with absence of the normal intranuclear cleft.

These MRI findings are much more typical of pyogenic than of tuberculous spondylitis [8]. In a comparative study of patients with suspected vertebral osteomyelitis, MRI had a sensitivity of 96%, a specificity of 92%, and an accuracy of 94% [6]. Gallium-67 and technetium-99m bone scintigraphy had a sensitivity of 90%, a specificity of 100%, and an accuracy of 94%

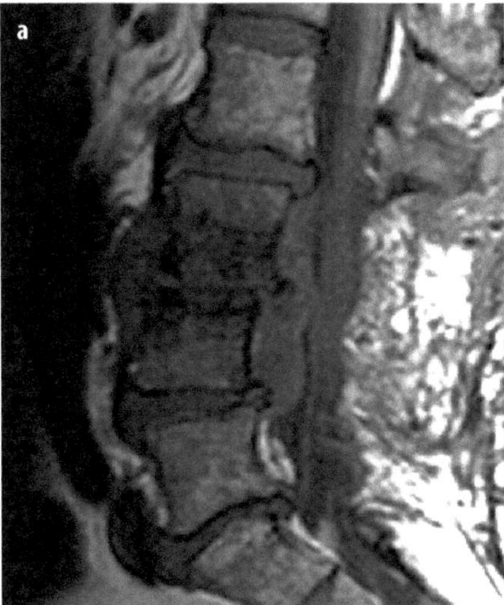

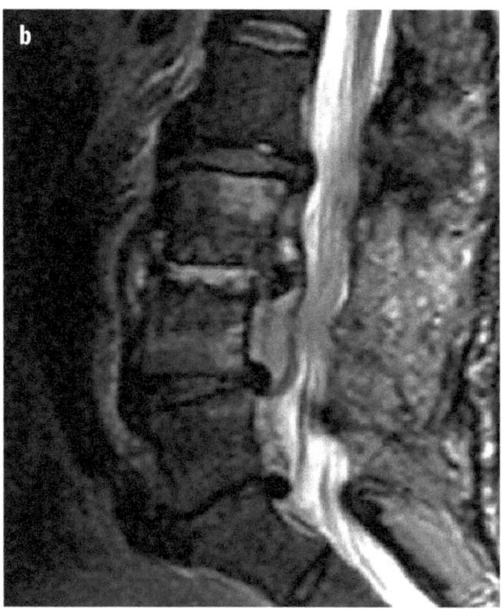

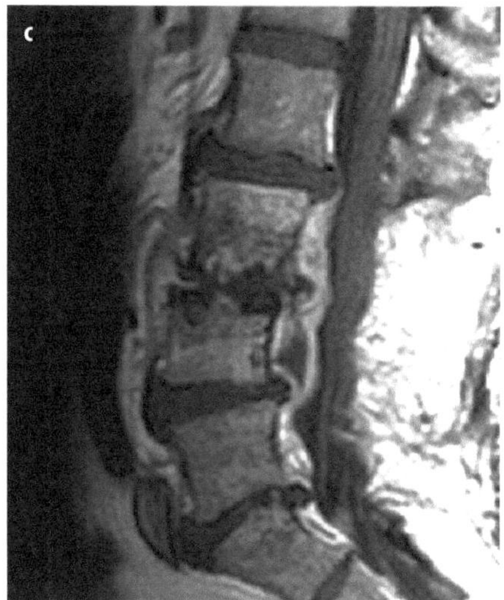

Fig. 1 a-c. Bacterial disc space infection and osteomyelitis. Sagittal T1- (**a**), T2- (**b**), and post-contrast T1- (**c**) weighted images show the typical findings of disc space infection with abnormal low T1 signal, disc T2 hyperintensity, and irregular endplate and disc enhancement. There is a large ventral epidural abscess at the L4 level

when these tracer studies were combined. In that study, MRI was as accurate and sensitive as radionuclide scanning for the detection of osteomyelitis.

The "classic" MRI changes of vertebral osteomyelitis include decreased signal of the disc and adjacent vertebral bodies on T1W images, increased non-anatomic signal of the disc on T2W images, increased signal of the adjacent vertebral bodies on T2W images, and enhancement of the disc and adjacent vertebral bodies. One study showed that 95% of DSI levels had typical T1W vertebral body changes, and 90% had increased non-anatomic signal of the disc on T2W images [9]. However, only 54% of the abnormal levels demonstrated increased signal of the vertebral bodies on T2W images. Thus, while 84% of patients demonstrated the typical T1 vertebral body, and T1 and T2 disc changes, only 49% demonstrated both the typical T1- and T2-weighted vertebral body and disc findings as originally described. T1W vertebral body, disc and endplate changes, and T2W imaging disc changes are the most reliable findings of DSI and vertebral osteomyelitis. When faced with the typical T1W vertebral body and disc changes, and T2W disc signal intensity changes of discitis, one should not be dissuaded from the MRI diagnosis of discitis with associated vertebral osteomyelitis by the absence of increased vertebral body signal on the T2W images. On plain films, 71% of patients with decreased or isointense signal of the body on T2W images had sclerosis, in contrast to 45% of patients with high signal of the body on T2W images. The T2 signal intensity of the vertebral body on MRI reflects the marrow space, while the sclerosis seen on plain films reflects the bony trabecula. Trabecular sclerosis may increase to such an extent that it will obliterate the marrow space, resulting in decreased signal intensity on T2W images.

The typical disk space infection presents no problem in diagnosis, provided both T1- and T2-weighted images are obtained. However, atypical-appearing disk space infections do exist and complicate a usually unequivocal diagnosis. One atypical form may be seen if DSI complicates a degenerated disk with an associated type II marrow change (i.e., increased signal from the endplates on T1W images). In these cases the T1W images may continue to show increased signal, in effect masking the usual characteristically confluent decreased intensity. The key MRI finding in these cases is the abnormal disk signal intensity on T2W images, something that does not occur in uncomplicated type II marrow change. Very early on in vertebral osteomyelitis, there may be decreased signal involving the endplates without an appreciable increase in signal from the bodies or disk on T2W images.

The differentiation of degenerative disease and tumor from vertebral osteomyelitis is easier on MRI than on radionuclide studies or plain radiographs. Degenerated disks show decreased signal intensity within their central portion on T2W images, which can be distinguished from the high signal of active inflammation. It may be difficult to differentiate metastatic disease, postoperative changes, or degenerative changes from osteomyelitis by scintigraphic means. These entities can usually be differentiated from osteomyelitis on MRI by the lack of confluent decreased signal of the vertebral body and disk on the T1W images. Likewise, metastatic disease can be distinguished from osteomyelitis by the lack of disk space involvement. Although rare instances of metastatic involvement of the disk have been reported, this continues to be a reliable sign of benign disease in the overwhelming majority of cases [10, 11]. In the initial stages of vertebral osteomyelitis, when the disk space is not yet involved, it may be difficult to exclude neoplastic disease or compression fracture from the differential diagnosis using only MRI. Follow-up studies are usually necessary to further define the nature of the lesion.

Boden et al. suggested that in the postoperative spine the triad of intervertebral disk space enhancement, annular enhancement, and vertebral body enhancement lead to the diagnosis of DSI, with the appropriate laboratory findings, such as an elevated sedimentation rate [12]. However, it is important to emphasize that there is a group of *normal* postoperative patients with annulus enhancement (at the surgical curette site), intervertebral disk enhancement, and vertebral endplate enhancement without evidence of DSI. In these cases, the intervertebral disk enhancement is typically seen as thin bands paralleling the adjacent endplates, and the vertebral body enhancement is enhancement associated with type I degenerative endplate changes. This pattern should be distinguished from the amorphous enhancement seen within the intervertebral disk with DSI.

The incidence of spinal epidural abscess ranges from 0.2 to 1.96 cases per 10,000 [13]. The incidence at the high end is seen in the more current literature. This apparent increase may relate to the general aging of the population as well as to the increasing number of spinal procedures and incidents of intravenous drug abuse. Risk factors for the development of epidural abscess include altered immune status, renal failure requiring dialysis, alcoholism, and malignancy. Although intravenous drug abuse is a risk factor for epidural abscess, HIV infection does not appear to play a role in the overall increasing incidence of the disease.

Staphylococcus aureus is the organism most commonly associated with epidural abscess, accounting for approximately 60% of the cases. It is ubiquitous, tends to form abscesses, and can infect immune-compromised as well as normal hosts. Other gram-positive cocci account for approximately 13% of cases and gram-negative organisms for approximately 15%. Clinical acute symptomatology classically includes back pain, fever, obtundation, and neurologic deficits. In chronic cases, there may be less pain and the patient's temperature is not elevated. The classic course of epidural abscess consists of four stages: spinal ache, root pain, weakness, and paralysis [14]. Acute deterioration from spinal epidural abscess, however, remains unpredictable. Patients may present with abrupt paraplegia and anesthesia. The cause for this precipitous course is unknown, but it is thought to be related to a vascular mechanism (epidural thrombosis and thrombophlebitis, venous infarction) [15, 16].

The primary diagnostic modality in the evaluation of epidural abscess is MR, which is as sensitive as CT myelography for epidural infection, but also allows the exclusion of other diagnostic choices, such as herniation, syrinx, tumor, and cord infarction [17]. MRI of epidural abscess demonstrates a soft-tissue mass in the epidural space with tapered edges and an associated mass effect on the thecal sac and cord (Fig. 2). The epidural masses are usually isointense to the cord on T1W images and show increased signal on T2W images. Post et al. recommended that in these ambiguous cases either CT myelography or perhaps Gd-DTPA enhancement is necessary for full elucidation of the abscess [18, 19].

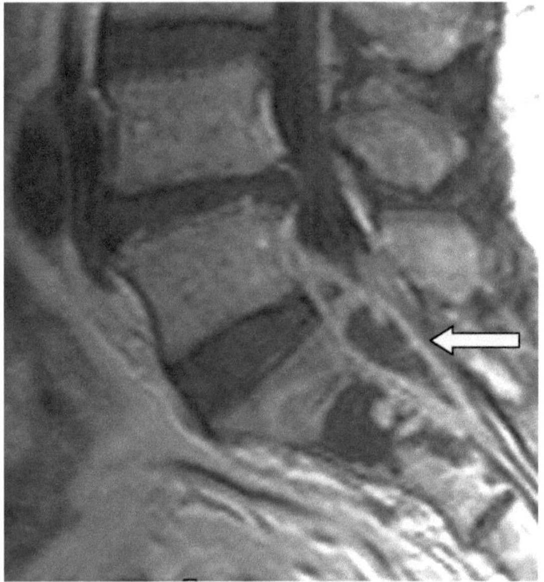

Fig. 2. Tuberculous osteomyelitis. Sagittal T1-weighted image following contrast shows irregular decreased enhancement involving the S1 and S2 bodies, and a large ventral epidural abscess with peripheral enhancement (*arrow*)

The patterns of Gd-DTPA enhancement of epidural abscess include: [1] diffuse and homogeneous, [2] heterogeneous, and [3] thin peripheral. Post et al. found that Gd-DTPA enhancement is a very useful adjunct for identifying the extent of a lesion when the plain MRI scan is equivocal, for demonstrating the activity of an infection, and for directing needle biopsy and follow-up treatment [19]. Successful therapy should cause a progressive decrease in enhancement of the paraspinal soft tissues, disk, and vertebral bodies.

Intramedullary Diseases

Multiple Sclerosis

The spinal cord is the site of much motor disability in multiple sclerosis (MS) patients, yet imaging of the spinal cord has always been subordinate to brain imaging in clinical investigations of this disease. None of the recent, large, therapeutic trials in MS patients included assessment of cord disease, even though brain MRI findings may be the primary objective determinant of disease activity. The reasons for the omission include a lack of established relationships between cord disease and disability in MS, the complexity and duration of MRI examinations when obtaining both brain and cord data, and technical difficulties in cord imaging due to the small size of the spinal cord, its orientation, and the presence of artifacts from pulsatile cerebrospinal flow (CSF) flow, as well as cardiac, respiratory, and oropharyngeal motion. Since some of the clinical disease activity in MS is related to the spinal cord, it is important to investigate cord disease activity to gain further insights into the nature of disability in these patients and to determine whether any objective improvements in brain and cord lesion burden that may be observed in a therapeutic trail are associated with changes in clinical disability scoring.

Patterns of Cord MS

Tartaglino et al. [20, 21] described in detail the MRI appearances of MS in the spinal cord. They found that the majority of focal plaques were less than two vertebral body lengths in size, occupied less than half the cross-sectional diameter of the cord, and were characteristically peripherally located with respects to a transverse, cross-sectional reference (Fig. 3). Approximately 60-75% of the spinal cord MS lesions are present in the cervical region, and more than half of the MS patients with cord plaques had multiple plaques. Of the patients with cord plaques, 90% had intracranial MS plaques. The vast majority of plaques did not significantly alter cord morphology. More than half of the cord plaques longer than two vertebral segments were accompanied by cord atrophy, or conversely, cord swelling. Cord swelling occurred only in relapsing-remitting MS patients and in patients with Devic's syndrome of optic neuritis and myelitis. In this syndrome (neuromyelitis optica), a long segment (up to nine vertebral body lengths), holo-cord signal abnormality with cord swelling, and mild, patchy gadolinium enhancement were seen. Weibe et al. [22] found that approximately 14% of cord plaques enhanced following gadolinium administration.

Cord MS Activity and Clinical Impairment

A study by Kidd et al. [23] with current MRI coil and sequence technologies revealed spinal cord lesions in nearly 75% of patients with clinically definite MS. Cord lesions are seen in every clinical subtype of MS. Approximately 10-15% of patients with spinal cord plaques have no intracranial disease. The cord lesion burden did not correlate with the brain lesion load. Cord atrophy, defined as a cross-sectional diameter less than 2 SD below normal for the specific cord level, is present in 40% of MS patients, and this determinant of atrophy is most relevant at the C5 level. There was a tendency for focal cord lesions to be more prevalent in normal-sized cords. Those patients with atrophy had a mean Expanded Disability Status Scale (EDSS) score that was significantly worse than in patients without atrophy. Losseff et al. [24] also found a statistically significant difference in cord cross-sectional area between MS patients and normal volunteers, and a significant correlation between the presence of cord atrophy and clinical disability.

Interestingly, Wiebe et al. [22] found that 12 of 25 newly detected cord plaques were not associated with any new clinical signs. Thus, a similar lack of precise clinical and

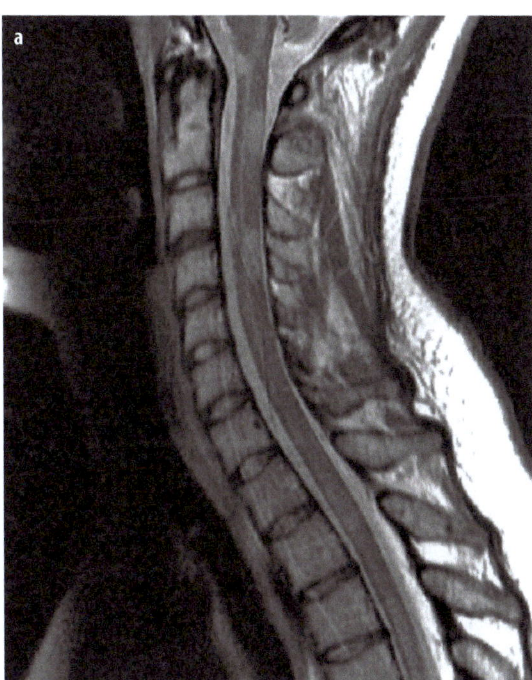

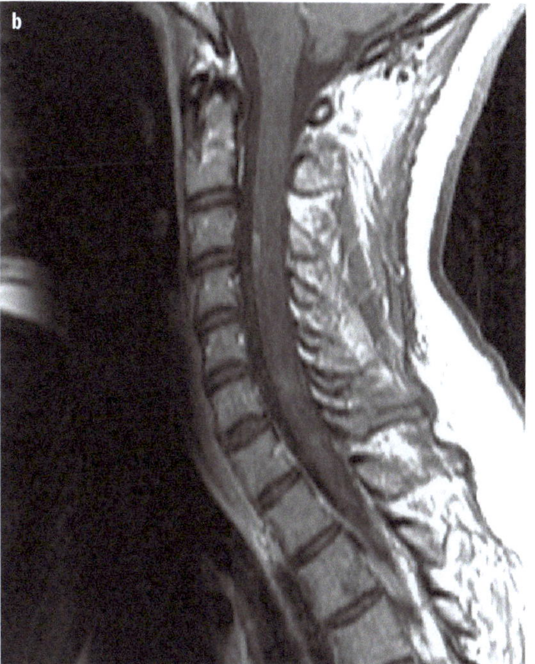

Fig. 3 a, b. Multiple sclerosis. Sagittal short tau inversion recovery (STIR) image shows multiple focal areas of T2 hyperintensity involving the cervical cord (**a**). Following contrast (**b**), the sagittal T1-weighted image shows several foci of cord enhancement consistent with areas of active demyelination

MRI correlation of anatomic localization of disease activity exists for spinal cord as well as brain MS. Lycklama a Nijeholt et al. [25] found that diffuse cord abnormalities were correlated with primary or secondary progressive clinical MS subtypes; diffuse disease was associated with cord atrophy and had a weak but significant correlation with clinical disability. Another study by Kidd et al. [26] in patients with primary progressive and secondary progressive MS showed no correlation between brain or spinal cord activity over 12 months and change in clinical disability, in a patient cohort in which 80% of the patients showed a change in EDSS ≥1 over the study period. The authors summarized by suggesting that serial imaging of the cord to detect new activity would not make a useful contribution to clinical therapeutic trials in patients with progressive MS.

Acute Transverse Myelopathy

Acute transverse myelopathy (ATM) is a monophasic, acute inflammatory process involving both halves of the spinal cord, producing paraplegia, a sensory impairment level, and sphincter dysfunction [27]. Longitudinal case series of ATM have revealed that approximately one-third of patients recover with little or no sequelae, one-third are left with a moderate degree of permanent disability, and one-third with severe disabilities.

The terms "acute transverse myelopathy" and "acute transverse myelitis" have often been used interchangeably in the literature, to some considerable confusion. Causes of acute transverse myelopathy includes inflammatory and non-inflammatory etiologies such as MS, viral infections, post-viral and post-vaccinial processes such as acute disseminated encephalomyelitis, collagen-vascular disorders such as systemic lupus erythematosis, vascular disorders, as in paraneoplastic syndrome or idiopathic [28-31]. There was a time when "acute transverse myelitis" was reserved for idiopathic cases, but currently "acute transverse myelopathy" is used to encompass the general clinical syndrome, whether or not the etiology is known. The MRI appearance is quite variable, with a large range in size of T2 hyperintense regions in the cord, although most commonly the lesions extend for three or four spinal segments. Unlike typical MS plaques, the area of high signal generally occupies more than two-thirds of the cross-sectional area of the cord on transverse images (Fig. 4). There is variable enlargement of the cord and variable enhancement patterns following gadolinium administration, including diffuse, patchy, and peripheral patterns [32]. Occasionally, ATM lesions mimic spinal cord tumors; thus, if the patient's clinical history is unrevealing, biopsy may be needed for diagnosis.

There is considerable interest in ATM as a clinically isolated syndrome in patients in whom the diagnostic criteria for MS are not yet fulfilled. MRI of the brain is a useful additional study. It revealed typical white matter changes of MS in approximately one-third of patients with ATM, and these patients had a high likelihood of developing clinically definite MS [28, 30]. Campi et al. [28] showed that patients with small, ovoid, enhancing spinal cord lesions without cord swelling were highly likely to develop clinically definite MS. Those with long segments of cord swelling, with inhomogeneous gadolinium enhancement, had no evolution to MS.

Inclusion criteria for acute transverse *myelitis* include [33]: (1) development of sensory, motor, or autonomic dysfunction attributable to the spinal cord; (2) bilateral signs and/or symptoms; (3) clearly defined sensory level; (4) exclusion of extra-axial compressive etiology by neuroimaging; (5) inflammation within the spinal cord demonstrated by CSF pleocytosis *or* elevated IgG index *or* gadolinium enhancement; and (6) progression to nadir between 4 h and 21 days following the onset of symptoms. For a diagnosis of "myelitis", there are notable exclusion criteria, including evidence of connective tissue diseases, CNS manifes-

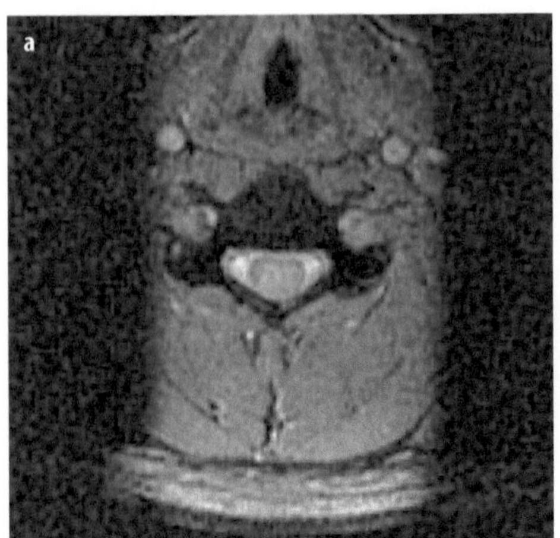

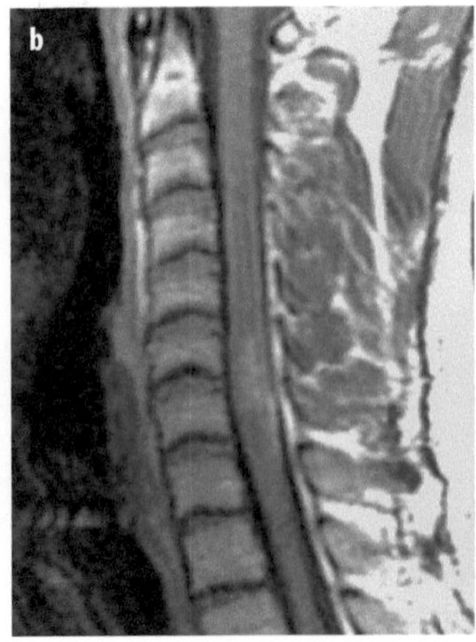

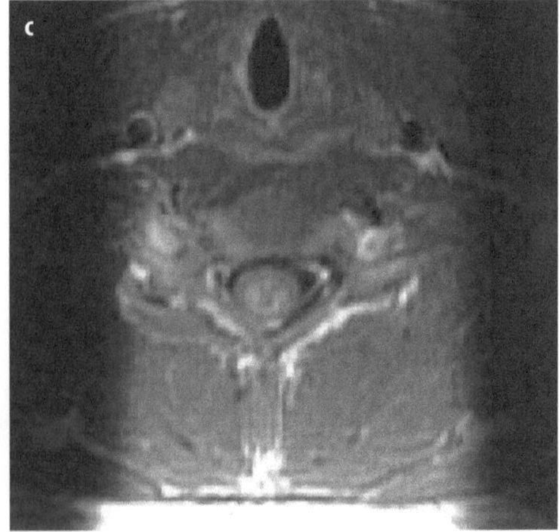

Fig. 4 a-c. Acute transverse myelitis. A 30-year-old patient with a monophasic episode of myelopathy. **a** Axial gradient echo image shows abnormal hyperintensity within the cervical cord. Enhanced T1-weighted sagittal (**b**) and axial (**c**) images show expansion and focal enhancement within the cervical cord at C6 and C7

tations of syphilis, Lyme disease, and human immunodeficiency virus (HIV), human T-cell lymphotrophic virus type 1 (HTLV-1), *Mycoplasma*, and other viral infections.

Neuromyelitis Optica (Devic's Syndrome)

Neuromyelitis optica (NMO) is an autoimmune, inflammatory disorder involving myelin of the neurons of optic nerves and spinal cord, with limited brain parenchymal involvement [34-37]. The classic imaging pattern is the presence of longitudinally extensive (>3 vertebral segments) T2 hyperintensity within the spinal cord and enhancement of the optic nerves (85% of cases) (Fig. 5).

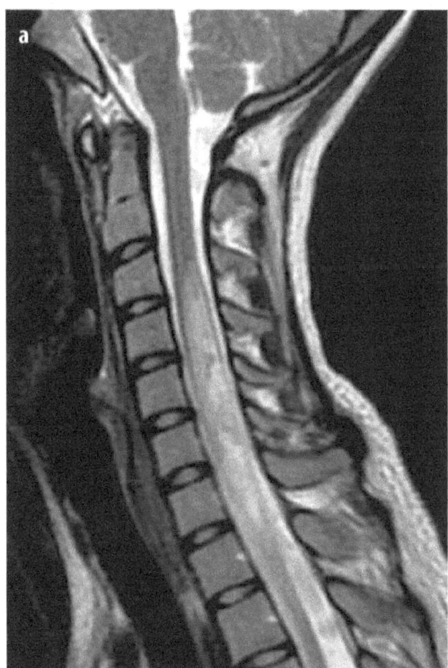

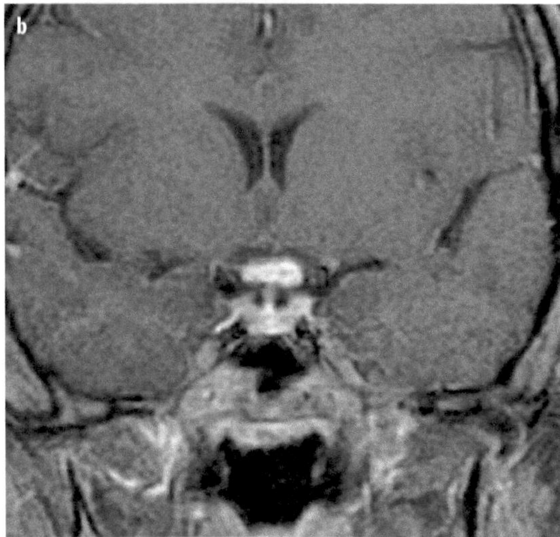

Fig. 5 a, b. Neuromyelitis optica. A 28-year-old female patient with optic neuritis and myelopathy. **a** Sagittal T2-weighted image shows a longitudinal extensive segment of T2 hyperintensity throughout the cervical cord. **b** Coronal T1-weighted image through the optic nerves shows diffuse enhancement of the optic chiasm

This disease has a clinical pattern distinct from that of MS in that it affects almost exclusively females, typically in the fourth decade, and leads to a more severe neurologic impairment. A previous infectious-inflammatory event may be involved in the pathogenesis of the disease, probably by triggering an autoimmune mechanism. The association of NMO with anti-DNA antibodies, systemic lupus erythematosus, Sjogren syndrome, and autoimmune thyroiditis has been shown.

Recently, a new serum autoantibody, NMO-IgG, has been detected that seems to distinguish between NMO and MS [38-40]. This test shows a 58-73% sensitivity and >90% specificity. Aquaporin-4, which is a water channel expressed in the brain, kidney, and stomach, is thought to be the target of NMO-IgG. Aquaporins are a family of trans-membrane channel proteins that are highly selective for the transport of water. These proteins function as bidirectional channels, facilitating the transport of water by diffusion along osmotic and hydrostatic gradients. AQP4 is the predominant water channel expressed in the brain; it is primarily an astroglial membrane protein, with highly polarized expression localized to astrocytic foot processes surrounding the cerebral capillary endothelium.

Revised NMO diagnostic criteria require optic neuritis, acute myelitis, and two of the following three characteristics: disease-onset brain MRI that is nondiagnostic for MS, contiguous spinal cord lesion, seen on MRI, and extending over three or more vertebral segments, and NMO-IgG seropositive status. Symptoms referable to CNS regions other than the optic nerve and spinal cord do not necessarily exclude the diagnosis of NMO [38].

AIDS

Spinal cord disease in AIDS is frequently overshadowed by other manifestations of the disease, however the incidence of spinal cord disease at autopsy is high [41]. There are several major categories of spinal cord disease in AIDS: those due to direct HIV infection (HIV myelitis); those due to opportunistic diseases or lymphoma; those associated with HIV, though of unclear etiology; and those related to vascular or metabolic disorders. HIV myelitis, which occurs in 5-8% of AIDS patients, is due to primary infection of the spinal cord, and is most often seen when the cerebral involvement is severe. There is inflammation with typical microglial nodules and multinucleated giant cells, predominately in the central gray region. Opportunistic infections of the spinal cord in AIDS include cytomegalovirus, fungal, toxoplasmosis, herpes simplex virus, varicella-zoster virus, tuberculosis, syphilis, and progressive multifocal leukoencephalopathy (PML).

Vacuolar myelopathy refers to a spongy degeneration in the spinal cord, predominately involving the posterior and lateral columns [41-43]. Vacuolar myelopathy is by far the most common spinal cord disease in AIDS, approaching an incidence of 50% in autopsy studies. It is a frequent cause of progressive ataxia and paraparesis in AIDS patients. The disease is most prominent in the mid-to lower thoracic cord, and is usually fairly symmetric in distribution over the cross-section of the cord. It is frequently most severe in the fasiculus gracilis. Histopathologically, there is prominent vacuolation of spinal white matter, with swelling within the myelin sheaths and splitting of lamellae. Axons may be normal, atrophic, or show secondary Wallerian degeneration. There is little active demyelination or inflammation, and there are some similarities to the changes seen in subacute combined degeneration. The fact that many AIDS patients are vitamin B12 deficient has resulted in speculation over possible etiologic links between the disorders, but this is not confirmed. MRI findings include cord atrophy in addition to symmetric hyperintensity in the dorsal columns on T2W images that can be traced over several spinal segments; less often, the lateral column is involved. There is no cord swelling or deformity, and, characteristically, there is no gadolinium enhancement. MRI findings of vacuolar myelopathy are generally distinctive, such that it can be differentiated from other spinal tract pathologies in AIDS, e.g., viral myelitis due to varicella-zoster virus, or cytomegalovirus radiculomyelitis, as discussed in the following section.

Viral Diseases

Varicella-zoster virus (VZV) infection in the CNS is rare in healthy populations, and it is also an infrequent opportunistic infection in patients with AIDS. Clinical recognition of the disease is difficult, because only one-third of patients present with the characteristic skin eruptions referred to as shingles. A neuropathologic study by Gray et al. [44] proposed five different patterns of CNS involvement in AIDS patients: multifocal leukoencephalitis, ventriculitis, acute meningomyeloradiculitis, focal necrotizing myelitis, and necrotizing angiitis involving leptomeningeal arteries with cerebral infarction. The multiple patterns of disease in the CNS from VZV infection suggest that there are multiple routes of spread to the CNS, including direct transneuronal and hematogenous routes, via CSF seeding, as well as the classically described reactivation of latent virus in the dorsal root ganglia that produces cutaneous shingles. This latter mechanism is likely in VZV myelitis, since it typically involves the posterior horn regions and spreads along axonal pathways primarily in the posterior columns. Pathologic changes of inflammation, demyelination, and hemorrhagic necrosis are seen. Thoracic cord involvement is most common, owing to the high frequency of thoracic-level dermatomal involvement in shingles. MRI reveals a swollen cord with patchy gadolinium enhancement, usually more posteriorly [44, 45] (Fig. 6). When VZV myelitis develops in association with cutaneous shingles, it typically is in the region of the cord corresponding to the involved dermatome, with possible focal enhancement of the corresponding dorsal root ganglia, nerve roots, and root entry zone. Myelitis may occur in conjunction with other CNS manifestations of VZV infection, such as leukoencephalitis.

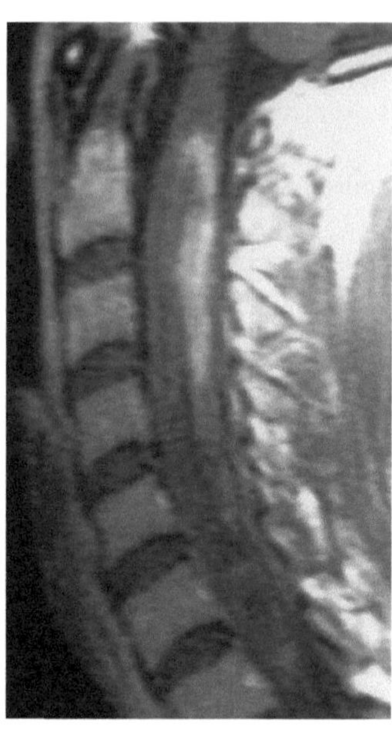

Fig. 6. Herpes myelitis. Sagittal T1-weighted image following contrast administration shows enlargement and diffuse enhancement of the cervical cord

Cytomegalovirus infection in the spinal cord produces a polyradiculomyelitis, which frequently involves the conus and nerve roots of the cauda equina [41, 46]. AIDS and other immune-compromised patients, as well as immune- competent individuals, may be affected. Typically, patients develop a flaccid paraparesis, saddle dysesthesia, and urinary retention. The paraparesis may be ascending, and a Guillian-Barre-like syndrome, associated with leg and/or back pain, may occur. CSF analysis reveals a polymorphonuclear pleocytosis. MRI reveals abnormal thickening, clumping, and enhancement of the nerve roots of the cauda equina, consistent with an inflammatory arachnoiditis. There is frequently abnormal peripheral pial and leptomeningeal enhancement over the spinal cord. The MRI pattern would suggest a differential diagnosis including carcinomatous and lymphomatous meningitis.

Poliomyelitis is a disease involving the anterior horn cells (lower motor neurons) in the ventral horns of the spinal cord. It classically produces an asymmetric, flaccid paralysis. Although poliomyelitis due to the natural polio virus has been virtually eradicated in Western countries, there are still several cases a year in the United States of vaccine-associated paralytic poliomyelitis, estimated to occur at a rate of approximately one per 2.5 million doses administered. In the acute infection, there is active inflammation, gliosis, and destruction of anterior horn cells. The characteristic MRI appearance described is that of local enlargement and abnormal signal in the ventral horns [47]. Chronically, the spinal cords of polio patients show loss of anterior horn cells, severe reactive gliosis, and persistent inflammation. There are rare, polio-like paralytic syndromes associated with other viruses, such as Coxsackie virus, echovirus, and enterovirus. A striking case of an acute paralytic syndrome secondary to Epstein-Barr virus encephalomyelitis was reported by Donovan et al. [48]. The patient exhibited striking inflammation and edema confined to the central gray of the cervical cord, as well as involvement of the cerebral gray matter structures in the basal ganglia and insula.

Infection with HTLV-1 can produce a slowly progressive myelopathy associated with spastic paraparesis [49]. The virus is highly endemic in Japan, Melanesia, the Caribbean, and some parts of Africa. HTLV-1-associated myelopathy (HAM) and tropical spastic paraparesis (TSP) are clinically, epidemiologically, and pathologically identical disorders. Patients usually have a slowly progressive course over several years, at which time MRI of the spinal cord reveals diffuse atrophy and abnormal signal intensity, most frequently involving the anterior and lateral columns. Rare patients have periods of rather acute progression of myelopathy, at which time mild cord swelling may be seen. Typically, there is peripheral gadolinium enhancement. Pathologically, there is loss of myelin and axons, with perivascular and parenchymal infiltration of inflammatory cells in white and gray matter tracts of the cord. Both HTLV-1 and HIV are human retroviruses that produce myelopathies; however, the clinicopathologic and MRI changes in HAM/TSP are quite different from those of vacuolar myelopathy in AIDS.

Bacterial Diseases

Bacterial spinal cord abscesses are relatively rare but can occur in septicemia, following spinal surgery, penetrating trauma, complicated meningitis, and associated with dysraphisms and dermal sinus tracts. The most common causative organisms are staphylococcal and streptococcus species. Cord swelling and edema are present, with a local, rim-enhancing collection in well-formed spinal cord abscesses. Unlike cerebral abscesses, whose temporal course of development is well-documented, the natural history of spinal cord abscesses is not well-described. Murphy et al. [50] observed evolutionary changes in the cord as infection progressed from myelitis to abscess formation. It is important to remember that patients may develop neurologic dysfunction prior to the development of a well-formed abscess, and thus the gadolinium enhancement characteristics of the disease may be variable [51].

Listeria monocytogenes may produce a primary meningoencephalomyelitis in healthy and in immune-compromised patients [52]. *Listeria* produces abscesses in the brainstem and upper cervical cord, as well as in the cerebral hemispheres. CSF analysis demonstrates a lymphocytic pleocytosis, but the organism is rarely discovered or cultured from CSF. Blood cultures may yield the gram-positive bacillus. *Listeria* meningoencephalomyelitis is a difficult clinical diagnosis, and fatal infections in patients with no predisposing factors have occurred.

Granulomatous Diseases

The pathologic and MRI findings characteristic of infectious granulomatous diseases, such as tuberculosis and syphilis, are similar to those of the major non-infectious granulomatous disease sarcoidosis. All of these entities can produce a granulomatous meningitis, myelitis, or radiculitis, and in any combination. Patients with tuberculous myelitis usually have evidence of primary or secondary tuberculous infection in the lungs, brain, or spine. Intramedullary tuberculomas may be solitary or multiple. They are generally well-defined, circumscribed lesions demonstrating avid gadolinium enhancement in a nodular or rim-enhancing fashion [29, 53, 54]. There is prominent cord edema and swelling, which may be related to cord ischemia secondary to vasculopathic changes.

Myelitis is a rare presentation of syphilis, and the granulomatous process has a predilection for the meninges, pial vessels, and sub-pial portions of the cord [55]. A swollen cord with patchy or nodular gadolinium enhancement is seen, especially in the cord periphery. Again, pathologic changes in the cord are thought to be due to a combination of granulomatous myelitis, and simultaneous cord ischemia due to granulomatous vasculitic changes.

Sarcoidosis is a multisystemic, idiopathic granulomatous disease that involves the CNS in approximately 5% of patients. Generally, patients with CNS sarcoidosis have evidence of pulmonary disease. Spinal sarcoidosis may involve the cervical and thoracic spinal cords as well as the intradural nerve roots. The acutely involved spinal cord is swollen, with variable patterns of enhancement following gadolinium administration, including uniform diffuse, multifocal patchy, nodular, or linear leptomeningeal enhancement [56].

Parasitic Diseases

Schistosomal infections are common worldwide, with endemic regions in Asia, the Caribbean, South America, and portions of Africa and Arabia. Since immigration has brought patients with schistosomal infections to North America, it is important for us to consider this disease here. Schistosomes are parasitic worms whose life cycle includes an asexual stage in an intermediate snail host, and an adult, sexual stage in vertebrate definitive hosts. Schistosomal larvae penetrate the skin of hosts who have been swimming in infested water. The larvae enter the lymphatic and venous systems, migrate to the lung and liver, mature, and take final residence in the mesenteric veins and vesical venous plexus. There are three schistosomes of clinical importance: *Schistosoma mansoni*, *S. haematobium*, and *S. japonicum*. Schistosomal myelitis is a relatively rare clinical manifestation of the disease, and *S. mansoni* is responsible for most cases. The organisms are thought to reach the spinal axis by migrating from pelvic and rectal veins into the paravertebral venous plexus, and finally to perimedullary veins. Schistosomal myelitis characteristically involves the conus, lower thoracic spinal cord, and cauda equina. Several basic patterns of spinal cord disease are seen, most commonly an intramedullary granulomatous mass, or an intradural-extramedullary granulomatous mass with compression of the conus [57]. Other forms include an acute transverse myelitis [58], which may be hemorrhagic and necrotizing [59], and an acute, anterior spinal artery syndrome. MRI reveals enlargement of the conus, occasionally somewhat irregular, nodular, or asymmetric, with increased signal intensity and patchy or nodular gadolinium enhancement. The appearance most frequently mimics a cord neoplasm. Schistosomal infection can be diagnosed by blood or CSF serology, and the ova may be recovered from the patient's stool. It is therefore important to elicit a clinical history of immigration from, or travel to endemic areas. This should prompt appropriate laboratory studies, enabling the diagnosis to be made without biopsy. Treatment with antiparasitic agents is usually curative, though occasionally laminectomy, myelotomy, and resection of the granulomatous mass are needed.

The parasitic disease toxoplasmosis is a common CNS pathogen in immune-compromised patients, but it rarely involves the spinal cord [41]. In AIDS patients, the spinal abscesses of toxoplasmosis usually present as enhancing intramedullary mass lesions, with extensive associated edema. Frequently, the presence of coexisting acute cerebral toxoplasma abscesses will suggest diagnosis of the spinal disease. Neurocysticercosis can involve the entire craniospinal axis, with cystic lesions in the brain, cord, and subarachnoid spaces [60, 61] (Fig. 7).

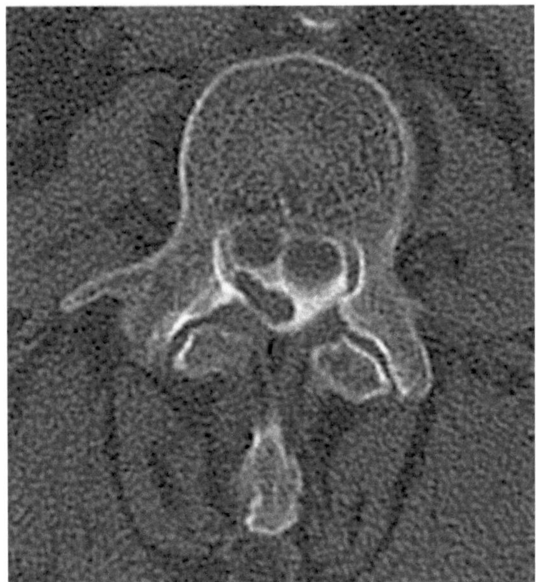

Fig. 7. Neurocysticercosis. Axial CT through the lumbar spine following intrathecal contrast administration shows several rounded filling defects within the lumbar subarachnoid space

Metabolic/Toxic Diseases

Subacute combined degeneration (SCD) is a complication of vitamin B12 deficiency, as may occur in pernicious anemia or with prolonged insufficient dietary intake. The pathologic changes of demyelination, axonal loss, and gliosis are seen in a roughly symmetric fashion, involving the dorsal and lateral columns of the thoracic and lower cervical cords. MRI may reveal increased signal intensity in the dorsal columns on T2W scans [62]. MRI has been less able to reveal the lateral column changes, even when present clinically. Interestingly, improvement in the MRI appearance has been described and corresponds to the improvement in clinical function following vitamin B12 supplementation. Nitrous oxide is a gaseous anesthetic agent also used as a propellant in the food industry; it is also abused as a recreational drug. Nitrous oxide toxicity can result in the identical pathophysiologic process as SCD, because nitrous oxide inactivates cobalamin (B12), which is essential in the metabolic processes that form and maintain myelin [63]. The myelopathy typically develops several weeks following exposure. Interestingly, myelopathy has been described in patients with normal B12 levels and high nitrous oxide exposure, as well as in patients with borderline B12 levels who have undergone surgical procedures in which nitrous oxide was the anesthetic agent. Again, abnormal signal intensity in the dorsal columns is seen.

Radiation Myelopathy

Radiation myelopathy is a complication of radiation therapy, most commonly seen in the cervical spinal cord of patients treated for head and neck malignancies with doses in the 50-70 Gy range [64, 65]. Radiation myelopathy is generally a subacute to chronic progressive myelopathy, with a variable latent period, generally several months to years following treatment. With the onset of clinical symptomatology, MRI reveals cord swelling, edema, and gadolinium enhancement, lasting for up to 8 months. During this phase, the histopathologic changes include edema, necrosis, demyelination, gliosis, and fibrinoid necrosis of small blood vessels. In patients with nasopharyngeal malignancies, the development of radiation myelopathy in the high cervical cord and medulla may be lethal. After approximately 8 months, the swelling gradually subsides, and progressive cord atrophy develops and eventually stabilizes over a few years in survivors. The pathologic gadolinium enhancement may persist even after the cord has become atrophic, but it has been shown to diminish over approximately 24 months. The cord damage frequently extends beyond the spatial distribution of the radiation exposure, although the main focus is always within the primary field.

References

1. Lisbona R, Rosenthal L (1977) Observations on the sequential use of Tc-99m phosphate complex and Ga-67 imaging in osteomyelitis, cellulitis, and septic arthritis. Radiology 123:123-129
2. Gelman MI, Coleman RE, Stevens PM et al (1978) Radiography radionuclide imaging and arthrography in the evaluation of total hip and knee replacement. Radiology 128:677-682
3. Weiss PPE, Mall JC, Hoffer PB et al (1979) Tc-99m methylene diphosphonate bone imaging in the evaluation of total hip prosthesis. Radiology 133:727-729
4. McAfee JG, Samin A (1985) In-111 labeled leukocytes: a review of problems in image interpretation. Radiology 155:221-229
5. Golimbu C, Firooznia H, Rafii M (1984) CT of osteomyelitis of the spine. AJR Am J Roentgenol 142:159-163
6. Modic MT, Feiglin DH, Piraino DW et al (1985) Vertebral osteomyelitis: assessment using MR. Radiology 157-166
7. Modic MT, Weinstein MA, Pavlicek W et al (1983) Nuclear magnetic resonance imaging of the spine. Radiology 148:757-762
8. deRoos A, Van Meerten EL, Bloem JL et al (1986) MRI of tuberculosis spondylitis. AJR Am J Roentgoenol 146:79-82
9. Dagirmanjian A, Schils J, Modic MT (1993) Vertebral osteomyelitis revisited. Radiology (Supplement) 189(P):193
10. Norman A, Kambolis CP (1964) Tumors of the spine and their relationship to the intervertebral disc. AJR Am J Roentgenol 92:1270-1274
11. Resnick D, Niwayama G (1978) Intervertebral disc abnormalities associated with intervertebral metastases: observation in patients and cadavers with prostatic cancer. Invest Radiol 13(3):182-190
12. Boden SD, Davis DO, Dina TS et al (1992) Postoperative diskitis: distinguishing early MR imaging findings from normal postoperative disk space changes. Radiology 184(3):765-771
13. Hlavin ML, Kaminski HJ, Ross JS, Ganz E (1990) Spinal epidural abscess: a ten-year perspective. Neurosurgery 27(2):177-184
14. Rankin RM, Flothow PG (1946) Pyogenic infection of the spinal epidural space. West J Surg Obstet Gynecol 54:320-323
15. Baker AS, Ojemann RG, Swartz MN, Richardson EP (1975) Spinal epidural abscess. N Engl J Med 293:463-468
16. Browder J, Meyers R (1941) Pyogenic infections of the spinal epidural space. Surgery 10:296-308
17. Angtuaco EJ, McConnell JR, Chadduck WM et al (1987) MR imaging of spinal epidural sepsis. AJNR Am J Neuroradiol 8:879-883
18. Post MJ, Quencer RM, Montalvo BM et al (1988) Spinal infection: evaluation with MR imaging and intraoperative US. Radiology 169:765-771
19. Post MJ, Sze G, Quencer RM et al (1990) Gadolinium-enhanced MR in spinal infection. J Comput Assist Tomogr 14(5):721-729
20. Tartaglino LM, Friedman DP, Flanders AE et al (1995) Multiple sclerosis in the spinal cord: MR appearance and correlation with clinical parameters. Radiology 195:725-732
21. Tartaglino LM, Flanders AE, Rapoport RJ (1994) Intramedullary causes of myelopathy. Semin Ultrasound CT MR 15:158-188
22. Wiebe S, Lee DH, Karlik SJ et al (1992) Serial cranial and spinal cord magnetic resonance imaging in multiple sclerosis. Ann Neurol 32:643-650
23. Kidd D, Thorpe JW, Thompson AJ et al (1993) Spinal cord MRI using multi-array coils and fast spin echo. Findings in multiple sclerosis. Neurology 43:2632-2637
24. Losseff NA, Webb SL, O'Riordan J et al (1996) Spinal cord atrophy and disability in multiple sclerosis. Brain 119:701-708
25. Lycklama A, Nijeholt GJ, Barkof F et al (1997) MR of the Spinal Cord in Multiple Sclerosis: Relation to clinical subtype and disability. AJNR Am J Neuroradiol 18:1041-1048
26. Kidd D, Thorpe JW, Kendall BE et al (1996) MRI dynamics of brain and spinal cord in progressive multiple sclerosis. J Neurol Neurosurg Psych 60:15-19
27. Choi KH, Lee KS, Chung SO et al (1996) Idiopathic transverse myelitis: MR characteristics. AJNR Am J Neuroradiol 17:1151-1160
28. Campi A, Filippi M, Comi G et al (1995) Acute transverse myelopathy: spinal and cranial MR study with clinical follow-up. AJNR Am J Neuroradiol 16:115-123
29. Gero B, Sze G, Sharif H (1991) MR Imaging of intradural inflammatory diseases of the spine. AJR Am J Roentgenol 12:1009-1019
30. Holtas S, Basibuyuk N, Fredriksson K (1993) MRI in acute transverse myelopathy. Neuroradiol 35:221-226
31. Mascalchi M, Cosottini M, Cellerini M et al (1998) MR of spinal cord involvement in Bechet's disease: case report. Neuroradiology 40:255-257
32. Pardatscher K, Fiore DL, Lavano A (1992) MR imaging of transverse myelitis using Gd-DTPA. J Neuroradiol 19:63-67
33. Transverse Myelitis Consortium Working Group (2002) Proposed diagnostic criteria and nosology of acute transverse myelitis. Neurology 59:499-505
34. Ghezzi A, Bergamaschi R, Martinelli V et al (2004) Clinical characteristics, course and prognosis of relapsing Devic's neuromyelitis optica. J Neurol 251:47-52
35. Wingerchuk DM, Lennon VA, Pittock SJ, Lucchinetti CF, Weinshenker BG (2006) Revised diagnostic criteria for neuromyelitis optica. Neurology 66:1485-1489
36. Weinshenker BG, Wingerchuk DM, Vukusic S et al (2006) Neuromyelitis optica IgG predicts relapse after longitudinally extensive transverse myelitis. Ann Neurol 59:566-569
37. Wingerchuk DM, Weinshenker BG (2003) Neuromyelitis optica: clinical predictors of a relapsing course and survival. Neurology 60:848-853
38. Wingerchuk DM (2007) Diagnosis and treatment of neuromyelitis optica. The Neurologist 13 (1)
39. Giovannoni G (2006) Neuromyelitis optica and anti-aquaporin-4 antibodies: widening the clinical phenotype. J Neurol Neurosurg Psychiatry 77:1001-1002
40. Bloch O, Manley GT (2007) The role of aquaporin-4 in cerebral water transport and edema. Neurosurg Focus 22(5):E3
41. Quencer RM, Post MJD (1997) Spinal cord lesions in patients with AIDS. Neuroimag Clin North Am 7:359-373
42. Sartoretti-Schefer S, Blattler T, Wichmann W (1997) Spinal MRI in patients with vacuolar myelopathy, and correlation with histopathological findings. Neuroradiology 39:865-869
43. Santosh CG, Bell JE, Best JJ (1995) Spinal tract pathology in AIDS: postmortem MRI correlation with neuropathology. Neuroradiology 37:134-138
44. Gray F, Belec L, Lescs MC et al (1994) Varicella zoster virus infection of the central nervous system in the acquired immune deficiency syndrome. Brain 117:987-999
45. Hirai T, Korogi Y, Hamatake S et al (1996) Case report: varicella zoster virus myelitis-serial MR findings. Br J Radiol 69:1187-1190
46. Hansman Whiteman ML, Dandapani BK, Shebert RT, Post MJD (1994) MRI of AIDS-related polyradiculomyelitis. J Comput Assist Tomogr 18:7-11
47. Malzberg MS, Rogg JM, Tate CM et al (1993) Poliomyelitis: hyperintensity of the anterior horn cells on MR images of the spinal cord. AJR Am J Roentgenol 161:863-865
48. Donovan WD, Zimmerman RD (1996) MRI findings of severe Epstein Barr virus encephalomyelitis. J Comput Assist Tomogr 20:1027-1029
49. Shakudo M, Inoue Y, Tsutada T (1999) HTLV-1 associated myelopathy: acute progression and atypical MR findings. AJNR Am J Neuroradiol 20:1417-1421
50. Murphy KJ, Brunberg JA, Quint DJ, Kazanjian PH (1998) Spinal cord infection: myelitis and abscess formation. AJNR Am J Neuroradiol 19:341-348

51. Friess HM, Wasenko JJ (1997) MR of staphylococcus myelitis of the cervical spinal cord. AJNR Am J Neuroradiol 18:455-458
52. King SJ, Jeffree MA (1993) MRI of an abscess of the cervical cord in a case of Listeria meningoencephalomyelitis. Neuroradiology 35:495-496
53. Sanchez Pernaute RS, Berciano J, Rebollo M et al (1996) Intramedullary tuberculoma of the spinal cord with syringomyelia. Neuroradiology 38:s105-s106
54. Yunten N, Alper H, Zileli M et al (1996) Tuberculous radiculomyelitis as a complication of spondilodiscitis: MR demonstration. J Neuroradiol 23:241-244
55. Nabatame H, Nakamura K, Matuda M (1992) MRI of syphilitic myelitis. Neuroradiology 34:105-106
56. Rieger J, Hosyen N (1994) Spinal cord sarcoidosis. Neuroradiology 36:627-628
57. Bennett G, Provenzale JM (1998) Schistosomal myelitis: findings at MR imaging. Eur J Radiol 27:268-270
58. Dupuis MJ, Atrouni S, Dooms GC et al (1990) MR imaging of schistosomal myelitis. AJNR Am J Neuroradiol 11:782-783
59. Silbergleit R (1992) Schistosomal granuloma of the spinal cord: evaluation with MR imaging and intraoperative sonography. AJR Am J Roentgenol 158:1351-1353
60. Leite CC, Jinkins JR, Escobar BE et al 1997) MR imaging of intramedullary and intradural-extramedullary spinal cysticercosis. AJR Am J Roentgoenol 169:1713-1717
61. Chang KH, Lee JH, Han MH, Han MC (1991) The role of contrast-enhanced imaging in the diagnosis of neurocysticercosis. AJNR Am J Neuroradiol 12:509-512
62. Timms SR, Cure JK, Kurent JE (1993) Subacute combined degeneration of the spinal cord: MR findings. AJNR Am J Neuroradiol 14:1224-1227
63. Pema PJ, Horak HA, Wyatt RH (1998) Myelopathy caused by nitrous oxide toxicity. AJNR Am J Neuroradiol 19:894-896
64. Wang PY, Shen WC, Jan JS (1995) Serial MRI changes in radiation myelopathy. Neuroradiol 37:374-377
65. Wang PY, Shen WC, Jan JS (1992) MR imaging in radiation myelopathy. AJNR Am J Neuroradiol 13:1049-1055

NUCLEAR MEDICINE SATELLITE COURSE
"DIAMOND"

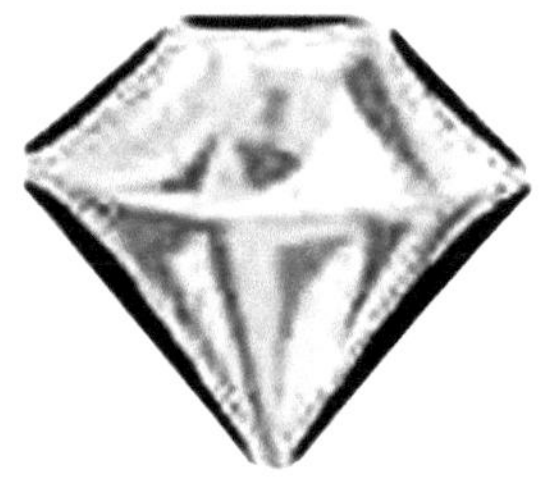

Positron Emission Tomography in the Evaluation of Brain Tumors

Alfred Buck

PET Center, University Hospital Zurich, Zurich, Switzerland

Introduction

Positron emission tomography (PET) has become a very valuable modality to evaluate different aspects of brain tumors. A good summary is given by two recent reviews [1, 2]. Simply stated, PET allows the quantitative measurement of radioactivity in a target volume based on the annihilation of positrons. The spatial resolution of state-of-the-art commercial PET scanners is in the order of 4-5 mm. Just as important for tumor evaluation is the tracer used, because it is the nature of the tracer which determines the biological properties of the healthy or diseased tissues that are measured. The useful clinical applications of PET in the evaluation of brain tumors are summarized in Table 1.

Grading of Gliomas

According to the system adopted by the World Health Organization, gliomas are classified from grade I to grade IV. Grade I and grade II gliomas are relatively benign, while grade IV corresponds to glioblastoma multiforme, one of the most malignant tumors. Histologically, there are three types of gliomas: astrocytomas, oligodendrocytomas, and mixed oligoastrocytomas.

Grading is important because it determines the management and the prognosis. In grade I and grade II tumors, a "wait and see" strategy can be considered, whereas in higher grades surgery is often mandatory. It would therefore be useful to have a non-invasive means to grade de-novo-detected brain lesions; but, unfortunately, none of the currently available non-invasive methods is accurate enough to obviate a biopsy. Although PET using 18F-fluorodeoxyglucose (FDG) is the most promising method to perform grading, its accuracy is too low. There are several reasons for this. One is that the grading system only holds for gliomas, and in newly detected brain lesions the tumor histology cannot be identified based on non-invasive imaging modalities such as magnetic resonance imaging (MRI). Another problem is that, for the same grade, oligodendrocytomas accumulate more FDG than astrocytomas. There are also low-grade tumors, such as pilocytic astrocytoma, which take up large amounts of FDG, and high grade tumors with only marginal FDG uptake. Sometimes the tumor rim in a glioblastoma is so thin that the true FDG uptake is severely underestimated. One other issue should be clarified: while FDG uptake is related to glucose metabolism, the quantitative relationship between the two is markedly different in healthy tissue vs. tumor tissue. Moreover, it has been convincingly demonstrated, that the increased FDG uptake in certain brain tumors is not associated with increased glucose metabolism [3].

Grading is more accurate in a recurring tumor in which the original histology was known. Often, the recurrence is of a higher grade than the original tumor.

Table 1. Indications for positron emission tomography (PET) evaluation of the brain

Indication	Tracer
Grading of gliomas	FDG
Separating necrosis from tumor	FDG, amino-acid analogs
Separating toxoplasmosis from lymphoma	FDG
Identification of optimal biopsy location	FDG

FDG[18], F-fluorodeoxyglucose

Separating Recurrent Tumor from Radiation Necrosis or Post-operative Changes

The idea behind this very good clinical application of PET is that there is no metabolism in dead tissue, such as a necrosis; therefore such lesions should be devoid of FDG in uptake studies. However, in practice, the situation is more difficult. The problem is the high physiologic FDG uptake of normal brain tissue. Radiation necrosis is characterized by decreased FDG accumulation, which is much more difficult to assess than foci of increased uptake (relative to normal brain tissue). This is most likely a reason for the wide spread between the sensitivity (81-

86%) and specificity (40-94%) for distinguishing tumor and necrosis [4]. As in most brain applications, co-registration of PET images with MRI is a must. In one published study, the sensitivity of detecting a radiation-necrosis-derived increase ranged from 65 to 86% when MRI was used for co-registration [5].

It seems that amino-acid analogs are more sensitive and more specific in identifying radiation necrosis. One of the most widely used of these tracers is ^{11}C-methionine. In a study involving 21 patients, this tracer correctly identified10 of 12 radiation injuries [6]. However, ^{11}C-labeled tracers are impractical due to their short half-life. In an experimental study in rats, we demonstrated that the ^{18}F-labeled compound fluoro-ethyl-tyrosine (FET) is very promising, since it did not accumulate in radiation injuries [7], but was instead avidly taken up by the tumors [8,9]. In another study, comprising 53 patients, the recurrence of gliomas was correctly diagnosed in 100% of the patients who were examined using the tracer FET [10].

Separation of Toxoplasmosis from Lymphoma

This application is most commonly used in HIV patients, in whom the correct diagnosis is essential for proper treatment. The diagnosis of lymphoma can be made with FDG PET [11]. Cerebral lymphomas are among the brain tumors with the highest tracer uptake. In contrast, toxoplasmosis lesions take up less FDG than normal gray matter.

Identification of the Optimal Biopsy Location

Stereotactic biopsies are the standard procedure in the evaluation of brain tumors. Since many brain tumors are very heterogeneous with respect to malignancy, it is important to take the biopsy from the most malignant part of the tumor. This part can be identified with either FDG [12,13], ^{11}C-methionine, or FET as the tracer. Often, the increased aggressiveness of a tumor is associated with increases in blood volume due to neoangiogenesis. This increased blood volume can be identified using MRI techniques, which are now increasingly applied to localize the ideal biopsy site [14,15]. However, it is probably the combination of MRI and PET that yields the best results. In one study [16], the specificity of MRI for detecting tumor was increased from 53 to 93% when the information obtained from FET PET was added.

References

1. Chen W (2007) Clinical applications of PET in brain tumors. J Nucl Med 48(9):1468-1481
2. Herholz K, Coope D, Jackson A (2007) Metabolic and molecular imaging in neuro-oncology. Lancet Neurol 6(8):711-724
3. Krohn KA, Mankoff DA, Muzi M et al (2005) True tracers: comparing FDG with glucose and FLT with thymidine. Nucl Med Biol 32(7):663-671
4. Langleben DD, Segall GM (2000) PET in differentiation of recurrent brain tumor from radiation injury. J Nucl Med 41(11):1861-1867
5. Chao ST, Suh JH, Raja S et al (2001) The sensitivity and specificity of FDG PET in distinguishing recurrent brain tumor from radionecrosis in patients treated with stereotactic radiosurgery. Int J Cancer 96(3):191-197
6. Tsuyuguchi N, Sunada I, Iwai Y et al (2003) Methionine positron emission tomography of recurrent metastatic brain tumor and radiation necrosis after stereotactic radiosurgery: is a differential diagnosis possible? J Neurosurg 98(5):1056-1064
7. Spaeth N, Wyss MT, Weber B et al (2004) Uptake of 18F-fluorocholine, 18F-fluoroethyl-L-tyrosine, and 18F-FDG in acute cerebral radiation injury in the rat: implications for separation of radiation necrosis from tumor recurrence. J Nucl Med 45(11):1931-1938
8. Wyss MT, Spaeth N, Biollaz G et al (2007) Uptake of 18F-Fluorocholine, 18F-FET, and 18F-FDG in C6 gliomas and correlation with 131I-SIP(L19), a marker of angiogenesis. J Nucl Med 48(4):608-614
9. Spaeth N, Wyss MT, Pahnke J et al (2006) Uptake of 18F-fluorocholine, 18F-fluoro-ethyl-L: -tyrosine and 18F-fluoro-2-deoxyglucose in F98 gliomas in the rat. Eur J Nucl Med Mol Imaging 33(6):673-682
10. Popperl G, Gotz C, Rachinger W et al (2004) Value of O-(2-[18F]fluoroethyl)- L-tyrosine PET for the diagnosis of recurrent glioma. Eur J Nucl Med Mol Imaging 31(11):1464-1470
11. Basso U, Brandes AA (2002) Diagnostic advances and new trends for the treatment of primary central nervous system lymphoma. Eur J Cancer 38(10):1298-1312
12. Hanson MW, Glantz MJ, Hoffman JM et al (1991) FDG-PET in the selection of brain lesions for biopsy. J Comput Assist Tomogr 15(5):796-801
13. Pirotte B, Goldman S, Massager N, et al (2004) Comparison of 18F-FDG and 11C-methionine for PET-guided stereotactic brain biopsy of gliomas. J Nucl Med 45(8):1293-1298
14. Aronen HJ, Pardo FS, Kennedy DN, et al (2000) High microvascular blood volume is associated with high glucose uptake and tumor angiogenesis in human gliomas. Clin Cancer Res 6(6): 2189-2200
15. Cha S, Knopp EA, Johnson G et al (2002) Intracranial mass lesions: dynamic contrast-enhanced susceptibility-weighted echo-planar perfusion MR imaging. Radiology 223(1):11-29
16. Pauleit D, Floeth F, Hamacher K et al (2005) O-(2-[18F]fluoroethyl)-L-tyrosine PET combined with MRI improves the diagnostic assessment of cerebral gliomas. Brain 128(Pt 3): 678-687

Imaging of Dementia

Karl Herholz

Wolfson Molecular Imaging Centre, The University of Manchester, Manchester, United Kingdom

Introduction

PET and SPECT are well-established tools to detect synaptic dysfunction in Alzheimer's disease (AD). SPECT tracers, such as Tc-99m-HMPAO, are used for imaging blood flow, while F-18-fluorodeoxyglucose (FDG) is used with PET for imaging cerebral glucose consumption (see reviews by [1, 2]). In normal subjects, regional glucose metabolism and blood flow are tightly coupled to neuronal function, while in neurodegenerative disease both are reduced due to regional synaptic dysfunction. Scans must be obtained under well-controlled standard conditions to avoid confounding effects by uncontrolled brain activation. Thus, while this review largely refers to FDG PET as the most accurate imaging tool to assess synaptic dysfunction in dementia, many aspects can also be addressed by blood-flow SPECT, albeit with somewhat lower accuracy [3].

Main Findings in Alzheimer's Disease

Over more than 20 years, multiple studies have demonstrated that glucose metabolism and blood flow are impaired in temporal-parietal association cortices, with the angular gyrus usually being the center of the metabolic impairment. Frontal association cortex may also be involved, but more variably so, usually to a lesser degree, and only during progression of AD. There may be a distinct hemispheric asymmetry, which usually corresponds to the predominant cognitive deficits (language impairment in the dominant and visuospatial disorientation in the subdominant hemisphere). In contrast to other dementia types, glucose metabolism in basal ganglia, primary motor and visual cortex, and cerebellum is usually well preserved. This pattern generally reflects AD clinical symptoms, with impairment of memory and associative thinking, including higher-order sensory processing and planning of action, but with relative preservation of primary motor and sensory function.

Voxel-based comparisons with normal reference samples clearly showed that the posterior cingulate gyrus and the precuneus are also impaired at an early stage of AD [4]. This is usually not directly obvious by mere inspection of FDG PET scans because metabolism in that area is above the cortical average in the normal brain at resting state [5], and with beginning impairment it returns to the level of surrounding cortex but does not become evident as a hypometabolic lesion. Thus, this important diagnostic sign is easily missed by standard visual interpretation of FDG PET brain scans. On the background of sufficient numbers of FDG PET scans in normal controls, it is increasingly becoming standard to base the interpretation of patient studies not merely on visual interpretation of tracer distribution, but also on quantitative mapping with reference to an appropriate normal sample [6-8].

Longitudinal Studies and Trials

Longitudinal studies have demonstrated the severity and extent of metabolic impairment in temporal and parietal cortex increases with dementia progression, and frontal reductions become more evident [9, 10]. The reduction of metabolism is in the order of 16-19% over 3 years in association cortices, which contrasts with an absence of significant decline in normal control subjects [11]. Asymmetrical metabolic impairment and associated predominance of language or visuospatial impairment tends to persist during the progression of AD [12, 13]. Based on these observations, FDG PET can serve as a surrogate marker in therapeutic trials [14]. If the change due to disease progression are monitored over 1 year using standard neuropsychological testing by MMSE and ADAS-cog, coefficients of variance (COV) around 100% are typically obtained for these changes, whereas PET measurements are subject to about 50% COV, thus doubling t-scores and reducing the required sample size by about 75% at the same study power [15, 16].

Mild Cognitive Impairment and Early Diagnosis of AD

Even at an asymptomatic stage, impairment of the regional cerebral metabolic rate of glucose consumption (rCMRglc) has been observed in individuals at high risk for AD due to family history of AD and possession of the ApoE 4 allele [17, 18] and this abnormality is seen decades before the likely onset of dementia [19]. In middle-aged and elderly asymptomatic ApoE 4-positive individuals, temporoparietal and posterior cingulate rCMRglc values decline by about 2% per year [20].

The first study noting the predictive power of posterior cingulate metabolism in patients with severe memory deficits for predicting progression was carried out by Minoshima et al. in 1997 [4]. This observation was followed by several studies indicating a high predictive power, with sensitivity and specificity above 80% for prediction of rapid progression. Recent studies found FDG PET clearly superior to ApoE 4 testing [21] and demonstrated that a normal FDG PET in mild cognitive impairment (MCI) indicates a low chance of progression within 1 year even if there is a severe memory deficit on neuropsychological testing [22].

Mesial temporal metabolic impairment has been observed as a general feature in patients with memory impairment, including but not limited to patients with MCI and AD [23-25]. Hippocampal and entorhinal metabolic impairment is difficult to assess visually on PET scans because of the small size, lower normal metabolism than neocortical association cortices, and partial volume effects due to early and significant hippocampal atrophy in MCI and AD. Nevertheless, predictive power for development of MCI has been demonstrated in a 3-year follow-up study of cognitively normal subjects [26].

Frontotemporal Lobar Degeneration

Several diseases feature frontotemporal dementia (FTD) as the most frequent manifestation and also more focal degenerative processes, such as primary progressive aphasia and semantic dementia [27]. Cerebral glucose metabolism is impaired mostly in the frontal cortex, especially in the mesial frontal cortex [28]. Frontolateral and anterior temporal cortices are often also impaired severely; this impairment is related to the clinical symptoms of aphasia or semantic memory deficits and may be very asymmetric [29, 30]. Milder metabolic changes often involve large parts of the brain [31]. The regional pattern of predominantly frontal impairment usually allows clear distinction from AD, although there may be overlap as AD can involve frontal regions as well and FTD may not spare the temporoparietal cortex. It was recently shown in a series of 45 patients with pathologically confirmed diagnosis that FDG PET can discriminate FTD from AD with more than 85% sensitivity and specificity [32].

Dementia with Lewy Bodies

Dementia with Lewy bodies (DLB) is clinically characterized by fluctuating consciousness, possible Parkinsonian motor features, and impairment of visual perception including hallucinations. The latter are the likely correlate of a reduction of glucose metabolism in primary visual cortex, described with FDG PET in DLB, in addition to an impairment of posterior association areas as in AD [33]. In contrast, metabolic activity in primary visual cortex is usually well-preserved in AD, but in practice the distinction may be difficult as metabolic activity in that area is subject to considerable variability and depends on examination conditions (eyes open or eyes closed). A more reliable imaging feature to differentiate DLB from AD is the impairment of dopamine synthesis and transport [34], which can be assessed with 18F-fluorodopa (as described later).

Imaging Amyloid Deposition

The development of PET tracers designed to label amyloid plaques in vivo is currently an area of great research interest. The deposition of amyloid-β (Aβ) is an early event in the pathogenesis of AD [35] and is central in the amyloid cascade hypothesis [36]. The first tracer to be used to label Aβ selectively in vivo was 11C-labeled thioflavin analogue, named for convenience Pittsburgh compound B (11C-PIB) [37]. It provides high sensitivity in detecting amyloid plaques and vascular amyloid in human brain in vivo [38-40]. Its clinical specificity for AD is currently being studied and it has been shown that patients with FTD do not show increased 11C-PIB binding [41].

A number of other compounds have been tested for amyloid imaging in humans, and most of them have properties similar to 11C-PIB without offering clear advantages so far [42]. One compound, 18F-FDDNP, binds to neurofibrillary tangles as well as to amyloid plaques and differentiates persons with MCI from those with AD and those with no cognitive impairment [43], but provides a substantially weaker imaging signal that 11C-PIB.

Imaging Neurotransmitter Systems

Major transmitter systems that are known to be impaired in AD are the cholinergic, serotonergic, and noradrenergic innervation of cerebral cortex. In Parkinson's disease (PD) and related dementia, the dopaminergic system is also impaired. The contribution of these systems to disease symptomatology has not yet been studied in depth in humans, and there are indications that impairment of these diffuse ascending projections may interact with the formation of pathological protein deposits, such as amyloid plaques and alpha-synuclein, in dementia [44, 45].

Cholinergic Receptors

The main receptor types for acetylcholine in the CNS are muscarinergic, with subtypes M1 and M2, and nicotinergic. Nicotinic receptors have attracted the most interest but available tracers still suffer from methodological limitations. 11C-nicotine has a high level of unspecific binding [46] and 18F-A-85380 suffers from very slow binding kinetics [47, 48]. There is reduced cortical binding of C-11-nicotine in AD [49].

As the cholinergic axons degenerate, acetylcholinesterase (AChE) activity is reduced [50]. Labeled analogues of acetylcholine that are also substrates for AChE can be used to measure and image the activity of the enzyme in vivo. These are C-11-N-methyl-4-piperidyl-acetate (MP4A, also known as AMP) [51], which is 94% specific for AChE in human brain, and C-11-N-methyl-4-piperidyl-propionate (MP4P, or PMP) [52]. There have been several studies measuring AChE activity and all of them found a reduction of cortical activity in AD [53-56], most severely affecting temporal cortex. The technique has also been used to measure drug-induced AChE inhibition in AD patients, which for all currently available cholinesterase inhibitors at standard clinical dose is in the range of 30 to 40% [57-59].

Dopamine

The most widely used PET tracer to examine dopamine synthesis and vesicular storage is 18F-fluorodopa [60], while dopamine transport can also be assessed with SPECT [61]. A deficit of dopamine synthesis and transport similar to PD has been found in DLB, even at a stage when Parkinsonism may not yet be prominent [34], while it is normal in patients with AD. In contrast to the cholinergic impairment which is severe in DLB but only mild in PD without dementia, the dopaminergic deficit does not appear to be related to dementia [62].

Conclusions

Brain PET using FDG is a firmly established technique for demonstration of regional functional impairment in neurodegenerative disease, while blood-flow SPECT addresses similar issues with somewhat lower accuracy. AD is associated with typical regional impairment of posterior cortical association areas, which allows very early diagnosis before clinical manifestation of dementia as well as monitoring of progression and treatment effects. DLB additionally involves metabolic impairment of primary visual cortex. Predominant impairment of frontal and anterior temporal regions is seen in FTD, primary progressive aphasia, and semantic dementia. New perspectives are being opened by tracers for imaging amyloid; these appear to be very sensitive to detect even preclinical AD cases, although confirmation of their specificity remains to be demonstrated. Tracers for measuring local AChE activity and the binding capacity of nicotinic and serotonergic receptors address neurotransmitter deficits in dementia. The impairment of dopamine synthesis that is characteristic for DLB can be demonstrated by 18F-fluorodopa PET and dopamine transporter SPECT.

References

1. Dougall NJ, Bruggink S, Ebmeier KP (2004) Systematic review of the diagnostic accuracy of 99mTc-HMPAO-SPECT in dementia. Am J Geriatr Psychiatry12:554-570
2. Herholz K (2003) PET studies in dementia. Ann Nucl Med 17:79-89
3. Herholz K, Schopphoff H, Schmidt M et al (2002) Direct comparison of spatially normalized PET and SPECT scans in Alzheimer disease. J Nucl Med 43:21-26
4. Minoshima S, Giordani B, Berent S et al (1997) Metabolic reduction in the posterior cingulate cortex in very early Alzheimer's disease. Ann Neurol 42:85-94
5. Gusnard DA, Raichle ME, Raichle ME (2001) Searching for a baseline: functional imaging and the resting human brain. Nat Rev Neurosci 2:685-694
6. Herholz K, Salmon E, Perani D et al (2002) Discrimination between Alzheimer dementia and controls by automated analysis of multicenter FDG PET. Neuroimage 17:302-316
7. Burdette JH, Minoshima S, Vander Borght T et al (1996) Alzheimer disease: improved visual interpretation of PET images by using three-dimensional stereotaxic surface projections. Radiology 198:837-843
8. Ishii K, Willoch F, Minoshima S et al (2001) Statistical brain mapping of 18F-FDG PET in Alzheimer's disease: validation of anatomic standardization for atrophied brains. J Nucl Med 42:548-557
9. Jagust WJ, Friedland RP, Budinger TF et al (1988) Longitudinal studies of regional cerebral metabolism in Alzheimer's disease. Neurology 38:909-912
10. Mielke R, Herholz K, Grond M et al (1994) Clinical deterioration in probable Alzheimer's disease correlates with progressive metabolic impairment of association areas. Dementia 5:36-41
11. Smith GS, de Leon MJ, George AE et al (1992) Topography of cross-sectional and longitudinal glucose metabolic deficits in Alzheimer's disease. Pathophysiologic implications. Arch Neurol 49:1142-1150
12. Grady CL, Haxby JV, Schlageter NL et al (1986) Stability of metabolic and neuropsychological asymmetries in dementia of the Alzheimer type. Neurology 36:1390-1392
13. Haxby JV, Grady CL, Koss E et al (1990) Longitudinal study of cerebral metabolic asymmetries and associated neuropsychological patterns in early dementia of the Alzheimer type. Arch Neurol 47:753-760
14. Heiss WD, Kessler J, Mielke R et al (1994) Long-term effects of phosphatidylserine, pyritinol, and cognitive training in Alzheimer's disease. A neuropsychological, EEG, and PET investigation. Dementia 5:88-98
15. Alexander GE, Chen K, Pietrini P et al (2002) Longitudinal PET evaluation of cerebral metabolic decline in dementia: a potential outcome measure in Alzheimer's disease treatment studies. Am J Psychiatry 159:738-745
16. Hirono N, Hashimoto M, Ishii K et al (2004) One-year change in cerebral glucose metabolism in patients with Alzheimer's disease. J Neuropsychiatry Clin Neurosci 16:488-492
17. Small GW, Mazziotta JC, Collins MT et al (1995) Apolipoprotein E type 4 allele and cerebral glucose metabolism in relatives at risk for familial Alzheimer disease. JAMA 273:942-947
18. Reiman EM, Caselli RJ, Yun LS et al (1996) Preclinical evidence of Alzheimer's disease in persons homozygous for the epsilon 4 allele for apolipoprotein E. N Engl J Med 334:752-758
19. Reiman EM, Chen K, Alexander GE et al (2004) Functional brain abnormalities in young adults at genetic risk for late-onset Alzheimer's dementia. Proc Natl Acad Sci USA 101:284-289
20. Small GW, Ercoli LM, Silverman DH et al (2000) Cerebral metabolic and cognitive decline in persons at genetic risk for Alzheimer's disease. Proc Natl Acad Sci USA 97:6037-6042

21. Drzezga A, Grimmer T, Riemenschneider M et al (2005) Prediction of individual clinical outcome in MCI by means of genetic assessment and (18)F-FDG PET. J Nucl Med 46:1625-1632
22. Anchisi D, Borroni B, Franceschi M et al (2005) Heterogeneity of brain glucose metabolism in mild cognitive impairment and clinical progression to Alzheimer disease. Arch Neurol 62:1728-1733
23. Heiss WD, Pawlik G, Holthoff V et al (1992) PET correlates of normal and impaired memory functions. Cerebrovasc Brain Metab Rev 4:1-27
24. Nestor PJ, Fryer TD, Smielewski P, Hodges JR (2003) Limbic hypometabolism in Alzheimer's disease and mild cognitive impairment. Ann Neurol 54:343-351
25. Mosconi L, Tsui WH, DeSanti S et al (2005) Reduced hippocampal metabolism in MCI and AD: automated FDG-PET image analysis. Neurology 64:1860-1867
26. de Leon MJ, Convit A, Wolf OT et al (2001) Prediction of cognitive decline in normal elderly subjects with 2-F-18-fluoro-2-deoxy-D-glucose positron-emission tomography (FDG PET). Proc Natl Acad Sci USA 98:10966-10971
27. Neary D, Snowden J, Mann D (2005) Frontotemporal dementia. Lancet Neurol 4:771-780
28. Salmon E, Garraux G, Delbeuck X et al (2003) Predominant ventromedial frontopolar metabolic impairment in frontotemporal dementia. Neuroimage 20:435-440
29. Diehl J, Grimmer T, Drzezga A, Riemenschneider M, Forstl H, Kurz A (2004) Cerebral metabolic patterns at early stages of frontotemporal dementia and semantic dementia. A PET study. Neurobiol Aging 25:1051-1056
30. Chawluk JB, Mesulam MM, Hurtig H et al (1986) Slowly progressive aphasia without generalized dementia: studies with positron emission tomography. Ann Neurol 19:68-74
31. Ishii K, Sakamoto S, Sasaki M et al (1998) Cerebral glucose metabolism in patients with frontotemporal dementia. J Nucl Med 39:1875-1878
32. Foster NL, Heidebrink JL, Clark CM et al (2007) FDG-PET improves accuracy in distinguishing frontotemporal dementia and Alzheimer's disease. Brain 130(Pt 10):2616-2635
33. Minoshima S, Foster NL, Sima AA et al (2001) Alzheimer's disease versus dementia with Lewy bodies: cerebral metabolic distinction with autopsy confirmation. Ann Neurol 50:358-365
34. Hu XS, Okamura N, Arai H et al (2000) 18F-fluorodopa PET study of striatal dopamine uptake in the diagnosis of dementia with lewy bodies. Neurology 55:1575-1577
35. Braak H, Braak E (1991) Neuropathological staging of Alzheimer-related changes. Acta Neuropathologica 82:239-259
36. Hardy JA, Higgins GA (1992) Alzheimer's disease: the amyloid cascade hypothesis. Science 256:184-185
37. Klunk WE, Engler H, Nordberg A et al (2004) Imaging brain amyloid in Alzheimer's disease with Pittsburgh Compound-B. Ann Neurol 55:306-319
38. Edison P, Archer HA, Hinz R et al (2007) Amyloid, hypometabolism, and cognition in Alzheimer disease: an [11C]PIB and [18F]FDG PET study. Neurology 68:501-508
39. Kemppainen NM, Aalto S, Wilson IA et al (2006) Voxel-based analysis of PET amyloid ligand [11C]PIB uptake in Alzheimer disease. Neurology 67:1575-1580
40. Nordberg A (2004) PET imaging of amyloid in Alzheimer's disease. Lancet Neurol 3:519-527
41. Rabinovici GD, Furst AJ, O'Neil JP et al (2007)11C-PIB PET imaging in Alzheimer disease and frontotemporal lobar degeneration. Neurology 68:1205-1212
42. Klunk WE, Lopresti B, Nebes RD et al (2006) Development and application of beta-amyloid imaging agents in Alzheimer's disease. In: Herholz K, Perani D, Morris CM (eds) The dementias: early diagnosis and evaluation. Dekker, New York, pp 279-310
43. Small GW, Kepe V, Ercoli LM et al (2006) PET of brain amyloid and tau in mild cognitive impairment. N Engl J Med 355:2652-2663
44. Heneka MT, Ramanathan M, Jacobs AH et al (2006) Locus ceruleus degeneration promotes Alzheimer pathogenesis in amyloid precursor protein 23 transgenic mice. J Neurosci 26:1343-1354
45. Braak H, Rub U, Schultz C, Del Tredici K (2006) Vulnerability of cortical neurons to Alzheimer's and Parkinson's diseases. J Alzheimers Dis 9:35-44
46. Nordberg A, Lundqvist H, Hartvig P et al (1995) Kinetic analysis of regional (S)(-)11C-nicotine binding in normal and Alzheimer brains – in vivo assessment using positron emission tomography. Alzheimer Dis Assoc Disord 9:21-27
47. Bottlaender M, Valette H, Roumenov D et al (2003) Biodistribution and radiation dosimetry of (18)f-fluoro-a-85380 in healthy volunteers. J Nucl Med 44:596-601
48. Mamede M, Ishizu K, Ueda M et al (2004) Quantification of human nicotinic acetylcholine receptors with 123I-5IA SPECT. J Nucl Med 45:1458-1470
49. Kadir A, Almkvist O, Wall A et al (2006) PET imaging of cortical 11C-nicotine binding correlates with the cognitive function of attention in Alzheimer's disease. Psychopharmacology (Berl) 188:509-520
50. Mesulam M, Giacobini E (2000) Neuroanatomy of cholinesterases in the normal human brain and in Alzheimer's disease. In: Cholinesterases and cholinesterase inhibitors. Martin Dunitz, London, pp 121-137
51. Namba H, Irie T, Fukushi K, Iyo M (1994) In vivo measurement of acetylcholinesterase activity in the brain with a radioactive acetylcholine analog. Brain Res 667:278-282
52. Kilbourn MR, Snyder SE, Sherman PS, Kuhl DE (1996) In vivo studies of acetylcholinesterase activity using a labeled substrate, n-[C-11]methylpiperdin-4-yl propionate ([C-11]PMP). Synapse 22:123-131
53. Kuhl DE, Koeppe RA, Minoshima S et al (1999) In vivo mapping of cerebral acetylcholinesterase activity in aging and Alzheimer's disease. Neurology 52:691-699
54. Iyo M, Namba H, Fukushi K et al (1997) Measurement of acetylcholinesterase by positron emission tomography in the brains of healthy controls and patients with Alzheimers disease. Lancet 349:1805-1809
55. Herholz K, Bauer B, Wienhard K et al (2000) In-vivo measurements of regional acetylcholine esterase activity in degenerative dementia: comparison with blood flow and glucose metabolism. J Neural Transm 12:1457-1468
56. Rinne JO, Kaasinen V, Jarvenpaa T et al (2003) Brain acetylcholinesterase activity in mild cognitive impairment and early Alzheimer's disease. J Neurol Neurosurg Psychiatry 74:113-115
57. Bohnen NI, Kaufer DI, Hendrickson R et al (2005) Degree of inhibition of cortical acetylcholinesterase activity and cognitive effects by donepezil treatment in Alzheimer's disease. J Neurol Neurosurg Psychiatry 76:315-319
58. Kaasinen V, Nagren K, Jarvenpaa T et al (2002) Regional effects of donepezil and rivastigmine on cortical acetylcholinesterase activity in Alzheimer's disease. J Clin Psychopharmacol 22:615-620
59. Kadir A, Darreh-Shori T, Almkvist O et al (2007) PET imaging of the in vivo brain acetylcholinesterase activity and nicotine binding in galantamine-treated patients with AD. Neurobiol Aging [Epub ahead of print]
60. Brooks DJ (1997) Advances in imaging Parkinson's disease. Curr Opin Neurol 10:327-331
61. McKeith I, O'Brien J, Walker Z et al (2007) Sensitivity and specificity of dopamine transporter imaging with 123I-FP-CIT SPECT in dementia with Lewy bodies: a phase III, multicentre study. Lancet Neurol 6:305-313
62. Hilker R, Thomas A, Klein JC et al (2005) Dementia in Parkinson's disease: functional imaging of cholinergic and dopaminergic pathways. Neurology 65:1716-1722

Clinical SPECT and PET for Management of Patients with Epilepsy

Koen Van Laere[1], Karolien Goffin[1], Wim Van Paesschen[2]

[1] Division of Nuclear Medicine, University Hospital Gasthuisberg, Leuven, Belgium
[2] Department of Neurology, University Hospital Gasthuisberg, Leuven, Belgium

Introduction

Epilepsy is a common chronic neurological disorder that is characterized by recurrent, unprovoked seizures and affects approximately 3% of the population. After the first seizure, about 80% of patients experience another seizure within the first 3 years. Some 60-70% of patients experience focal or partial seizures, and 30-40% generalized seizures. Epilepsy is controlled with medication in around 70% of cases. When seizures are medically intractable, resection of the epileptogenic cortex may be considered.

Several brain-imaging modalities with different spatial and temporal resolutions are available for in vivo studies of patients with epilepsy. Combinations of these imaging modalities that integrate their strengths while eliminating one or more of their individual weaknesses may provide new and superior information [1]. Here we address the role of radionuclide functional imaging techniques that incorporate single photon emission computed tomography (SPECT) and positron emission tomography (PET) to localize the ictal onset zone, seizure propagation pathways, and functional deficit zones in patients with intractable partial epilepsy who are candidates for epilepsy surgery.

Presurgical Assessment of Patients with Refractory Epilepsy

Presurgical evaluation starts with a complete seizure history, physical and neurological examination, routine scalp electroencephalography (EEG), and high-resolution magnetic resonance imaging (MRI) of the brain to assess structural abnormalities [2]. These investigations are complemented by video-EEG monitoring, which allows evaluation of the clinical features of seizures, as well as interictal and ictal EEG, ictal SPECT injection, interictal 2-[^{18}F]fluoro-2-deoxy-d-glucose (FDG) PET, and neuropsychological examination.

The presurgical evaluation of patients with refractory partial epilepsy is aimed at determining whether a patient has a single epileptogenic focus and at localizing the epileptogenic zone. The epileptogenic zone is the cortical region that is indispensable for the generation of seizures and which has to be removed in order to render a patient seizure-free. The epileptogenic zone is a theoretical construct defined in terms of different cortical zones [3]. The seizure-onset zone is the region where the seizure actually originates, whereas the symptomatogenic zone is the (sub)cortical region producing ictal symptoms.

Several recent studies have stressed that both ictal perfusion SPECT and FDG PET can give additional information in the presurgical evaluation of patients with refractory partial epilepsy. Moreover, this information is independent of the results of other investigations.

Ictal SPECT is the only imaging modality that can define in a reliable and consistent manner the ictal onset zone. The epileptogenic lesion can be visualized on morphological imaging such as MRI. The functional deficit zone is the part of the cortex with an abnormal function in between seizures, due to morphological or functional factors, or to both [4]. Interictal FDG PET is probably the best imaging method to assess the functional deficit zone. Epilepsy surgery has the best results if the above-defined cortical zones are concordant, i.e., they point towards the same cortical region, provided that there is no overlap with eloquent cortex. The latter question can be addressed by means of functional MRI (fMRI) activation paradigms.

The nature of the epileptic lesion and the completeness of the resection are important prognostic factors. Surgery renders seizure-free up to 60-90% of patients with unilateral temporal lobe epilepsy (TLE) [5] and up to 70% of patients with a focal cortical malformation [6].

Ictal and Interictal Perfusion SPECT Imaging

Ictal SPECT perfusion cannot be performed reliably without video-EEG monitoring. It is therefore only available in tertiary care hospitals with an epilepsy surgery program and a dedicated nuclear medicine department. It is the only imaging modality able to visualize the ictal onset zone.

During epileptic activity, hyperperfusion of the seizure onset zone occurs because of an autoregulatory response to the local neuronal hyperactivity. For ictal SPECT perfusion imaging, mostly [^{99m}Tc]-labeled compounds are used, such as [^{99m}Tc]-ethyl cysteinate dimer (ECD) or [^{99m}Tc]-hexamethylpropyleneamine oxime (HMPAO). They are characterized by fast (a few tens of seconds) cerebral uptake proportional to blood flow and trapping into neurons (and astrocytes) by intracellular conversion to polar metabolites, resulting in a "frozen" or fixed image that remains stable (i.e., without regional redistribution or washout) up to 4 h post-injection. Thus, when one of these perfusion SPECT tracers is injected intravenously (IV) immediately after the start of a seizure, hyperperfusion at the ictal onset zone can be captured such that the ictal SPECT images reflect the perfusion changes occurring in the early phase of the seizure (Fig. 1).

However, the time resolution of ictal perfusion SPECT is relatively poor compared with the kinetics of most frequently occurring seizure types. After injection of the radioligand in an arm vein, it takes 15-20 s for the compound to reach the brain, and only around 70% of the radioligand is taken up during first-pass. Therefore, an ictal perfusion SPECT image usually displays both the ictal onset zone and the seizure propagation pathways.

In all current published studies in which ictal perfusion SPECT was used, it has been common practice to consider the region with the largest and most intense hyperperfusion as the ictal onset zone; however, these regions may also represent areas of ictal propagation. In patients with TLE, propagation of seizure activity to the contralateral temporal lobe, ipsilateral insula, basal ganglia, and frontal lobe often occurs, but propagation to the parieto-occipital region has also been described. In a study of ictal perfusion patterns associated with single, MRI-visible focal dysplastic lesions (FDLs), we described three patterns of hyperperfusion [7]. In pattern 1, hyperperfusion was most intense at the FDL. Pattern 2 showed an hourglass pattern, in which the least intense lobule overlapped with the FDL, and the most intense occurred at a distance, representing propagation. Pattern 3 was a variant of pattern 2, showing a complicated multilobulated propagation pattern. Propagation patterns were most often found in frontal lobe seizures. Fukuda and colleagues [8] reported the results of very early ictal perfusion SPECT (i.e., injections within 5 s after seizure onset) in patients with frontal lobe epilepsy. In 11 of 18 patients, ictal perfusion SPECT findings were concordant with other investigations, such as invasive EEG studies. In on-

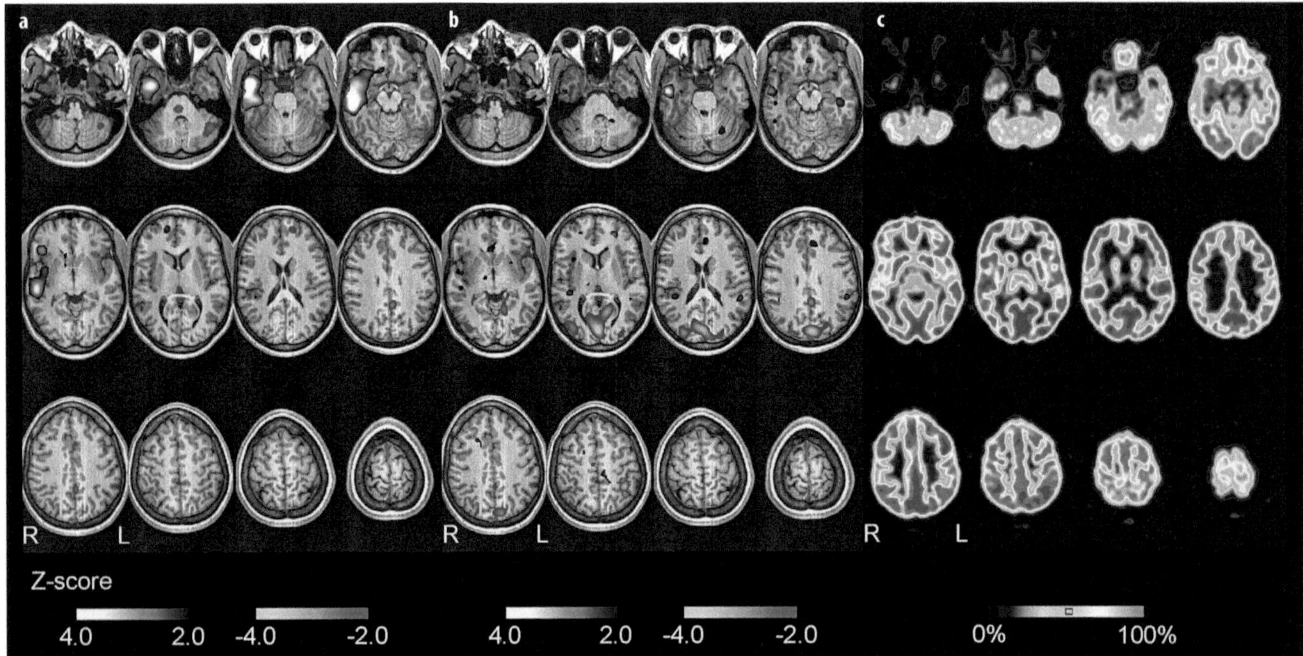

Fig. 1 a-c. Subtraction ictal SPECT co-registered to MRI (SISCOM) image and effect of timing of injection in a 21-year-old, right handed female patient with suspected refractory mesial temporal lobe epilepsy (TLE). Magnetic resonance imaging (MRI) shows right hippocampal sclerosis. Interictal EEG: abundant slow activity and peaks over the right temporal lobe. Clinical: temporal lobe auras and complex partial seizures (lateralizing: dystonia left, automatisms of the right hand, turning of the head to the right). Postictal aphasia. Ictal EEG shows anterotemporal right recruitment of the theta rhythm. Single photon emission computed tomography (SPECT) SISCOM images show: **a** First injection: start 36 s after first clinical manifestation; total duration of seizure 82 s. **b** First injection: start 60 s after first clinical manifestation; total duration of seizure 102 s. **c** coregistered [^{18}F]fluoro-2-deoxy-d-glucose (FDG) PET. Treatment consisted of resection of the anterior two-thirds of the temporal neocortex hippocampus and corpus amygdaloideum. Anatomopathological confirmation of hippocampal sclerosis. Patient was still seizure-free after 1 year

ly three of these 11 (27%), hyperperfusion was localized within the epileptic focus; in the remaining eight (73%), areas of hyperperfusion extended to other regions.

In a comprehensive study of factors affecting the pattern of hyperperfusion of ictal perfusion SPECT in neocortical epilepsies, Lee and colleagues [9] found that an injection delay of less than 20 s after seizure onset was necessary for correct localization. These observations also imply that the earlier the injection is given during a seizure, the more likely the largest and most intense ictal perfusion SPECT cluster represents the true ictal onset zone, and not seizure propagation (Fig. 1b). Contralateral spread of ictal activity is often restricted to a region homotopic to the ictal onset zone, resulting in a "mirror" image.

The accuracy of ictal SPECT analysis is highest when ictal perfusion images are compared to interictal perfusion data. Methodologically, this can be done by traditional side-by-side visual evaluation, but computer-aided voxel-based coregistration techniques, such as subtraction ictal SPECT co-registered to MRI (SISCOM) and ictal-interictal SPECT difference image (ISAS), are fast, accurate, and routinely available [10].

For SISCOM analysis, interictal and ictal SPECT scans are coregistered using an automatic registration algorithm based on mutual information. The interictal image is then subtracted from the ictal one. The difference image is smoothed and transformed into a *z*-score map using the mean and the standard deviation of the differences in all brain voxels. The mean image of the ictal and interictal coregistered images can be used for coregistration to the patient's MRI. The same transformation is then applied to the *z*-map. For the functional overlay, different thresholds can be used to assess the most probable differences and propagated seizure activity, which may be at a lower *z*-threshold.

The interpretation of automatically generated SISCOM data is often easy and straightforward [10]. SISCOM analysis has been shown to be more sensitive and specific in detecting the epileptic onset zone than visual assessment and provides an objective way to study individual propagation patterns [7, 10], especially in extratemporal epilepsies and when fast seizure propagation after an early tracer injection is present. As a caveat, SISCOM may generate false-negatives due to subclinical seizure activity at the moment of tracer injection of interictal SPECT imaging [9]. Therefore, EEG monitoring should be routinely performed during the interictal injection.

In principle, perfusion changes occurring after the termination of a seizure can also be assessed by injection of the tracer in the early postictal (1-60 s after seizure termination) or late postictal (1-10 min after seizure termination) phase. The postictal phase is characterized by a postictal switch, when hyperperfusion at the seizure-onset zone changes into hypoperfusion. This switch takes place about 60 s after seizure termination. When tracer is injected in the first 100 s after the end of the seizure, hyperperfusion persists in >60% of patients, while hypoperfusion is found in all patients when tracer is injected later than 100 s after seizure termination [11]. In patients with TLE, early postictal SPECT had a sensitivity of 75% in localizing the seizure onset zone. According to McNally and colleagues, postictal SPECT in which injections are administered soon after seizures are very poor at localizing a single region based on either perfusion increases or decreases, often because the changes were similar in multiple brain regions [12].

Interictal Glucose Metabolism Imaging with FDG PET

Brain glucose metabolism, as an indirect measure of neural activity, can be studied using PET scanning of the glucose analog FDG, which after phosphorylation, accumulates in neuronal cells. FDG uptake thus represents the regional metabolic rate of glucose consumption (rCMRglu) of the tissue.

While FDG PET is usually evaluated visually, in many tertiary centers the pixelwise comparison of the patient's image to an age-matched reference database is routinely performed in an automated manner, thereby providing an objective evaluation of the changes in glucose metabolism reducing observer variability. Automated analysis is especially useful in patients with extratemporal epilepsy [13]. In patients with TLE, automated quantification of the maximal metabolic asymmetry in the temporal lobes has been reported to allow observer-independent increases in accuracy [14].

Interictal brain FDG PET scanning can provide useful localizing information regarding the epileptogenic focus. Classically, the brain region with the most profound hypometabolism is considered to contain the epileptogenic zone. Using this hypothesis, Lee and coauthors found an overall diagnostic sensitivity of 44% for FDG PET in detecting the area of seizure onset in a group of patients with different forms of refractory partial epilepsy and normal MRI findings [15]. The accuracy of FDG PET localization was greatest in patients with neocortical TLE. Indeed, an area of interictal temporal lobe hypometabolism ipsilateral to the side of the seizure focus can be found in 60-90% of patients with TLE [13, 16], even in those without structural lesions on MRI (Fig. 2). In extratemporal epilepsy, a literature review resulted in a mean detection rate of hypometabolism relevant to the focus in around 67% of patients [16]. In these patients, the sensitivity of FDG PET in detecting the epileptogenic focus increased from 30-40% to 67% by using three-dimensional stereotactic surface projections (SSP) instead of visual assessment [13].

FDG PET detected the epileptogenic zone in >90% of children with focal cortical dysplasia and epilepsy and provided information additional to that obtained with other investigations regarding the epileptogenic zone in 77% of children with refractory epilepsy. Accordingly, management was changed in 50% of the patients [17].

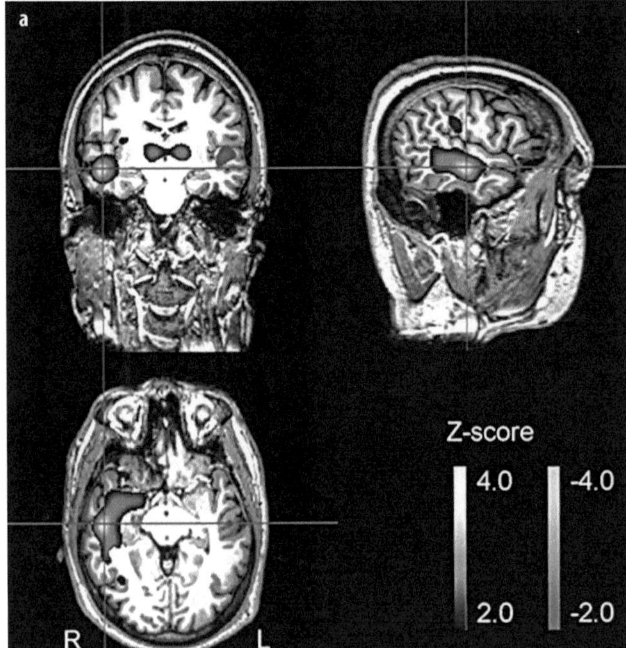

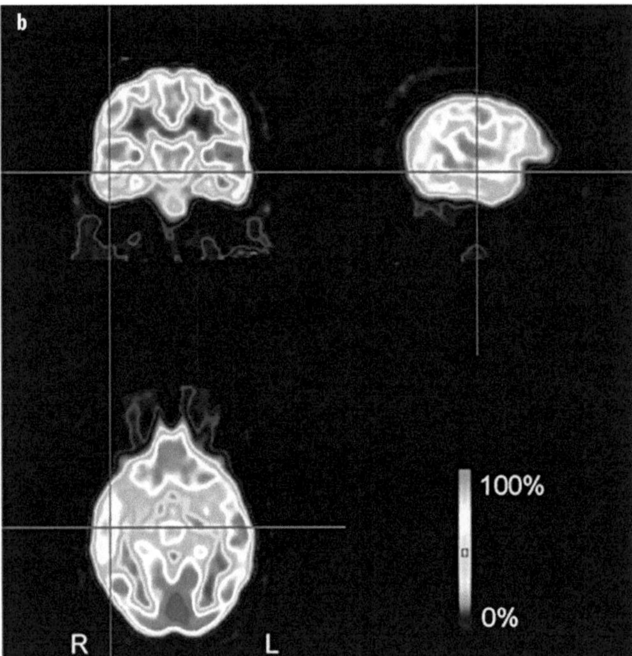

Fig. 2 a, b. SISCOM (**a**) and FDG PET (**b**) images of a 29-year-old male patient with refractory partial epilepsy since the age of 7. His seizures were characterized by version of the head to the right with secondary generalization. 3T MRI including fluid-attenuated inversion recovery (FLAIR) was normal. Interictal EEG showed multifocal disturbances (left temporal and right frontopolar). The ictal SPECT injection was administered 26 s after the first clinical manifestation, and 20 s before the secondary generalization. Total seizure duration was 94 s. No operation was performed since the MRI was normal and there was no consistent focus localisation. Invasive dural grids are placed on the SISCOM location

Surgical Outcome

Lobar localization of the ictal focus by FDG PET correlates significantly with a seizure-free surgical outcome, as does concordance between two or more presurgical evaluations [15]. Also, the extent of hypometabolism can help to predict whether a good surgical outcome can be achieved: in patients with TLE, unilateral temporal hypometabolism is correlated with a better surgical outcome than is the case with more extended hypometabolism. Over 75% of patients with TLE and hypometabolism selective to the ipsilateral temporal cortex are completely seizure-free after surgery. This is in contrast to the 45% of patients with extratemporal cortical hypometabolism confined to the ipsilateral cerebral hemisphere and the 20% of patients with hypometabolism in the contralateral cerebral cortex who are completely seizure-free after surgery [18].

Functional Deficit Zone and Surround Inhibition

Hypometabolism on FDG PET has been ascribed to factors such as neuronal loss, diaschisis, inhibitory processes, reduction in synaptic density, and decreased blood-brain barrier glucose transporter activity. Recent studies have, however, provided new insights into the pathophysiology of hypometabolism. In partial epilepsy, hypometabolism on PET is often more extensive than the pathological abnormality [16]. In patients with TLE, hypometabolism in the ipsilateral temporal lobe is often associated with hypometabolism in the ipsilateral orbitofrontal and prefrontal cortex. This frontal hypometabolism can even be more pronounced than the temporal hypometabolism [19] (Fig. 3). We have speculated that frontal hypometabolism can be attributed to surround inhibition in the areas of seizure propagation, which acts as a dynamic defense mechanism against seizure propagation. Frontal hypometabolism may also be responsible for the deficits in frontal executive functions that are often observed in patients with TLE. Depression, often present in patients with TLE, is also associated with hypometabolism in the frontal lobe [20].

The frontal hypometabolism seen on PET in cases of mesial TLE is a dynamic seizure-related process. Longitudinal changes in cortical glucose hypometabolism have been reported in children with refractory epilepsy on the basis of comparison of two sequential FDG PET scans performed 7-44 months apart. The change in seizure frequency in the period between the two PET scans correlated positively with the change in the extent of cortical glucose hypometabolism. There was enlargement in the area of hypometabolism on the second PET scan when the seizure frequency was persistent or increased whereas the area of hypometabolism decreased with improved seizure control [21]. Similar results were found when pre- and postoperative FDG PET scans were compared in patients with TLE caused by hippocampal

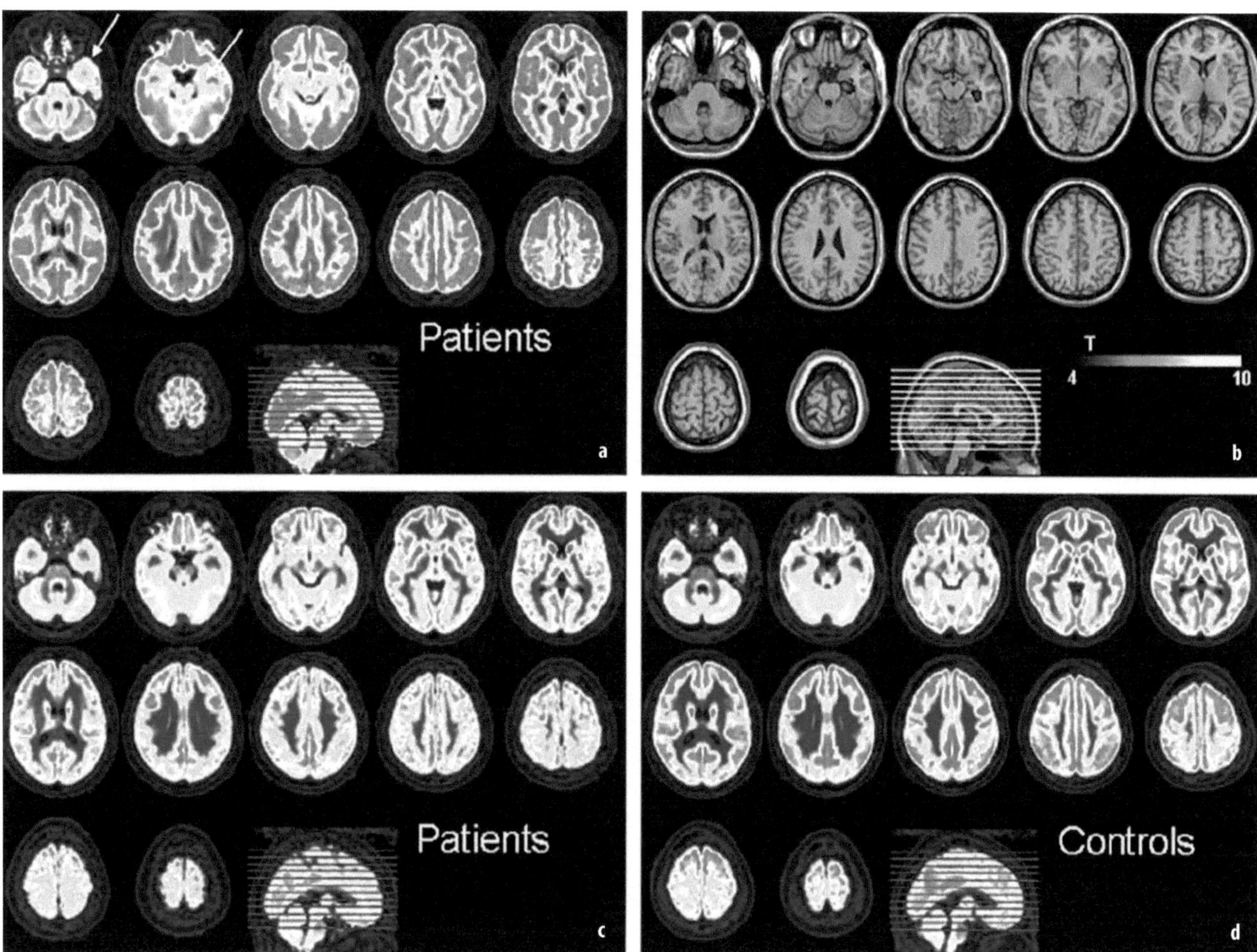

Fig. 3 a-d. Frontal lobe hypometabolism in a patient with mesial temporal lobe epilepsy with hippocampal sclerosis (mTLE-HS). **a** Mean image of the normalized FDG PET across a group of patients with TLE due to HS shows that the ipsilateral temporal lobe (*white arrows*) is more hypometabolic than the contralateral side and appears to be the most hypometabolic region in the brain. **b** SPM T-map (uncorrected *p* value <0.001) shown on the MRI of a single subject in MNI space confirms that a significant asymmetry in interhemispheric metabolism is only found in the temporal lobes. Mean images of the normalized FDG PET across patients with TLE (**c**) and controls (**d**), displayed using the same color table, show a striking hypometabolism in the frontoparietal lobes in patients compared to controls. The hypometabolism in the epileptic temporal lobe is less striking than the changes in the extratemporal regions

sclerosis (HS) who were seizure-free after surgery. Increases in metabolism were seen after surgery in the propagation pathways of ictal and interictal epileptic discharges, such as temporal stem white matter, inferior precentral gyrus, and anterior cingulate gyrus in the ipsilateral hemisphere. The hypometabolism in these areas was likely to be functional, seizure-related, and reversible.

Partial Volume Effects

Measuring small brain structures such as the cortical ribbon will lead to an underestimation of the tracer activity due to the limited resolution (approximately 4-5 mm) of current PET scanners. This partial volume effect (PVE) can lead to spurious hypometabolic regions, resulting in an increased number of false-positively predicted hypometabolic regions. Moreover, if the finite spatial resolution of the imaging system is not accounted for, there may be spillover of activity to neighboring regions, leading to misinterpretation of the extent of the hypometabolic regions. Several algorithms are available for partial volume correction, either post-hoc (e.g. PVEOut) [22] or during reconstruction (e.g., an anatomy-based maximum-a-posteriori iterative reconstruction algorithm; A-MAP) [23]. Partial volume correction improves the detection accuracy of small hypometabolic lesions in FDG PET images of the brain compared to conventional analysis [23].

Imaging of Specific Neurotransmitter Systems

Although not routinely performed, imaging of receptors and other CNS processes reflecting metabolic or proliferative pathways allows extraction of additional diagnostic and prognostic information in selected series of epilepsy patients [24].

[^{11}C]-Methionine PET can reliably detect primary or recurrent glioma with high sensitivity and high negative predictive value. Dysembryoplastic neuroepithelial tumors (DNET) can cause refractory partial epilepsy; they have a much more benign course than gliomas. Differentiation of DNET from gliomas on the basis of MRI characteristics may not be reliable. Rosenberg and colleagues [25] reported that normal MET PET findings in patients with an epileptogenic and non-rapidly progressing brain tumor are suggestive of DNET, whereas a markedly increased tumor MET uptake makes this diagnosis unlikely.

High uptake of α-[^{11}C]-methyl-L-tryptophan (AMT) on PET occurs in a subset of epileptogenic tubers, consistent with the location of seizure focus. Kagawa and colleagues [26] analyzed the surgical outcome of children with tuberous sclerosis complex in relation to AMT PET results. Their findings suggested that resection of tubers with increased AMT uptake is highly desirable to achieve seizure-free surgical outcome in children with tuberous sclerosis complex and intractable epilepsy.

Hammers and colleagues [27] performed a retrospective [^{11}C]-flumazenil (FMZ) PET study in 15 patients with refractory mesial temporal lobe epilepsy with hippocampal sclerosis (mTLE-HS) and 13 control subjects. A periventricular increase in FMZ binding, implying heterotopic neurons, was observed in three of 13 controls (23%), three of eight patients (38%) with Engel class IA outcome (i.e., completely seizure-free), and four of seven patients (57%) who were not completely seizure-free. Although these periventricular increases correlated with poorer outcome, individual predictions of postoperative outcome were difficult in view of the poor sensitivity and specificity of the method.

Interictal PET studies using [^{11}C]-carfentanyl [28], which is selective for the α opioid peptide receptor, have shown increased binding in the lateral temporal neocortex on the side of the epileptogenic focus in patients with TLE.

Picard and colleagues [29] studied nicotinic receptor density using [^{18}F]-F-A-85380, a high-affinity agonist of α4α2 nicotinic acetylcholine receptors, in patients with autosomal dominant nocturnal frontal lobe epilepsy. Patients had increased densities in the epithalamus, ventral mesencephalon, and cerebellum, and decreased densities in the right dorsolateral prefrontal region, implicating these changes in the pathophysiology of autosomal dominant frontal lobe epilepsy.

In studies with using [^{18}F]-FCWAY, a 5-HT1A receptor antagonist, serotonin 1A receptors (5-HT1A) were shown to be reduced in patients with TLE. Theodore and colleagues [30] reported that reductions of 5-HT1A receptor binding in mesial temporal structures and the insula remained significantly reduced after partial volume correction.

Multimodality Imaging

Supplementary clinical information can be gained by coregistration of ictal SPECT, SISCOM, and MRI, since these different imaging modalities provide complementary information [1]. Beyond these techniques, coregistration of ictal perfusion SPECT, PET, structural MRI, fMRI, diffusion-tensor imaging (DTI), EEG and magneto-encephalography (MEG) in one multimodality imaging platform could provide a very powerful tool to systematically study the relationships between the epileptic lesion (MRI), irritative zone (MEG and interictal EEG), ictal onset zone (ictal perfusion SPECT and ictal EEG), functional deficit zone (FDG PET), eloquent cortex (fMRI), and the connectivity between the different cortical regions (DTI) [3].

There is mounting evidence that multimodality imaging combining FDG PET, ictal perfusion SPECT, and MEG in combination with MRI has increased the number of patients being considered for epilepsy surgery and obviated the need for invasive EEG studies. In cryptogenic neocortical epilepsy with FDG PET, ictal perfusion SPECT, and interictal/ictal EEG, concordance with two or more presurgical evaluations is significantly related to a seizure-free outcome. Studies consisting of coregistered combinations of FDG PET, MRI, and DTI to distinguish epileptogenic tubers and cortex in patients with tuberous sclerosis complex showed that epileptogenic tubers had larger volumes of FDG PET hypometabolism and increased apparent diffusion coefficients (ADC). Moreover, the severity of FDG PET hypometabolism was found to correlate with interictal regional delta slowing in TLE, suggesting related underlying pathophysiological mechanisms for metabolic and electrical dysfunction in TLE.

Conclusions

Ictal perfusion SPECT and interictal FDG PET imaging remain important first-line tools in the localization of the ictal onset zone, seizure propagation pathways, and the functional deficit zone in the presurgical evaluation of patients with refractory partial epilepsy. Automated image processing techniques, novel reconstruction techniques, and multimodal imaging are likely to provide more objective results, although careful interpretation by close collaboration between the nuclear medicine, radiology and neurology departments remains necessary. Continuous improvement in our understanding of the biological processes causing perfusion and metabolic changes in epilepsy will improve the diagnostic sensitivity of the many functional imaging tools.

References

1. Cherry SR (2006) Multimodality in vivo imaging systems: twice the power or double the trouble? Annu Rev Biomed Eng 8:35-62

2. Li LM, Fish DR, Sisodiya SM et al (1995) High resolution magnetic resonance imaging in adults with partial or secondary generalised epilepsy attending a tertiary referral unit. J Neurol Neurosurg Psychiatry 59(4):384-387
3. Rosenow F, Lüders H (2001) Presurgical evaluation of epilepsy. Brain 124(Pt 9):1683-1700
4. Elger CE, Helmstaedter C, Kurthen M (2004) Chronic epilepsy and cognition. Lancet Neurol 3(11):663-672
5. Wiebe S, Blume WT, Girvin JP, Eliasziw M (2001) A randomized, controlled trial of surgery for temporal-lobe epilepsy. N Engl J Med 345(5):311-318
6. Cohen-Gadol AA, Ozduman K, Bronen RA et al (2004) Long-term outcome after epilepsy surgery for focal cortical dysplasia. J Neurosurg 101(1):55-65
7. Dupont P, Van Paesschen W, Palmini A et al (2006) Ictal perfusion patterns associated with single MRI-visible focal dysplastic lesions: implications for the noninvasive delineation of the epileptogenic zone. Epilepsia 47(9):1550-1557
8. Fukuda M, Masuda H, Honma J et al (2006) Ictal SPECT analyzed by three-dimensional stereotactic surface projection in frontal lobe epilepsy patients. Epilepsy Res 68(2):95-102
9. Lee SK, Lee SY, Yun CH et al (2006) Ictal SPECT in neocortical epilepsies: clinical usefulness and factors affecting the pattern of hyperperfusion. Neuroradiology 48(9):678-684
10. O'Brien TJ, So EL, Mullan BP et al (1998) Subtraction ictal SPECT co-registered to MRI improves clinical usefulness of SPECT in localizing the surgical seizure focus. Neurology 50(2):445-454
11. Avery RA, Spencer SS, Spanaki MV et al (1999) Effect of in jection time on postictal SPET perfusion changes in medically refractory epilepsy. Eur J Nucl Med 26(8):830-836
12. McNally KA, Paige AL, Varghese G et al (2005) Localizing value of ictal-interictal SPECT analyzed by SPM (ISAS). Epilepsia 46(9):1450-1464
13. Drzezga A, Arnold S, Minoshima S et al (1999) 18F-FDG PET studies in patients with extratemporal and temporal epilepsy: evaluation of an observer-independent analysis. J Nucl Med 40(5):737-746
14. Lin TW, de Aburto MA, Dahlbom M et al (2007) Predicting seizure-free status for temporal lobe epilepsy patients undergoing surgery: prognostic value of quantifying maximal metabolic asymmetry extending over a specified proportion of the temporal lobe. J Nucl Med 48(5):776-782
15. Lee SK, Lee SY, Kim KK et al (2005) Surgical outcome and prognostic factors of cryptogenic neocortical epilepsy. Ann Neurol 58(4):525-532
16. Casse R, Rowe CC, Newton M et al (2002) Positron emission tomography and epilepsy. Mol Imaging Biol 4(5):338-351
17. Ollenberger GP, Byrne AJ, Berlangieri SU et al (2005) Assessment of the role of FDG PET in the diagnosis and management of children with refractory epilepsy. Eur J Nucl Med Mol Imaging 32(11):1311-1316
18. Choi JY, Kim SJ, Hong SB et al (2003) Extratemporal hypometabolism on FDG PET in temporal lobe epilepsy as a predictor of seizure outcome after temporal lobectomy. Eur J Nucl Med Mol Imaging 30(4):581-587
19. Nelissen N, Van Paesschen W, Baete K et al (2006) Correlations of interictal FDG-PET metabolism and ictal SPECT perfusion changes in human temporal lobe epilepsy with hippocampal sclerosis. Neuroimage 32(2):684-695
20. Salzberg M, Taher T, Davie M et al (2006) Depression in temporal lobe epilepsy surgery patients: an FDG-PET study. Epilepsia 47(12):2125-2130
21. Benedek K, Juhasz C, Chugani DC et al (2006) Longitudinal changes in cortical glucose hypometabolism in children with intractable epilepsy. J Child Neurol 21(1):26-31
22. Quarantelli M, Berkouk K, Prinster A et al (2004) Integrated software for the analysis of brain PET/SPECT studies with partial-volume-effect correction. J Nucl Med 45(2):192-201
23. Baete K, Nuyts J, Van Laere K et al (2004) Evaluation of anatomy based reconstruction for partial volume correction in brain FDG-PET. Neuroimage 23(1):305-317
24. Koepp MJ, Woermann FG (2005) Imaging structure and function in refractory focal epilepsy. Lancet Neurol 4(1):42-53
25. Rosenberg DS, Demarquay G, Jouvet A et al (2005) [11C]-Methionine PET: dysembryoplastic neuroepithelial tumours compared with other epileptogenic brain neoplasms. J Neurol Neurosurg Psychiatry 76(12):1686-1692
26. Kagawa K, Chugani DC, Asano E et al (2005) Epilepsy surgery outcome in children with tuberous sclerosis complex evaluated with alpha-[11C]methyl-L-tryptophan positron emission tomography (PET). J Child Neurol 20(5):429-438
27. Hammers A, Koepp MJ, Brooks DJ, Duncan JS (2005) Periventricular white matter flumazenil binding and postoperative outcome in hippocampal sclerosis. Epilepsia 46(6):944-948
28. Mayberg HS, Sadzot B, Meltzer CC et al (1991) Quantification of mu and non-mu opiate receptors in temporal lobe epilepsy using positron emission tomography. Ann Neurol 30(1):3-11
29. Picard F, Bruel D, Servent D et al (2006) Alteration of the in vivo nicotinic receptor density in ADNFLE patients: a PET study. Brain 129(Pt 8):2047-2060
30. Giovacchini G, Toczek MT, Bonwetsch R et al (2005) 5-HT 1A receptors are reduced in temporal lobe epilepsy after partial-volume correction. J Nucl Med 46(7):1128-1135

Magnetic Resonance Essentials for Correlative Imaging of the Brain with PET and SPECT

Karl-Olof Lövblad

Neuroradiology Unit, Radiology Department, HUG, Geneva University Hospital, Geneva, Switzerland

Introduction

Imaging of the brain has become an increasingly complex but also more complete undertaking that lies at the crossroads of many medical specialities. Indeed, anatomical, physiological, and pathological information can be obtained by the combination of multiple imaging parameters that will provide the essential details needed for tissue characterization. Thus, Radiology and Nuclear Medicine are two specialties that can be viewed not as concurrent entities but as mutually beneficial ones, as technology has made giant leaps in both these areas in the last decades. Thus, increasingly, these specialties have cooperated in the work-up of patients with neurological diseases.

Knowledge of anatomy based on computed tomography (CT) and magnetic resonance imaging (MRI) is necessary not only for simple correlation with available examinations but also for combined examinations such as positron emission tomography (PET)-CT, single photon emission tomography (SPECT)-CT or even PET-MRI. Recently, the ability of MRI to offer high anatomical resolution has been improved such that it has become a functional and a physiological method. This chapter aims to provide the necessary background to correlate findings on PET and SPECT with MRI.

MRI Techniques

While CT still has a privileged place, mainly in emergency situations, MRI is used mostly for the work-up of patients with diseases of the central nervous system. Indeed, since it does not use ionizing radiation but magnetic fields, it can be repeated many times without any side effects to the patient.

MRI requires the presence of a strong static magnetic field; today's clinical scanners may reach strengths of up to 3.0 T (Fig. 1). Specific coils are used for imaging of body

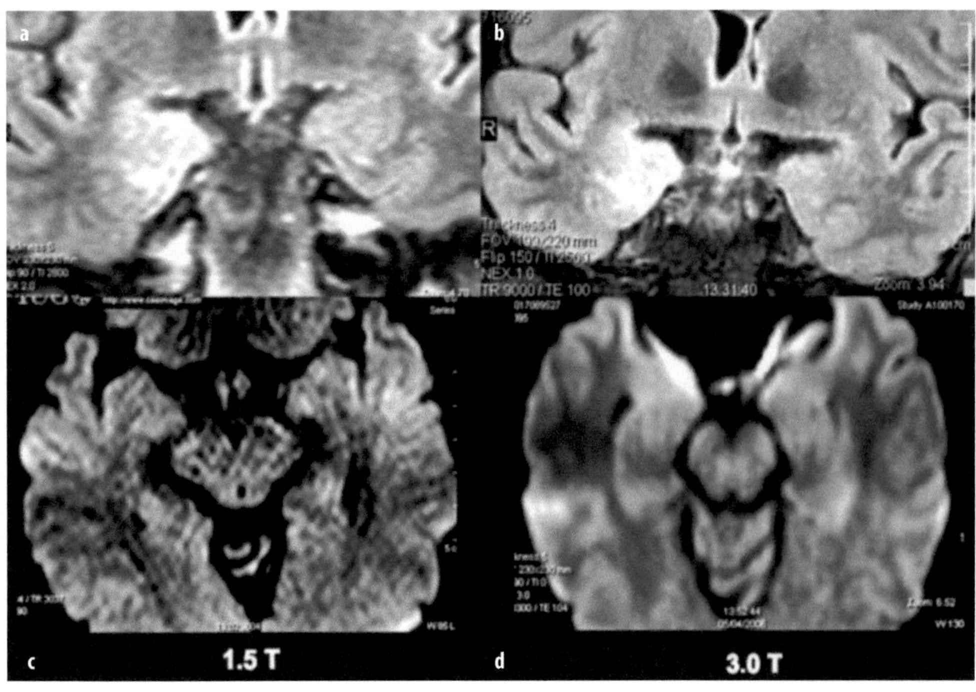

Fig. 1 a-d. MR imaging at 3T: FLAIR and diffusion images obtained at 1.5T (**a**, **b**) and 3T (**c**, **d**) in a patient with right-sided temporal lobe epilepsy. The images at 3T show the improved anatomic detail, especially on the FLAIR image

parts; in the case of the brain, a head coil is used. In recent years, progress has been made in reducing imaging time by the development of faster sequences and coils that allow parallel imaging. This has led to a considerable reduction in scanning time and thus an improvement in patient comfort.

MRI has quickly established itself as an indispensable tool for the diagnosis and management of neurological diseases. Developments in software and hardware [1] as well as in contrast media have played an important role. The multitude of MRI sequences allows the clinician and the radiologist to acquire information regarding several parameters of the organ examined, resulting in improved tissue characterization.

Magnetic resonance has a few contraindications that are still valid, such as patients with severe claustrophobia and reactions to the presence of some of the metallic devices and stimulators [2].

MR Sequences

A MR examination is comprised of many sequences during which different parameters are tested regarding the water content of the tissue. Due to the fact that each sequence is acquired over 3-5 min, a complete MR examination lasts between 30 and 45 min, depending on the information sought by the clinician. The standard MR sequences that are used are: T1, T2, FLAIR, and T2* (Figs. 2-4). MRI can be acquired in a multiplanar fashion, with images reconstructed directly in the required orientation without to the need for secondary reconstructions.

Conventional MR Sequences

T1- and T2-weighted images are standard workhorses of MRI, as they provide the basic orientation with respect to anatomic and pathologic information. Cerebrospinal fluid (CSF) is bright (white; hyperintense) on T2-weighted images, as are most structures containing water. On T1-weighted images, CSF is dark (hypointense), while blood (methemoglobin) (Fig. 4), melanin, fat, high protein content, calcifications, and contrast are white.

Fluid level attenuated inversion recovery (FLAIR) images allow water in the parenchyma to be differentiated from water in the ventricles. This is clearly important in inflammatory diseases such as multiple sclerosis (MS) but also in order to assess tumor extension. These sequences mainly provide the same information as T2 images [3].

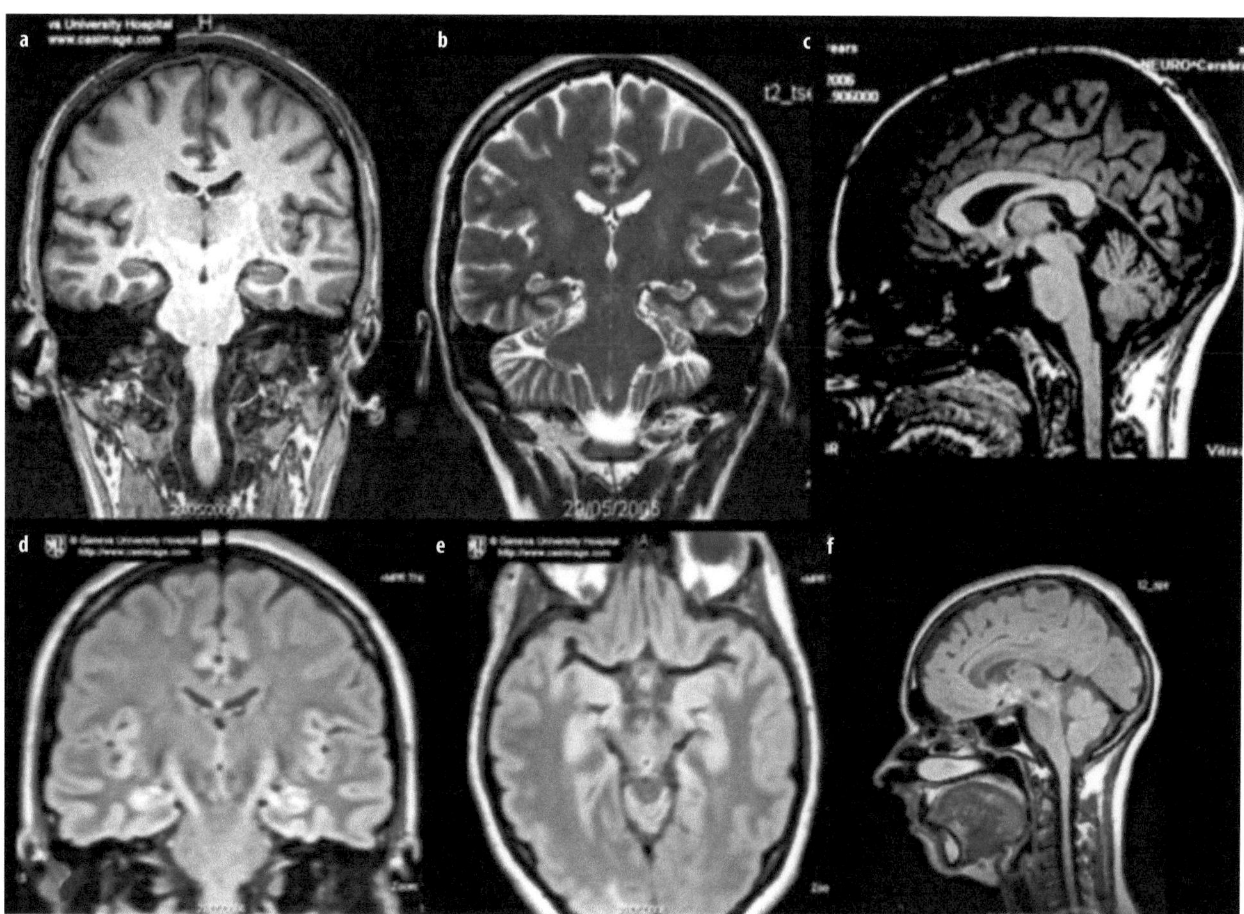

Fig. 2 a-f. Coronal T1 (**a**), coronal T2 (**b**) and sagittal T1 (**c**), coronal FLAIR (**d**), axial (**e**), and sagittal (**f**) FLAIR

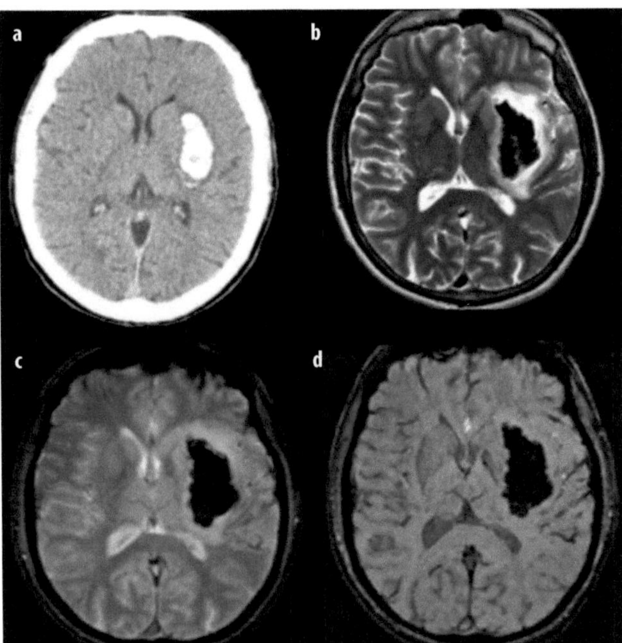

Fig. 3 a-d. Susceptibility imaging. CT of a patient with a left-sided hematoma in the basal ganglia. CT shows typically hyperdense hematoma (**a**); on T2, this lesion is inhomogeneously hypodense (**b**), while on standard T2* image (**c**) there is important signal loss, which is even stronger on the susceptibility-weighted image (**d**)

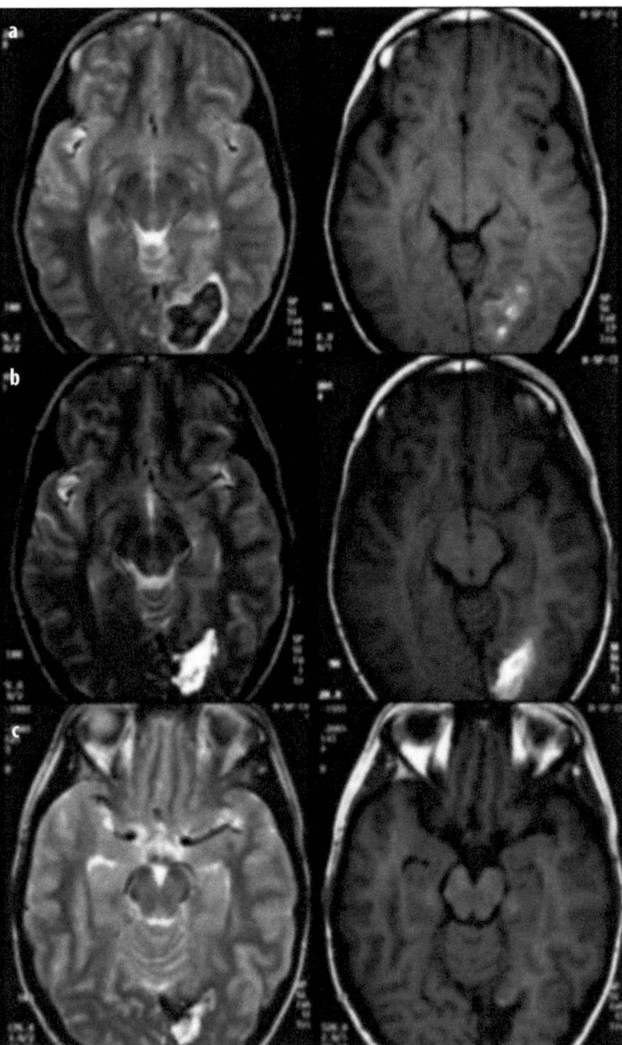

Fig. 4 a-c. Follow-up MR in a young patient with a left-sided occipital hematoma. (**a**) In the early stage there is hypointensity on T2 (left), while T1 is slightly hyper- and iso-intense. (**b**) In the subacute stage, the hematoma is bright on both T1 and T2-weighted images. (**c**) In the late stage, it is hypointense on T1 and hyperintense on T2, reflecting liquefaction

T2*, called gradient-echo or susceptibility imaging, provides low anatomic contrast but has a high sensitivity for changes in the local magnetic field. This will provoke decreases in signal intensity due to the presence of calcification or blood. A recent development, susceptibility-weighted imaging (SWI), enables 3D T2* imaging to be carried out, with a high degree of sensitivity for such alterations (Fig. 3) [4].

Diffusion and Perfusion Techniques

These two fast techniques became available together with echo-planar imaging [5]. Diffusion imaging is very sensitive to the motion of molecules in a given tissue [6, 7]. This has been used with success in the detection of acute brain ischemia [8-14]. Indeed, diffusion can detect the early onset of cytotoxic edema, as it is accompanied by a decrease in diffusion due to the redistribution of water from extra- to intra-cellular compartments [15]. Diffusion imaging thus allows the quantification of water motion in a given tissue. It has been used for numerous other applications, such as epilepsy [16, 17], tumor progression, and brain development.

A further modification of diffusion imaging is diffusion tensor imaging, in which information is obtained not only about diffusion alterations but also about the direction and strength of these movements. This results in the generation of fractional anisotropy maps and allows secondary tractography to be carried out [2, 16]. This new method has shown potential applications in the evaluation of brain tumors, particularly, analysis of the integrity of corticospinal tracts and other white matter bundles, and thus the effect of the tumor on white matter tracts [15].

The coupling of diffusion imaging with perfusion imaging yields a protocol that allows the assessment of tissue injury as well as the underlying hemodynamic state. Perfusion imaging is additionally used for the follow-up of brain tumors. In this technique, a paramagnetic contrast agent, such as a gadolinium chelate [20], is injected. Alternatively, the endogenous contrast of labeled spins, the so-called spin-labeling technique, can be used [22-24]. However, most perfusion techniques provide information relative to blood flow and volume rather than quantitative data.

MR angiography can be performed either with or without contrast medium. It is most commonly used in intracranial studies together with time-of-flight techniques. Extracranial evaluations require the use of contrast medium [25].

MR spectroscopy can be used for the follow-up for brain tumors [26, 27]. The technique provides a measure of local metabolite concentrations. In the presence of a brain tumor, levels of the neuronal tracer *N*-acetyl-aspartate (NAA) are reduced whereas choline (Cho) levels are increased, i.e., there is a decrease in the NAA/Cho ratio. Additionally, the presence of lactate and lipids is a marker of malignancy.

Functional MR (fMRI) techniques take advantage of the sensitivity of T2* images to changes in local susceptibility, and have thus been used to acquire images of local activation during the performance of a specific task [28]. This has the advantage as being performed in the same setting as the anatomic reference MRI. Functional MR is being used clinically both for the assessment of brain function before and after treatment (e.g. before operation of brain tumours) as well as to assess higher brain functions for pure research purposes.

Contrast Materials

The most frequently used contrast materials are gadolinium chelates, which alter the magnetic field. On T1-weighted images this effect is seen as an increase in signal intensity. In oncologic studies, T1-weighted images covering the whole brain in three planes are required. Isotropic 3D T1-weighted imaging can be carried out, with reconstructions in any plane (Fig. 5). In tissues with high T1 signal intensities, fat-suppression techniques can be additionally employed. Recently, due to rising concerns about systemic nephrogenic fibrosis, patients should undergo screening of renal function before contrast agent is administered.

Image fusion can be performed using a variety of workstations. A virtual space is created that allows coregistration of the data sets obtained from PET or SPECT with three-dimensional sequences such as 3D-T1 or 3D-FLAIR. To some degree, image fusion has been rendered obsolete by new hybrid technologies, such as PET-CT and SPECT-CT, and even by MR PET, which is currently in development and available at selected centers.

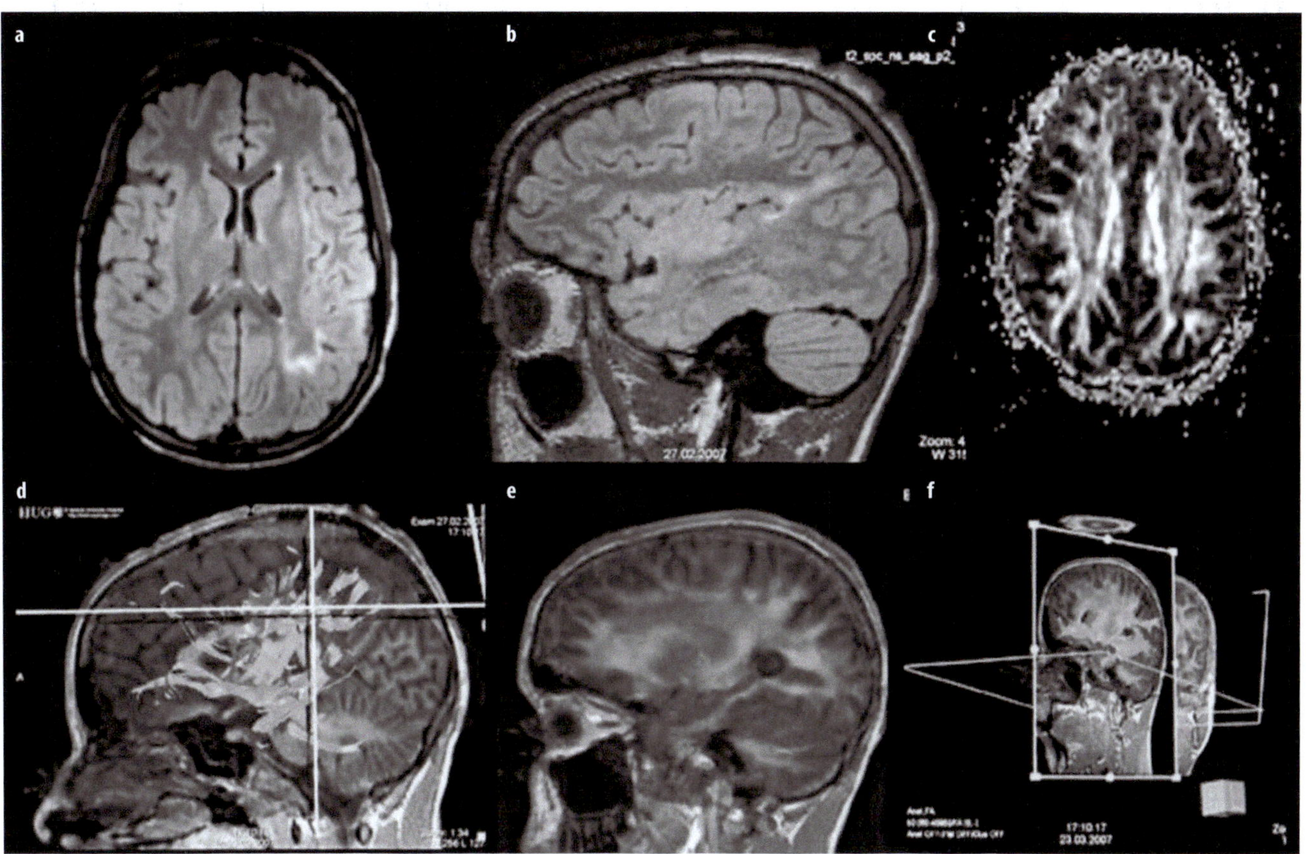

Fig. 5 a-f. Three-dimensional FLAIR imaging allows coregistration with other modalities for image fusion: (**a**) Axial FLAIR reconstruction, (**b**) sagittal FLAIR. (**c**) Axial fractional anisotropy image in the same patient from whom tractography was reconstructed (**d**). The images were superposed on those from 3D FLAIR (**e**) and incorporated into a 3D space (**f**)

Common Neuroradiological Pathologies

Epilepsy

Epileptic syndromes are classified into symptomatic or cryptogenic forms. Symptomatic epilepsy has many possible causes, such as trauma and tumors. This type of epilepsy is often detected very well with MR techniques, especially high-resolution ones [29]. In the evaluation of temporal lobe epilepsy, coronal, axial and sagittal thin slices are obtained along the axis of the hippocampus using a combination of T1 and FLAIR images. If a tumoral cause of the epilepsy is suspected, contrast-enhanced images can be additionally acquired (Fig. 6).

Tumors

In the management of oncologic diseases, the combined use of MRI and nuclear medicine methods is indispensable. Indeed, MRI provides exquisite anatomic detail and tissue characterization, as detailed above, while PET, for example, provides supplementary functional metabolic data. Usually an oncologic protocol will comprise precontrast axial T1 and T2-weighted images as well as FLAIR imaging (usually in the coronal plane), followed by tri-planar T1-weighted images after injection of contrast (Figs. 7-10). Perfusion imaging can be done with contrast before the post-contrast images are acquired, as can spectroscopy.

Brain tumors are classified according to their location: extra-axial, intra-axial, or intraventricular. Extra-axial tumors tend to be meningiomas and neurinomas.

When a benign lesion is suspected, their imaging appearance provides valuable data: meningiomas are typically seated with a broad base on the meninges, have a dural tail, and tend to enhance strongly after contrast; neurinomas are more inhomogeneous (Fig. 8).

Gliomas tend not to enhance when they are of low grade. The appearance of a higher-grade glioma is accompanied by contrast enhancement due to rupture of the blood-brain barrier (grade III, Fig. 9) and necrosis (grade IV, Fig. 10).

Cerebrovascular Diseases: Stroke, Carotid Artery Stenosis, and Others

While CT has maintained an important role in the acute management of cerebrovascular diseases, MRI is clearly superior for the follow-up of these patients. CT has the advantage of being able to reliably demonstrate the presence of intracerebral hemorrhage. Perfusion CT and CT angiography allow complete follow-up. In addition, these techniques can be used to demonstrate vascular occlusion and hypoperfusion.

Diffusion perfusion techniques have an important role in the assessment of patients with acute or chronic cerebrovascular disorders. Full cerebrovascular protocols will

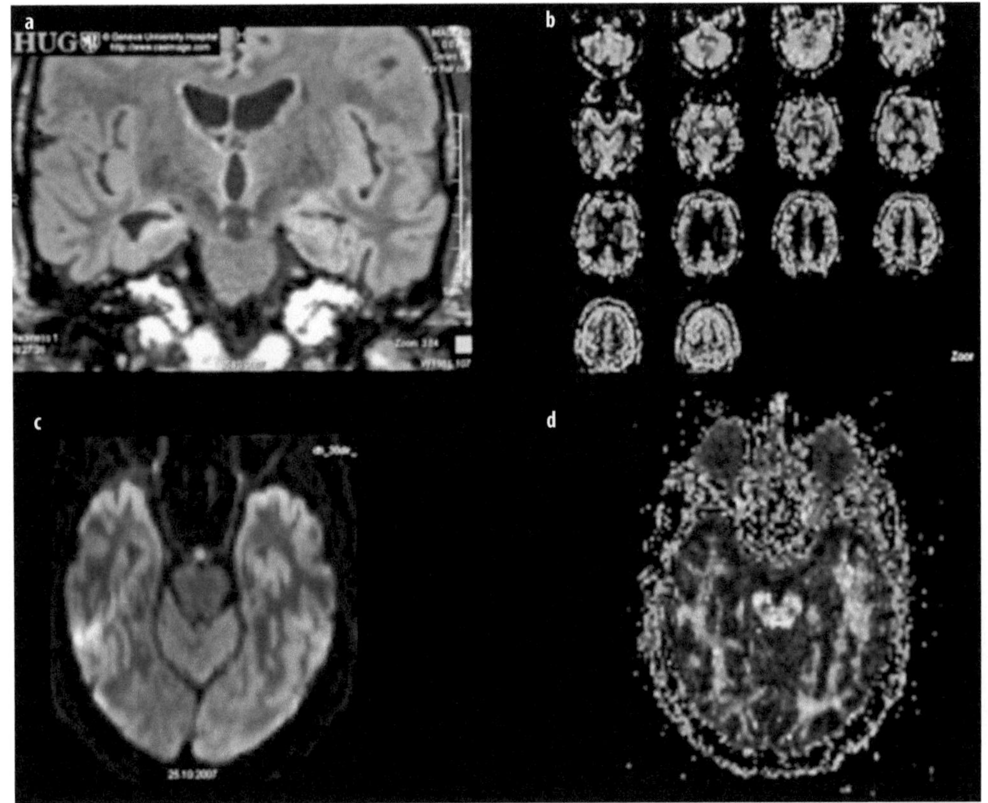

Fig. 6 a-d. Patient with right-sided hippocampal sclerosis. Atrophy and hyperintensity of the right hippocampus are seen on the coronal FLAIR image (**a**), with hypoperfusion seen on the perfusion images (**b**). Slight hyperintensity is shown on the diffusion image (**c**) along with a decrease of the fractional anisotropy (**d**)

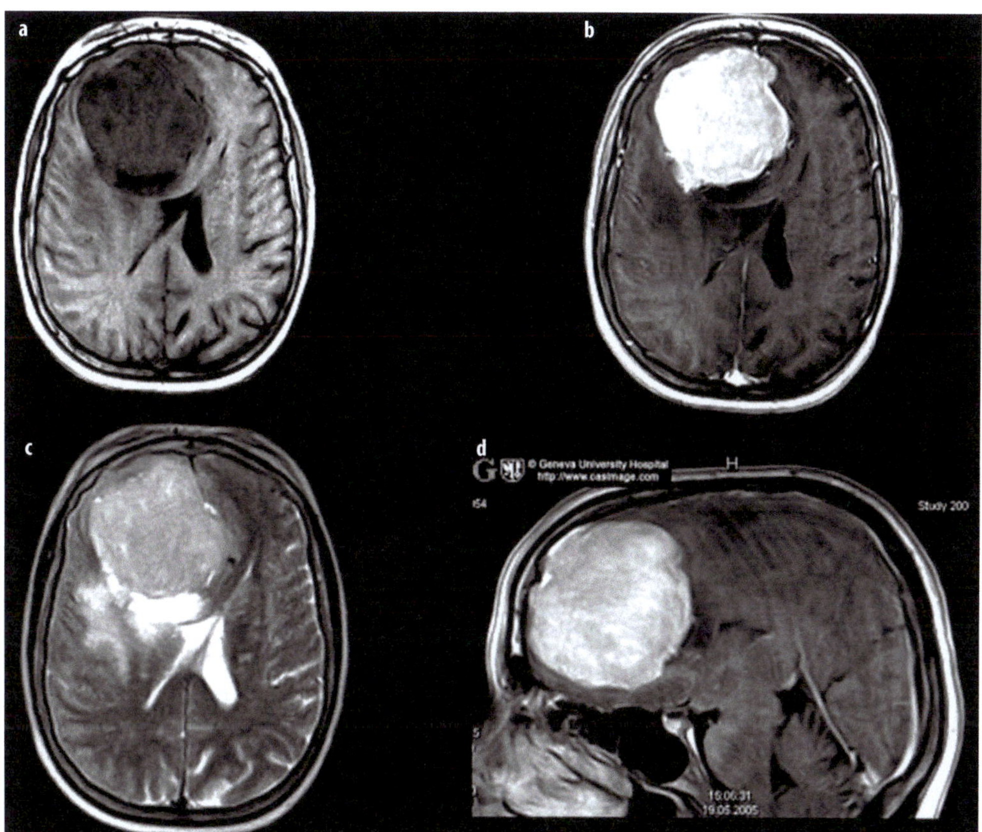

Fig. 7 a-d. Frontal meningioma. This lesion is hypointense on T1 (**a**), hyperintense on T2-weighted images (**c**), and enhances strongly (**b**, **d**)

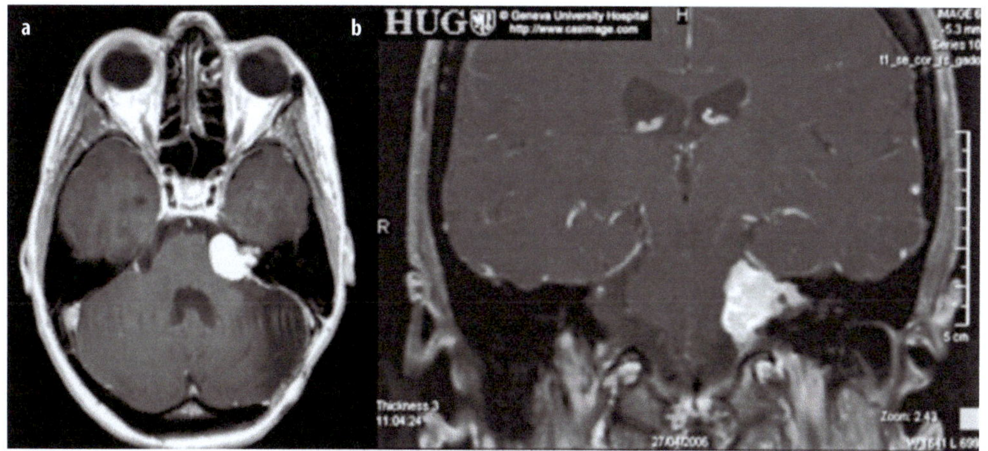

Fig. 8 a, b. Left-sided schwannoma of the vestibular nerve. Post-contrast T1 images in the axial (**a**) and coronal planes (**b**) show that the intrameatal tumour enhances strongly

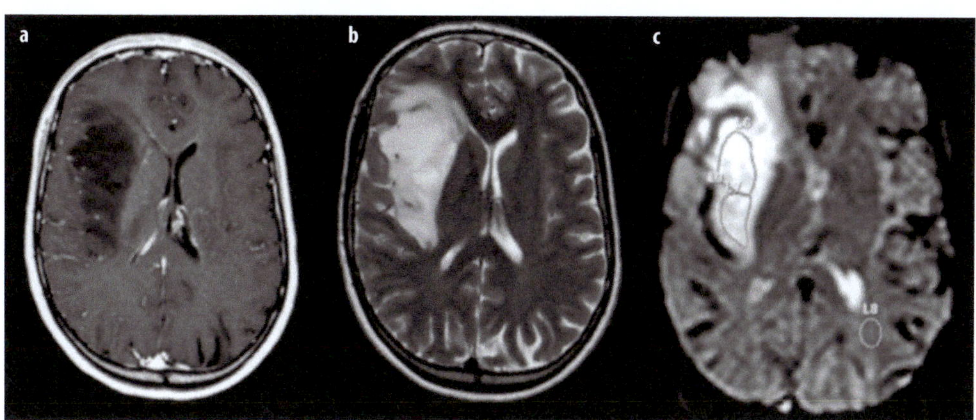

Fig. 9 a-c. Low grade glioma in the right insular region. The lesion is hypointense and does not enhance (**a**) on T1-weighted images: it is hyperintense on T2-weighted images (**b**), and perfusion is decreased (**c**)

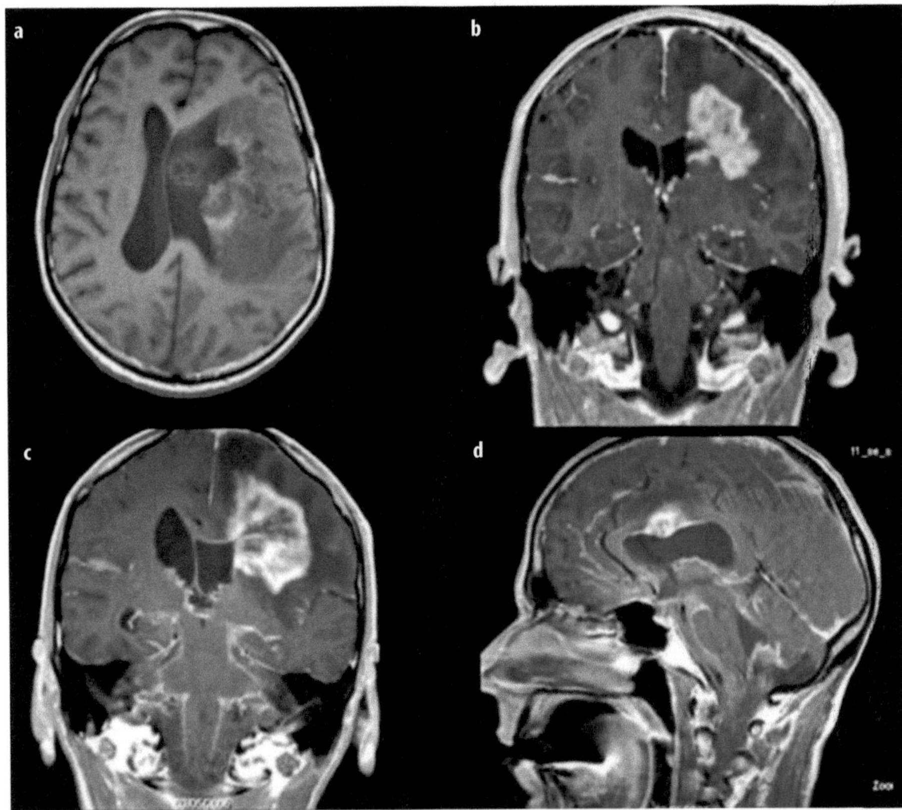

Fig. 10 a-d. Glioblastoma multiforme: There is a centrally necrotic (**a**) and peripherally enhancing (**b, c**) tumour in the left hemisphere which also infiltrates the corpus callosum (**d**)

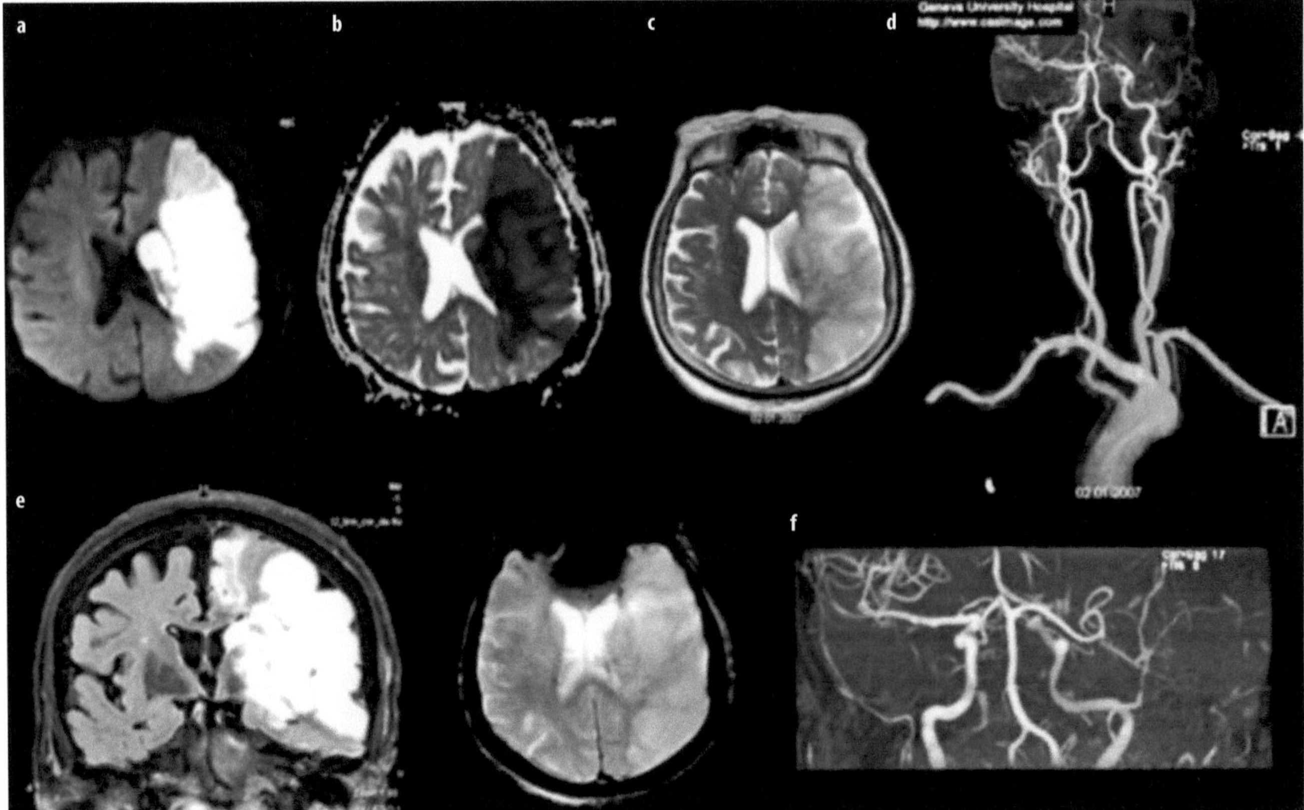

Fig. 11 a-f. Multi-modality imaging in a patient with acute stroke: the diffusion image shows a hyperintensity in the left MCA territory (**a**), along with a decrease of signal on the ADC image (**b**). On T2 the lesion is slightly visible (**c**). MR angiography shows no occlusion of the neck vessels (**d**) but an interruption of the left MCA (**g**). Changes are seen on the coronal FLAIR image (**e**) but there is no hemorrhage on the T2* image (**f**)

consist of T-weighted images, diffusion and perfusion imaging, MR angiography, including time-of-flight (TOF) intracranially and with contrast to visualize the extracranial carotids, as well as T2* and post-contrast T1-weighted images (Fig. 11).

While acute hemorrhage may be difficult to interpret, MRI is an excellent method in the follow-up of hematomas, since it is able to demonstrate the cascade of signal intensity changes that occur due to the degradation of hemoglobin.

Conclusions

Magnetic resonance methods allow tissue characterization by generating high-resolution sequences, which in turn provide detailed anatomic resolution. The armamentarium of imaging methods has been improved drastically by the development of functional MRI techniques, such as diffusion, perfusion, spectroscopy, PET, and SPECT . While these methods have their drawbacks and limitations, they nonetheless nearly always provide the anatomical, metabolic, and functional information sought by clinicians.

References

1. Sodickson DK, Griswold MA, Jakob PM (1999) SMASH imaging. Magn Reson Imaging Clin N Am 7(2):237-54
2. Shellock FG (2002) Magnetic resonance safety update 2002: implants and devices. J Magn Reson Imaging 16(5):485-496
3. Mills RJ, Young CA, Smith ET (2007) 3D MRI in multiple sclerosis: a study of three sequences at 3 T. Br J Radiol 80(953):307-320
4. Haacke EM, Xu Y, Cheng YC, Reichenbach JR (2004) Susceptibility weighted imaging (SWI). Magn Reson Med 52(3):612-618
5. Edelman RR, Wielopolski P, Schmitt F (1994) Echo-planar MR imaging. Radiology 192(3):600-612
6. Le Bihan D, Breton E, Lallemand D et al (1986) MR Imaging of intravoxel incoherent motions: application to diffusion and perfusion in neurologic disorders. Radiology 161: 401-407
7. Le Bihan D, Mangin JF, Poupon C et al (2001) Diffusion tensor imaging: concepts and applications. J Magn Reson Imaging 13(4):534-546
8. Lövblad KO, Baird A, Schlaug G et al (1997) Ischemic lesion volumes in acute stroke by diffusion-weighted magnetic resonance imaging correlate with clinical outcome. Ann Neurol 42:164-170
9. Lövblad KO, Baird AE (2006) Actual diagnostic approach to the acute stroke patient. Eur Radiol 16(6):1253-1269
10. Lövblad KO, Laubach HJ, Baird AE et al (1998) Clinical experience with diffusion-weighted MR in patients with acute stroke. AJNR Am J Neuroradiol 19(6):1061-1066
11. Sorensen AG, Buonano FS, Gonzalez RG et al (1996) Hyperacute stroke: Evaluation with combined multisection diffusion-weighted and hemodynamically-weighted echo-planar MR imaging. Radiology 199: 391-401
12. 24. Sorensen AG, Wu O, Copen WA, Davis TL, Gonzalez RG, Koroshetz WJ, Reese TG, Rosen BR, Wedeen VJ, Weisskoff RM (1999) Human acute cerebral ischemia: detection of changes in water diffusion anisotropy by using MR imaging. Radiology 212(3):785-792
13. Warach S, Gaa J, Siewert B et al (1995) Acute human stroke studies by whole brain echo planar diffusion-weighted magnetic resonance imaging. Ann Neurol 37:231-241
14. Warach S, Ives JR, Schlaug G et al (1996) EEG-triggered echo-planar functional MRI in epilepsy. Neurology 47(1):89-93
15. Moseley ME, Cohen Y, Mintorovitch J et al (1990) Early detection of regional cerebral ischemia in cats: comparison of diffusion- and T2-weighted MRI and spectroscopy. Magn Res Med 14 330-346
16. El-Koussy M, Mathis J, Lovblad KO et al (2002) Focal status epilepticus: follow-up by perfusion- and diffusion MRI. Eur Radiol 12(3):568-574
17. Heiniger P, el-Koussy M, Schindler K et al (2002) Diffusion and perfusion MRI for the localisation of epileptogenic foci in drug-resistant epilepsy. Neuroradiology 44(6):475-480
18. Assaf BA, Mohamed FB, Abou-Khaled KJ et al (2003) Diffusion tensor imaging of the hippocampal formation in temporal lobe epilepsy. AJNR Am J Neuroradiol 24(9):1857-1862
19. Melhem ER, Mori S, Mukundan G et al (2002) Diffusion tensor MR imaging of the brain and white matter tractography. AJR Am J Roentgenol 178(1): 3-16
20. Lu S, Ahn D, Johnson G, Cha S (2003) Peritumoral diffusion tensor imaging of high-grade gliomas and metastatic brain tumors.AJNR Am J Neuroradiol 24(5):937-941
21. Rosen BR, Belliveau JW, Vevea JM, Brady TJ (1990) Perfusion imaging with NMR contrast agents. Magn Reson Med 14(2):249-265
22. Detre JA, Alsop DA (1999) Perfusion magnetic resonance imaging with continuous arterial spin labeling: methods and clinical applications in the central nervous system. Eur J Radiol 30:115-124
23. Wang J, Zhang Y, Wolf RL et al (2005) Amplitude-modulated continuous arterial spin-labeling 3.0-T perfusion MR imaging with a single coil: feasibility study. Radiology 235:218-228
24. Wang Z, Wang J, Connick TJ et al (2005) Continuous ASL (CASL) perfusion MRI with an array coil and parallel imaging at 3T. Magn Reson Med 54:732-737
25. Remonda L, Senn P, Barth A et al (2002) Contrast-enhanced 3D MR angiography of the carotid artery: comparison with conventional digital subtraction angiography. AJNR Am J Neuroradiol 23(2):213-219
26. Alimenti A, Delavelle J, Lazeyras F et al (2007) Monovoxel 1H magnetic resonance spectroscopy in the progression of gliomas. Eur Neurol 58(4):198-209
27. Law M, Yang S, Wang H et al (2003) Glioma grading: sensitivity, specificity, and predictive values of perfusion MR imaging and proton MR spectroscopic imaging compared with conventional MR imaging. AJNR Am J Neuroradiol 24(10):1989-1998
28. Belliveau JW, Kennedy DN Jr, McKinstry RC et al (1991) Functional mapping of the human visual cortex by magnetic resonance imaging. Science 254(5032):716-719
29. Urbach H (2005) Imaging of the epilepsies. Eur Rad 15:494-500

Extrapyramidal Syndromes: PET and SPECT

Klaus Tatsch

Department of Nuclear Medicine, University Hospital – Großhadern, Ludwig-Maximilians-University Munich, Munich, Germany

Introduction

Extrapyramidal syndromes or diseases belong to the most common neurologic illnesses. Since new and promising therapeutic options are currently under development, there is a substantial demand for functional imaging procedures that have the potential to identify the pathologic changes of those illnesses. This chapter gives an overview of the current major positron emission tomography (PET) and single photon emission computed tomography (SPECT) applications in this context.

Among the extrapyramidal syndromes Parkinson's disease (PD) and atypical parkinsonian syndromes (PS) such as multiple system atrophy (MSA), progressive supranuclear palsy (PSP), and corticobasal degeneration (CBD) are the clinically most relevant diagnoses. Dementia with Lewy bodies (DLB) also plays an increasing role. In patients suffering from those illnesses, the establishment of an early and accurate diagnosis impacts management, helps to avoid wrong treatment decisions, and may allow the selection of candidate patients for therapeutic trials involving newly developed drugs. Clinically, extrapyramidal diseases are characterized by disturbances in motor function, such as tremor, rigidity, bradykinesia, and postural abnormalities. Structural imaging approaches, such as computed tomography (CT) and magnetic resonance imaging (MRI), have limited value in the early diagnosis of extrapyramidal diseases, as in most instances structural abnormalities can be seen only when the disease is advanced, if at all. Conversely, among the other approaches, such as assessment of perfusion or metabolism, PET and SPECT allow the assessment of various aspects of dopaminergic neurotransmission, which is helpful in the differential diagnosis of extrapyramidal diseases. However, before differential diagnosis among these diseases becomes an issue, parkinsonism and tremor conditions that are not associated with neurodegeneration but may mimic "true" parkinsonism (e.g., drug-induced and psychogenic parkinsonism; essential, drug-induced, psychogenic tremor) have to be reliably ruled out.

Imaging Techniques

Since the pathologies of extrapyramidal diseases involve the dopaminergic system, PET and SPECT investigations of the latter contribute significantly in establishing the correct diagnosis. Presynaptic nigrostriatal terminal function can be assessed with radioligands suitable for imaging at least three different functions, aromatic amino acid decarboxylase activity (PET: fluorodopa), vesicular monoamine transporter type 2 (PET: dihydrotetrabenazine), and the plasma membrane dopamine transporter (PET and SPECT: cocaine analogues). Imaging of postsynaptic dopamine receptors has focused on the D2-like receptor system [PET: raclopride, (desmethoxy)fallypride; SPECT: iodobenzamide, iodobenzofuran, epidepride]. Dopaminergic synapses and neurotransmission are schematically illustrated in Fig. 1, which also highlights the targets for the more widely used PET and SPECT tracers to assess this system. Apart from the dopaminergic system, other approaches, e.g., assessment of brain metabolism with 2-deoxy-2-[fluorine-18] fluoro-D-(FDG) PET or the determination of functional deficits in organs other than the brain, such as cardiac sympathetic denervation [PET: hydroxyephedrine (HED), SPECT: metaiodobenzylguanidine(MIBG)] may also aid in the further classification of extrapyramidal diseases.

Parkinson's Disease

The predominant pathology in PD, which accounts for about 70-80% of extrapyramidal diseases, is the loss of dopaminergic neurons that project from the substantia nigra pars compacta in the midbrain to the striatum (putamen and caudate nucleus). Typically the projections to the posterior putamen are affected earlier and to a greater extent than those to the caudate. The loss of neurons results in a dopaminergic deficit, which is believed to provoke most of the clinical symptoms. The diagnosis of PD is most often established clinically based on the criteria of the UK Parkinson's Disease Society Brain Bank criteria, including positive response on

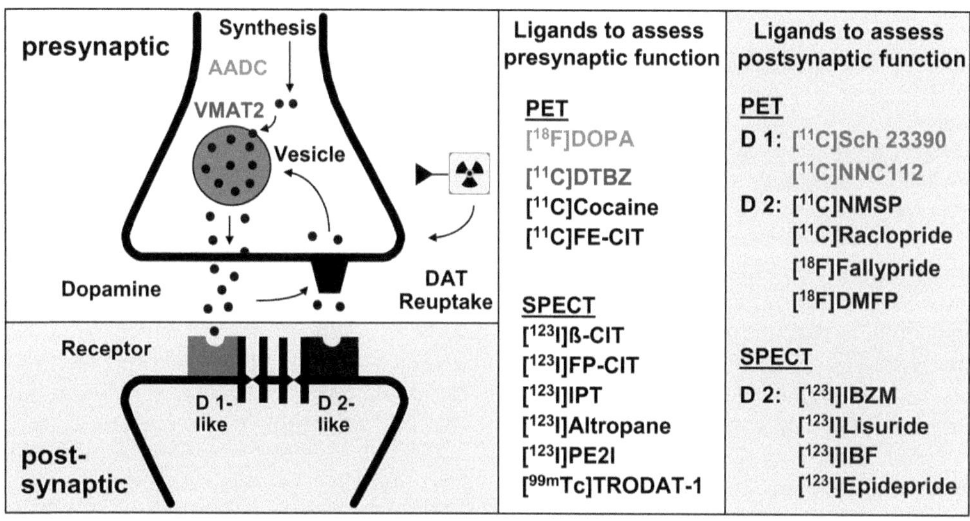

Fig. 1. Simplified scheme of the dopaminergic synapse and dopaminergic neurotransmission, illustrating also the presynaptic and postsynaptic targets for PET and SPECT ligands. The most often used tracers are listed

dopaminergic medication as an important criterion. However, since PD shares several important features with other disorders, there is evidence that clinically established diagnoses may be wrong in early and even late stages of the disease. When the diagnosis is unclear, neuroimaging with PET or SPECT may help to clarify the diagnosis.

The biochemical hallmark of PD is the degeneration of the presynaptic nigrostriatal nerve fibers, whereas the postsynaptic side bearing the receptors remains – at least initially – intact. Functional imaging with presynaptic terminal measures therefore show reduced radioligand uptake in the striatum of PD patients, with a more pronounced decrease in the (posterior) putamen than in the caudate, and usually an asymmetry with more severe affection of the striatum contralateral to the side with the predominant clinical symptoms (Fig. 2). Significant correlations between disease severity and disability stages with the extent of the reduction of presynaptic terminal measures have been reported. In addition, studies in patients with early PD and those with hemi-PD (Hoehn and Yahr stage I) have concordantly shown a bilateral deficit in dopamine function. Interestingly, these findings were not only observed in the striatum and especially the putamen corresponding to the symptomatic limbs but also in the contralateral putamen associated with the still asymptomatic side of the body. These results strongly suggest that these types of studies are capable of discriminating patients with early PD from healthy subjects and may also be suitable for detecting preclinical disease, e.g., in familial PD. In addition, longitudinal studies have documented their usefulness in intraindividually determining disease progression. The annual rate of decline of the respective outcome measure in PD patients has been shown to range from 5 to 13% in early PD patients, whereas in those with longer disease duration the annual decline of presynaptic outcome measures was lower (2-3%). In atypical PS, annual progression is much faster; for example, in MSA patients values around 15% per year have been reported. Imaging of presynaptic functions has also been used in clinical trials as an endpoint measure of potential disease-modifying therapies. Both fluorodopa PET and β-CIT SPECT studies have shown that the respective outcome measure indicated a milder decline in patients receiving therapy with a dopamine agonist compared to L-DOPA. Currently, there is an intense and somewhat controversial discussion whether these data can be used to prove the potentially neuroprotective effects of a particular medication.

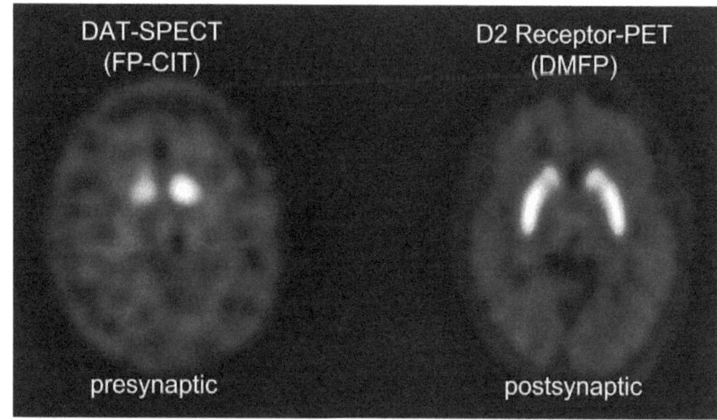

Fig. 2. Patient with Parkinson's disease (PD). Presynaptic dopamine transporter (DAT) imaging clearly reveals reduced striatal binding, with more severe affection of the (*posterior*) putamen and an asymmetry with disadvantage to the right side which is contralateral to the predominant clinical findings (*left sided*). Postsynaptic D2 receptors show not only preserved but even up-regulated binding, which is more accentuated in the posterior putamen than in the anterior putamen and caudate. Note the asymmetry, with higher binding in the right striatum which is inversely related to the more severe presynaptic deficit at this location

PET and SPECT with D_2-receptor antagonists have also been extensively used to study the postsynaptic striatal D_2-receptor availability of PD patients. Uniformly, at least in earlier stages of the disease, elevated D_2-receptor binding has been reported in the striatum contralateral to the more affected limb. Characteristically, in these cases binding is higher in the putamen than in the caudate, and even higher in the posterior than in the anterior putamen (Fig. 2). This up-regulation has been interpreted as the brain's attempt to compensate for the dopaminergic deficit due to presynaptic nerve cell loss and may be considered characteristic of PD; in most other extrapyramidal diseases, the postsynaptic side is also affected by neurodegeneration and herewith displays reduced D_2-receptor density.

Whether changes in glucose metabolism and perfusion may be helpful in establishing the diagnosis of PD is controversially discussed, even though distinct patterns have been reported. In early PD, studies have shown increased regional metabolic rates of glucose in the striatum and thalamus. The use of modern processing tools, such as anatomical standardization with pixelwise evaluation or discriminant and network analyses, have reported promising results in discriminating PD patients from controls and from those with atypical PS.

The diagnosis of PD may be further supported by pathologic results of HED PET and MIBG SPECT scans, which address cardiac sympathetic terminal innervation. Autonomic abnormalities in PD have been ascribed to postganglionic sympathetic nerve dysfunction, which is depicted by those imaging techniques. In this respect, PD patients differ from those with atypical PS, in whom normal or only mild reduction of cardiac uptake is present. Pathologically, atypical PS involves a central and preganglionic denervation that is not targeted by the mentioned tracers. Thus, cardiac HED and MIBG imaging distinguishes between PD patients and healthy subjects and patients with atypical PS.

SWEDDs

Recent studies using PET and SPECT imaging in PD clinical trials have found that a distinct subgroup of subjects who were thought to have early PD presented with normal scans. These patients are referred to as SWEDDs (subjects with scans without evidence of dopaminergic deficit). Up to now SWEDDs have been mentioned in three large-scale clinical trials: the CALM-PD-CIT, ELL-DOPA, and REAL-PET. The combined data of those studies resulted in a rate for SWEDDs of 11% (45 of 410 PD subjects), consistent with reported rates in the clinical literature of misdiagnosis of early PD by movement-disorder specialists. One possible and self-evident conclusion, therefore, would be that SWEDDs may simply reflect clinically misdiagnosed PD patients. Furthermore, follow-up data have shown that SWEDDs maintain this feature over time and herein clearly differ from typical PD subjects. Thus, SWEDDs may comprise a distinct population within the above-mentioned clinical trials, and it has been questioned whether these subjects have PD or an alternative diagnosis. A histopathologic diagnosis obtained in SWEDDs might be the clue to unraveling this mystery, unfortunately it is still lacking.

Multiple System Atrophy

This sporadic progressive neurodegenerative disorder may account for up to 10% of patients with extrapyramidal diseases. Clinically, MSA is characterized by varying degrees of parkinsonism, cerebellar ataxia, and autonomic dysfunction. Depending on the predominant phenotype of the motor disorder, MSA is mainly classified into a parkinsonian type (MSA-P) and a cerebellar type (MSA-C). Pathologic studies of both groups of patients have demonstrated neuronal degeneration and gliosis in the basal ganglia, brainstem, cerebellum, and spinal cord. In MSA, glucose metabolism and regional cerebral blood flow are reportedly reduced in the striatum, cerebellum, and in some cortical structures. This reduced metabolism in the striatum might help to distinguish MSA from PD patients. With respect to neurotransmission, MSA is characterized by a degeneration of the pre- and postsynaptic dopaminergic system. Accordingly, PET and SPECT investigations with the respective presynaptic and postsynaptic tracers show reduced binding (Fig. 3). The major difference between MSA and PD, therefore, is the presence of pathologic findings on the postsynaptic level. On the presynaptic level, diagnostic discrimination between MSA and PD is not reliably possible.

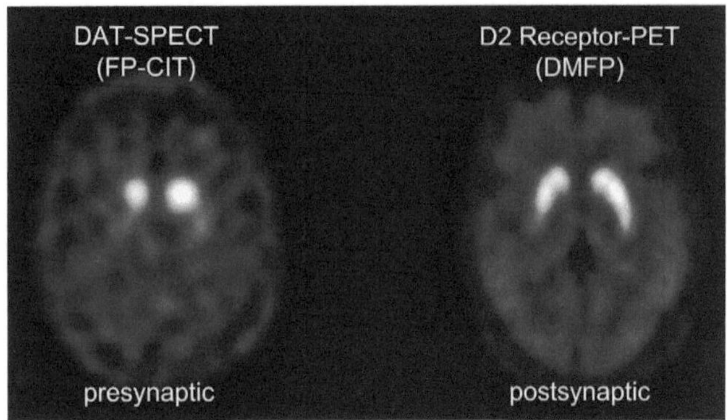

Fig. 3. Patient with multiple system atrophy (MSA). Presynaptic DAT and postsynaptic D2 receptor images concordantly show reduced binding of the respective tracers and more severe affection of the right side. The pathologic imaging results reflect degeneration of both presynaptic and postsynaptic fibers of the dopaminergic system within the striatum. Note that presynaptic imaging alone would not distinguish between PD (see Fig. 2) and MSA (as an example of atypical PS). Only at the postsynaptic level is there a marked difference between PD (no neurodegeneration) and atypical PS (neurodegeneration)

Progressive Supranuclear Palsy

This rapidly progressing degenerative disease belongs to the family of tauopathies. Clinically, PSP is characterized by parkinsonism with bradykinesia and rigidity, postural instability and a pseudobulbar syndrome with dysarthria and dysphagia. The key feature of PSP, the supranuclear palsy of vertical gaze, is rarely present at disease onset and usually appears later. Histopathologic findings show cell loss, gliosis, and the accumulation of tau proteins in different brain regions, such as brainstem and basal ganglia with the cortex being usually spared. Decrements of glucose metabolism in the midline frontal regions and in the brainstem have been postulated as the main distinguishing features of PSP vs. MSA and PD. Hypometabolism in the superior frontal cortex, insula, and caudate nucleus, together with relative hypermetabolism in cortical motor areas, the parietal cortex, and the thalamus have also been reported. According to this pattern, PSP patients could be differentiated from MSA and PD patients with an accuracy of 85-92%. Since neurodegeneration in PSP affects both the pre- and postsynaptic dopaminergic system, the respective PET and SPECT findings are similar to those in MSA subjects, i.e., showing a marked reduction on both levels. Therefore, PSP patients can neither with pre- nor postsynaptic tracers be reliably distinguished from those with MSA. However, as in MSA, the presence of pathologic PET and SPECT findings on the postsynaptic level allows discrimination between PSP and PD.

Corticobasal Degeneration

In this asymmetric progressive neurodegenerative disease, cortical and subcortical involvement is present together with motor and cognitive dysfunctions. CBD patients often initially present with apraxia and parkinsonian symptoms (akinetic rigid type), which usually do not respond to dopaminergic therapy. Dystonia and alien limb phenomenon are further frequently observed symptoms. Pathology reveals asymmetric frontoparietal neuronal loss and gliosis, nigral degeneration, and variable subcortical involvement. This results in markedly asymmetric cortical hypometabolism of glucose, affecting primary sensorimotor (frontoparietal) cortex, insula, striatum, and thalamus. Since corticobasal ganglionic degeneration involves the striatal presynaptic and possibly also the postsynaptic dopaminergic system, PET and SPECT studies of the latter should show pathologic results. Concordantly, reduction in striatal fluorodopa uptake down to 25% of normal values was described. In addition, SPECT studies have also revealed a marked decrease in dopamine transporter binding. Generally, a clear asymmetry was noted, with predominant affection of the striatum contralateral to clinical symptoms. Both the caudate and putamen seem to be similarly affected. Reports on postsynaptic receptor status in CBD are rare and somewhat conflicting, describing preserved as well as diminished striatal binding.

Exclusion of Neurodegenerative Extrapyramidal Disease

One important question for clinicians is whether patients with equivocal or unclear symptoms suffer from extrapyramidal disease or have other disorders that are not associated with neurodegeneration. Sometimes, clinical symptoms indicative of parkinsonism or tremor conditions may mimic "true" parkinsonism but are not associated with dopamine terminal dysfunction. Whereas assessment of glucose metabolism or regional cerebral blood flow is of little help in this context, imaging of presynaptic terminal function with PET and SPECT has shown to be highly accurate in confirming or excluding nigrostriatal degeneration. With these techniques, for example, patients with PD and atypical PS have been clearly distinguished from healthy controls, as well as from patients with drug-induced or psychogenic parkinsonism, essential tremor, and other tremor syndromes, and from those with dopa-responsive dystonia. One example is shown in Fig. 4. Since dopamine terminals are not involved in the latter groups, normal presynaptic terminal function has been reported in those cases.

Vascular Parkinsonism

The diagnosis of vascular parkinsonism (VP) is often established clinically in conjunction with the results of morphologic imaging. The latter has provided circum-

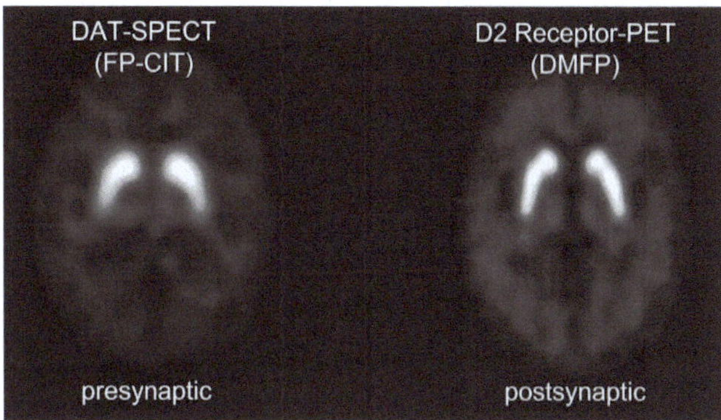

Fig. 4. Patient with essential tremor. Presynaptic images show normal striatal binding, thus indicating the absence of neurodegenerative parkinsonism. Presynaptic imaging can be used to highly reliably confirm or exclude a neurodegenerative parkinsonian syndrome. As expected, postsynaptic D2 receptor binding in essential tremor is normal as well. In this disorder, therefore, the binding pattern of presynaptic and postsynaptic dopaminergic functions cannot be distinguished from those in healthy controls

stantial support for the concept of VP together with histopathologic evidence of small-vessel disease as a cause of VP. Based on clinical and histopathologic findings, two types of VP can be identified: one with insidious onset and vascular lesions diffusely located in the watershed areas (VPi) and another comprising acute onset and strategic infarcts in areas involved in the striato-thalamo-cortical circuit (VPa). A recent study described a significant presynaptic dopaminergic deficit in both VPi and VPa patients compared to controls. The image pattern was similar to that observed in PD, with the exception that the asymmetry index comparing right to left striatal binding was lower than in PD; this finding suggested more symmetric involvement in VP, and particularly VPi subjects. The latter is consistent with the notion that disease in the vascular group is more diffusely distributed (as also supported by the evidence of diffuse small-vessel disease on MRI) than in PD. In some VPa patients "punched out" striatal uptake was seen, corresponding to areas of focal infarction. Understandably, in those cases striatal asymmetry was more marked. In general, data in the literature do not consistently report deficits of presynaptic functions in VP but also normal findings. These inconsistencies suggest that VP is a heterogeneous group with subtypes and/or stages in which presynaptic function may be preserved.

Dementia with Lewy Bodies

Neurodegenerative dementia is an increasingly common disorder, with Alzheimer's disease (AD) and DLB accounting for most cases. Unfortunately, some overlap in clinical presentations among the two diseases may lead to diagnostic confusion. However, accurate clinical detection is therapeutically important, because a considerable number of DLB patients will show good responsiveness to cholinesterase inhibitors but also extreme sensitivity to side effects of neuroleptic drugs. Clinical features aiding in the diagnosis of DLB and AD have shown an acceptable high specificity (> 90%) for the diagnosis of DLB, but an unacceptably low sensitivity (mean: 49%, range 0-83%). Thus, there is a need to improve the diagnosis of DLB in vivo.

Several studies have addressed the changes in cerebral perfusion and glucose metabolism in neurodegenerative dementias, and distinct patterns have been suggested to identify and distinguish between the various types. Even though the methodology has improved over the years and more refined data analyses, e.g., those based on voxelwise comparison with normal data bases, have been introduced into clinical routine practice, there is still some doubt whether these techniques allow individual patients to be correctly diagnosed. Indeed, approaches addressing a striking biological difference between DLB and AD, i.e., the severe nigrostriatal degeneration and consequent loss of presynaptic dopaminergic terminal functions that occurs in DLB, but not to any significant extend in AD, may currently be the most appropriate adjunct to clinical assessment. Today, this is substantiated by concordant ante-mortem and post-mortem findings. Autoradiographic studies concordantly stated that it is possible to distinguish DLB from AD by addressing targets of presynaptic dopaminergic functions. At the same time single-site and multi-center studies have proven that, independent of the technology used (SPECT or PET) and the target addressed (dopamine turnover, DAT, VMAT2), the highly significant differences in findings between DLB and AD always allow the two groups to be distinguished with a high accuracy during the lifetime of these patients. In those studies reporting numbers, the sensitivities and specificities in relation to clinical diagnoses based on the established consensus criteria ranged from 78 to 86%, and 85 to 100%, respectively. More importantly, imaging findings correlated even better with those at autopsy (sensitivity 88%, specificity 100%). Corresponding data for imaging postsynaptic dopamine receptors are comparatively rare, less conclusive, and thus suggest a very limited role for this purpose. Of note, presynaptic measures may be extended by adding complementary information derived from other imaging techniques; for example, the combination of two parameters from different studies, such as FDG and dihydrotetrabenazine, in the assessment of metabolic abnormalities in conjunction with nigrostriatal dopaminergic function may improve discrimination between different groups of demented patients.

Other Extrapyramidal Syndromes

Huntington's disease (HD) is an autosomal-dominant neurodegenerative disorder that is clinically characterized by progressive cognitive impairment, neuropsychiatric symptoms, and abnormalities of movement including chorea and akinetic rigidity. Histopathologically, one hallmark of HD is neuronal loss and gliosis in the striatum. Accordingly, PET and SPECT studies show a substantial decrease in striatal perfusion and glucose metabolism as well as severely compromised presynaptic and postsynaptic dopaminergic functions. Wilson's disease (WD) is also a genetically determined disorder (autosomal recessive) that is characterized by a deficiency of biliary copper excretion, resulting in pathologic copper deposition in various organs including the brain. The latter is accompanied by extrapyramidal symptoms including parkinsonism. Similar to HD, patients with WD also present with compromised binding to presynaptic and postsynaptic dopaminergic targets in the striatum and present – apart from the concomitant involvement of other brain areas – with clearly reduced striatal metabolism and perfusion. Both HD and WD are generally diagnosed clinically and genetically, with the role of functional imaging being restricted to research applications.

Suggested Reading

Booij J, Tissingh G, Winogrodzka A, van Royen EA (1999) Imaging of the dopaminergic neurotransmission system using single-photon emission tomography and positron emission tomography in patients with parkinsonism. Eur J Nucl Med 26:171-182

Brooks DJ (2000) Morphological and functional imaging studies on the diagnosis and progression of Parkinson's disease. J Neurol 247:11-18

Brooks DJ (2004) Neuroimaging in Parkinson's disease. NeuroRx 1:243-254

Eckert T, Barnes A, Dhawan V et al (2005) FDG PET in the differential diagnosis of parkinsonian disorders. Neuroimage 26:912-921

Feigin A, Lewis D, Huang CR et al (2005) Parkinsonian patients without evidence of a dopaminergic deficit: an F-dopa and FDG PET study. Neurology 64:A234-A235

Gerschlager W, Bencsits G, Pirker W et al (2002) [123I]beta-CIT SPECT distinguishes vascular parkinsonism from Parkinson's disease. Mov Disord 17:518-523

Koch W, Hamann C, Radau PE, Tatsch K (2007) Does combined imaging of the pre- and postsynaptic dopaminergic system increase the diagnostic accuracy in the differential diagnosis of parkinsonism? Eur J Nucl Med Mol Imaging 34:1265-1273

McKeith I, O'Brien J, Walker Z et al (2007) Sensitivity and specificity of dopamine transporter imaging with 123I-FP-CIT SPECT in dementia with Lewy bodies: a phase III, multicentre study. Lancet Neurol 6:305-313

Morrish PK, Rakshi JS, Bailey DL et al (1998) Measuring the rate of progression and estimating the preclinical period of Parkinson's disease with F-18 dopa PET. J Neurol Neurosurg Psychiatry 64:314-319

Piccini P, Whone A (2004) Functional brain imaging in the differential diagnosis of Parkinson's disease. Lancet Neurol 3:284-390

Pirker W, Holler I, Gerschlager W et al (2003) Measuring the rate of progression of Parkinson's disease over a 5-year period with beta-CIT SPECT. Mov Disord 18:1266-1272

Plotkin M, Amthauer H, Klaffke S et al (2005) Combined 123I-FP-CIT and 123I-IBZM SPECT for the diagnosis of parkinsonian syndromes: study on 72 patients. J Neural Transm 112:677-692

Ravina B, Eidelberg D, Ahlskog JE et al (2005) The role of radiotracer imaging in Parkinson disease. Neurology 64:208-215

Scherfler C, Schwarz J, Antonini A et al (2007) Role of DAT SPECT in the diagnostic work-up of parkinsonism. Mov Disord 22:1229-1238

Seibyl J, Jennings D, Tabamo R, Marek K (2004) Neuroimaging trials of Parkinson's disease progression. J Neurol 251 Suppl 7:vII9-vII13

Seibyl J, Jennings D, Tabamo R, Marek K (2005) Unique roles of SPET brain imaging in clinical and research studies. Lessons from Parkinson's disease research. Q J Nucl Med Mol Imaging 49:215-221

Tatsch K (2008) Imaging of the dopaminergic system in differential diagnosis of dementia. Eur J Nucl Med Mol Imaging DOI 10.1007/s00259-007-0702-0

Thobois S, Jahanshahi M, Pinto S et al (2004) PET and SPECT functional imaging studies in Parkinsonian syndromes: from the lesion to its consequences. Neuroimage 23:1-16

Zijlmans J, Evans A, Fontes F et al (2007) [(123)I] FP-CIT spect study in vascular parkinsonism and Parkinson's disease. Mov Disord 22:1278-1285

SPECT/CT of the Spine

Torsten Kuwert

Clinic of Nuclear Medicine, Friedrich-Alexander-University of Erlangen-Nürnberg, Erlangen, Germany

Introduction

The lecture reviews typical cases of skeletal single-photon emission computed tomography (SPECT)/spiral CT of the spine to familiarize the reader with this new hybrid imaging technology. The following issues are covered: (1) anatomy of the cervical, thoracic, and lumbar spine; (2) SPECT/CT appearance of malignant disease; and (3) SPECT/CT appearance of benign disorders, including osteoarthritis, inflammation, and normovariants.

Skeletal scintigraphy is one of the most frequently performed procedures in nuclear medicine. For this examination, Tc-99m-labeled polyphosphonates are used. Usually, a whole-body image of tracer distribution is registered several hours after injection of the tracer, which in some cases is preceded by earlier data acquisition. Skeletal uptake of the polyphosphonates in the later phases represents bone metabolism, whereas earlier images of tracer distribution allow an evaluation of perfusion as well as the diagnosis of expansion of the extravascular space. The latter variables are usually increased in inflammation so that three-phase bone scintigraphy yields information on the floridity of skeletal lesions. For skeletal scintigraphy, planar views are always registered. They may be supplemented by SPECT, which allows a more precise localization of foci of abnormal tracer uptake.

Bone scintigraphy has a high sensitivity for detecting ossseous lesions. In particular, its sensitivity for this purpose is considerably higher than that of planar radiography. Nevertheless, its specificity is quite low. Therefore, in the case of increased tracer uptake, further imaging procedures are required to establish a definite diagnosis. Procedures used in this context are magnetic resonance imaging (MRI) or X-ray computerized tomography (CT). MRI is unique in the sense that it excellently visualizes soft tissue. It is, however, far more expensive than CT.

For several years, hybrid systems integrating dual-headed gamma cameras and CT scanners in one gantry have been commercially available. These systems differ especially with regard to the technical performance of their CT component. The first hybrid cameras introduced into the marketplace used low-quality CT devices operating at very low mAs-products, in the order of 2.5 mAS. These systems allow a fairly precise localization of foci of abnormal tracer uptake, but their capacity to provide detailed anatomical information is limited. In 2005, hybrid systems incorporating helical CT scanners became available. Currently, several SPECT/spiral CT systems are marketed, differing with regard to the number of their CT detectors (2-16). These systems offer CT images of diagnostic quality and may thus be considered the current gold standard of SPECT/CT.

Hybrid cameras have distinct advantages over stand-alone machines, since both examinations can be performed directly one after another without an unnecessary time delay. Time to definite diagnosis can therefore be greatly shortened. Numerous studies have shown that SPECT/CT is significantly more accurate than stand-alone SPECT. This is true for tumor scintigraphies as well as skeletal scintigraphy, as evidenced in the literature cited below.

SPECT/CT for Staging Malignant Disease

The staging of malignant disease using skeletal scintigraphy suffers from comparatively low specificity, since benign disorders such as spondylarthrosis exhibit also increased uptake of polyphosphonates. The addition of CT to SPECT is expected to compensate for this shortcoming (Fig. 1). So far, three SPECT/CT papers have addressed this issue:

In 2004, Horger and coworkers demonstrated the significantly increased specificity of skeletal SPECT/low-dose non-spiral-CT in classifying 104 lesions in 47 cancer patients who exhibited indeterminate findings on conventional planar imaging [1]. This study is particularly valuable considering that the reference gold standard for the final classification of lesions was either histological confirmation or extended clinical follow-up, and thus independent from the results obtained by SPECT/CT.

Römer and coworkers employed a SPECT/CT camera equipped with a two-slice spiral CT in order to classify 52 lesions in 44 cancer patients; the lesions had been defined as indeterminate on skeletal SPECT imaging [2]. These authors reported that SPECT/CT enabled correct classification of the scintigraphic abnormalities in 92% of the subjects studied.

Utsunomiya and coworkers used a hardware setup comparable to that of a hybrid SPECT/CT camera, transferring

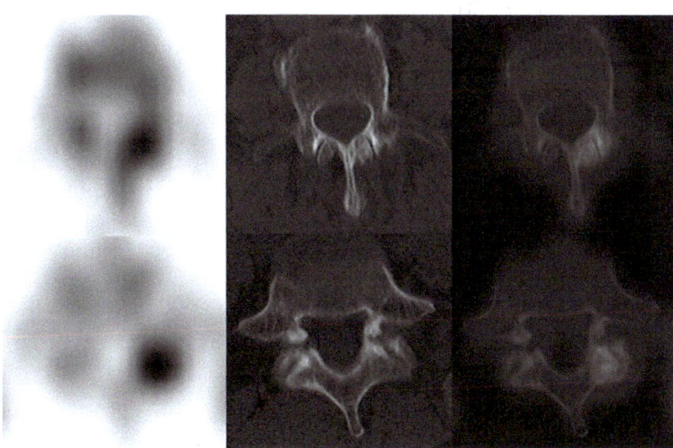

Fig. 1. *Upper row* SPECT, CT, and fused images of a lumbar vertebra in a breast-cancer patient. Increased uptake of Tc-99m-polyphosphonates is due to an arthrosis of the facet joint. *Lower row* Analogous images in another breast-cancer patient. Although the SPECT appearance of the lesion is quite similar to that in the first patient, the CT overlay proves it to be a small osteolysis

the patient positioned on the same table in an identical position from a stand-alone SPECT camera to the gantry of an 8-slice CT [3]. Their study of 45 patients confirmed the significant increase in diagnostic accuracy gained by coregistration of these two modalities. Furthermore, they also showed that coregistration performs significantly better than side-by-side viewing of the two sets of images (SPECT and CT, respectively) at the same workstation.

Based on the evidence summarized above, it is clear that skeletal SPECT/CT is the new nuclear medical gold standard in the search for osseous metastases and that this approach makes conventional scintigraphy for this purpose obsolete. Unsettled issues include the quality of the CT integrated into the hybrid system needed for this purpose, as well as the relative diagnostic accuracy of this approach compared to whole-body MRI and PET using [^{18}F]FDG or ^{18}F-fluoride [4]. Although these options appear attractive, a cost-effectiveness analysis is needed to support the role of SPECT/CT in this context.

Skeletal SPECT/CT in Orthopedic Disease

Until approximately 20 years ago, planar X-ray and skeletal scintigraphy were the imaging procedures of choice in patients with benign orthopedic disease. Although MRI has brought a dramatic change to the predominance of radionuclide imaging in this field, skeletal scintigraphy still holds the promise of sensitively depicting functional alterations of bone. However, difficulties in precisely localizing abnormalities of bone metabolism relative to the complex anatomy of the skeleton have greatly weakened the clinical role of scintigraphy, despite its much lower costs compared to MRI.

In principle, SPECT/CT would be suited to overcome these problems, as demonstrated in several case reports (e.g., [5, 6]) (Fig. 2). However, so far, only one study has

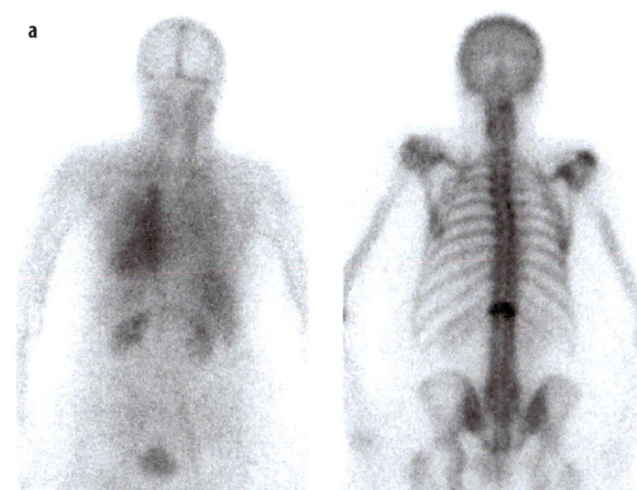

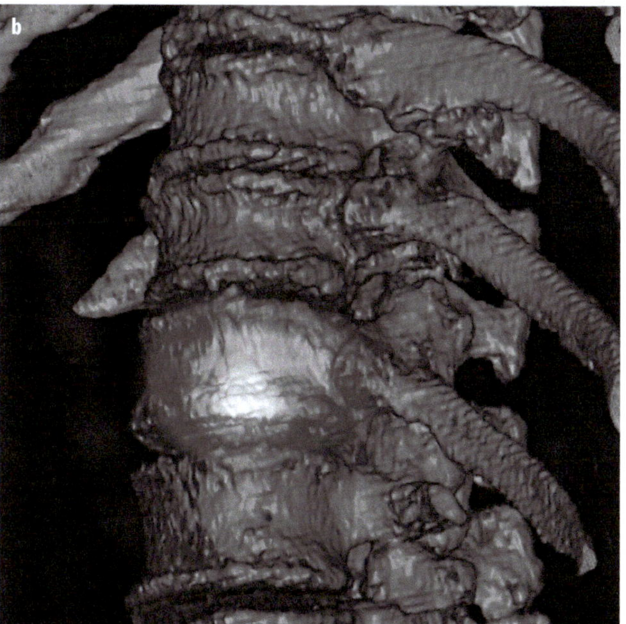

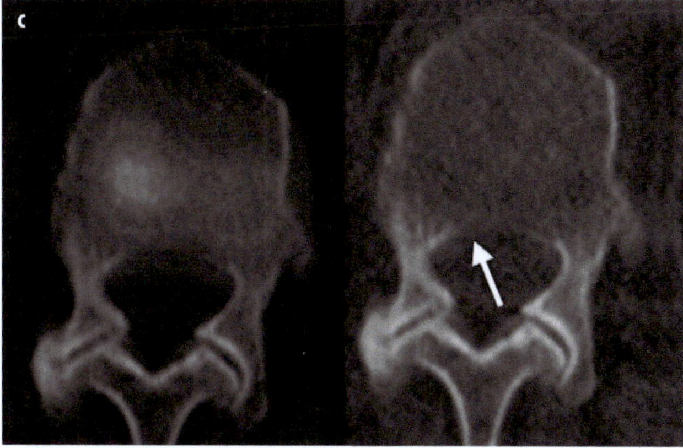

Fig. 2 a-c. Early and late planar skeletal scintigrams of a 74-year-old patient (**a**) after trauma. Note the enhanced uptake of Tc-99m-polyphosphonates in a vertebral body of the lower thoracic spine. 3D-volume rendering of the SPECT/CT fusion (**b**) shows that the lesion is in the twelfth vertebral body. Inspection of the fused tomograms (**c**) proves it to be a fracture. Moreover, the one-stop shop examination discloses the lesion to be unstable, since the posterior corticalis is involved (*arrow*), necessitating immediate surgery

systematically studied the clinical benefit of skeletal SPECT/CT in non-oncological diseases.

Using a SPECT/multi-slice non-spiral CT, Even-Sapir and coworkers analyzed skeletal image data from 89 consecutively studied, non-oncological patients [7]. These patients had non-specific lesions on planar skeletal scintigraphy for which correlation with morphological imaging was considered necessary. The indications for radionuclide bone imaging were pain in 61, prior trauma in seven, suspected infection or inflammation in six, and fever of unknown origin in the remaining two patients. The gold standard for final classification was consensus opinion among the readers, which represented a possible limitation of the study since it was not independent of SPECT/CT itself. Hybrid imaging enabled a definite diagnosis to be reached in 59% of the patients studied, obviating the need to perform additional imaging. In another 30% of patients, SPECT/CT provided information relevant for further diagnostic workup. The authors therefore concluded that SPECT/CT is a clinically relevant component of the diagnostic process in patients with non-oncological disease who are referred for bone scintigraphy.

Clearly, additional studies are needed to define the exact role of skeletal SPECT/CT in orthopedic disease. Nevertheless, the already available evidence may be taken as proof of principle, illustrating the considerable potential of SPECT/CT also in this regard.

References

1. Horger M, Eschmann SM, Pfannenberg C et al (2004) Evaluation of combined transmission and emission tomography for classification of skeletal lesions. AJR Am J Roentgoenol 183:655-661
2. Römer W, Nömayr A, Uder M et al (2006) SPECT-guided CT for evaluating foci of increased bone metabolism classified as indeterminate on SPECT in cancer patients. J Nucl Med 47:1102-1106
3. Utsunomiya D, Shiraishi S, Imuta M et al (2006) Added value of SPECT/CT fusion in assessing suspected bone metastasis: comparison with scintigraphy alone and nonfused scintigraphy and CT. Radiology 238:264-271
4. Even-Sapir E (2005) Imaging of malignant bone involvement by morphologic, scintigraphic, and hybrid modalities. J Nucl Med 46:1356-1367
5. Römer W, Olk A, Hennig FF, Kuwert T (2005) Assessment of aseptic loosening of the acetabular component in a total hip replacement with Tc-99m-DPD-SPECT/ spiral-CT hybrid imaging. Nuklearmedizin 44:N58-N60
6. Wüst W, Kuwert T, Grunewald M et al (2007) Skeletal SPECT/CT of the peripheral extremities – interdisciplinary approach in orthopaedic disorders – first clinical results. Central Europ J Med 2:499-510
7. Even-Sapir E, Flusser G, Lerman H et al (2007) SPECT/multislice low-dose CT: a clinically relevant constituent in the imaging algorithm of nononcological patients referred for bone scintigraphy. J Nucl Med 48:319-324

Role of Imaging in Thyroid Disease

Christoph A. Meier

Department of Internal Medicine, Triemli Hospital, Zurich, Switzerland

Introduction

The diagnosis of specific thyroid disorders is currently carried out with magnetic resonance imaging (MRI), computed tomography (CT), radioiodine scintigraphy and positron emission tomography (PET) scanning, as well as ultrasound. Each of these imaging modalities has specific indications, which have changed considerably over the past decade. Specifically, radioiodine scintigraphy, although still an invaluable tool in the differential diagnosis of hyperthyroidism, has lost some of its importance and has been replaced by ultrasonography, particularly in the diagnostic work-up of thyroid nodules and the follow-up of patients with thyroid cancer. This chapter discusses the contribution of the various imaging techniques in the context of specific thyroid disorders in adults.

Hypothyroidism

The diagnosis of primary (i.e., of thyroidal origin) hypothyroidism is made on the basis of decreased thyroid hormone levels and increased serum thyroid-stimulating hormone (TSH) concentrations. The constellation of an increased TSH level and normal free T4 concentrations is referred to as "subclinical hypothyroidism", which occurs in up to 20% of postmenopausal women.

The most frequent cause of thyroid underfunction in the Western world is the occurrence of chronic lymphocytic (Hashimoto's) thyroiditis, resulting in painless progressive destruction of thyroid tissue. The other frequent causes, such as thyroidectomy or prior radioiodine treatment, are usually apparent from the patient's history and physical examination (presence of a scar on the neck). Hence, in the vast majority of patients with newly diagnosed hypothyroidism, no additional blood tests (such as anti-TPO or anti-Tg antibodies) or imaging are necessary. The only exceptions are children (thyroid dysgenesis and ectopy, dyshormonogenesis) and adults with the rare variant of hypertrophic Hashimoto's thyroiditis; in this latter situation ultrasound can sometimes be useful in the assessment of the volume and progression of the goiter, as well as in the exclusion of significant nodules requiring further investigation (see below).

Hyperthyroidism

Primary hyperthyroidism is diagnosed by the constellation of elevated free T4 and total T3 levels in the presence of lowered or suppressed, i.e. undetectable, TSH concentrations. The differential diagnosis encompasses thyroid autonomy (uni- or multinodular), Graves' disease (Basedow hyperthyroidism), and thyroiditis.

The clinical presentation often allows the etiological diagnosis in younger patients, since the presence of a diffuse goiter with symptoms and signs of an endocrine ophthalmopathy are virtually diagnostic for Graves' disease. However, this is much more difficult in older patients, in whom thyroid autonomy is most frequently at the origin of thyroid overfunction. Moreover, thyroiditis as a cause of hyperthyroidism is important to rule out, since these patients do not respond to anti-thyroid drugs. While the diagnosis of subacute (de Quervain's) thyroiditis can be readily made on clinical grounds without any imaging (hyperthyroidism with neck pain and signs of systemic inflammation, sometimes including fever and leukocytosis), silent thyroiditis is painless and can only be diagnosed by radioiodine scanning. Hence, with the exception of young patients with a clinical presentation typical for Graves' disease, most patients with newly diagnosed hyperthyroidism should undergo thyroid scintigraphy, which allows a precise diagnosis of the underlying etiology:

- Reduced or no uptake is compatible with thyroiditis or an ectopic source of thyroid hormones (factitia or struma ovarii).
- Increased (or inadequate 'normal' uptake in view of a suppressed TSH level) and homogeneous uptake, sometimes with a visible pyramidal lobe, is diagnostic for Graves' disease.
- Unifocal or multifocal uptake allows the diagnosis of thyroid autonomy.

However, even after thyroid scintigraphy, some uncertainty may persist. For example, patients with diffuse but slightly patchy uptake of tracer may have a diffuse micronodular autonomy or Graves' disease in the context of a pre-existing multinodular goiter. Nevertheless, this distinction is most often semantic, since the treatment options are usually the same.

Thyroid scintigraphy for hyperthyroidism should be performed before anti-thyroid treatment is started. The most convenient tracer is technetium-99m pertechnetate, although I-123 has its place when a retrosternal goiter is suspected or an uptake measurement is required to determine the dose of therapeutic I-131. It must be emphasized that thyroid scanning should not be performed in pregnant women or in a patient who was recently exposed to excess doses of iodine (amiodarone treatment, contrast medium), as in the latter case the result will be a blank scan.

Evaluation of Thyroid Nodules

Thyroid nodules are very frequent findings and their prevalence steadily increases with age. However, clinically significant thyroid cancer is a rare malignancy and death from thyroid cancer is even less common, with an estimated annual mortality in the US population of 0.25 per 100,000. Moreover, the ever-increasing discovery of thyroid nodules by high-resolution radiological imaging procedures performed for other indications raises the problem of how such lesions should be investigated in a cost-effective and safe manner in order to identify the rare patient who indeed has a clinically significant malignancy.

In the following, the clinical criteria prompting the evaluation of thyroid nodules are described, as is the currently recommended diagnostic approach, which principally relies on fine-needle aspiration (FNA) biopsies. The clinical implications of the different cytological diagnoses are discussed, with special emphasis on the management of indeterminate microfollicular lesions. Finally, the evidence for and against suppressive thyroid hormone therapy for benign thyroid nodules and multinodular goiters is reviewed, especially regarding high-risk patients with prior external radiation therapy involving the neck region.

Frequency of Thyroid Nodularity

Thyroid nodules, either solitary or within a multinodular gland, are very frequent occurrences. In autopsy series, 30-60% of thyroids are found to harbor nodules, with nearly 40% of these nodules being >2 cm in diameter. With modern ultrasonographic techniques, which are able to detect thyroid nodules of a few millimeters, the frequency of nodularity was estimated at 16-67% in unselected subjects. From such population studies it becomes apparent that thyroid nodules are extremely frequent in the normal population, and their prevalence increases with advancing age. Starting at the age of 20, the prevalence of nodules detected by palpation increases by 1% for each decade of age, and by 10% per decade if the nodules are detected by ultrasound. About half of such patients present with a solitary nodule, while the other half harbors multiple nodules. When palpation is used as the mode of detection, nodules are found in 5-20% of the normal population; most of the nodules are >1 cm in diameter, which is usually the threshold for detection by physical examination. As for the nodules detected by ultrasonography, nearly 50% of patients with a clinically solitary nodule in fact have a multinodular gland on echographic examination. The prevalence of thyroid nodules and multinodular goiters strongly depends on iodine intake; thus, it is lower in iodine-replete areas, such as the USA. However, even in iodine-sufficient regions, clinically detectable nodular thyroids or sporadic goiters are present in up to 4-7% of the population.

Etiology of Thyroid Nodules and Risk for Malignancy

Histologically, most thyroid nodules are either a cystic or solid adenoma or a colloid nodule, both of which represent various stages of nodule formation and degeneration within a nodular thyroid gland. Indeed, 30% of nodules consist of a mixture of solid and cystic components, with pure thin-walled cysts being very rare. Graves' disease and chronic lymphocytic Hashimoto's thyroiditis can give rise to nodules, as may subacute de Quervain's thyroiditis or an infection. Less than 10% of palpable thyroid nodules are malignant, and with the increasing use of FNA biopsy to evaluate ever smaller lesions, this figure is closer to 5%. The risk of a concomitant thyroid cancer within a longstanding multinodular gland has been well-investigated and is similar to that in a solitary thyroid nodule, i.e., <5-10%. Over 80% of the malignancies present in palpable nodules are papillary cancers, followed by follicular cancers and the much rarer anaplastic carcinomas. Non-epithelial cancers such as thyroid medullary carcinoma and thyroid lymphomas are even less frequent, the latter being associated with Hashimoto's thyroiditis.

The low prevalence of thyroid cancer within palpable nodules contradicts the prevalence of cancers in autopsy and surgical series with careful histological analysis, describing foci of mostly papillary cancers in up to 17% and 13% of the glands, respectively. If one estimates that 20% of the population has a multinodular thyroid and that 5% of these patients harbor a thyroid cancer, the estimated prevalence in the general population is around 10 per 1,000. However, the prevalence of clinically relevant thyroid malignancies is only 0.025-0.050 cases per 1,000 persons, strongly suggesting that less than one of 200-400 histological microcarcinomas leads to clinically relevant disease. Hence, the histological definition of a thyroid cancer does not always predict the clinically relevant malignant biological behavior of the lesion within the life span of the patient. This is particularly true for non-palpable thyroid lesions (<1 cm in diameter) that are incidentally detected by radiological or ultrasonographic procedures for other indications and which harbor cancers as frequently as larger nodules. Clinicians should always keep in mind these fundamental epidemiological figures when trying to exclude cancer in a given nodule. It has been estimated that, among the US population, 10-18 million persons have palpable nodules, a number that rises to 75-125 million persons when ultrasound detection is used. However, only 12,000 thyroid cancers are diagnosed in the US, with 1,000 persons dying as a consequence of thyroid cancer per year.

Clinical Presentation of Thyroid Nodules

The size and nodularity of the thyroid gland increases over time such that the presence of a nodular gland is often first detected either by the patients themselves or by the physician during either a routine physical examination or a radiological examination of the neck. Most patients with nodular goiters are asymptomatic and the medical concerns essentially revolve around three questions: (1) the presence of thyroid dysfunction, (2) the presence of a malignancy, and (3) the likelihood of a progressive increase in size of the nodule ultimately leading to symptoms. Some patients present with a rapidly enlarging, and sometimes painful, thyroid mass, which may reflect the degeneration of and hemorrhage into a previously undetected adenomatous nodule or cancer. Alternatively, this type of mass may indicate the presence of an aggressive malignancy, particularly anaplastic carcinoma or lymphoma.

Which Nodules Should Be Evaluated for Malignancy?

Most experts would agree that palpable solitary nodules >1 cm in diameter should be investigated in euthyroid patients. This limit is justified by the very low recurrence rate and the virtually absent mortality for individuals with differentiated thyroid cancers <10 mm in size. Since the presence of an autonomous nodule, Graves' disease, or Hashimoto's thyroiditis may result in erroneous cytological diagnoses, it is important for the clinician to rule out hyper- or hypothyroidism by measuring a serum TSH level before proceeding further with the evaluation of a nodule. The prevalence of multinodular glands in elderly persons from marginally iodine-sufficient regions (such as certain parts of Europe) is still considerable, and the risk for a malignancy in these patients in the absence of additional risk factors is no higher than that observed for patients with a solitary nodule. Accordingly, a reasonable approach consists of evaluation of the dominant nodule in a multinodular gland of a euthyroid patient, with "dominant" referring to either the largest nodule or the one that has recently increased significantly in size. In elderly patients with multinodular goiters but without a history of radiation exposure before adolescence and without recent changes in the size of the existing nodules or the appearance of new lesions, we usually only evaluate nodules >1.5 cm, while following their evolution clinically. It would be erroneous to assume that the best quality of care is delivered by evaluating all thyroid nodules, including by FNA, irrespective of their size and their clinical context (multinodular gland, age of the patient, radiation history), since the probability of the presence of a cytologically "suspicious" (i.e., microfollicular) lesion is 20%. Moreover, most of these patients will eventually undergo a thyroidectomy to exclude the presence of a follicular cancer, which is present in 10-20% of all microfollicular lesions. Hence, once the decision is made to aspirate a nodule, the patient has an a priori probability of 10-20% for a thyroidectomy, which is unnecessary in 80-90% of patients! From these considerations and the clinical irrelevance of most occult papillary microcarcinomas, it can be concluded that nodules <1 cm in diameter (or <1.5 cm within a multinodular goiter) do not require further evaluation in most patients; instead, these lesions can be followed clinically unless the patient presents with specific risk factors for malignancy (such as local or distant metastases of unknown origin, family history of thyroid cancer, or irradiation before adolescence). This strategy applies to thyroid "incidentalomas", i.e., nodules that are discovered on an imaging study (usually an ultrasound) ordered for a non-thyroid disease or as part of the evaluation of a clinically solitary apparent thyroid nodule. Thyroid incidentalomas have also been detected in patients undergoing PET using the radiotracer fluorodeoxyglucose (FDG). Normally, the thyroid gland is not visualized on whole-body FDG-PET scan, but incidental diffuse or focal increased uptake has been reported in large series in 0.6% and 1.6% of cases, respectively. Diffuse uptake is indicative of a benign process (thyroiditis) whereas focal uptake is associated with a significantly increased risk of thyroid cancer (30-50% in those selected for FNA). This latter pattern of uptake may warrant further investigation, depending on the general and oncological status of the patient.

While the above discussion is appropriate for patients with nodules <4 cm in diameter, patients with non-functioning lesions above this size should undergo surgery in most cases. This approach is justified by the high potential of such nodules to become locally symptomatic and the difficulty in confidently excluding a malignancy, present in more than 40% of lesions of this size, by aspiration cytology. FNA in such nodules could give a higher rate of false-negative cytology, potentially due to sampling issues.

Finally, patient preferences must be taken into account; for example, when choices must be made between clinical follow-up, biopsy, and surgery. Clinicians must not forget that death from cancer is a rare event and that microscopic cancers seldom lead to significant disease.

Diagnostic Approach to a Thyroid Nodule

Classically, thyroid scanning with radioiodine was used to distinguish between benign, hot nodules, with further evaluation being reserved for cold lesions. However, this approach is fraught with various problems: (1) 80-85% of the nodules are cold, requiring further work-up anyway, and, moreover, these autonomous hot nodules can also be identified in patients on the basis of a low TSH serum level; (2) thyroid scintigraphy may be falsely reassuring for cold nodules <2 cm in diameter, since the overprojection of normal thyroid tissue may mimic the presence of a functioning nodule; and (3) the use of ^{99m}Tc pertechnetate is practical and economical, but in 3-8% of cases it can result in false-positive capture of the tracer. For these reasons together with the perfection of the technique and interpretation of thyroid cytology, the current preferred approach is biopsy of the nodule by FNA (Fig. 1). A thyroid scan is only indicated in the small fraction of patients with a low or low-normal TSH, as FNA can safely be avoided if the nodule is clearly scintigraphically "hot". Besides the clinical reasons discussed above, this strategy is also more cost-effective, since a minority of the patients (<10%) will undergo both FNA and a thyroid scan, compared to 90% in whom the reverse is true. The experience of the physician performing the FNA and of the cytopathologist is crucial to obtain proper sampling of the nodule and a correct cytological diagnosis.

Fine-Needle Aspiration

After exclusion of hypo- or hyperthyroidism by measuring the patient's TSH level, FNA biopsy is the first and most important diagnostic procedure in the evaluation of a thyroid nodule. Aspiration cytology of the thyroid has an overall diagnostic accuracy of >95%, with a sensitivity of typically >95% and a specificity >95% even in multinodular glands. The interpretation of FNA biopsies is summarized in Table 1. Here, only a brief summary of the clinically relevant conclusions is discussed. The cytopathology laboratory should classify the sample into one of four categories, each of which is distinct in terms of nodule etiology, but similar regarding the subsequent management. This FNA-based approach has been shown to reduce the number of unnecessary thyroidectomies while increasing the cancer yield in those patients who undergo surgery. Table 1

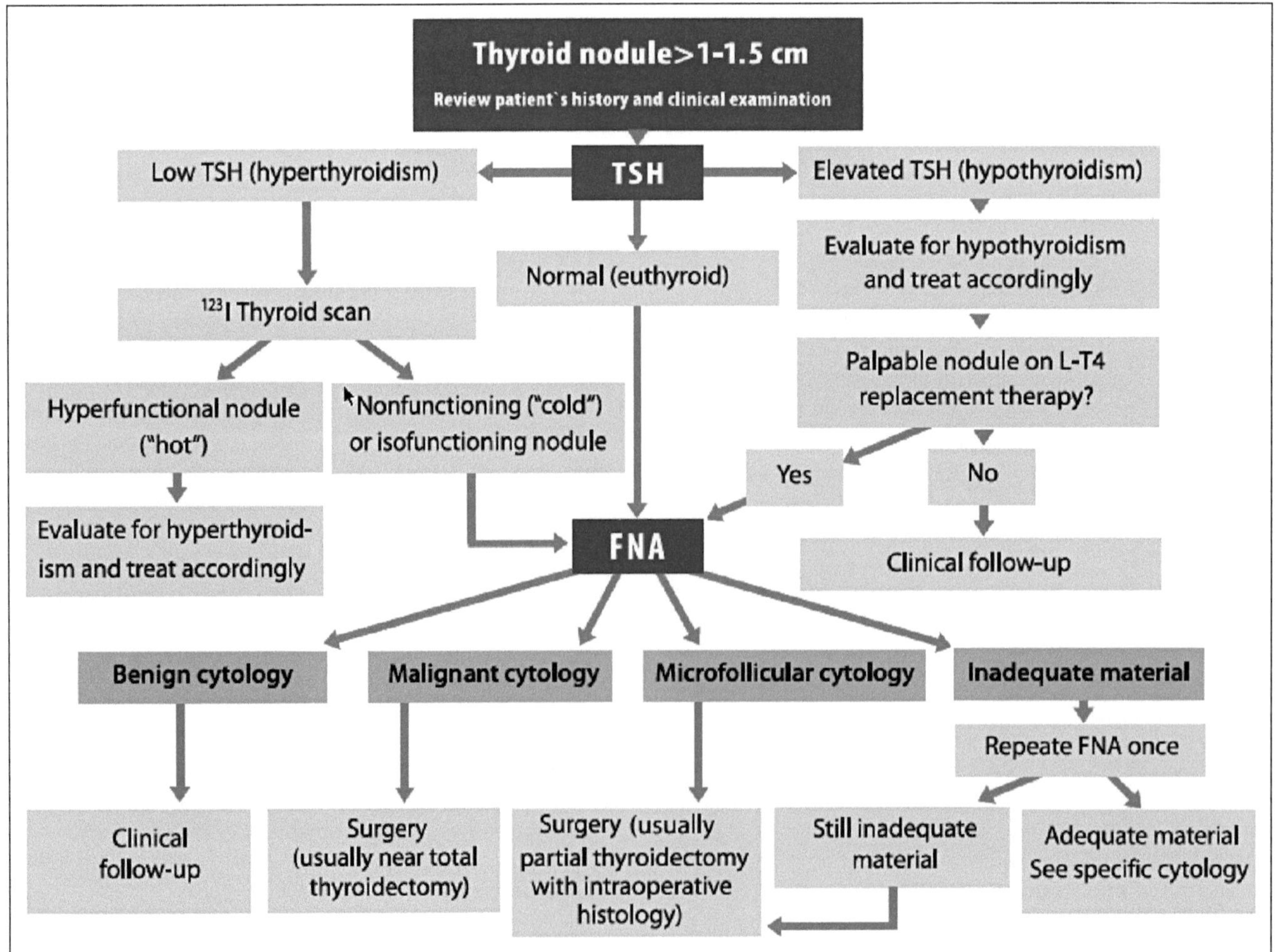

Fig. 1. Management of solid thyroid nodules

Table 1. Diagnostic categories for thyroid FNA

Clinical relevance	Cytology	Management
Benign	Macrofollicular	Clinical follow-up
Malignant	Papillary cancer (or other cancers types, such as anaplastic carcinoma, medullary carcinoma, lymphoma)	Surgery (specific management for the anaplastic carcinoma and thyroid primary lymphoma)
Suspect	Microfollicular (=follicular neoplasm)	Surgery
Inadequate	Insufficient material	Repeat FNA

FNA, Fine-needle aspiration

gives an overview of cytological diagnosis after FNA and corresponding probabilities of malignant and benign histological diagnoses.

Unsatisfactory Sample

Between 5 and 20% of samples are unsatisfactory with respect to cellularity, although there are no universally accepted criteria that define the adequacy of a specimen. Material considered adequate may vary from a minimum of five groups of cells to as many as ten groups on each of two slides. According to the often-quoted definition of Hamburger, a sample must contain "at least six clusters of benign cells on each of two slides prepared from separate aspirates, for a diagnosis of benign". The percentage of inadequate samples is largely dependent on the experience of the physician performing the aspiration and on the criteria used to judge adequacy, but even in the most experienced hands the rate of non-diagnostic biopsies is around 5%. Other factors that increase the number of unsatisfactory samples are dilution of aspirated thyrocytes (either by blood in vascularized nodules or by fluid in cystic lesions) and lesions technically difficult to biopsy. While the presence of a degenerated fibrotic or colloid nodule makes sampling difficult, it is important to emphasize that samples with insufficient material do not provide reassurance and the procedure will need to be repeated. Indeed, in one surgical series around 10% of operated nodules with previous non-diagnostic biopsies turned out to be cancers. Performing more than one aspiration during the first FNA decreases the rate of unsatisfactory samples. Repeat FNA is worthwhile because it provides adequate sampling in 50-70% of patients.

Benign Lesion

Around 70% of all aspirates are interpreted as being of a benign macrofollicular nature, reflecting the presence of an adenomatous or colloid nodule. Once the presence of a malignant lesion in a dominant nodule has been ruled out by FNA, such patients should be followed clinically. Since the false-negative rate for a malignancy is usually <5%, re-biopsy is not warranted unless the nodule changes significantly in size.

Malignant Lesion

A reading of the biopsy sample as malignant occurs in about 5% of the aspirated nodules. A papillary thyroid cancer is present in the vast majority of these patients and, due to its specific cytological features, the diagnosis can be made with >90-95% sensitivity and specificity. Hence, surgery is warranted in such patients without further tests or imaging. In rare cases, the cytology suggests the presence of anaplastic cancer, medullary carcinoma, a metastasis, or lymphoma. While the false-positive rate for the diagnosis of papillary cancer as determined by FNA biopsies is typically <5%, the cytological features of aspirates from autonomous benign nodules may mimic those present in follicular cancers (microfollicular lesions, see below), emphasizing that the biopsy of nodules in hyperthyroid patients should be avoided. Finally, the lymphocytic infiltrates found in Hashimoto's thyroiditis may erroneously indicate the presence of a thyroid lymphoma. Consequently, the latter diagnosis requires careful evaluation by the pathologist using flow cytometry.

Microfollicular Lesion

A microfollicular lesion (also called "follicular neoplasms", or simply, "suspicious") is reported in 10-20% of aspirated thyroid nodules, leaving the clinician with the differential diagnosis of a follicular adenoma or a follicular cancer, the latter being present in <10-20% of microfollicular lesions. The cancer rate may be even lower than 10%, depending on the cytological criteria used to define microfollicular lesions. Since the cytological features of aspirates from autonomous benign nodules can mimic those present in follicular cancers (microfollicular lesions), it is important that the thyroid nodule be cytologically evaluated only after the euthyroid state of the patient has been ascertained. Thus, in hyperthyroid patients with a low TSH, a radioiodine scan should be obtained, and an FNA should only be done if the nodule is scintigraphically cold (see above). It is generally recommended that patients with microfollicular lesions undergo a partial thyroidectomy with intraoperative histology, which will allow the procedure to be extended to a near-total thyroidectomy if vascular or capsular invasion is found, i.e., a follicular cancer is diagnosed. However, given the relatively low a priori likelihood for the presence of a malignancy in such lesions (typically 10-20%), this approach should be individualized, for example in elderly patients with increased surgical risk or a shortened life expectancy. In such patients, the history of the nodule's growth, its size, and the presence of cervical lymph nodes allow a more refined, albeit subjective, assessment of the risk of malignancy, which should be balanced against the operative risk. It should also be kept in mind that careful clinical follow-up of such surgically high-risk patients (e.g., by ultrasonographic measurements of the nodule's size after 3, 6, and 12 months and then every 6-12 months) should allow the detection of most, but certainly not all, clinically relevant malignant lesions, and thus a reevaluation of the indication for surgery.

The management of patients with microfollicular lesions, 80-90% of whom undergo unnecessary thyroidectomy, will likely be improved by the advent of novel immunological and molecular markers.

Cystic Lesion

Upon aspiration or ultrasound examination, a thyroid nodule may turn out to be cystic rather than solid. Pure cysts lined by epithelial cells are very rare and the vast majority of thyroid cystic lesions contain a solid component, resulting from the degeneration of a solid lesion, most frequently a benign adenoma or a papillary cancer. Roughly 30% of thyroid nodules feature a cystic component, ranging from a small area to a predominant cystic part with a minimal solid aspect in the cyst wall. The finding of a cystic component in a thyroid lesion does not give any information on the nodule's potential for malignancy. The risk is neither increased nor reduced. Consequently, cystic nodules should, as a rule, be managed in the same way as purely solid nodules, although as shown in Fig. 2, some particularities of these lesions should be noted.

Additional Tests

Thyroid Scan

With the advent of FNA biopsies, the importance of thyroid scans in the evaluation of nodular thyroids has been greatly reduced. However, it still plays a role in patients with a low or low-normal TSH level, indicating developing thyroid autonomy and hence the possible presence of a toxic adenoma, which is associated with microfollicu-

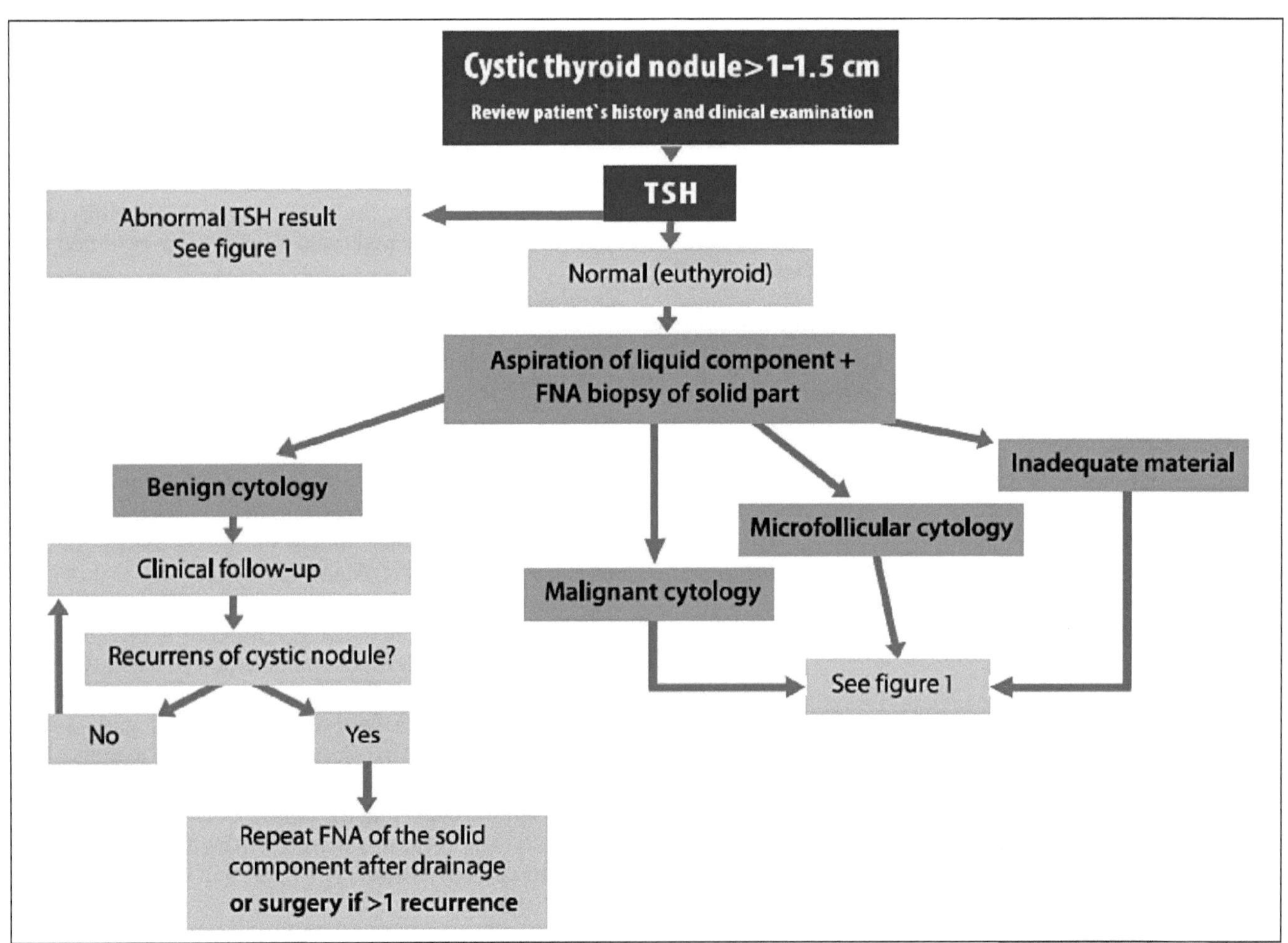

Fig. 2. Management of cystic thyroid nodules

lar cytology. In such patients, a thyroid scan can exclude the presence of a truly autonomous thyroid nodule, appearing "hot" on a ^{123}I scan, as these nodules are almost never malignant. Since the use of ^{99m}Tc pertechnetate results in the false-positive capture of tracer in 3-8% of thyroid cancers, ^{123}I is the preferred isotope for this examination. ^{123}I is devoid of this problem because it requires an intact organification step after trapping.

As noted above, in patients with nodules <2 cm, the overprojection of normally functioning thyroid tissue may hide the presence of a cold nodule. Alternatively, an autonomous nodule not yet resulting in a suppressed TSH level may display no enhancement of tracer uptake compared to the surrounding follicles (indeterminate scan). Only the finding of a clearly "hot" (hyperfunctional) nodule is reassuring and such a nodule need not be biopsied.

Ultrasonography

The precise role of ultrasonography in the initial evaluation of nodular thyroids is controversial and its routine use is not universally recommended. Certain ultrasonographic features have been associated with malignancy (hypoechogenicity, microcalcifications, irregular margins, and intranodular vascularization) while others are suggestive of benignity (coarse calcifications, thin and well-defined halo, regular margin, and low or absent intranodular flow). However, the echographic criteria and their accuracy for determining the benign or malignant nature of a nodule are insufficient even in the opinion of clinicians who use it systematically. In one study, no single echographic sign was predictive for malignancy in patients with non-palpable nodules, although the combination of hypoechogenicity with another ultrasound "malignancy" sign could be effective in selecting high-risk nodules for FNA. The utility and reproducibility of these echographic signs remain to be confirmed in other centers before their widespread use can be recommended. The ultrasound examination is highly operator-dependent and adds to the cost of the evaluation of a thyroid nodule without providing clinically relevant decisional support in most patients with a palpable nodule.

Recent studies evaluating the use of ultrasound reached unexpected conclusions. Papini et al. evaluated prospectively 494 patients with non-palpable nodules referred for ultrasound examination and ultrasound-guided FNA. The authors found 31 cancers among the 402 patients with adequate samples (8%) and the incidence was similar in nodules measuring 8-10 mm compared with nodules of 11-15 mm. Eleven of these cancers showed extracapsular invasion (36%). While these results might be interpreted as justifying a more aggressive approach toward nodules <10 mm, one has to keep in mind the very low incidence of clinically significant cancers. If the results of this study were extrapolated to the whole US population, with as many as 50% of patients having thyroid nodules on ultrasound examination, more than *2 million* Americans should be living with an "invasive" thyroid cancer, whereas the true US annual incidence of thyroid cancer and death from thyroid cancer are much lower (around 12,000 and 1,000 per year, respectively). Possible explanations for these findings are: (1) a referral bias in the population examined and (2) the possibility that the cancers, although showing capsular invasion, might not have had an aggressive clinical behavior. In a study evaluating the usefulness of ultrasonography in the management of nodular thyroid disease, the authors found that it altered clinical management in 63% of patients (109 of 173); however, they compared their echographic findings to the examinations of the referring physicians, 61% of whom were primary-care physicians. Furthermore, some of the changes in management would probably not have been judged necessary at other centers.

Nonetheless, ultrasonography may be an important tool in determining the origin of an unclear neck mass, as well as in assisting in the diagnosis of a multinodular gland and the definition of the "dominant" nodule, which requires cytological evaluation. Similarly, the ultrasound-guided FNA biopsy of incidentally discovered, but non-palpable thyroid nodules >1 cm is helpful in obtaining a representative specimen and may more generally be considered when a repeat FNA has to be performed because of an inadequate first sample. However, we are unconvinced that the *systematic* use of thyroid ultrasound significantly improves patient care beyond that provided through clinical management by a physician with expertise in nodular disease. Thyroid ultrasound might, in fact, not only increase costs but also augment patient anxiety with the disclosure of incidental and insignificant findings, a phenomenon known as "labeling".

Calcitonin Level

Medullary carcinoma of the thyroid (MTC) is a rare tumor derived from the neuroendocrine thyroid C cells. These tumors are hereditary (MEN type 2A or rarely type 2B, familial MTC) in 20% of cases, while the majority of are sporadic. Metastatic cervical adenopathy at diagnosis is present in 50% of patients with sporadic disease; the 10-year disease-specific survival is about 50% for patients older than 40 years. More than 50% of cases are diagnosed only after a surgical procedure has been performed to rule out a differentiated thyroid carcinoma. Except for families with inherited tumor syndromes, MTCs are present in <0.5% of thyroid nodules, corresponding to about 5% of all thyroid cancers. In order to detect these sporadic cases earlier and to perform the appropriate surgical intervention, some groups have advocated screening serum calcitonin in those patients with thyroid nodular disease. Calcitonin is secreted by the thyroid C cells and is a sensitive marker of MTC. In one series from France, of 1,167 solitary nodules, 16 medullary cancers (1.4%) were present, three of which were detected by FNA. Nearly 60% of these medullary cancers were <1 cm in size. Although only 25% of them were detected by cytology, calcitonin levels were elevated in nearly 90%. This has led to the claim that serum calcitonin should be routinely measured in patients with thyroid nodules. However, 20 of the 1,151 patients without medullary cancer also had elevated serum calcitonin concentrations, resulting in a false-positive rate of 59% for this test. A recent prospective series from Italy of 10,864 patients found 44 cases of MTC with only three false-positive tests. This is the lowest rate of false-positive tests (6.4%) so far published in a prospective study. In the series from Vierhapper, the rate of false-positive tests for basal calcitonin was 81% and still 57% after pentagastrin stimulation. The reasons for these differences are unclear but might be due to different cut-offs or to the selection of the populations screened. Systematic screening could therefore diagnose indolent forms of MTC earlier (with an "apparent" benefit), while truly aggressive MTC would still present at an advanced stage. Given the high probability for a false-positive result that would lead to a thyroidectomy despite a reassuring cytological result, as well as the unknown clinical relevance of sporadic medullary microcarcinomas, most experts would currently not recommend the routine measurement of basal serum calcitonin levels. However, any cytological suspicion of an MTC should prompt immunocytological staining for calcitonin on FNA, which has excellent sensitivity and specificity.

In the event of a patient with an elevated calcitonin serum level who is referred for surgery, the calcitonin level should be confirmed with a validated assay and reference range. In case of a borderline abnormal result, a pentagastrin stimulation test should be administered and the patient evaluated for an alternative cause of a false-positive result, such as renal failure. FNA should then be performed with appropriate immunohistochemical staining for calcitonin. However, it should be kept in mind that the serum level of calcitonin may result from an occult medullary carcinoma different from the nodular lesion that prompted the initial evaluation.

Thyroglobulin Levels

It is important to note that the measurement of thyroglobulin levels is not helpful for the exclusion of a thyroid cancer, since there is substantial overlap between thyroglobulin levels in patients with any thyroid disorder (particularly multinodular disease) and thyroid cancer. However, in a patient presenting with metastatic disease of unknown origin and a nodular thyroid, measurement of the thyroglobulin level can be a helpful tool in the exclusion of a differentiated thyroid cancer as the underlying malignancy.

Thyroid Cancer

The advent of more sensitive thyroglobulin measurements, recombinant human TSH (rhTSH), and ultrasound have profoundly altered the follow-up of patients with thyroid cancer. An extensive discussion of thyroid cancer is beyond the scope of this syllabus. Briefly, radioiodine whole-body scanning is no longer routinely recommended, while the measurement of rhTSH-stimulated thyroglobulin levels and neck ultrasonography has assumed a prominent place (for details, see the current guidelines from the American, British and European Thyroid Associations, as well as from the National Comprehensive Cancer Network from the U.S.).

Suggested Reading

Alexander EK, Heering JP, Benson CB et al (2002) Assessment of nondiagnostic ultrasound-guided fine-needle aspirations of thyroid nodules. J Clin Endocrinol Metab 87:4924-4927

Belfiore A, La Rosa GL (2001) Fine-needle aspiration biopsy of the thyroid. Endocrinol Metab Clin North Am 30:361-400

Burguera B, Gharib H (2000) Thyroid incidentalomas. Prevalence, diagnosis, significance, and management. Endocrinol Metab Clin North Am 29:187-203

Hegedus L (2001) Thyroid ultrasound. Endocrinol Metab Clin North Am 30:339-360

Meier CA (2000) Thyroid nodules: pathogenesis, diagnosis and treatment. Baillieres Best Pract Res Clin Endocrinol Metab 14:559-575

Papini E, Guglielmi R, Bianchini A et al (2002) Risk of malignancy in nonpalpable thyroid nodules: predictive value of ultrasound and color-Doppler features. J Clin Endocrinol Metab 87:1941-1946

Schoder H, Yeung HW (2004) Positron emission imaging of head and neck cancer, including thyroid carcinoma. Semin Nucl Med 34:180-197

Sherman SI (2003) Thyroid carcinoma. Lancet 361:501-511

Tan GH, Gharib H (1997) Thyroid incidentalomas: management approaches to nonpalpable nodules discovered incidentally on thyroid imaging. Ann Intern Med 126:226-231

Topliss D (2004) Thyroid incidentaloma: the ignorant in pursuit of the impalpable. Clin Endocrinol (Oxf) 60:18-20

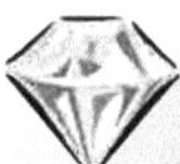

PET/CT Staging and Restaging of ENT Tumors, Pitfalls

Klaus Strobel

Department of Nuclear Medicine, University Hospital, Zurich, Switzerland

Introduction

Head and neck squamous cell carcinoma (HNCC) is the sixth most common cancer worldwide. Accurate staging is crucial for therapy planning. Patients with small tumors and without nodal and distant metastases (T1/T2N0M0) have a good chance to be cured. Nodal metastases or distant metastases at initial presentation worsen the prognosis significantly. Because alcohol and nicotine abuse are important risk factors for head and neck cancers, these patients often develop second primaries, especially in the upper aerodigestive tract (up to 5-10% of cases). PET and PET/CT play an emerging role in staging of patients with HNCC. FDG-PET/CT is increasingly used for radiation therapy planning in combination with intensity-modulated therapy (IMRT). Nearly all PET/CT studies in patients with HNCC involve the use of FDG, which is the focus of this article.

The "Zurich-PET/CT Protocol" for Imaging ENT Cancers

We favor a "one-stop shop" imaging protocol for patients with ENT cancers: 60 min after the injection of 250-370 MBq FDG, a low-dose (40 mAs) non-enhanced CT from the head to the legs is obtained for attenuation correction and anatomic correlation with PET data. PET of the same region is carried out in the next step, followed by a diagnostic "full-dose" CT of the neck. In this last step, intravenous administration of contrast media (power injector) is administered as it is usually done in neuroradiology departments. Images are reconstructed in all planes and analyzed by readers with double board certification in radiology and nuclear medicine. This approach provides the ENT surgeon with all the necessary information and is comfortable for the patient.

Physiologic FDG uptake and its pitfalls

FDG is not tumor-specific; instead it also accumulates in various regions of the head and neck without an underlying pathology, so called physiologic uptake [1]. To avoid misinterpretation, PET/CT readers must be aware of these effects. Physiologic FDG uptake occurs in the lymphatic tissue of Waldeyer's ring, in the oropharynx, in the nasopharynx (Fig. 1), in the tonsils, and at the base of the tongue. Low FDG uptake can be found regularly in the salivary glands. Muscular uptake depends on the activation of the muscles before or during the uptake period and is often seen at the tip of the tongue (Fig. 2), extra-ocular muscles, larynx, masticatory muscles, sternocleidomastoid muscles, or scalenus muscles [2]. In general, physiologic uptake is low to moderate and symmetric (Fig. 3). Asymmetric strong uptake should raise the suspicion for a pathologic lesion. In patients with laryngeal nerve palsy, compensatory glottic muscle activity is observed on the healthy side. Infection can be another reason for pathologic non-tumor-related FDG uptake. Before radiation therapy, patients with neck cancer undergo dental restoration; surgical intervention can cause focal FDG uptake at the resected side of the mandible or maxilla.

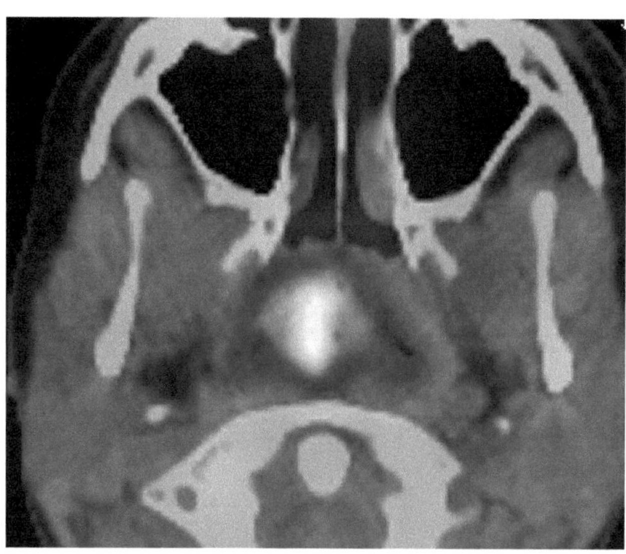

Fig. 1. Physiologic FDG uptake in the lymphoid tissue of a young patient

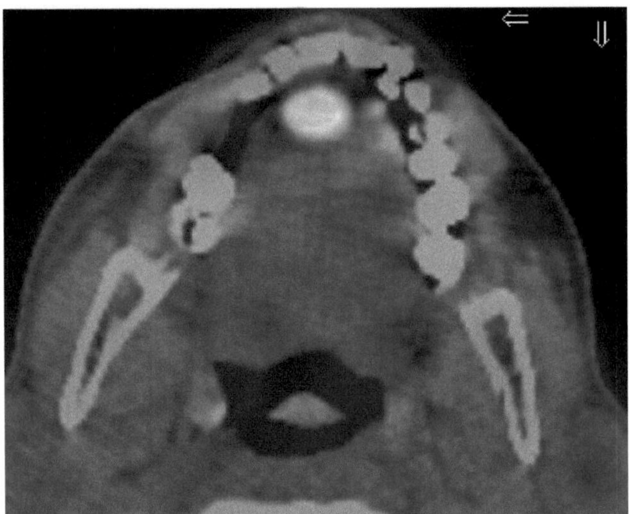

Fig. 2. Physiologic FDG-uptake at the tip of the tongue

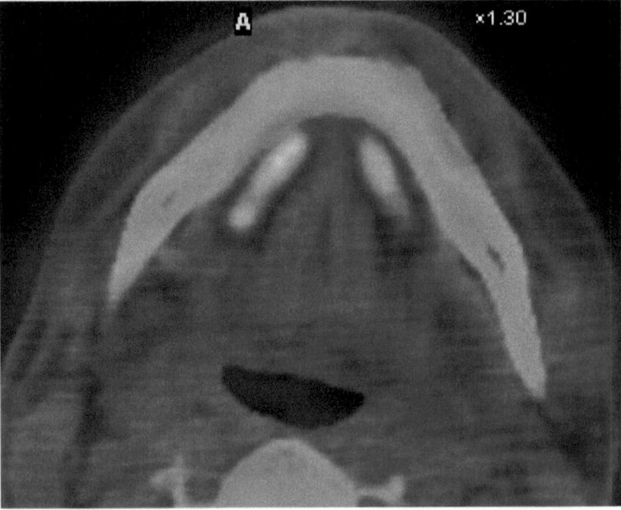

Fig. 3. Physiologic FDG uptake in the submandibular glands and mylohyoid muscles

Primary Tumor Staging

T-Staging

Imaging should help to determine the extent of the primary tumor, especially with regard to the involvement of important adjacent structures such as the skull base or the carotids. FDG-PET/CT in ENT tumors is limited to small invasive tumors with superficial spread, such that the tumor mass may not be large enough to show FDG uptake [3]. Perineural spread can also be difficult to see with PET alone. Intracranial extension of tumors may be difficult to differentiate from physiological brain activity. Because of these limitations, adequate T-staging always needs additional contrast-enhanced CT or MRI, performed in one session or with stand alone scanners and side by side reading [4].

N-Staging

The assessment of the nodal status is an important goal of PET/CT. The presence of regional lymph-node metastases worsens the prognosis and affects patient management (Fig. 4). Also, the number of involved lymph nodes, their location, and extracapsular spread are prognostically relevant findings. With CT and MRI, lymph nodes are primarily chararcterized based on size criteria. Contrast enhancement and central necrosis are additional but not reliable criteria for diagnosing malignant lymph nodes. Even fine-needle puncture (FNP) has a relevant false-negative rate in lymph-node staging. In comparative studies, PET was found to have a higher sensitivity and specificity for nodal staging than ultrasound, MRI, and CT [5]. In our experience, the most accurate lymph-node staging is done by combining the findings of FNP and contrast-enhanced PET/CT. Additional administration of intravenous contrast helps to identify necrotic or cystic neck nodes, which may show no FDG-uptake due to the small number of viable tumor cells (Fig. 5). The CT part of the study also helps to identify FDG-active

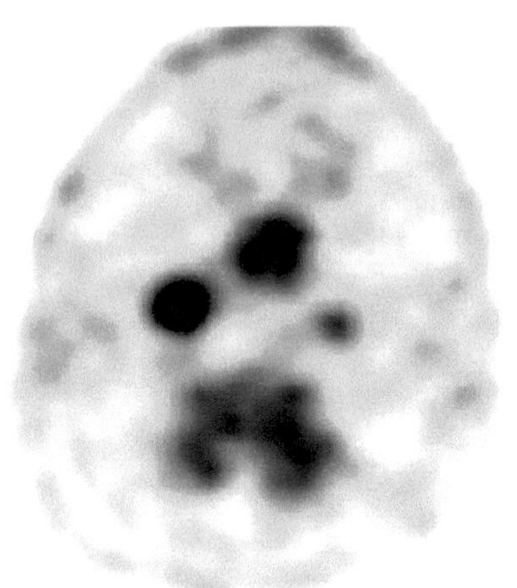

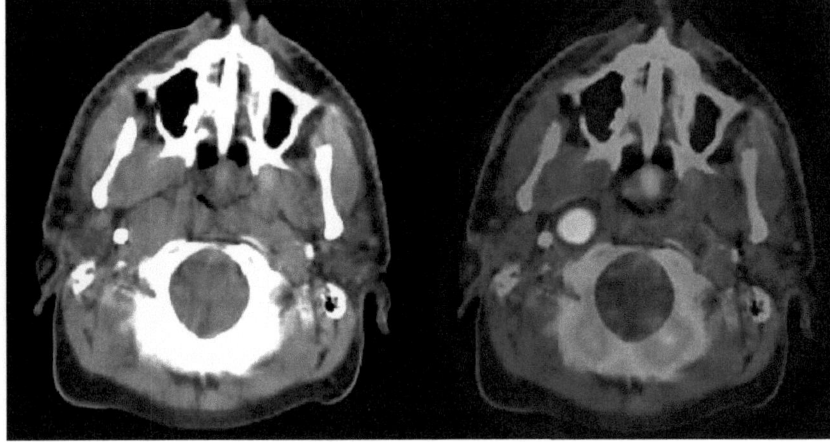

Fig. 4. Nasopharyngeal cancer with bilateral retropharyngeal lymph-node metastases (Rouvier's lymph nodes)

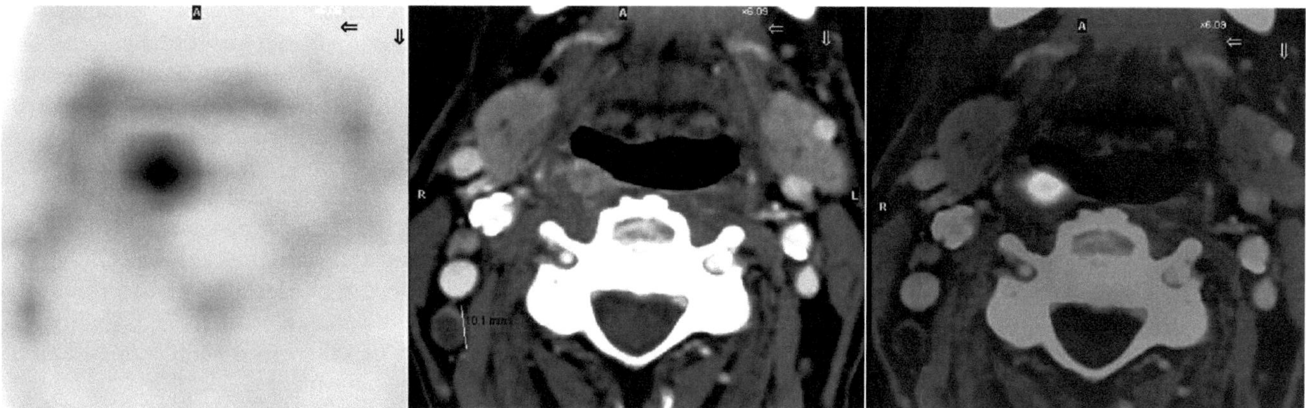

Fig. 5. Hypopharyngeal cancer with ipsilateral FDG-negative necrotic lymph-node metastasis

small lymph nodes directly adjacent to the primary tumor, which might be difficult to differentiate with PET alone.

M-Staging

At the time of diagnosis, 10% of ENT cancer patients have M1 disease. The probability of distant metastases increases with the size of the primary tumor and the presence of lymph-node metastases. Because PET/CT is a whole-body method, it allows the detection of metastases in every possible site. The combination of PET with CT makes this a very sensitive approach for detecting small lung metastases. If PET/CT is performed routinely in these patients, ultrasound of the abdomen or conventional bone scans are superfluous.

Synchronous Second Primary Malignancies

Due to the genetic predisposition and the high prevalence of nicotine and/or alcohol abuse in the population, head and neck cancer patients have a relatively high propensity for synchronous second primaries (Fig. 6). These second cancers occur in other ENT regions, the lung and the esophagus. They are often not suspected and significantly alter the treatment strategy. Based on the experience and literature reports, second primaries can be detected in up to 5-10% of patients [6, 7]. If an unsuspected lung lesion is solitary, the probability of a second primary lung cancer is high (Fig. 7). If there are multiple well-defined round lung lesions, lung metastases of the head and neck primary are more likely. Again, the morphologic appearance of the lesion in the CT part of the study helps to clarify the diagnosis. Although pan-endoscopy is regularly performed for staging head and neck tumors, it is surprising that even unexpected large esophageal cancers missed by rigid endoscopy can be detected easily with PET/CT. One reason is that some of these squamous cell cancers grow submucosally, without visible alteration of the mucosa.

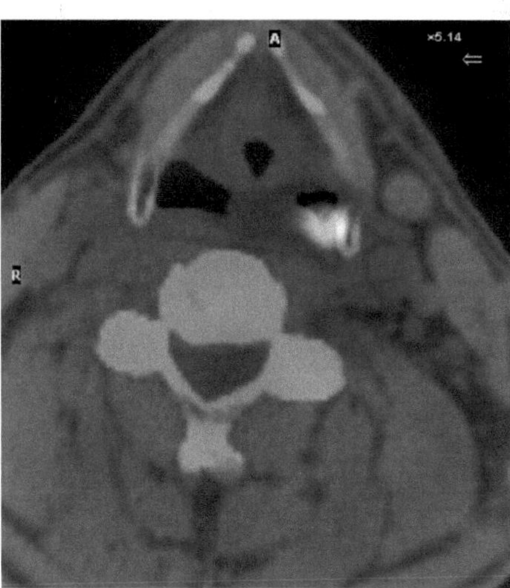

Fig. 6. Piriform sinus cancer overlooked with endoscopy but confirmed with second-look endoscopy

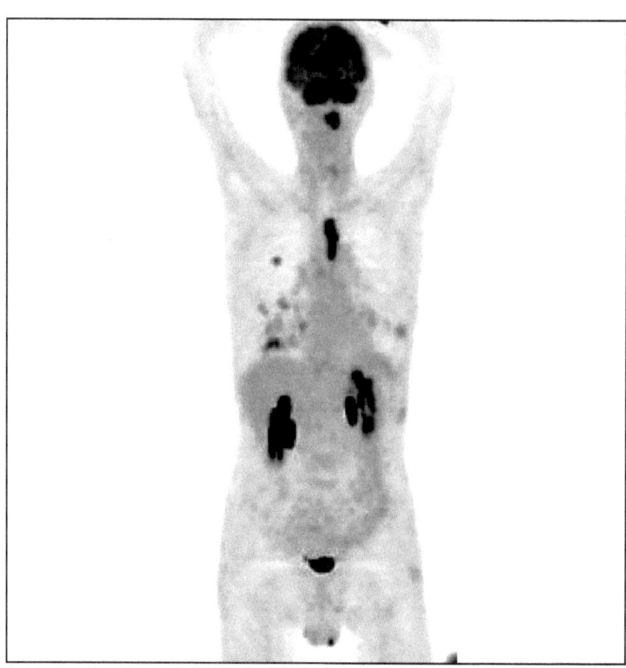

Fig. 7. Detection of a secondary unknown esophageal cancer in a patient with ENT cancer and multiple lung metastases

Carcinoma of Unknown Primary (CUP) Syndrome

Cervical metastases are a common manifestation of occult head and neck cancers. This condition accounts for approximately 1-2% of head and neck cancers. Small primaries of the tonsils, tongue base, nasopharynx, and piriform sinus can initially be overlooked in clinical examination (Fig. 8). The detection rate of unknown primaries undetected with other modalities is approximately 20-30% [8]. Although FDG-uptake in primary tumors is usually greater than in the most metabolically active normal structures, there might be an overlap between tumor and physiologic FDG uptake.

Therapy Response Evaluation

Treatment options in head and neck cancer patients include surgery, radiotherapy, chemotherapy, or combinations thereof. CT and MRI findings depend on structural changes and therefore might be unreliable for therapy response evaluation because of treatment related inflammation and nonspecific contrast enhancement [9]. The metabolic response to therapy may precede changes in tumor volume. Reduction in FDG uptake appears to coincide with a decline in the number of viable tumor cells. An analysis of the PET literature regarding the detection of residual and recurrent head and neck tumors after radiation and/or chemoradiation gives an average sensitivity and specificity of 86 and 73% compared with 56 and 59% for CT and/or MRI [10]. The time interval between end of therapy and PET/CT imaging is crucial to avoid false-positive findings that are due to inflammation. Based on the literature, the time interval after therapy should be at least 6 or, better, 8 weeks after the end of therapy to obtain accurate results [11]. The great value of PET/CT in the therapy response situation is the very high negative predictive value; in other words, a PET/CT scan without pathologic FDG uptake reliably excludes a persistent primary tumor or recurrence so that patients can be safely followed without intervention. Because of the relatively low positive predictive value, a positive PET finding after therapy needs to be confirmed with biopsy before management decisions are made.

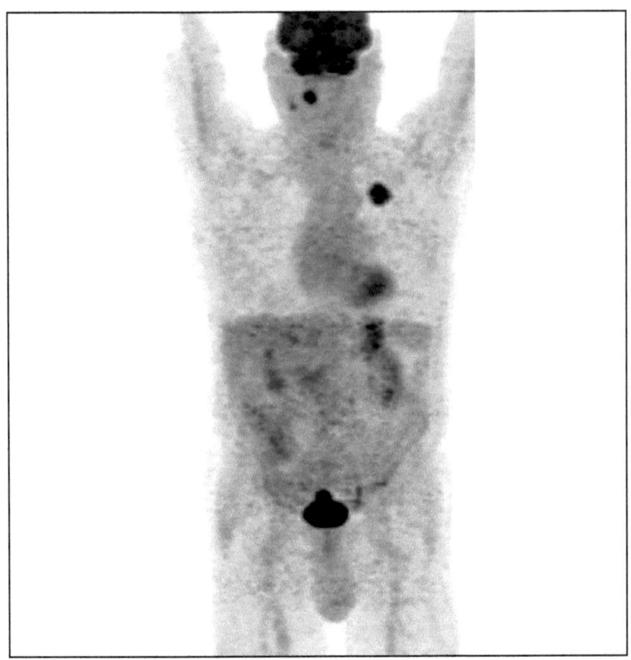

Fig. 8. Detection of an unknown lung cancer in the left upper lobe in a patient with ENT cancer

Restaging for Recurrence

It is critical to detect recurrences early because early-stage recurrences are better treatable and have a better prognosis than advanced recurrences. Again, morphologic modalities such as CT and MRI might be unreliable because of treatment-related alterations like flaps, bone grafts, and bone plates, as well as unspecific contrast enhancement. Although some false-positive PET findings may be unavoidable, a recurrence is ruled out reliably with an entirely negative PET/CT scan. Date on the use of PET/CT for the surveillance of high-risk patients are promising but not sufficient to derive recommendations for follow-up with PET/CT [12].

Radiotherapy Planning

Intensity-modulated therapy is increasingly used in patients with head and neck cancers. FDG-PET/CT data can be employed in radiation therapy planning by importing the PET/CT data into the treatment algorithm [13-15]. Target volumes may be significantly modified when PET/CT data are incorporated into radiation treatment planning, increasing in normal-sized FDG-active nodules and decreasing in necrotic nodes. Radiation therapy will be modified significantly if unknown distant metastases are detected in the treatment-planning PET/CT scan. Before PET/CT can be used as a routine tool, several problems have to be solved; for example, contouring therapy volumes with PET/CT is not yet standardized. Outcome data are still missing or very limited [16].

References

1. Goerres GW, Von Schulthess GK, Hany TF (2002) Positron emission tomography and PET CT of the head and neck: FDG uptake in normal anatomy, in benign lesions, and in changes resulting from treatment. AJR Am J Roentgenol 179:1337-1343
2. Yeung HW, Grewal RK, Gonen M et al (2003) Patterns of (18)F-FDG uptake in adipose tissue and muscle: a potential source of false-positives for PET. J Nucl Med 44:1789-1796

3. Popperl G, Lang S, Dagdelen O et al (2002) Correlation of FDG-PET and MRI/CT with histopathology in primary diagnosis, lymph node staging and diagnosis of recurrency of head and neck cancer. Rofo 2002; 174:714-720 [German]
4. Schoder H, Yeung HW, Gonen M et al (2004) Head and neck cancer: clinical usefulness and accuracy of PET/CT image fusion. Radiology 231:65-72
5. Adams S, Baum RP, Stuckensen T et al (1998) Prospective comparison of 18F-FDG PET with conventional imaging modalities (CT, MRI, US) in lymph node staging of head and neck cancer. Eur J Nucl Med 25:1255-1260
6. Schwartz DL, Rajendran J, Yueh B et al (2003) Staging of head and neck squamous cell cancer with extended-field FDG-PET. Arch Otolaryngol Head Neck Surg 129:1173-1178
7. Schwartz LH, Ozsahin M, Zhang GN et al (1994) Synchronous and metachronous head and neck carcinomas. Cancer 74:1933-1938
8. Rusthoven KE, Koshy M, Paulino AC (2004) The role of fluorodeoxyglucose positron emission tomography in cervical lymph node metastases from an unknown primary tumor. Cancer 101:2641-2649
9. Lowe VJ, Dunphy FR, Varvares M et al (1997) Evaluation of chemotherapy response in patients with advanced head and neck cancer using [F-18]fluorodeoxyglucose positron emission tomography. Head Neck 19:666-674
10. Klabbers BM, Lammertsma AA, Slotman BJ (2003) The value of positron emission tomography for monitoring response to radiotherapy in head and neck cancer. Mol Imaging Biol 5:257-270
11. Goerres GW, Schmid DT, Bandhauer F et al (2004) Positron emission tomography in the early follow-up of advanced head and neck cancer. Arch Otolaryngol Head Neck Surg 130:105-109
12. Lowe VJ, Boyd JH, Dunphy FR et al (2000)Surveillance for recurrent head and neck cancer using positron emission tomography. J Clin Oncol 18:651-658
13. Ciernik IF, Dizendorf E, Baumert BG et al (2003) Radiation treatment planning with an integrated positron emission and computer tomography (PET/CT): a feasibility study. Int J Radiat Oncol Biol Phys 57:853-863
14. Davis JB, Reiner B, Huser M et al (2006) Assessment of 18F PET signals for automatic target volume definition in radiotherapy treatment planning. Radiother Oncol 80:43-50
15. El-Bassiouni M, Ciernik IF, Davis JB et al (2007) [18FDG] PET-CT-based intensity-modulated radiotherapy treatment planning of head and neck cancer. Int J Radiat Oncol Biol Phys 69:286-293
16. Rothschild S, Studer G, Seifert B et al (2007) PET/CT staging followed by Intensity-Modulated Radiotherapy (IMRT) improves treatment outcome of locally advanced pharyngeal carcinoma: a matched-pair comparison. Radiat Oncol 2-22

PEDIATRIC SATELLITE COURSE
"KANGAROO"

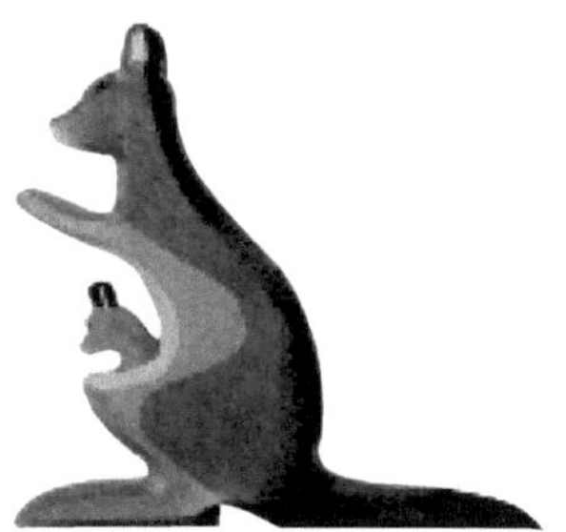

Pediatric Neuroradiology

William S. Ball

Biomedical Engineering, Children's Hospital Medical Center, University of Cincinnati College of Medicine, Cincinnati, OH, USA

Introduction

There is nothing mystical about imaging in children. It differs from imaging in adults for three reasons: (1) Many of the more common diseases of the brain and spine encountered in children are different from those that occur in adults; there are also many diseases in children that are seldom if ever seen in adults. (2) The appearance of disease in children is often modified by the process of progressive maturation whereas in mature adults disease is often modified by the process of regressive aging – two very different processes pathophysiologically. (3) Even when "adult" diseases begin in childhood, they often appear very different by the time the child reaches maturity. The radiologist's familiarity with these differences will allow him or her to successfully and competently perform imaging studies in children. A detailed discussion of these differences is beyond the scope of this chapter. Instead, some of the more controversial issues within the more common types of disease occurring in children under the age of 16 years will be presented here.

Congenital Malformations from the Perspective of Embryology

Modern neuroimaging techniques allow the separation of congenital anomalies from encephaloclastic injury of the brain. Here, an abnormality that arises during the process of neurulation, ventral induction, neuronal proliferation, histogenesis, and/or migration is defined as being congenital in origin. Patterns of injury that originate in utero within the last trimester are the direct result of a known or unknown insult and generally differ in appearance from the more classic forms of a congenital malformation. Are they to be considered congenital by virtue of arising in utero, or should they be recognized more as a pattern of injury and considered as an encephaloclastic event? These and other issues that divide congenital malformations from an encephaloclastic event are complex. Congenital anomalies such as neurocutaneous syndromes may be part of a diffuse syndrome (Fig. 1) or they may be isolated, as in absence of the corpus callosum (Fig. 2). Many isolated malformations seem to be the result of a single in-utero insult, e.g. of vascular or infectious origin, that leads to an injury during a specific time in development (i.e., schizencephaly). Are these true congenital malformations or simply another form of encephaloclas-

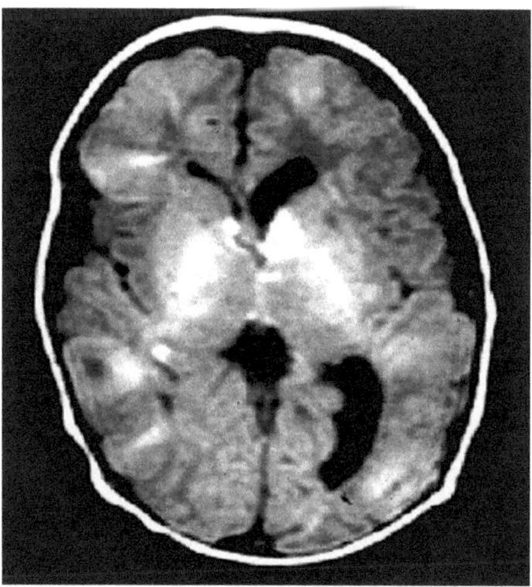

Fig. 1. Tuberous sclerosis. As with all of the neurocutaneous syndromes, this disorder embryologically represents a primary disorder of cell proliferation and differentiation

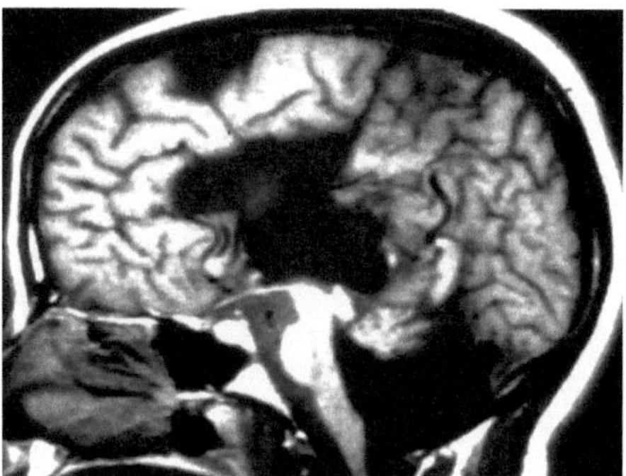

Fig. 2. Agenesis of the corpus callosum. Most often, this congenital maldevelopment is found in association with other abnormalities, but may also present as a dominant or isolated anomaly

tic injury? Other CNS malformations are classified as congenital by virtue of their being linked to a known genetic abnormality, by their association with a specific syndrome, by a familial pattern of expression, or by developmental anomalies in other organ systems. The definition of congenital malformation vs. "brain damage" is not always clear and is often confusing. Perhaps the best approach is to simply define events as having occurred either in utero or postnatal, based on the injury patterns vs. clinical timing of the birthing process, but even this approach is not as simple as it may seem. An understanding of normal embryology and development will provide the radiologist with the best opportunity to understand malformations and abnormal development of the brain.

Intracranial Hemorrhage and Hypoxic-Ischemic Encephalopathy in the Neonate

Intracranial hemorrhage is a leading cause of central nervous system morbidity and mortality in neonates. Numerous factors have been linked to intracranial hemorrhage: gestational age, low birth weight, "birth trauma", hypoxia and/or ischemia, respiratory distress syndrome, abnormalities in coagulation, hypercarbia, hyperosmolarity, metabolic acidosis, mechanical ventilation, patent ductus arteriosus (PDA), bicarbonate administration, and hypotension, to name but a few.

The appearance of intracranial hemorrhage on cross-sectional imaging takes many forms. The bleeding may be intraventricular, intra-axial or extra-axial. Intra-axial hemorrhage may be intraparenchymal or subependymal. Extra-axial hemorrhage can be epidural, subdural, or subarachnoid depending on its relationship to the surrounding leptomeninges, but is less common in the neonate. Frequently, specific patterns of hemorrhage will repeat themselves often enough to allow their recognition and classification according to anatomic location, common natural history, or pathophysiology. The "classic" example of such a hemorrhage is the germinal matrix hemorrhage, found in premature infants. Other forms of hemorrhage in the preterm infant include hemorrhagic periventricular leukomalacia and hemorrhagic venous infarction. Of all the factors that are said to be linked to intracranial hemorrhage, gestational age provides the most consistent means for classifying many of the patterns found on neuroimaging. Far more intracranial hemorrhages occur as a result of the complications of prematurity than as a result of birth trauma. By contrast, in the term infant, hemorrhage is more likely to be related to trauma or, less often, to coagulopathies, systemic manifestations of other disorders, and vascular injury or malformation.

What is meant by the term "hypoxic-ischemic encephalopathy"? Any meaningful discussion using this term must be preceded by a definition of hypoxic-ischemic encephalopathy (HIE). Even so, HIE means different things to different people. The neurologist, neonatologist, and perinatologist may consider HIE a clinical diagnosis only, supported solely by specific clinical indicators of multi-organ system failure. The neuroradiologist may suggest a diagnosis of HIE based on imaging studies and drawing from prior experience, correlating current findings with the same or similar findings in children with known hypoxic and/or ischemic brain injury. To the neurophysiologist, HIE describes a series of metabolic alterations, arising from either a lack of oxygenation or blood flow, which have an effect on brain tissue, irrespective of any specific etiology. Finally, the neuropathologist may require histologic evidence, regardless of the clinical features or imaging findings, in order to make the diagnosis of HIE. Here, the term "hypoxic/ischemic encephalopathy" indicates a pathophysiologic event without considering the cause or etiology of the hypoxia or ischemia. Thus, HIE is a direct result of either a lack of oxygen or a lack of blood supply, the effect of which may or may not be documented on imaging studies.

How sensitive are imaging studies in detecting CNS injury as a result of either hypoxia or ischemia; and, how well does imaging correlate with motor delay, neurocognitive dysfunction, or mental retardation (Fig. 3)? These are two questions frequently asked for which there are only partial answers. Whereas imaging often correlates well with gross motor and sensory neurologic dysfunction, marked limitations remain in correlating imaging findings with clinical development, neurocognitive deficits, and mental retardation.

Metabolic/Neurodegenerative Disorders

The many degenerative pathologic processes that involve the central nervous system (CNS) in children are classified as primary metabolic, or neurogenerative, disorders and as secondary disorders related to metabolic dysfunction in response to neurotoxic agents.

Metabolic and neurodegenerative disorders, which are often grouped together, are frequently responsible for the abnormal growth and development manifesting early or late in childhood. Common to all of these conditions are their injurious effect on normal CNS maturation at a time of maximal growth and development. While the classifications of these diseases vary, the scheme described by Valk and Van der Knapp, which is based on an abnormal cellular morphology and/or function of the lysosome, peroxisome, or mitochondria, is useful for discussion, as these three defects account for the majority of the common neurogenerative disorders likely to be encountered in the pediatric population.

Lysosomal disorders encompass a wide variety of cellular enzyme (hydrolase) deficiencies, all of which lead to an abnormal accumulation of undigested material (lipid, carbohydrates, or mucopolysaccarides) within

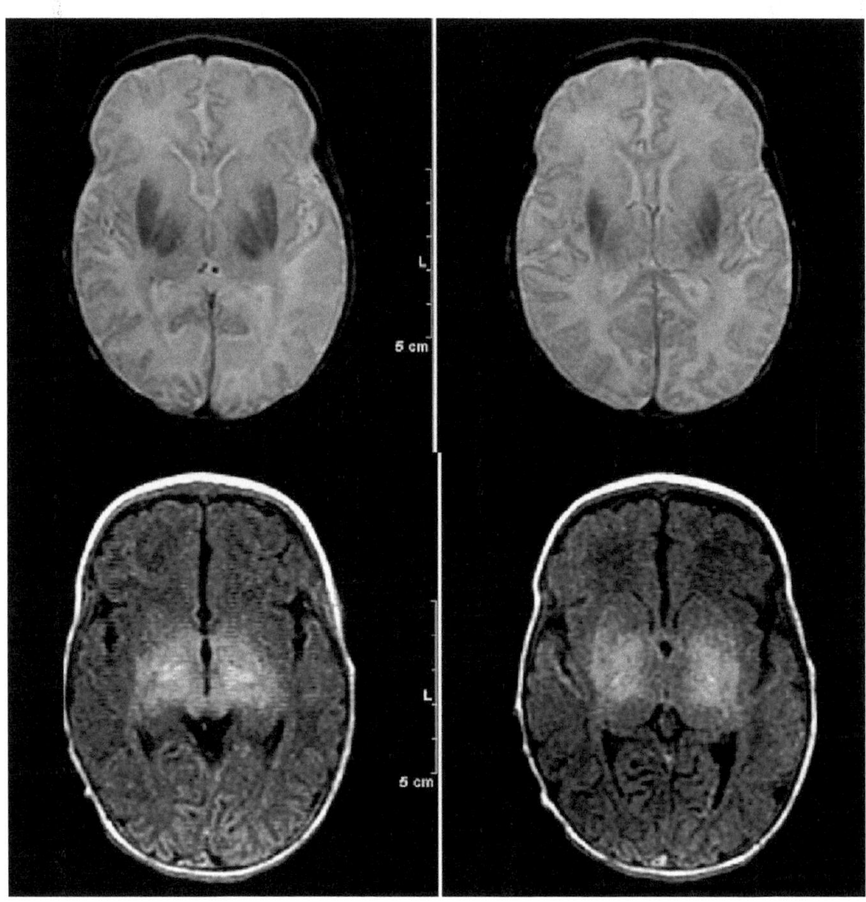

Fig. 3. Neonatal hypoxic-ischemic encephalopathy. Abnormal signal on both T1- (*below, left and right*) and T2-weighted images (*above, left and right*) can be identified in the posterior putamen and ventrolateral thalamus bilaterally. APGAR scores were 1 at 1 min, and 4 at 5 min

lysosomes, the subsequent rupture of these organelles into the cytoplasm of the cell, and eventual cellular dysfunction. The lysosome contains hydrolytic enzymes but also serves as a storage organelle that plays an important function in the phagocytosis of unwanted cellular particulates. Conditions primarily affecting the white matter are the sphingolipidoses, such as metachromatic leukodystrophy (Fig. 4) and globoid cell leukodystrophy (Krabbe's disease); whereas the mucolipidoses (I-cell disease), lipidoses (Niemann-Pick disease), and mucopolysaccharidoses predominately involve only gray matter or both white and gray matter.

The peroxisome is another cellular organelle that is home to a host of enzymes critical to proper cellular function, including the oxidation of long-chain-fatty-acids, the synthesis of bile acids, the formation of plasmalogens, glycerol ether lipid synthesis and amino-acid metabolism. Morphologic abnormalities (absence, de-

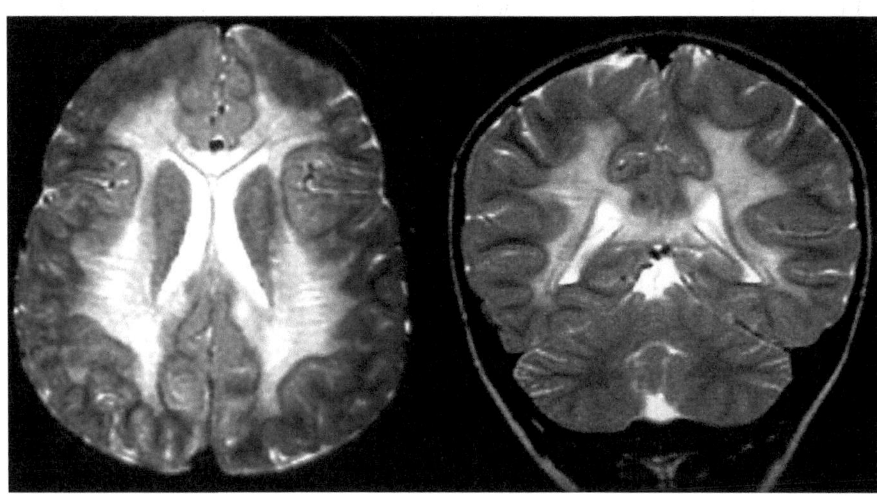

Fig. 4. Metachromatic leukodystrophy. Diffure symmetrical hypomyelination is present in this 3-year-old as seen on the axial (*left*) and coronal (*right*) images. Note the sparing of the subcortical white matter

creased size, or deficient numbers) or specific enzyme defects lead to a variety of clinical syndromes, the peroxisomal disorders, which includes Zellweger's syndrome, neonatal and X-linked adrenoleukodystrophy (ALD), and adrenomyeloneuropathy.

Finally, abnormalities in the mitochondria and in respiratory oxidation such as occur with enzyme deficiencies may involve the Kreb's cycle and cytochrome-electron transfer system, leading to an inability to provide sufficient quantities of ATP. Abnormal accumulation of lactate, pyruvate, and alanine in blood, serum, CSF, brain, and muscle may be found in many of these disorders as a result of alterations in the pyruvate dehydrogenase complex. Clinical features vary considerably among these disorders, and the frequent overlap in signs and symptoms leaves the biochemical, pathologic, and neuroimaging alterations as the only means for diagnosis. Among the more common of these disorders are MELAS (mitochondrial myopathy, encephalopathy, lactic acidosis, and stroke) syndrome, MERRF (myoclonus epilepsy associated with ragged-red fibers), and disorders of electron transport.

Other useful classification schemes are that of metabolic disease associated with macrocrania (Canavan's disease, Alexander's disease), and those presenting in neonates, such as the organic acidurias and uric acid abnormalities. Today, neurotoxicity is most commonly encountered in the form of chemotherapy- and radiation-induced injury secondary to treatment of childhood neoplasms.

Trauma

Non-accidental trauma, in contrast to trauma caused by accidents, is a childhood disease with no similar process in adults. Cranial abuse is the leading cause of morbidity and mortality in children <5 years of age. The physical manifestations depend on the mechanism of injury: direct blows to the calvarium produce lacerations, calvarial fractures, intracranial hemorrhage, and/or parenchymal injury; the combination of violent shaking (applied rotational force) and direct impact (translational force), known as the shaken-baby-impact syndrome, produces white-matter shearing injury, subdural hematomas, and hemorrhagic contusions; strangulation and/or suffocation lead to HIE.

Calvarial fractures are present in 45-55% of physically abused children. Fractures that are multiple, bilateral, cross suture lines, depressed, or diastatic are common but are not diagnostic, of abuse. Conventional radiographs are most likely to reveal a fracture; however, CT is the imaging modality of choice in the evaluation of intracranial complications.

Intracranial injury typically takes the form of extra-axial hemorrhage, hemorrhagic parenchymal contusions, white-matter shearing injury, or HIE (Fig. 5). Subdural hematomas may be multiple, vary in size, and located anywhere over the cerebral or cerebellar convexities. A posterior interhemispheric subdural hematoma is suggestive, but not pathognomonic of abuse. MR is more sensitive than CT in the detection of subdural hematomas located high over the convexity, in the anterior and middle cranial fossae, and infratentorial space; and for aging hematomas as well. Nonetheless, CT remains the imaging modality of choice in the detection of an acute subdural hematoma requiring surgical attention. Shearing injury to the deep white matter and corpus callosum, and intraparenchymal cortical contusions are common. Hypoxic/ischemic injury is the result of violent shaking, suffocation, or strangulation and leads to devastating consequences. On CT, the appearance is that of diffuse low attenuation of gray and white matter in contrast to the persistent isodensity of the basal ganglia (reversal sign) or cerebellum (white cerebellar sign). The findings represent both diffuse edema as well as cortical necrosis. The end result is typically that of either diffuse atrophy or cystic encephalomalacia.

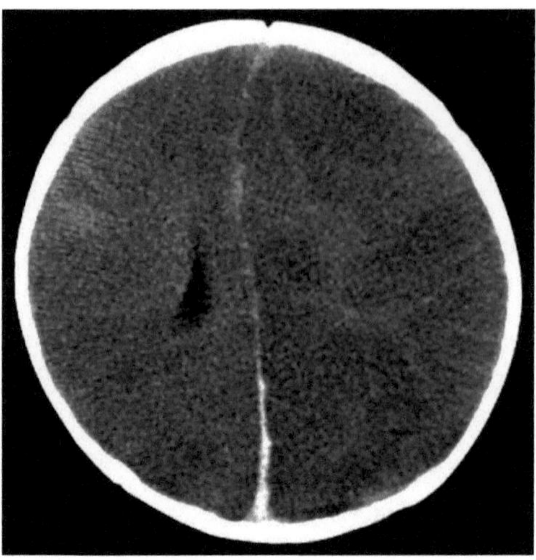

Fig. 5. Non-accidental trauma. There is diffuse hypodensity to both the white and gray matter. An interhemispheric subdural hematoma is also present

Cerebrovascular Disease in Childhood

Cerebrovascular disease in children covers many etiologies, including congenital vascular malformations, traumatic vascular injury, aneurysms, vasculitis/angiitis, and cerebrovascular occlusive disease.

Vascular malformations are generally classified as true arteriovenous malformations, cavernous or venous angiomas, and congenital hereditary telangiectasias. Hereditary telangiectasias are mainly found at autopsy, are usually of little clinical significance, and go unrecognized on imaging. True arteriovenous malformations are composed of a compact tangle of arteries and veins within a nidus. They are fed by normal dural and/or cerebral vessels and further characterized by the lack of intervening vessels of resistance, i.e., the capillaries. Cavernous malformations or angiomas can be identified on imaging in children by the presence of one of three patterns: A less common CT appearance is that of a solitary mass with calcification that often makes the lesion appear slightly dense. Enhancement is characteristically lacking, as is also significant mass effect. A second pattern, often associated with a familial pattern of occurrence, is that of multifocal lesions of very low signal on T2-weighted images due to the presence within the angioma of hemosiderin from previous hemorrhage. Identification of this type of cavernous angioma can be improved by using a gradient T2* acquisition technique. These lesions cannot actually be seen prior to hemorrhage. The third and final pattern is that of a mass associated with acute hemorrhage in which there is considerable mass effect. Differentiation from a hemorrhagic neoplasm may be difficult.

Aneurysms involving the cerebral vasculature in children are much less common than in adults. A true aneurysm represents a dilatation of a blood vessel in which the wall is still composed of all three layers, whereas a false aneurysm may result in an interruption of the wall layers with similar results. The distribution of aneurysms in childhood is similar to that in adults, with perhaps a slightly greater incidence in the region of the basilar tip. Aneurysms in children differ somewhat in their appearance from those in adults, For example, many aneurysms in childhood are quite large (>2.5 cm) and may actually present with mass effect (cranial nerve palsy) rather than with distal ischemia. Aneurysms may be associated with various syndromes including polycystic kidney disease and coarctation of the aorta.

Cerebrovascular occlusive disease is far more common in children than previously recognized (Fig. 6). The causes include trauma, infection, sickle cell disease and other hemoglobinopathies, alterations within the fibrinolytic system, complications of therapy (e.g., radiation, chemotherapy), cardiac disorders, primary CNS angiitis, autoimmune vascular disorders, and metabolic disease. Stroke is generally defined as either embolic or thrombotic in origin. Embolic disease in childhood is most often the result of cardiac disease, trauma, or vasculitis. Cardiac disorders associated with embolic stroke arise from cyanotic cardiac conditions, mitral valve prolapse, cardiomyopathies, infections, arrhythmias, and neoplasms. Therefore, the evaluation of acute stroke without a known underlying disorder must include careful evaluation of the heart by echocardiography or MR imaging. Spontaneous thrombosis of the carotid or vertebrobasilar systems is a well-described entity that may or may not be associated with a history of trauma. Trauma, if present, may seem to be trivial but can nevertheless have devastating consequences. Fibromuscular disease and Takayasu's arteritis are rare causes of childhood embolic disease that can be carefully sought for by MR angiography and color Doppler ultrasound.

Thrombotic disease is far more common in children. Vascular injury, hypercoagulable states, and clotting disorders all may result in thrombosis and stroke in childhood. Vascular injury leading to stroke occurs with radiation, trauma, homocystinuria and sickle cell disease. Dehydration, dyslipoproteinemia, protein-C deficiency, sickle cell disease, paraneoplastic disorders, cyanotic cardiac conditions, and polycythemia may result in a hypercoagulable state and thus induce stroke in the pediatric age group. Imaging is primarily of importance in the confirmation of a clinical stroke, to determine the extent of injury, and to classify the stroke as bland or hemorrhagic, which may affect therapy. MR is more sensitive than CT in detecting the early changes of infarction.

Moya Moya represents an obliterative vasculitis of the distal internal carotid arteries and the proximal middle and anterior cerebral vessels. Causes include idiopathic,

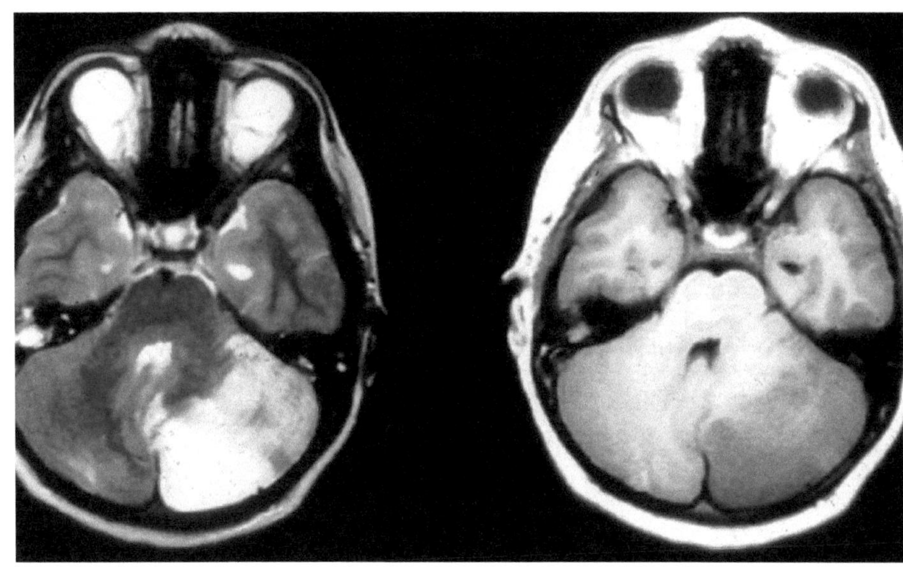

Fig. 6. Acute cerebellar stroke. This acute vascular occlusion is evident on both the T2- (*left*) and T1-weighted (*right*) images, followed an allergic reaction to a bee sting

sickle cell disease, neurofibromatosis, and Downs's syndrome. In Japanese, "Moya Moya" literally means "like a puff of smoke", in reference to the angiographic appearance of collateral flow in the lenticulostriate vessels. While cerebral angiography is definitive, the utility of MR angiography and color Doppler ultrasound in the diagnosis of this disorder was recently reported. On conventional MR, multifocal white matter signal changes consistent with watershed infarctions are present. Classic wedge-shaped infarctions are also common. Prominent perivascular spaces indicative of collateral flow can be seen in the basal ganglia region of the globus pallidus and putamen.

Suggested Reading

Ball WS (1991) Magnetic resonance imaging of the infant brain. Semin Ultrasound CT MR. 12:379-409

Ball WS, Prenger EC, Ballard ET (1992) Neurotoxicity of radio/chemotherapy in children: pathologic and mr correlation. AJNR Am J Neuroradiol 13:761-776

Barkovich AJ, Norman D (1989) Absence of the septum pellucidum: a useful sign in the diagnosis of congenital brain malformations. AJNR Am J Neuroradiol 9:1107-1114

Barkovich AJ, Truwit CL (1990) Brain damage from perinatal asphyxia: correlation of MR findings with gestational age. AJNR Am J Neuroradiol 1:1087-1096

Byrd SE, Osborn RE, Bohan TP, Niadich TP (1989) The CT and MR evaluation of migrational disorders of the brain. Pediatr Radiol 19:219-222

Byrd SE, Osborn RE, Radkowski MA et al (1988) Disorders of midline structures: holoprosencephaly, absence of corpus callosum, and Chiari malformation. Semin Ultrasound CT MR 9:201-215

Flodmark O, Roland EH, Hill A, Whitfield MF (1987) Periventricular leukomalacia: radiologic diagnosis Radiology 162:119-124

Graves VB, Duff TA (1990) Intracranial arteriovenous malformations: current imaging and treatment. Invest Radiol 25:952-960

Kjos BO, Umansky R, Barkovich AJ (1990) Brain MR imaging in children with developmental retardation of unknown cause: results in 76 cases. AJNR Am J Neuroradiol 1:1035-1040

Nowell MA, Grossman RI, Hackney DB et al (1988) MR imaging of white matter disease in children. AJR Am J Roentgenol 151:359-365

Pavlakis SG, Gould RJ, Zito JL (1991) Stroke in children. Adv Pediatr 38:151-179

Pollei SR, Boyer RS, Crawford S et al (1988) Disorders of migration and sulcation. Semin Ultrasound CT MR 9:231-246

Rorke LB (1990) Demystifying malformations. AJNR Am J Neuroradiol 11:675

Sato Y, Yuh WTC, Smith WL et al (1989) Head injury in child abuse: evaluation with MR imaging. Radiology 173:653-657

Tzika AA, Ball, Jr WS, Vigneron DB et al (1993) Childhood adrenoleukodystrophy: assessment with proton MR spectroscopy. Radiology 189:467-480

Valk J, van der Knaap MS (1989) Magnetic resonance of myelin, myelination, and myelin disorders. Springer-Verlag, New York, p 82

Wilson DA, Steiner RE (1986) Periventricular leukomalacia: evaluation with MR imaging. Radiology 160:507-511

Withers HR, Peters LJ, Kogelnik HS (1980) The pathobiology of late effects of irradiation. In: Meyn RE, Withers HR (eds) Radiation biology in cancer research. Raven, New York, pp 439-448

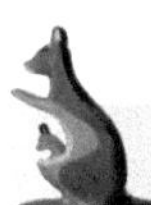

Ultrasonographic Evaluation of the Spinal Sac and Its Content in Neonates and Infants

Ingmar Gassner

Department of Paediatrics, Section of Paediatric Radiology, University Hospital Innsbruck, Innsbruck, Austria

Introduction

In newborns and young infants, sonography allows detailed depiction of the spinal cord. Ultrasonography of the intraspinal contents is included in the screening evaluation of neonates with suspected spinal dysraphism (cutaneous lesions of the back, deformities of the spinal column, neurologic disturbances), and with syndromes with known risk for spinal-cord compression. Spinal sonography is also important in the evaluation of birth-related spinal cord injury.

Ultrasonography with high frequency transducers can demonstrate the entire spectrum of intraspinal pathologic conditions and should therefore be the imaging modality of choice for investigation of the spinal cord in newborns.

Normal Anatomy

At term, the vertebrae are made up completely of cartilage and typically contain three ossification centers. A single midline ossification center occupies the center of the future vertebral body. The paired neural ossification centers lie within the lateral elements and neural arches. These incompletely ossified posterior spinal arches create an acoustic window that permits transmission of the sonographic beam. The spinal cord also can be well visualized in patients who have bony defects created by surgical laminectomy.

Longitudinal scans show the spinous processes. The posterior dura mater appears as an echogenic line paralleling the posterior subarachnoid space, which lies between the dura mater and the spinal cord and is anechoic.

The spinal cord is visualized as a relatively hypoechoic cylindrical structure with echogenic anterior and posterior walls and a central echogenic complex representing the central end of the anterior median fissure. It is surrounded anteriorly by the anechoic anterior subarachnoid space and echogenic vertebral bodies. The width of the spinal cord varies and is broadest in the cervical and lumbar regions corresponding to the origin of the nerves that supply the extremities. At the level of the first or second lumbar vertebral bodies, the cord tapers to form the conus medullaris (Fig. 1). Occasionally, a dilatation, often transient, of the central canal of the lumbar spinal cord is seen (Fig. 2). On transverse images, the posterior dura mater appears as an echogenic band. The spinal cord, beneath the posterior subarachnoid space, appears as a round to oval structure with a central echogenic complex. Nelson and colleagues showed, quite convincingly, that the central echogenicity arises from the interface between myelinated ventral white commissure and the central end of the anterior median fissure. The central canal in normal infants is, in fact, overgrown with glial fibrils and is variably present at different levels.

The dentate ligament passes laterally from the equator of the cord and can be seen in part of the thoracic spinal canal. The dorsal and ventral roots pass toward the neural foramen. The paravertebral muscles appear as sonolucent scimitars that lie alongside the echogenic laminae. At the thoracolumbar junction the cord is surrounded by echogenic nerve roots. At the very tip of the conus medullaris, sonograms may display an "X" pattern, which represents the more vertically oriented nerve roots that descend as paired columns (Fig. 3). Occasionally, the filum terminale shows after birth a transient cystic dilatation adjacent to the tip of the conus (Fig. 4). Below this level, the filum terminale may sometimes be imaged in the midline posteriorly; in other cases, the arrangement of the roots is more variable and the filum cannot be discerned separately.

With real-time sonography, vascular pulsations within the cord and cauda equina can be demonstrated. In addition, anterior-posterior motion of the cord can be noted during episodes of crying, while longitudinal movement of the spinal cord can be observed with flexion-extension neck motion.

The normal conus medullaris lies at about the level of the L1-L2 vertebral bodies. Extension of the cord more caudally is an indication of a tethered cord. The position of the conus can be best identified by identifying sonographically the promontory and counting the vertebral bodies cranially (Fig. 1). At the craniocervical junction, sagittal sonograms display the medulla, pons, cervical cord, cisterna magna, vermis or tonsils (Fig. 5).

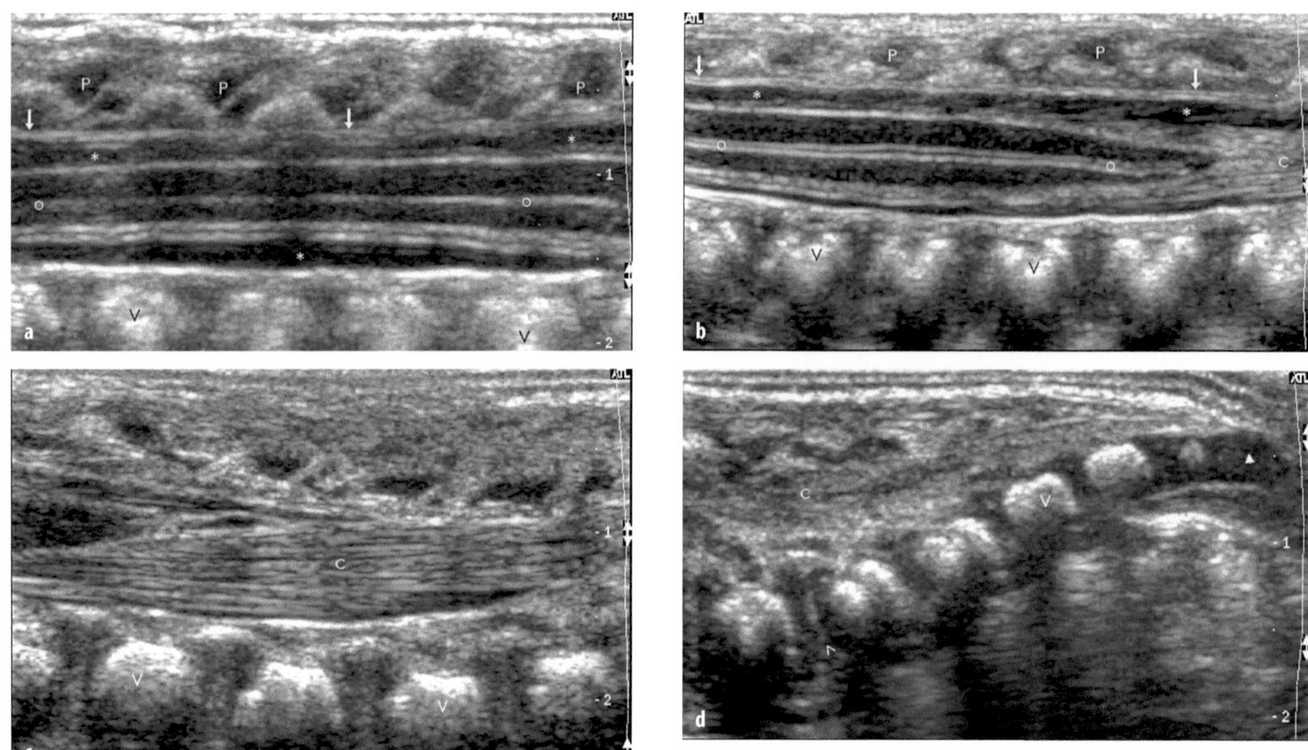

Fig. 1 a-d. Normal longitudinal anatomy of the spinal cord. **a** Thoracic region; **b** intumescentia lumbosacralis; **c** conus medullaris and cauda equina; **d** sacrum and coccyx. *P*, Hypoechoic cartilaginous spinous processes; *V*, echogenic vertebral bodies; ↓, posterior dura mater; ∗, posterior subarachnoid space; *o*, central echogenic complex; *C*, cauda equina; ∧, promontory; ▲, nonossified coccyx

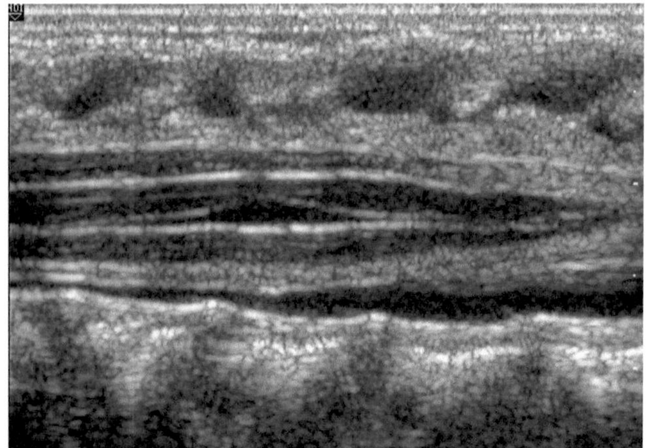

Fig. 2. Dilatation of the central canal of the distal cord, longitudinal scan

Spinal Dysraphism

Spinal dysraphism is defined as incomplete or absent fusion of midline mesenchymal, bony, and neural structures. To appreciate the different types of spinal dysraphism, an understanding of the development of the bony spine and spinal cord is of paramount importance. During normal development, the neural plate forms a groove in the midline and this groove forms folds laterally. The neural plate closes at its midpoint dorsally and then proceeds to close from this midpoint in both a cranial and caudal direction.

When there is premature disjunction of neural ectoderm from cutaneous ectoderm, the surrounding mesenchyme gains access to the inner surface of the neural tube. When mesenchyme comes in contact with this primitive ependymal lining, the mesenchyme is induced to become fat. This is believed to be the process underlying the formation of spinal lipomas. Complete nondisjunction of cutaneous ectoderm from neural ectoderm results in the formation of myelomeningoceles.

Bone abnormalities associated with spinal dysraphism involve multiple vertebrae. Spina bifida, which means cleft into two parts, is characterized by incomplete fusion of the neural arch. There is absence of all or parts of the laminae, spinous processes, and other parts of the posterior elements. Associated segmental changes of the vertebral bodies, such as hemivertebrae, butterfly vertebrae, and block vertebrae, are usually present.

Children with spinal dysraphism may present with a back mass, abnormal cutaneous manifestations of the back (hemangioma, hairy tuft, nevus, sinus tract), gait disturbance, club foot, and bowel and bladder incontinence. Classifications of spinal dysraphism are based either on the

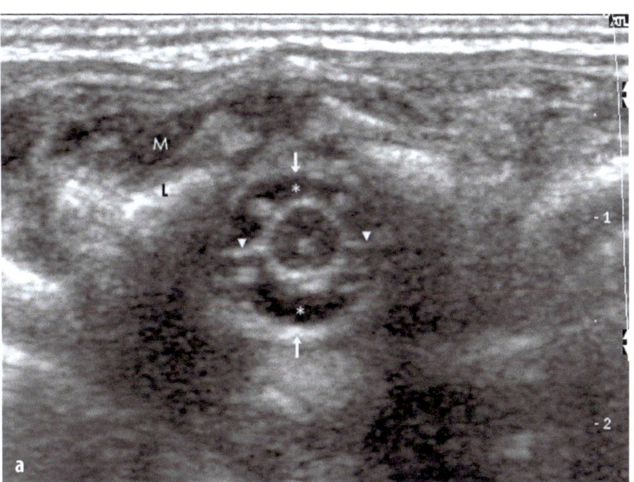

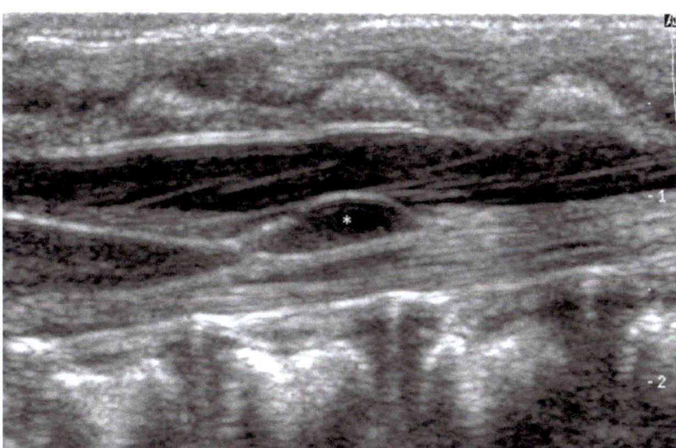

Fig. 4. Cystic dilatation of the filum terminale (*) adjacent to the tip of the conus, longitudinal scan

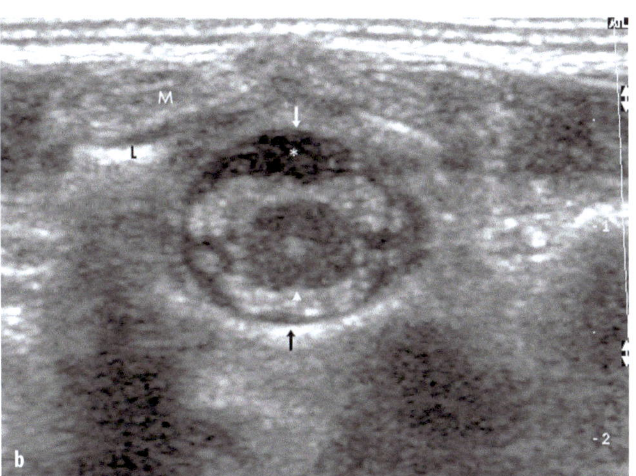

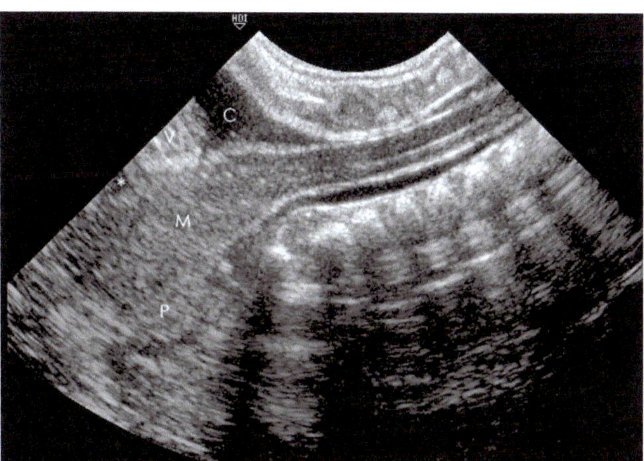

Fig. 5. Normal longitudinal anatomy of craniocervical junction. *P*, Pons ; *M*, medulla oblongata; *V*, cerebellar vermis; *, fourth ventricle; *C*, cerebellomedullary cistern

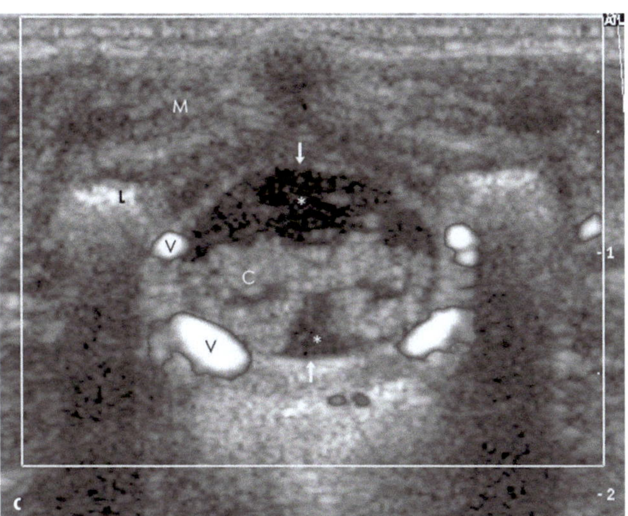

Fig. 3 a-c. Normal transverse anatomy of the spinal cord. **a** Thoracic region; **b** intumescentia lumbosacralis; **c** conus medullaris and cauda equina. *M*, Muscle; *L*, laminae; ↓, dura mater; *, subarachnoid space; ▼, dentate ligaments; ▲, anterior median fissure; *C*, cauda equina; *V*, epidural veins

specific derangement of embryonic development or on the clinical or neuroradiological appearance. Clinically spinal dysraphism can be classified into three categories based on the presence or absence of a back mass: (1) Spinal dysraphism may be associated with a back mass that is not covered by skin; the anomalies are the myelomeningocele and myelocele. (2) There may be a skin-covered back mass; the anomalies in such patients are the lipomyelomeningocele, myelocystocele, and posterior meningocele. (3) Spinal dysraphism without an associated back mass (occult spinal dysraphism) encompasses the largest group of anomalies: diastematomyelia, dorsal dermal sinus, spinal lipoma, tight filum terminale, anterior sacral meningocele, lateral thoracic meningocele, hydromyelia, split notochord syndrome, and caudal regression syndrome.

A myelomeningocele is a back mass of exposed spinal cord, without a covering of skin, that resembles the primitive neural plate. The spinal cord is split dorsally, splayed open (myeloschisis), and herniated through a large posterior dysraphic defect in the bone and dura onto the back. Also herniated onto the back with the exposed spinal cord is cerebrospinal fluid, with pia and arachnoid layers. This exposed herniated sac protrudes beyond the surface plane of the back and the cord is tethered at this level.

The myelocele is similar to the myelomeningocele except that its herniated sac of exposed spinal cord is flush with the plane of the back. Since this pathology is visible, there is little reason to study these patients prior to corrective closure of the back. However, there is a real need to study the associated anomalies, in particular hydrocephalus.

Children with a myelomeningocele have associated anomalies of the brain; in 99% of there is a Chiari II malformation. Other, rare anomalies are dysgenesis of the corpus callosum and dysplasia of the calvaria (*Lückenschädel*), meninges, cerebral hemispheres, and cerebellum. These children may also have hydromyelia, arachnoid cyst of the spinal canal, and diastematomyelia.

Lückenschädel, or craniofenestria, is characterized by marked thinning of the occipital or parietal bones and is identified in Chiari malformations examined in affected infants < 6 months of age, after which time the defect becomes unrecognizable.

The falx can be thinned or absent, allowing interdigitation of the medial surfaces of the two cerebral hemispheres.

A characteristic diencephalic appearance is that of a large massa intermedia.

Chiari II malformation is characterized by the downward herniation of portions of the medulla oblongata, fourth ventricle, and inferior cerebellum into the upper cervical canal, often with a cervicomedullary kink (Fig. 6).

Fig. 6. Chiari-II-Malformation with caudally displaced thick vermian peg (↓), longitudinal scan

Arachnoid cysts accompanying dysraphic myelodysplasias probably result from developmental deficiencies in the formation of the arachnoid or dura.

Hydromyelia is present in between 29 and 77% of patients with myelomeningoceles. It may be focal or involve the entire central canal, from the cervicomedullary junction down to the placode (Fig. 7). Untreated, hydromyelia can cause the rapid development of scoliosis.

After myelomeningocele repair, the spinal cord will lie toward the center or ventral half of the spinal canal when the patient is in prone position; however, this is abnormally low. The emerging nerve roots will emerge nearly horizontally and segmentally rather than being drawn into a cauda equina. With real-time scanning, the cord and roots will be seen to pulse and "dance". Such motions of the cord and roots indicate freedom from tethering. Absence of this normal cord motion is strong evidence of tethering.

Lipomyelo(meningo)celes are lipomas that extend in continuity from the subcutaneous plane to the spinal cord through a focal midline dehiscence in the fascia, muscle, bone, and dura. In these patients, the posterior half of the spinal cord is cleft and the lipoma inserts into that cleft

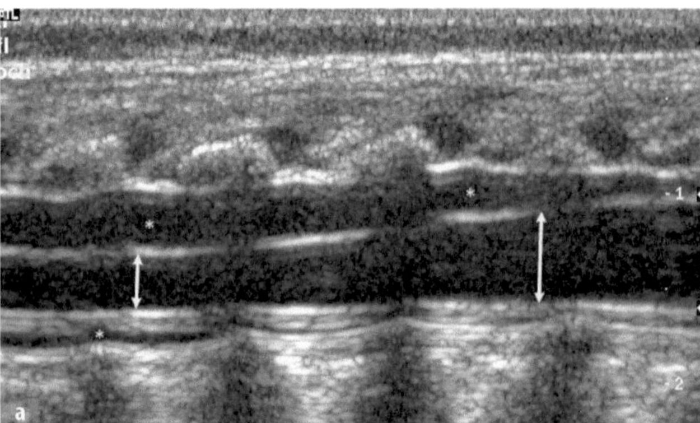

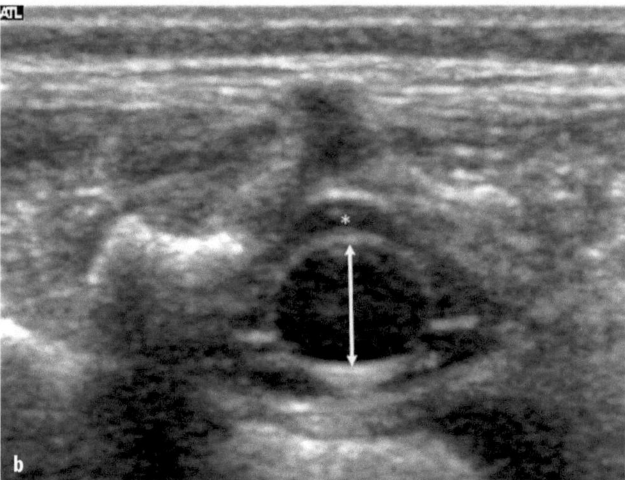

Fig. 7. Myelomeningocele with hydromyelia. **a** Longitudinal scan; **b** transverse scan through the thoracic spine. The central canal is enormously dilated (↕). Subarachnoid space (∗) with dentate ligaments

on the dorsal surface of the cord and then may ascend within the central canal of the cord. The lipoma tethers the cord inferiorly.

In lipomyelomeningocele an expanded subarachnoid space bulges posteriorly through the spina bifida into the subcutaneous plane, whereas in lipomyelocele there is no bulging of the meninges. The cord typically remains wholly within the spinal canal. Sonographically, lipomyelo(meningo)celes typically present as large subcutaneous masses of highly echogenic fat that extend from the subcutaneous plane into the spinal canal through a posterior spina bifida. The normally sonolucent subcutaneous fat plane is disrupted focally at the site of the lipoma. The position of the spinal cord is low.

The term diastematomyelia refers to a sagittal division of the spinal cord into two hemicords, not necessarily symmetric, each of which contains a central canal, one dorsal horn (giving rise to a dorsal nerve root) and one ventral horn (giving rise to a ventral nerve root). Each hemicord is surrounded by a layer of pia. The division may involve the entire thickness of the cord or may only affect the anterior or posterior half of the cord (partial diastematomyelia). Partial divison is frequently observed in the transitional zones superior and inferior to an area of complete diastematomyelia. A septum consisting of bone, fibrous and/or cartilaginous tissue is frequently present between the hemicords. When a septum is present, each hemicord is surrounded by its own dura-arachnoid sheath. In the absence of a septum, a single sheath surrounds the hemicords. The two hemicords reunite caudal to the cleft in most patients. Occasionally, the cleft will extend unusually low and the hemicords remain distinct, with two separate conus medullares and two fila terminalia. The conus medullaris typically lies in an abnormally low position. Thickening of the filum terminale is often seen.

The spinal column is nearly always abnormal in patients with diastematomyelia. Spina bifida and scoliosis are present, the interpediculate distance is widened. As noted above, anomalies of the vertebral bodies including hemivertebrae, butterfly vertebrae, block vertebrae, and decreased disc height are observed. The presence of a bony spur is not necessary for the diagnosis of diastematomyelia.

Patients with diastematomyelia commonly manifest abnormal cutaneous stigmata on the skin of the back, such as large hairy tuft, hemangioma, nevus, and pilonidal cyst. Axial sonograms show two separate hemicords lying side by side. The intersegmental laminar fusion creates a thick bony plate that obscures the region of greatest interest. Sagittal views of the spine are less useful for documentation of this condition because the two hemicords cannot be imaged simultaneously.

The "tight filum terminale syndrome", also known as the "tethered cord syndrome", refers to the low position of the conus medullaris (below the L2-L3 level) associated with a short, thickened filum. The filum has a diameter > 2 mm at the L5-S1 level. The filar thickening is usually fibrous but may often be fatty, fibrofatty, or, less often, cystic (Fig. 8). The symptoms in this syndrome are due to stretching of the spinal cord with vascular insufficiency in the conus medullaris. Patients can become symptomatic at any age. Occasionally, there is filar thickening with a normal conus level, including filar lipoma or fibrolipoma as an otherwise incidental finding.

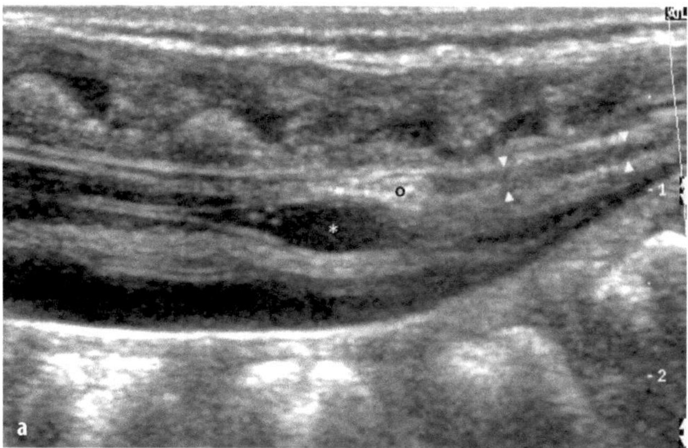

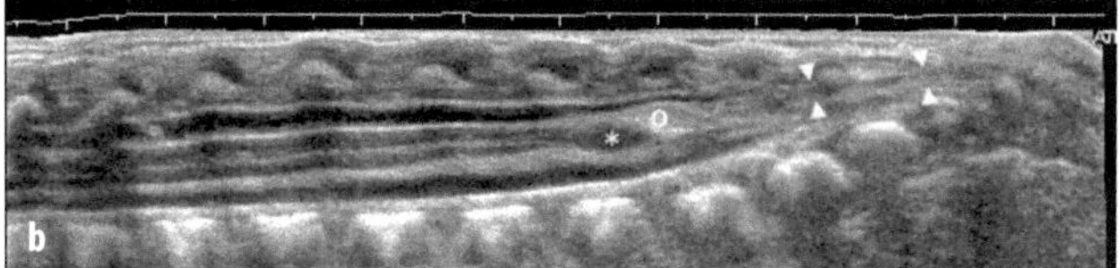

Fig. 8 a, b. Dermal sinus with an epithelial tubular tract (▼) extending from the sacrococcygeal skin surface upward into the spinal canal. It terminates in an epidermoid (*o*) and tethers the low-lying conus. There is also cystic dilatation of the central canal (*). **a** Longitudinal scan; **b** extended field-of-view

Caudal Regression Syndrome

This refers to a spectrum of caudal cell mass disorders that result in a range of caudal spinal, anorectal, urogenital, and lower limb abnormalities. At one extreme of the syndrome, there is lumbosacral agenesis, fused lower extremities, anal atresia, and abnormal genitalia. At the other extreme, there may be foot deformity, motor and sensory impairment of the lower limb, other hindgut and genitourinary anomalies, and neurogenic bladder. The spinal anomalies range from partial or unilateral sacral agenesis to sacral or lumbosacral agenesis. The spinal cord anomalies are either a high lying plump conus or a tethered cord with an elongated and caudally stretched conus. When the cord is not tethered, the terminus of the spinal cord has a characteristic blunted or chisel-shaped appearance, with greater preservation of the dorsal sensory portion of the conus. The conus terminates abruptly at T11 or T12 as if the normal distal "tip" were absent (Fig. 9). The distal central canal may be slightly or substantially dilated. When the cord is tethered, it is difficult to determine where the conus medullaris ends and the filum terminale begins.

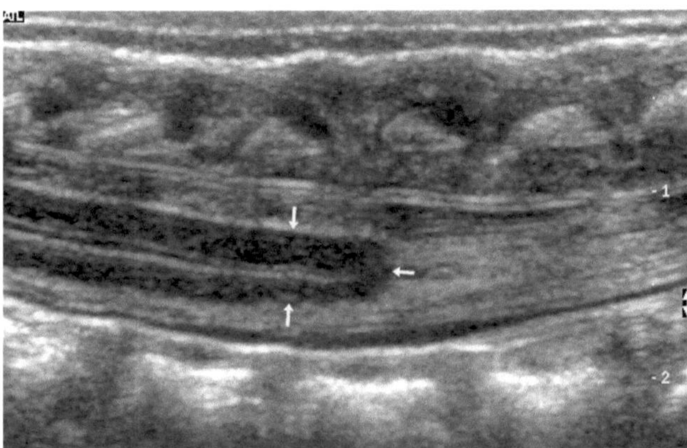

Fig. 9. Imperforate anus with osseous sacral anomaly. Longitudinal scan of the distal thoracic spine. The high-lying terminus of the cord (↓) has a blunted shape (without the normal tapering)

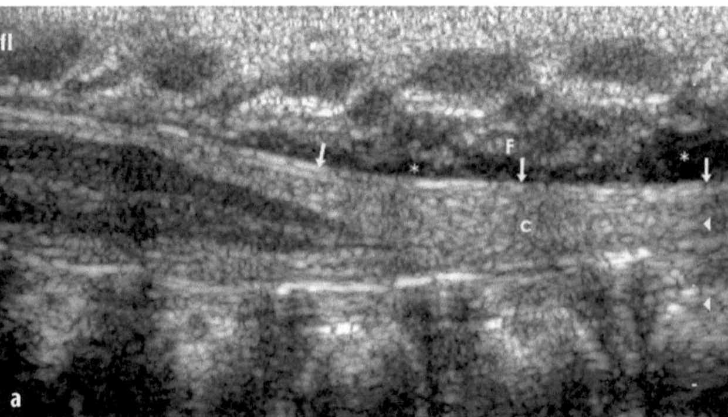

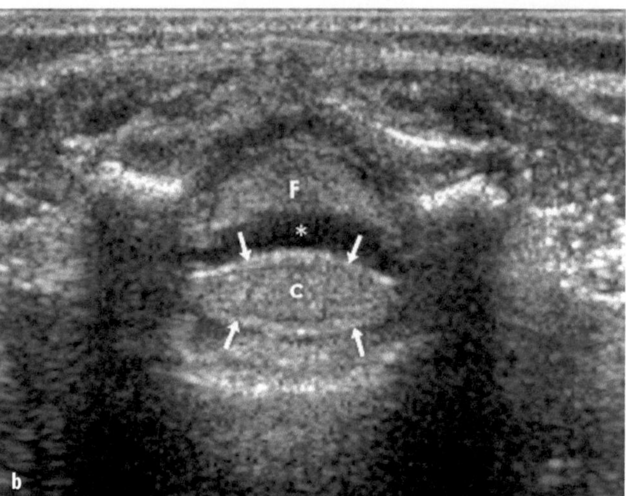

Fig. 10 a, b. 27-day-old male neonate born at term with cerebrospinal fluid leakage after lumbar puncture. Longitudinal(**a**), and axial (**b**) sonograms of the lumbar spine show epidural cerebrospinal fluid collection (*) with markedly compressed subarachnoid space and bundled cauda equina (*C*). Shifted dura mater (↓). Floating fat (*F*) shows characteristic wave form structure on longitudinal and triangular structure on axial sonogram

Trauma to the Spine and Spinal Cord in the Neonate

In such patients there is almost always obstetrical trauma. The most common predisposing factor is hyperextension of the cervical spine caused by intrauterine fetal malposition (brow, face, or breech presentation). Typically, three main pathologic patterns of injury occur, either alone or in combination: (1) meningeal damage with epidural hemorrhage, the most common manifestation of spinal injury in the newborn; (2) laceration and avulsion of spinal nerve roots; and (3) laceration and distortion of the cord, ranging from edema to focal hemorrhage and necrosis to complete transection. The cervical and/or upper thoracic cord is most commonly injured. High-resolution real-time ultrasound is very useful in identifying these injuries.

Cerebrospinal fluid leakage into the epidural space is a frequent complication of lumbar puncture in neonates and must be differentiated from cerebrospinal fluid leakage due to perinatal meningeal injury (Fig. 10).

Another serious birth trauma is occipital osteodiastasis. The area of fetal cranium that is disrupted readily is the syndesmosis between the squamous and lateral parts of the occipital bone. The lower margin of the squamous occipital bone forms the posterior boundary of the foramen magnum, centrally, and is closely related to the occipital sinuses, on each side, near their junctions with the lateral aspects. Traumatic separation results in displacement and forward rotation of the lower edge of the squamous occipital bone. The sharp edge of the bone may shear through the dura and occipital sinuses, causing gross subdural hemorrhage in the posterior fossa and sometimes laceration of the cerebellum. The injury occurs most often during manipulations to deliver the child's head in a breech delivery. Occipital osteodiastasis is almost certainly the most frequent cause of the rare but bizarre occurrence of multiple cerebral emboli within pulmonary and other vessels following delivery. Damage to the dural sinus and cerebellum would allow the cerebellar tissue to be squeezed or sucked into the sinus.

Suggested Reading

Normal Anatomy

Beek FJ, Bax KM, Mali WP (1994) Sonography of the coccyx in newborns and infants. J Ultrasound Med 13(8):629-634

Beek FJ, de Vries LS, Gerards LJ, Mali WP (1996) Sonographic determination of the position of the conus medullaris in premature and term infants. Neuroradiology Suppl 1:S174-S177

Dick EA, de Bruyn R (2003) Ultrasound of the spinal cord in children: its role. Eur J Radiol 13:552-562

Di Pietro MA (2005) The pediatric spinal canal. In: Tortori-Donati P, Rossi A (ed) Pediatric Neuroradiology. Springer, Berlin, Heidelberg, New York, pp 1589-1615

Di Pietro MA (1993) The conus medullaris: normal US findings throughout childhood. Radiology. 188(1):149-153

Gusnard DA, Naidich TP, Yousefzadeh DK, Haughton VM (1986) Ultrasonic anatomy of the normal neonatal and infant spine: correlation with cryomicrotome sections and CT. Neuroradiology 28(5-6):493-511

Kriss VM, Kriss TC, Coleman RC (2000) Sonographic appearance of the ventriculus terminalis cyst in the neonatal spinal cord. J Ultrasound Med 19(3):207-209

Nelson MD Jr, Sedler JA, Gilles FH (1989) Spinal cord central echo complex: histoanatomic correlation. Radiology 170(2):479-481

Rypens F, Avni EF, Matos C et al (1995) Atypical and equivocal sonographic features of the spinal cord in neonates. Pediatr Radiol 25:429-432

Zieger M, Dörr U (1988) Pediatric spinal sonography. Part I: Anatomy and examination technique. Pediatr Radiol 18(1):9-13

Spinal Dysraphism

Byrd SE, Darling CF, McLone DG (1991) Developmental disorders of the pediatric spine. Radiol Clin North Am 29(4):711-752

Gerscovich EO, Maslen L, Cronan MS et al (1999) Spinal sonography and magnetic resonance imaging in patients with repaired myelomeningocele: comparison of modalities. J Ultrasound Med 18(9):655-664

Könner C, Gassner I, Mayr U, Kreczy A (1990) Zur Diagnose der Diastematomyelie mittels Ultraschall. Klin Pädiatr 202(2):124-128

Korsvik HE, Keller MS (1992) Sonography of occult dysraphism in neonates and infants with MR imaging correlation. Radiographics 12:297-306

Kriss VM, Desai NS (1998) Occult spinal dysraphism in neonates: assessment of high-risk cutaneous stigmata on sonography. AJR Am J Roentgenol 171(6):1687-1692

Naidich TP, McLone DG, Mutluer S (1983) A new understanding of dorsal dysraphism with lipoma (lipomyeloschisis): radiologic evaluation and surgical correction. AJR Am J Roentgenol 140(6):1065-1078

Robinson AJ, Russell S, Rimmer S (2005) The value of ultrasonic examination of the lumbar spine in infants with specific reference to cutaneous markers of occult spinal dysraphism. Clin Radiol 60:72-77

Tortori-Donati P, Rossi A, Cama A (2000) Spinal dysraphism: a review of neuroradiological features with embryological correlations and proposal for a new classification. Neuroradiology 42(7):471-491

Tortori-Donati P, Rossi A, Biancheri R et al (2001) Magnetic resonance imaging of spinal dysraphism. Top Magn Reson Imaging 12:375-409

Unsinn KM, Geley T, Freund MC, Gassner I (2000) US of the spinal cord in newborns: spectrum of normal findings, variants, congenital anomalies, and acquired diseases. Radiographics 20(4):923-938

Caudal Regression Syndrome

Appignani BA, Jaramillo D, Barnes PD, Poussaint TY (1994) Dysraphic myelodysplasias associated with urogenital and anorectal anomalies: prevalence and types seen with MR imaging. AJR Am J Roentgenol 163:1199-1203

Beek FJ, Boemers TM, Beek FJ et al (1995) Spine evaluation in children with anorectal malformations. Pediatr Radiol Suppl 1:S28-S32

Trauma to the Spine and Spinal Cord

Babyn PS, Chuang SH, Daneman A, Davidson GS (1988) Sonographic evaluation of spinal cord birth trauma with pathologic correlation. AJR Am J Roentgenol 151(4):763-766

Coley BD, Murakami JW, Koch BL et al (2001) Diagnostic and interventional ultrasound of the pediatric spine. Pediatr Radiol 31:775-785

Filippigh P, Clapuyt P, Debauche C, Claus D (1994) Sonographic evaluation of traumatic spinal cord lesions in the newborn infant. Pediatr Radiol 24(4):245-247

Fotter R, Sorantin E, Schneider U et al (1994) Ultrasound diagnosis of birth-related spinal cord trauma: neonatal diagnosis and follow-up and correlation with MRI. Pediatr Radiol 24(4):241-244

Kiechl-Kohlendorfer U, Unsinn KM, Schlenck B et al (2003) Cerebrospinal fluid leakage after lumbar puncture in neonates: incidence and sonographic appearance. AJR Am J Roentgenol 181(1):231-234

Towbin A (1970) Central nervous system damage in the human fetus and newborn infant. Mechanical and hypoxic injury incurred in the fetal-neonatal period. Am J Dis Child 119(6):529-542

Towbin A (1969) Latent spinal cord and brain stem injury in newborn infants. Dev Med Child Neurol 11(1):54-68

Wigglesworth JS, Husemeyer RP (1977) Intracranial birth trauma in vaginal breech delivery: the continued importance of injury to the occipital bone. Br J Obstet Gynaecol 84(9):684-691

Transfontanellar Gray Scale and Doppler Ultrasonography in Newborns

Corinne Veyrac, Magali Saguintaah, Catherine Baud, Alain Couture

Department of Pediatric Radiology, Hopital Arnaud de Villeneuve, Montpellier, France

Brain ultrasound (US) plays an important role in the detection and management of neonatal disease. It is a non-invasive, non-irradiating, reproducible procedure that can be performed at bedside, in the intensive care unit, or on an intubated ventilated newborn. In this article, we focus on the role of brain ultrasonography in perinatal brain injury.

The Preterm Infant

Intraventricular-Periventricular Hemorrhagic Disease

The positive diagnosis of intraventricular-periventricular hemorrhagic disease is based on morphological imaging, which is highly sensitive since hemorrhagic lesions show a strong hyperechogenicity.

Intraventricular vs. Germinal Matrix Hemorrhage

When the amount of intraventricular bleeding is large enough, its morphological diagnosis is easy. The highly echogenic image is obviously located within the ventricular lumen. The role of US is to appreciate the amount of blood and severity of injury. However, a minimal intraluminal hemorrhage may be confused with a large germinal matrix hemorrhage, which has a quite different prognosis. Color Doppler provides diagnostic information in the Sylvian aqueduct through colored signals (alternately coded in red and blue), which reflect the presence of small particles in the cerebrospinal fluid (CSF) that produce turbulent flow in CSF pathways. The most sensitive area is the narrowest portion of the aqueduct. The colored signal may be detected spontaneously but is more common with patient activity, e.g., sucking, crying, leg movements. It may also be produced by maneuvers that are easy to perform in a ventilated sedated newborn, such as abdominal palpation or intermittent compression of the anterior fontanelle. This finding lacks specificity, since it may be observed in post-infectious ventriculitis but is especially informative in the context of the preterm newborn.

Periventricular Hemorrhagic Infarction

When sonography shows a large strongly echogenic area, round or fan-shaped, lateral to the external angle of the lateral ventricle and associated with a large ipsilateral intraventricular hemorrhage (IVH), the diagnosis of periventricular hemorrhagic infarction (PVHI) is made. The volume of periventricular infarct should be assessed. Almost all of the hemispheric white matter may be involved, resulting in extensive macrocystic destruction. Conversely, the infarct may remain focal and small. It progressively cavitates, decreases in size, and becomes confluent with the ventricular lumen.

PVHI probably results from compression or obstruction of the terminal vein – which drains the white matter via the medullary veins – by a large IVH. In normal infants, and on the normal side of the brain, the terminal vein is always easily shown by color Doppler, whereas with PVHI flow in the terminal vein is not detectable. The disappearance of venous flow precedes the imaging of the periventricular infarct. Thus, one goal of the examination is to look for terminal vein flow when a large clot is visible in order to predict the subsequent occurrence of PVHI, which is considered to be a grade IV hemorrhage. In patients with large intraventricular bleeding and patent terminal vein flow, PVHI will not occur.

Other types of white matter damage may be encountered in association with IVH, especially periventricular leukomalacia, which has a different pathogenesis, sonographic appearance, and neurodevelopmental outcome.

IVH-PVH and Transfontanellar Doppler Ultrasonography in Preterm Infants

The pathogenic mechanisms that are responsible for hemorrhagic damage are multi-factorial, but are mainly the result of intravascular factors. The assessment of cerebral blood flow (CBF) velocities by pulsed Doppler is now possible and has been applied to detect conditions associated with a high risk of hemorrhage. Perlman et al. described a Doppler pattern, called fluctuant Doppler, that is characterized by beat-to-beat variability along the spectrum. These fluctuations are mainly observed when an infant breathes out of synchrony with the ventilator and are considered to be due to the loss of cerebral autoregulation, with direct transmission of arterial blood pressure variations to the cerebral blood circulation, as a pressure-passive state. Other circumstances may have the same effect, such as upper airway obstruction, occurrence of pneumothorax, maneuvers of routine care, and rapid volume expansion. A correlation between the fluctuating pattern and subsequent development of IVH, and between the elimination of this pattern and a decreased incidence of IVH has been documented. These studies underlined the importance for pediatricians to avoid the occurrence of these high-risk situations, such that nowadays identification of a fluctuant Doppler trace has become extremely rare.

Normal values of CBF velocities have been determined in preterm and full-term neonates. Arterial velocities increase with age. They are significantly higher at term than at 32 weeks gestation (Fig. 1) while the resistive index (RI) does not significantly differ between these two age groups. This is one of the arguments that highlight the great importance of measuring the velocities, and not only RI. In extremely premature infants, the normal values are lower.

It is important to keep in mind that a hemodynamic assessment should always be correlated with the systemic hemodynamic state and postnatal age of the patient as well as the blood gas concentrations. Hypoxia and hypercapnia are strong vasodilators that induce increases in diastolic velocities and decreases in RI. When a normal newborn is stimulated (e.g., by cutaneous stimulation), the heart rate first increases, the peak-systolic velocity does not change, but end-diastolic velocity and, as a consequence, time-average velocity significantly increase, resulting in a decrease in RI. Velocities return to normal later than the end of stimulation. This is normal autoregulation. The same changes occur after a transient bradycardia or hypoxia.

Thus, the main role of Doppler sonography, especially when the examination is performed early after birth but before day 3, is to detect hemodynamic situations associated with a high risk of ischemic-hemorrhagic injury. These situations include a fluctuating Doppler spectrum, severe increases in CBF velocities, mainly diastolic with low RI (high blood flow), and severe decreases in CBF velocities (low blood flow).

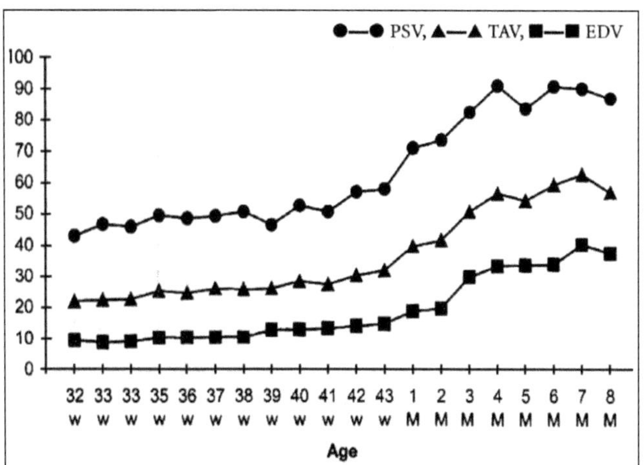

Fig. 1. Normal values of cerebral blood flow (CBF) velocities in the anterior cerebral artery. *PSV*, Peak systolic velocity; *TAV*, time-average velocity; *EDV*, end-diastolic velocity

Post-Hemorrhagic Ventricular Dilatation

This condition affects approximately 36% of preterm infants with IVH but resolves in 65% of affected infants. The diagnosis is based on morphological sonography, which demonstrates the onset of ventricular dilatation and determines its progression or regression. It also differentiates non-communicating tetraventricular dilatation (with rounded 4th ventricle and brainstem compression) from a communicating dilatation (with a triangular-shaped 4th ventricle and clearly visible cisterna magna).

Pulsed Doppler sonography provides additional information by demonstrating an increased RI in the presence of increased intracranial pressure (ICP). Intracranial hypertension is associated with reduced end-diastolic velocity and increased RI, which may exceed 1. Another cause of this abnormal pattern, such as patent ductus arteriosus, should be excluded first. Progressive hydrocephalus is strongly correlated with a high RI, but when the dilatation is only slowly progressive, clinical and hemodynamic data may be discordant or inconclusive. Taylor et al. proposed increasing the sensitivity of Doppler investigation by applying fontanellar compression. Indeed, in a healthy infant, when pressure is exerted on the anterior fontanelle, ICP rises, end-diastolic velocity decreases, and RI increases. However, when intracranial volume is already increased, as in hydrocephalic infants, the pressure-volume relationship is altered and simple manual fontanelle compression induces excessive changes in CBF velocities. Taylor's group proposed an index, called delta-RI, defined as fontanelle compression RI-baseline RI/baseline RI. These authors showed that delta-RI was <30% in infants who did not require shunt placement, but >45% in infants who did require shunt placement. Determination of delta-RI, when correlated with other available data, may be used for deciding on therapeutic intervention; for example, repeated CSF removal (efficacy of CSF withdrawal and delay between two such punctures).

To summarize, US permits the positive diagnosis of the damage and documents its severity; demonstrates some hemodynamic disturbances indicative of a high risk of hemorrhage; and plays a primary role in the follow-up and management of post-hemorrhagic ventricular dilatation.

Periventricular Leukomalacia

Early Sonographic Aspects of Periventricular Leukomalacia

The sonographic diagnosis of PVL is based on the detection of an abnormal echogenicity of the periventricular white matter and is recognized as difficult. Parenchymal echodensities may be evident, but show a variable pattern: lateral extension with spiculated margins, high hyperechogenicity with sharp margins, organization in clusters, butterfly appearance, and extensive density scattered with punctuations. The distribution of the lesion should be considered, either bilateral and diffuse, or focal and nodular. However, periventricular echodensities may be less obvious, with a hazy pattern, spiculated margins, or only punctate densities within white matter of normal echogenicity.

These appearances should be distinguished from features that are encountered in extremely preterm neonates, usually before 28 weeks of gestation. Echogenic stripes may be observed parallel to the external wall of the ventricles but without other parenchymal abnormalities. They remain unchanged during the first weeks of follow-up and are probably related to a layer of migrating cells.

In some situations, the echodensity of posterior white matter is difficult to appreciate, for example with post-hemorrhagic dilatation. Accessory windows should be investigated, such as posterior or mastoid fontanelles, or even the coronal suture.

Periventricular Echodensities: PVL or Not?

The first argument is the development of cysts. When macrocysts appear, with their progressive confluent extension, the diagnosis is easy, but nowadays this is a rare occurrence. Most often, these are microcysts, which are more difficult to detect, even if surrounded by hyperechogenic white matter. They appear between day 8 and day 25, after any type of echodensity. Their recognition is important since they are correlated with abnormal clinical outcome.

Usually, no cyst is detected. The severity and extension of echodensities may determine the diagnosis, as well as their pattern, especially the presence or absence of parenchymal distortion. However, the main criterion is the duration of the echodensities. Early normalization (<7 days) is associated with a favorable outcome, while late persistence of an abnormal aspect is associated with motor sequelae. However, there is widespread agreement that magnetic resonance imaging (MRI) is more sensitive than US for evaluating white matter damage.

Other Types of Acute Intracranial Damage in Preterm Infants

Despites their rare occurrence, gangliothalamic ischemic damage, cortical necrosis, subpial hemorrhage, and infratentorial bleeding may occur in preterm infants. These conditions are described in the section on hypoxic-ischemic encephalopathy of the full-term infant.

Delayed Ischemic-Hemorrhagic Damage

This occurs mainly in unstable or extremely premature infants (<25 weeks gestation) especially after acute septic events. PVL, multi-focal hemorrhagic infarcts, ischemic damage of the corpus callosum (with transient enlargement and subsequent volume reduction), and acute subarachnoid or subpial hemorrhage with underlying parenchymal necrosis all may be encountered. Thus, sonographic follow-up of the preterm brain should be prolonged, even if there has been no evidence of ischemic-hemorrhagic damage during the neonatal period; this is especially true when there are intervening acute events.

Late Sonographic Examination

We routinely perform the final US examination when the infant reaches term. This is to detect persistent ventricular enlargement, pericerebral fluid effusion and decreased volume of the corpus callosum, any of which may indicate white matter damage and a decrease in cerebral volume.

The Full-Term Infant

The neuropathological lesions that result from hypoxic-ischemic encephalopathy are multiple and frequently associated: parasagittal injury, subcortical leukomalacia, cortical necrosis, gangliothalamic ischemia, PVL, and brainstem ischemia.

Hypoxic-Ischemic Encephalopathy and Gray-Scale Imaging

A positive sonographic diagnosis is difficult because the lesions are mildly hyperechogenic, only slightly different from the echogenicity of normal parenchyma. When the first examination is performed very soon after birth, it usually shows a diffusely dense echogenic brain, with shadowing of the sulci and fissures. At this stage, Doppler studies are of particular interest since they provide additional information and greatly improve the early diagnosis.

Sonographic follow-up is carried out using high-frequency probes, which generate a high-resolution image and thus demonstrates either the normalization of brain parenchyma or the presence of anatomical lesions, which commonly appear from day 2 to day 7.

In subcortical leukomalacia, the white matter echogenicity is increased, resulting in enhanced cortico-subcortical differentiation and sharp boundaries between gray and white matter.

Conversely, in diffuse corticosubcortical ischemic damage there is no gray-white matter differentiation.

Parasagittal ischemia is characterized by a wedge-shaped hyperechogenicity in the parasagittal areas.

Selective cortical necrosis is classically difficult to diagnose by sonography, except when located beneath the anterior fontanelle. It appears as an echodense focal area or hyperechoic ribbon centered by a sulcus. These are usually asymmetrically distributed multi-focal lesions, in which normal hypoechogenic cortex is associated with echodense cortical patches.

The diagnosis of gangliothalamic ischemia is much easier as the lesions appear as well-delineated echodensities within the thalamus and/or basal ganglia. The ischemic foci may be very small.

Periventricular leukomalacia has already been described.

Brainstem ischemia is exceptionally demonstrated by sonography. We have seen only one patient whose brainstem was considerably swollen and displayed homogeneously increased echogenicity.

Hypoxic-Ischemic Encephalopathy and Doppler Studies

Hypoxic-ischemic encephalopathy results from CSF disturbances, some of which may be detected by pulsed Doppler when the examination is performed early after birth. Two particular hemodynamic patterns should be searched for: luxury perfusion and low blood flow.

Luxury perfusion refers to postasphyxial reperfusion. It corresponds to a state of vasodilatation with high CBF and is correlated with a poor neurological outcome. The Doppler spectrum is characteristic, since end-diastolic and time-average velocities are highly increased, resulting in a decreased RI. In our cohort of 82 patients with grade II or grade III encephalopathy, RI was always less than 0.50. This alteration was observed as early as the first day of life and lasted as long as until day 6. Arterial velocities were generally higher in grade III than in grade II injuries while RI values were similar in the two groups.

Low blood flow is characterized by a significant drop in arterial velocities. RI may be normal, increased, or decreased. Once more, such findings demonstrate the importance of measuring CBF velocities.

The difficulty of using the results of brain Doppler in clinical practice is the tremendous variability in the patient's day-to-day hemodynamic status. A full-term infant with neurological distress may present with: a characteristic pattern of low blood flow at day 1, a characteristic pattern of luxury perfusion at day 2, and a progressive return to normal hemodynamic status at day 3 or 4.

Arterial Infarction

Several factors predisposing to arterial infarction are recognized, such as congenital heart disease, cardiac catheterization, cardiac surgery, and a hypercoagulable state, but idiopathic infarctions are frequent. Early sonography may be normal. Moderate hyperechogenicity appears later in a territory of systemic arterial distribution. Color Doppler may demonstrate the absence of blood flow in a main artery.

Sequential sonographic follow-up is able to show the recovery of arterial flow and eventual cavitation of the infarcted territory.

Complications of Twin to Twin Transfusion

Some lesions may be already cystic at birth, but other are still hyperechogenic and will cavitate subsequently. The diagnosis is suspected in a monochorionic twin gestation in front of corticosubcortical peripheral lesions, often bilateral, with a parieto-occipital location.

Subpial, Subarachnoid Hemorrhage

This condition is marked by underlying cortical necrosis. It appears as a focal rounded hyperechogenic area, with a peripheral lobar location. On follow-up, the lesion becomes heterogeneous, with several layers exhibiting different echogenicities. There is also a rapid decrease in parenchymal volume.

Infratentorial Hemorrhage

Sonographic detection of this condition is rare, and MRI is the method of choice. On US, large lesions may appear as hyperechogenic areas, usually laterally placed. The subdural space or/and cerebellar hemispheres are involved. Infratentorial hemorrhage is often associated with IVH and sometimes with supratentorial ventricular dilatation.

To summarize, in hypoxic-ischemic encephalopathy, morphological sonography provides a reliable, but often delayed diagnosis. Hemodynamic assessment may detect luxury perfusion or low blood flow before the anatomical lesions can be demonstrated.

Conclusions

The use of sonography and Doppler US are of great interest in the diagnosis and prognostic evaluation of ischemic-hemorrhagic neonatal injuries. However, high-resolution sonography is required (with the use of high-frequency probes); color and pulsed Doppler should be combined with gray-scale sonography. Doppler analysis should always be correlated with the patient's clinical history and systemic hemodynamic condition, as well as the blood gas concentrations. The sonographer should be experienced in neonatal sonography and be able to recognize subtle alterations.

Is there an optimal moment for US examination? If the diagnosis of ischemic-hemorrhagic lesions is the only goal, brain sonography performed at day 4 or day 5 is often sufficient. However, if the goal is to detect at-risk situations, earlier examinations are required.

Finally, sonography should be repeated, not only to confirm and follow-up a detected lesion but also to diagnose new damage especially in patients who in the meantime have experienced an acute event, such as sepsis or acute hemorrhage.

Suggested Reading

Andre P, Thebaud B, Delavaucoupet J et al (2001) Late-onset cytic periventricular leukomalacia in premature infants: a threat until term. Am J Perinatol 18:79-86

Childs Am, Cornette L, Ramenghi LA et al (2001) Magnetic resonance and cranial ultrasound characteristics of periventricular white matter abnormalities in newborn infants. Clin Radiol 56:647-655

Couture A, Veyrac C, Baud C (1994) Echographie cérébrale du foetus au nuoveau-né. Imagerie et hémodynamique. Sauramps, Montpellier

Couture A, Veyrac C (2001) Transfontanellar Doppler imaging in neonates. Springer, Berlin-Heidelberg-New York

Daneman A, Epelman M, Blaser S Jarrin JR (2006) Imaging of the brain in full-term neonates: does sonography still play a role? Pediatrs Radiol 36:636-646

De Vries LS, Eken P, Groenendaal F et al (1993) Correlation between the degree of periventricular leukomalacia diagnosed using cranial ultrasound and MRI later in infancy in children with cerebral palsy. Neuropediatrics 24:263-268

De Vries LS, Roelants-van Rijn AM Rademaker KJ et al (2001) Unilateral parenchymal haemorrhagic infarction in the pereterm infant. Eur J Pediatr Neurol 5:139-149

Guzzetta F, Deodato F, Rando T (2000) Brain ischemic lesions of the newborn. Clid's Nerv Syst 16:633-637

Huang AH, Robertson RL (2004) Spontaneous superficial parenchymal and leptomeningeal hemorrhage in term neonates, AJNR Am J Neuroradiol 25:469-475

Jongelin BR, Badawi N, Kurinczuk JJ et al (2002) Cranial ultrasound as a predictor of outcome in term newborn encephalopathy. Pediatr Neurol 26:37-42

Lai FF, Tsou KY (1999) Transient periventricular echodensities and evelopmental outcome in preterm infants. Pediatr Neurol 21:797-801

Limperopoulos C, Benson CB, Bassan H et al (2005) Cerebellar hemorrhage in the preterm infant: ultrasonographic findings and risk factors. Pediatrics 116:717-724

Perlman JM, McMeanmin JB, Volpe JJ (1983) Fluctuating cerebral blood flow velocity in respiratory distress syndrome. Relation to the development of intraventricular hemorrhage. N Engl J Med 309:204-209

Perlman JM, Goodman S, Kreusser KL, Volpe JJ (1985) Reduction in intraventricular hemorrhage by elimination of fluctuating cerebral blood flow velocity in preterm infants with respiratory distress syndrome. N Engl J Med 312:1253-1257

Taylor GA, Madsen J (1996) Neonatal hydrocephalus: hemodynamic response to fontanelle compression. Correlation with intracranial pressure and need for shunt placement. Radiology 201:685-689

Townsend SF, Rumack CM, Thilo EH et al (1999) Late neurosonographic screening is important to the diagnosis of periventricular leukomalacia and ventricular enlargement in preterm infants. Pediatr Radiol 29:347-352

Volpe JJ (1995) Neurology of the newborn. 3rd edn. Saunders, Philadelphia

Winkler P (1992) Color-coded echographic flow imaging and spectral analysis of CSF in meningitis and hemorrhage. Part I: clinical evidence. Pediatr Radiol 22-24-30

Diagnostic Imaging of Primary Pediatric Brain Tumors

Tina Young Poussaint

Harvard Medical School and Department of Radiology, Division of Neuroradiology, Children's Hospital Boston, Boston, MA, USA

Introduction

Pediatric brain tumors are the most common type of solid tumor among children, the second most frequent childhood malignancy after leukemia [1], and the leading cause of death from solid tumors in this population. The incidence of brain tumors in children younger than 20 years of age was 27.4 cases per million children according to the NCI's *Surveillance Epidemiology and End Results* (SEER) cancer statistics reported in 2004 [2]. Approximately 9% of tumors included in the *Central Brain Tumor Registry of the United States* (CBTRUS) were diagnosed in children under the age of 20 [3].

Imaging Evaluation

Magnetic Resonance Imaging

Magnetic resonance imaging (MRI) is the leading modality for evaluating a child with a suspected brain tumor. It has unique multi-planar capabilities that offer detailed anatomical information with superior resolution and sensitivity. MRI is typically used for making a preoperative diagnosis and for guiding treatment planning, including image-guided therapies such as surgery, chemotherapy, and radiotherapy. In addition, it is used for tumor follow-up; for evaluating disease progression; and for assessing both treatment response and effects such as leukoencephalopathy, second tumor development, ischemic and hemorrhagic vasculopathy, and mineralization. Craniospinal MRI with gadolinium is useful in evaluating the degree to which a tumor has disseminated in the cerebrospinal fluid (CSF) pathways. With respect to the circle of Willis (the circle of arteries that supply blood to the brain) or the dural venous sinuses, (venous channels found between layers of dura mater in the brain) standard MRI, magnetic resonance venography and magnetic resonance angiography may depict the extent of vascular involvement. Conventional aniography is effective in the preoperative endovascular treatment of tumors.

Advanced MRI techniques include magnetic resonance diffusion imaging, magnetic resonance perfusion imaging and magnetic resonance spectroscopy, which separately and in combination, can elucidate and characterize the physiologic characteristics of pediatric brain tumors [4]. Magnetic resonance perfusion imaging, which is complementary to conventional MRI, is currently used to evaluate cerebral perfusion dynamics by analyzing hemodynamic parameters, including relative cerebral blood volume, relative cerebral blood flow, and transit time. The techniques used to perform perfusion imaging include T2*-weighted dynamic susceptibility, arterial spin labeling techniques, and T1-weighted dynamic contrast-enhanced perfusion techniques. These techniques use either exogenous tracer agents, such as paramagnetic contrast material, or endogenous tracer agents, such as magnetically labeled blood (arterial water) [5].

Of the several perfusion methods, the most common is dynamic, contrast-enhanced perfusion imaging with gadopentetate dimeglumine (Gd-DTPA) using echoplanar gradient-echo sequences. This technique yields useful information in the imaging of pediatric tumors that occur in the supratentorium, with less useful results for very small tumors, hemorrhagic tumors, or calcified tumors [6]. Dynamic T1-weighted contrast-enhanced perfusion techniques are employed to assess microvascular permeability in tumors. Kinetic modeling of dynamic signal changes can produce estimates of regional fractional blood volume and microvascular permeability (Kps), which is an indicator of blood-brain barrier disruption and correlates with angiogenesis [7]. This technique has been used in clinical trials of anti-angiogenesis drugs [8]. Arterial-spin labeling (ASL) is a magnetic resonance perfusion technique that does not use an intravenous contrast agent and has been applied in patients with brain tumors. The perfusion contrast in the image results from the subtraction of two successively acquired images: one *with* and the other *without* proximal labeling of arterial water spins, with a magnetic gradient used to invert the magnetization of inflowing blood [9]. Magnetic resonance perfusion techniques can be applied to grading tumors, evaluating margins, and helping to distinguish tumor recurrence from treatment effects such as radiation necrosis.

Echoplanar magnetic resonance diffusion techniques have been used to characterize tumor tissue [10], distinguish between tissue types, and gauge the response to treatment [11]. Diffusion tensor imaging characterizes the rate and direction of white matter diffusion by providing visualization of fiber tract direction and integrity, a feature that aids in presurgical planning and in assessing treatment-induced white matter changes in children [12, 13].

Proton nuclear magnetic resonance spectroscopy (MRS) provides additional complimentary metabolic information beyond standard anatomic MRI. Techniques include single voxel and multi-voxel MRS with 2D and 3D acquisitions. Proton nuclear MRS allows the monitoring of important brain metabolites such as *N*-acetyl aspartate (NAA), creatine (Cr), choline (Cho), and lactate (Lac), and offers unique metabolic features that can identify tumor tissue, grade tumors, differentiate tumor types, guide stereotactic biopsies, and distinguish active tumor from scar or radiation necrosis [4].

Functional MRI (fMRI), a term generally applied to brain activation imaging, effectively captures local or regional changes in cerebral blood flow that accompany stimulation or activation of sensory (e.g., visual, auditory), motor, or cognitive centers. In addition, fMRI can identify eloquent regions of the pediatric brain when surgical resection of a brain tumor is planned. In such cases, the blood oxygenation level dependent (BOLD) technique, which is dependent on the state of oxygenation of hemoglobin during brain activity, is often utilized. Magnetic source imaging (MSI), which integrates anatomical data from conventional MRI with electrophysiological data from magnetoencephalography, may also help guide the surgical approach to brain tumors. Magnetoencephalography is a technique that measures magnetic fields associated with intracellular current flows within neurons.

Computed tomography (CT) is useful in assessing acute neurological presentations as well as evidence of hemorrhage. It is often applied to evaluate the extent of tumoral calcification and involvement of the bony cortex in lesions primary to the sinuses, temporal bone, skull base, and calvarium. Ultrasound often serves as a useful intraoperative guide for intracranial and intraspinal lesions. Surgical and radiation therapy planning is guided by stereotactic MRI and CT, the open magnet, and intraoperative magnets [14]. Three-dimensional reconstruction of fused images is essential to the delivery of accurate radiosurgery, radiotherapy, and image-guided surgery.

Molecular imaging includes modalities such as single photon emission computed tomography (SPECT) and positron emission tomography (PET). These techniques use radiotracers that can assess metabolic activity in brain tumors and distinguish tumor from radiation necrosis or scar. Most recently, radiotracers such as fluorodeoxyglucose (FDG) have been used in children; however, new radiotracers on the horizon, such as ^{18}F-fluorothymidine (FLT) and ^{18}F-DOPA, may have a role in metabolic assessment and treatment evaluation of these tumors.

Classification of Brain Tumors

Most pediatric brain tumors are primary in origin. Metastases from outside the brain, meningiomas, Schwann-cell tumors, and pituitary tumors, while rare in children, are common in adults [15]. Pediatric brain tumors are typically classified according to histology (i.e., tissue types), the grades of which have been recently updated by the World Health Organization [16]. Using the WHO classification system as a guide, the essential features of common primary brain tumors in childhood are covered in this chapter, with an emphasis on tumors located in the cerebral hemispheres and pineal, posterior fossa, sellar, and suprasellar regions.

Tumors of the Cerebral Hemispheres

Astrocytomas

The majority of tumors of childhood (25%) occur in the cerebral hemispheres [3]. Included among these tumors are pilocytic astrocytoma, diffuse fibrillary astrocytoma, anaplastic astrocytoma, and glioblastoma multiforme, which are graded from I to IV [16]. Gliomas represent 65% of all malignant tumors in children ages 0-14 and account for 56% of all tumors.

Pilocytic astrocytomas represent 21% of all brain tumors in children between the ages of 0 and 14 years [3]. These tumors typically occur in the optic pathway system, basal ganglia, thalami, cerebral hemispheres, cerebellum, and brainstem; some may have an associated cyst. Pilocytic astrocytomas are well demarcated, are T2-hyperintense, have little vasogenic edema, and show marked enhancement after gadolinium. On perfusion imaging, high cerebral blood volume that mimics that of high-grade tumors may be observed in pilocytic astrocytomas [17]; and on diffusion imaging, apparent diffusion coefficient (ADC) values higher than those commonly noted in ependymomas and medulloblastomas in the posterior fossa are found [18]. The utility of single-voxel MRS in depicting elevation of the Cho peak in pilocytic astrocytomas has also been demonstrated.

Higher grades of malignancy are usually heterogeneous in magnetic resonance signal intensity, with ill-defined margins, edema, hemorrhage, necrosis, mass effect, and irregular enhancement (Fig. 1). Diffusion imaging studies in astrocytomas have demonstrated a significant negative correlation between ADC values and WHO astrocytic tumor grades for tumor grades II-IV [4]. With the exception of perfusion findings in pilocytic astrocytomas, low-grade astrocytomas have a significantly lower average regional cerebral blood volume (rCBV) than high-grade astrocytomas, such as anaplastic astrocytomas or glioblastoma multiforme [19]. MRS is able to measure the high Cho to Cr ratio characteristic of high-grade gliomas.

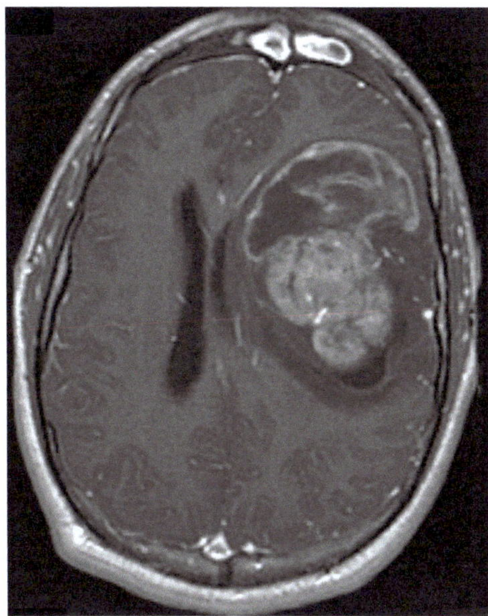

Fig. 1. Glioblastoma multiforme in an 18-year-old male patient. Axial T1 MRI with gadolinium shows a heterogeneous enhancing mass in the left frontal lobe. Note the regions of cyst and necrosis, mass effect on the left lateral ventricle, and midline shift to the right

Supratentorial Primitive Neuroectodermal Tumors

These embryonal cerebral WHO grade IV tumors occur in children with a mean age of 5.5 years [16]. Supratentorial PNET are typically large in size, with sharp margins; on imaging, they can be either heterogeneous in appearance with a cyst, calcification, or hemorrhage, or solid and homogeneous (Fig. 2). PNET are included in the differential diagnosis of large, heterogeneous supratentorial tumors including ependymoma and atypical teratoid/rhabdoid tumors. The genetic alterations within these tumors differ, however, from those identified in PNET that occur in the posterior fossa such as medulloblastoma.

Fig. 2. Supratentorial primitive neuroectodermal tumor (PNET) in a 3-year-old girl. Axial T1 image with gadolinium demonstrates a minimally enhancing heterogeneous mass in the right frontal lobe

Supratentorial Ependymomas

Classified as WHO grade II lesions histologically, supratentorial ependymomas occur in both adults and children. On CT, these tumors are heterogeneous with calcification and cyst formation; on MRI, they are seen as heterogeneous with cysts, calcification, and occasional hemorrhage with irregular, heterogeneous enhancement (Fig. 3). Of particular note, supratentorial ependymomas also show loss of chromosome 9 on cytogenetic studies, which may provide a genetic marker for the disease [16].

Subependymal Giant Cell Astrocytomas

Subependymal giant cell astrocytomas (SEGA) are generally viewed as part of tuberous sclerosis complex (TSC), a multi-system genetic disease that affects 1-2 million individuals worldwide according to the National Institutes of Health/National Institute of Neurological Disorders and Stroke (NIH/NINDS). This complex is linked to mutations in two genes, TSC1, located on chromosome 9, and TSC2, located on chromosomes 16, which encode the proteins hamartin and tuberin, respectively. Neuroimaging findings include subependymal and cortical tubers, white

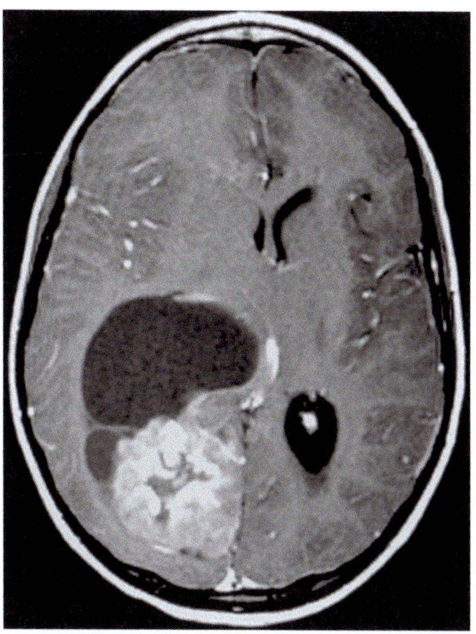

Fig. 3. Supratentorial ependymoma in a 7-year-old boy. Axial T1 image with gadolinium demonstrates a cystic and solid mass in the right parietal lobe, with mass effect on the right lateral ventricle and a mild midline shift to the right

matter lesions, and subependymal giant cell astrocytomas. Subependymal giant cell tumors are of mixed glioneuronal lineage and are associated with subependymal nodules that have symptoms such as hydrocephalus, interval growth, or papilledema. These tumors are seen in approximately 10% of patients with TS [20]. They arise from the lateral ventricle near the foramen of Monro and present with obstructive hydrocephalus in children and young adults, between the ages of 10 and 30. SEGA are often calcified on CT; on MRI, they are hypointense or isointense on T1-weighted images and isointense to hyperintense on T2-weighted sequences. Following contrast, these tumors uniformly enhance and are often associated with subependymal nodules and cortical tubers.

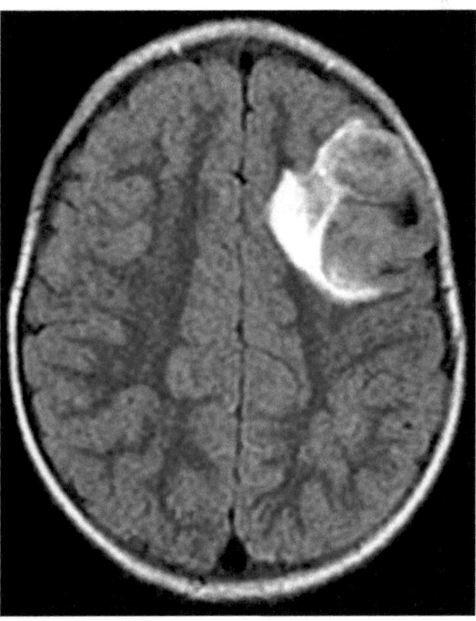

Fig. 4. Dysembryoplastic neuroepithelial tumor (DNT) in a 3-year-old with seizures. Axial FLAIR image demonstrates a mass within the left frontal lobe, with an incomplete medial rim of T2 hyperintensity and thickening of the cortex

Neuronal and Mixed Neuronal-Glial Tumors

Tumors in this category include gangliocytoma, desmoplastic infantile astrocytoma and ganglioglioma, ganglioglioma, dysembryoplastic neuroepithelial tumor (DNT), central neurocytoma, paraganglioma, and cerebellar liponeurocytoma [16]. Three of these (DNT, ganglioglioma, and desmoplastic infantile astrocytoma) are described below.

Dysembryoplastic Neuroepithelial Tumor

This tumor is a supratentorial glial-neuronal WHO grade I mass associated with intractable, partial complex seizures in children and young adults. DNTs most often present in a supratentorial location, with more than 60% found in the temporal lobe and approximately 30% found in the frontal lobe. They are often associated with cortical dysplasias. On CT, the tumors are hypodense and may remodel the inner table of the skull; on MRI, T2-weighted images are hyperintense, but associated vasogenic edema in the surrounding tissues is lacking and there is only occasional nodular enhancement. DNTs typically demonstrate either a complete or incomplete hyperintense rim seen on the FLAIR images (Fig. 4), which may signal the presence of loose peripheral neuroglial elements and may serve as a marker to differentiate these tumors from other tumors, such as low grade gliomas, oligodendrogliomas, and gangliogliomas [21].

Ganglioglioma

The current WHO classification system defines ganglioglioma as a well-differentiated neoplasm composed of mature neural (ganglion cells) and glial elements, with both components being neoplastic. These tumors typically correspond to either WHO grade I or II and are most often found in temporal lobe epilepsy patients. In order of frequency, gangliogliomas are found in the temporal lobe, the parietal lobe, the frontal lobe, the occipital lobe, the third ventricle, and the hypothalamus. Occasionally, the cerebellum, brainstem, and spinal cord are also affected.

On CT, these tumors tend to be low in attenuation, with 35-50% demonstrating some evidence of calcification. Contrast enhancement is typically noted in the solid component of the lesion; when the tumor is located peripherally, erosion of the adjacent of inner table of calvarium may be apparent.

On MRI, the appearance of ganglioglioma tends to be variable and nonspecific. They typically appear hypointense to isointense relative to gray matter on short TR images and hyperintense to gray matter on long TR images. They also tend to be solid or mixed solid and cystic in nature; the solid elements usually enhance.

Desmoplastic Infantile Ganglioglioma

Desmoplastic infantile gangliogliomas/astrocytomas are rare intracranial tumors that, by definition, contain abnormal ganglion and glial cells and have a prominent desmoplastic stroma. They are categorized as WHO grade I neuronal or glioneuronal tumors and occur most often in children 1-24 months of age.

These tumors exclusively develop supratentorially, with a predilection for the frontal and parietal lobes. They may also present in the temporal lobes but very rarely in the occipital lobes. Multi-lobe involvement is common. On standard CT scans, these tumors typically appear as large cystic lesions with superficially solid, slightly hyperdense components that enhance strongly after contrast administration. Calcification and hemorrhage are uncommon. On standard MRI examinations, desmoplastic infantile gangliogliomas typically present with large cystic components that are hypointense on T1-weighted images and hyperintense on T2-weighted images. A smaller, solid peripheral component, generally isointense to gray matter on T1- and T2-weighted images, enhances intensely after gadolinium injection.

Choroid Plexus Tumors

Choroid plexus papilloma and choroid plexus carcinoma are the most common choroid plexus tumors in childhood. Choroid plexus tumors represent 2-4% of brain tumors in children; of these, 10-20% occur in the first year of life [16]. The median age of presentation of these tumors is 1.5 years for the lateral and third ventricle [22].

Choroid Plexus Papilloma

In children, choroid plexus papillomas are intraventricular tumors that arise in the lateral ventricle, often the trigone, whereas, in adults they are found in the fourth ventricle. On CT, a lobulated intraventricular mass with calcification and homogenously intense enhancement is typically noted. MRI features include T1 isointense to hypointense signal with T2 hypointensity and intense contrast enhancement. On MRS, choroid plexus papillomas exhibit a significantly higher level of the metabolite, myoinositol, but lower Cr and Cho levels than in choroid plexus carcinomas [23, 24]. These tumors may also be associated with Aicardi syndrome, which is an X-linked disorder characterized by dysgenesis of the corpus callosum, infantile spasms, and chorioretinal lacunae [25]. Cortical migration abnormalities can also be seen in these patients.

Choroid Plexus Carcinoma

Choroid plexus carcinomas represent 20-40% of choroid plexus tumors, with the majority arising in children. They are heterogeneous on MRI, with irregularly enhancing margins extending beyond the margin of the ventricle, and are associated with edema and mass effect (Fig. 5). Both choroid plexus papilloma and carcinoma can seed the CSF pathways.

On MRS, choroid plexus carcinomas have elevated Cho levels compared to choroid plexus papillomas [23] and lower Cr and Cr/total Cho ratios than other pediatric brain tumors [24].

Pineal Region Tumors

Tumors of the pineal region include germ cell tumors, non-germinomatous germ cell tumors, pineal parenchymal cell tumors, astrocytomas, meningioma, metastases, vascular malformations, lipoma, epidermoid/dermoid tumors, arachnoid cysts, and pineal cysts. Clinical presentation includes hydrocephalus secondary to compression of the cerebral aqueduct, diplopia, and Parinaud syndrome, which is characterized by paralysis of upward gaze.

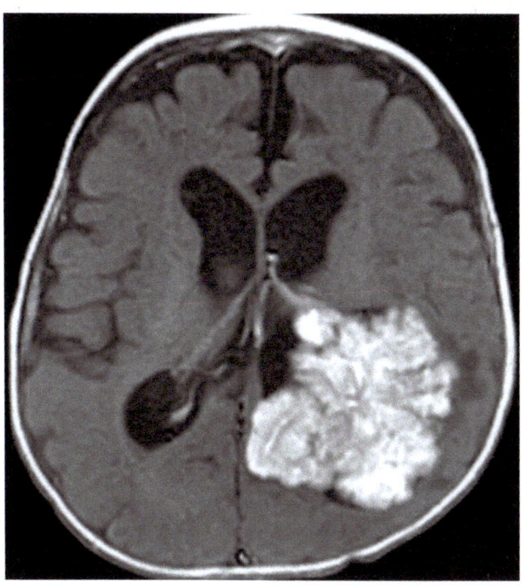

Fig. 5. Choroid plexus carcinoma in a 4-month-old girl. Axial T1 image with gadolinium demonstrates a large, avidly enhancing mass in the trigone and body of the left lateral ventricle, with vascular flow voids and surrounding parenchymal vasogenic edema

Pineal Germ Cell Tumors

Two-thirds of all masses in the pineal region masses are germ cell tumors. Of these, germinoma is most common, and is usually seen in the pineal region, suprasellar region, basal ganglia, and thalamus, in decreasing order of frequency. Nongerminomatous germ cell tumors, which are less common, include teratoma, choriocarcinoma, endodermal sinus tumor, embryonal carcinoma, and mixed germ cell tumors.

On CT, these lesions are well-defined and slightly hyperdense. On MRI, they are T1-hypointense, T2-isointense to hyperintense, and markedly enhancing (Fig. 6).

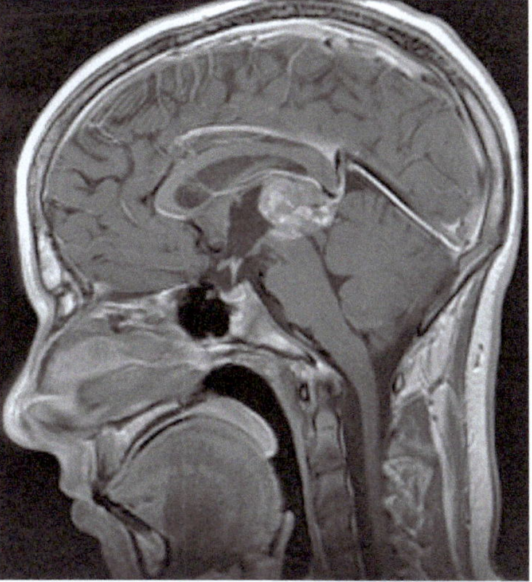

Fig. 6. Pineal germinoma in a 16-year-old boy. Sagittal T1 image with gadolinium demonstrates an enhancing mass in the pineal region and extending into zthe posterior aspect of the third ventricle

There is usually no associated cyst or calcification. CSF seeding is not uncommon. There may be an associated suprasellar lesion, although it is often unclear whether this represents a metastatic or a synchronous lesion. Pineal germ cell tumors are highly radiosensitive.

Teratomas contain components of all three germ cell layers. On CT and MRI, the mass often contains fat, bone, cartilage, or teeth, with heterogeneous density and intensity characteristics.

Pineal Parenchymal Tumors

Pineal parenchymal cell tumors include pineoblastoma and pineocytoma. Pineoblastoma is a malignant, primitive embryonal tumor (WHO grade IV) of the pineal gland with a predilection to develop in children and to seed the CSF pathways. Pineoblastoma may be found in association with bilateral retinoblastoma. On CT, the mass is heterogeneous and large with isodense or hyperdense features. On MRI, this tumor is hypointense to isointense on T1-weighted images and isointense to hyperintense on T2-weighted images, with marked enhancement. There may be associated calcification, hemorrhage, and necrosis. Both types of tumors have a poor prognosis and are usually associated with CSF dissemination.

Posterior Fossa Tumors

The common posterior fossa tumors of childhood include medulloblastoma, cerebellar astrocytoma, brainstem glioma, and ependymoma. Less frequently diagnosed posterior fossa tumors in children are atypical teratoid/rhabdoid tumors, hemangioblastoma, dermoid-epidermoid tumors, acoustic schwannomas, meningioma, teratoma, and skull base tumors.

Medulloblastoma

Medulloblastoma is the most common childhood tumor of the posterior fossa. These tumors are molecularly distinct from supratentorial PNETs. In 50% of cases there is a loss of chromosome 17p. Signaling pathways implicated in the formation of these tumors include sonic hedgehog pathway, the WNT/WG pathway, and the receptor kinase family ErbB. Pathologically, these lesions have been characterized as classic, large cell, melanotic, anaplastic, and desmoplastic. Medulloblastomas have been associated with syndromes including basal cell nevus syndrome, Turcot syndrome, and Li-Fraumeni syndrome.

Medulloblastomas usually arise in the midline within the vermis, with growth into the fourth ventricle. In adults and older children, the tumor is found laterally in the cerebellar hemispheres. On CT, it is typically characterized as hyperdense; on MRI, the tumor is viewed on T1-weighted images as hypointense and on T2-weighted images as hypointense to gray matter (Fig. 7a). Homogenous enhancement is usually seen following gadolinium administration (Fig. 7b). The craniospinal axis must be screened with gadolinium-enhanced MRI to identify leptomeningeal enhancement and seeding. Medulloblastomas demonstrate restricted diffusion due to high cellularity within the tumor (Fig. 7c) [18]. In addition, MRS of untreated medulloblastomas has demonstrated taurine concentrations that are significantly higher than in other types of untreated tumors [24].

Cerebellar Astrocytomas

Astrocytomas of the cerebellum are often diagnosed as pilocytic astrocytomas, which consist classically of a cerebellar mass with a large cyst and a solid tumor nodule. The tumor may be located at midline or in the cerebellar hemi-

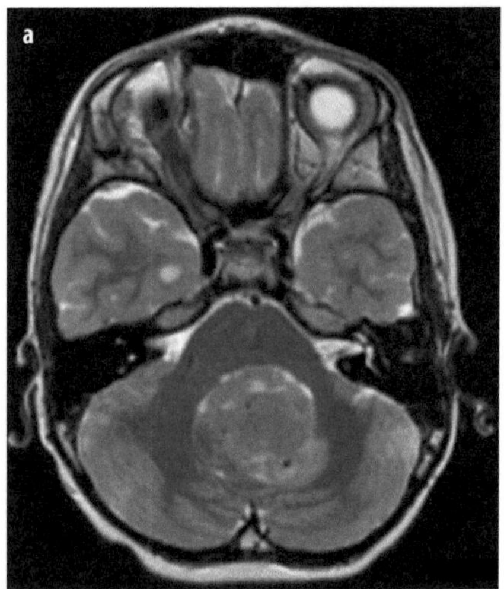

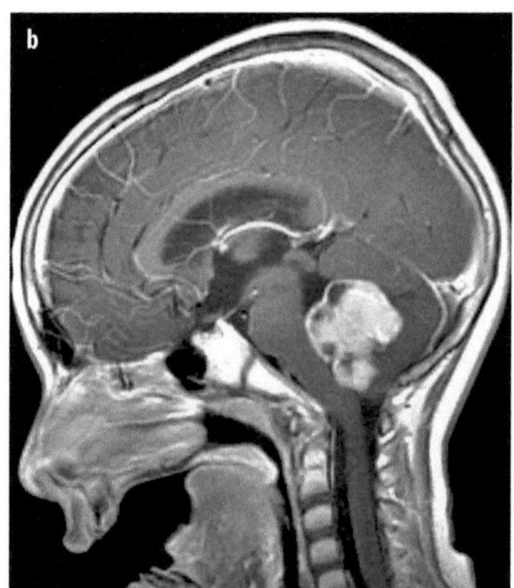

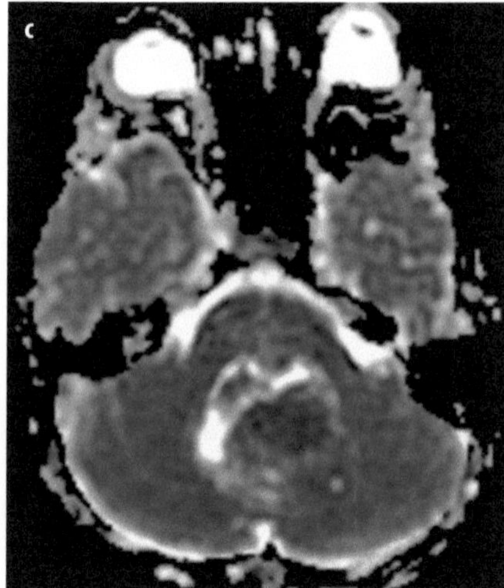

Fig. 7 a-c. Medulloblastoma in a 7-year-old boy. **a** Axial T2 image demonstrates a T2-hypointense mass in the fourth ventricle. **b** Sagittal T1 image with gadolinium demonstrates the homogeneously enhancing fourth ventricular mass. **c** Apparent diffusion coefficient (ADC) map demonstrates restricted diffusion in the fourth ventricular mass

spheres. The spectrum of imaging appearances, however, may include cystic, solid, or a mixture of cystic and solid presentations. Macrocysts or microcysts can form and the tumor can be grossly cystic or solid. On CT and MRI, a cyst with enhancement of the solid nodular component is typically found (Fig. 8). The solid, enhancing component of cerebellar pilocytic astrocytomas has greater ADC values than other pediatric cerebellar tumors such as ependymoma, rhabdoid tumor, and medulloblastoma [18].

Brainstem Tumors

Brainstem tumors include pontine, medullary, and midbrain tumors. They are categorized according to where they develop and whether they are diffuse or focal. The imaging features of brainstem tumors are described below.

Pontine Tumors

Focal gliomas (i.e., focal pontine tumors) in the pons are uncommon. They have circumscribed T2 hyperintensity with marked enhancement and generally have a better prognosis than diffuse pontine gliomas. Diffuse pontine gliomas typically present with ataxia, multiple cranial nerve palsies, and long tract signs. In the presence of this tumor, the pons typically expands by more than 50%; the glioma may extend superiorly or inferiorly into the midbrain or medulla. These tumors represent 15-20% of all CNS tumors in childhood and account for most deaths in children with brain tumors [26]. On CT, these lesions are isodense to low density; on MRI, they are isointense to hypointense on T1- and hyperintense on T2-weighted images. Diagnosis is typically made on the basis of the hyperintense T2 signal within the brainstem. Enhancement is minimal or absent. MRS has shown utility in evaluating the short-term response to therapy as well as in assessing the relative success/failure of treatment over time [27].

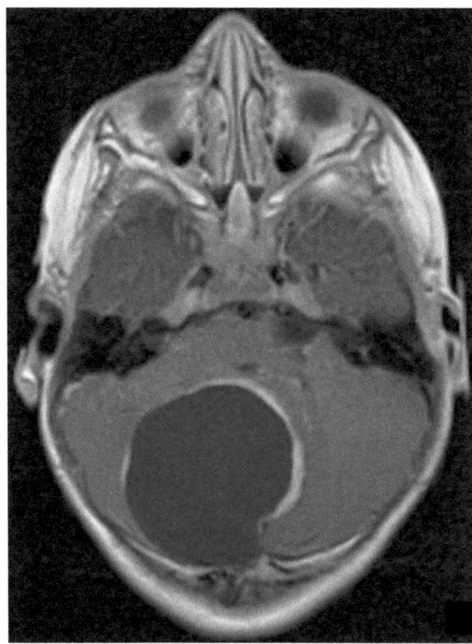

Fig. 8. Cerebellar pilocytic astrocytoma in a 22-month-old male. Axial T2 image with gadolinium shows a cystic mass with peripheral medial enhancement in the right cerebellum and obliterating the fourth ventricle

Medullary Tumors

Cervicomedullary astrocytomas are a subset of brainstem tumors with a good prognosis. These tumors originate in the upper cervical cord, are dorsally exophytic, and grow upward toward the obex into the medulla. They are well-demarcated with enhancement and are often pilocytic astrocytomas. Diffuse medullary tumors are centered in the medulla and may extend rostrally or caudally into the pons and cervical cord. The prognosis for these lesions is poorer than that of cervicomedullary astrocytomas.

Midbrain Tumors

Included among tumors in this category are focal or diffuse midbrain lesions and tectal tumors. Tectal tumors are often low grade pilocytic astrocytomas, present with obstructive hydrocephalus, and usually do not require treatment beyond CSF diversion such as third ventriculostomy or shunting. On MRI, the lesions are usually isointense on T1-weighted images and hyperintense on non-enhanced T2-weighted images. In one study, lesions with a volume less than 4 cm^3 were likely to follow a benign course. All large lesions, defined as having a volume >10 cm^3 at presentation, eventually required treatment [28].

Ependymomas

Ependymomas are the fourth most common posterior fossa tumor in children, following medulloblastoma, cerebellar astrocytoma, and brainstem glioma. These tumors originate from ependymal cells lining the ventricles and typically grow out of the fourth ventricle via the foramina of Luschka and Magendie into the cisterna magna, basilar cisterns, and cerebellopontine angles, and then through the foramen magnum into the upper cervical canal around the spinal cord. On CT, the tumor is of mixed density with punctate calcification in 50% of cases in which there is variable enhancement. On MRI, ependymomas are heterogeneous, reflecting a combination of solid component, cyst, calcification, necrosis, edema, or hemorrhage. On T1-weighted images, they are usually hypointense; on T2-weighted images, the mass is often isointense to gray matter with two types of foci evident: a dark T2 signal related to calcification or blood, or a bright T2 signal related to the presence of a cyst or necrosis within the tumor. Following contrast administration, there is heterogeneous enhancement in the tumor.

Atypical Teratoid/Rhabdoid Tumors

Atypical teratoid/rhabdoid tumors (ATRTs), most commonly found in young children, are classified as WHO grade IV tumors. Most of them are characterized by an inactive hSNF5/INI1 gene and have a propensity to seed CSF pathways. These tumors can be infratentorial or supratentorial in location; on imaging, they may have features identical to those of medulloblastoma. The prognosis for an ATRT is poor.

Acoustic Schwannomas

Acoustic schwannomas are uncommon in early childhood; however, between the ages of 18 and 22, the patient can present with hearing loss as a manifestation of neurofibromatosis type 2 (NF-2). NF-2 is a rare disorder, affecting 1 in 40,000 people, according to the NIH/NINDS. Patients with this disorder present with bilateral vestibular schwannomas, meningiomas, and ependymomas. On MRI, these lesions are cerebellopontine-angle masses that enhance intensely with gadolinium.

Hemangioblastoma

Hemangioblastomas are rare tumors corresponding to WHO grade I. They can be sporadic but commonly occur as a manifestation of von Hippel Lindau syndrome, which is an autosomal dominant disorder associated with retinal, cerebellar, and spinal hemangioblastomas, pancreatic cysts, pheochromocytomas, renal cysts, endolymphatic cell tumors, and renal cell carcinoma. It is caused by a defect in the tumor suppressor gene on chromosome 3p25-p26. CNS hemangioblastomas typically present clinically during the second decade of life and thus are rarely seen in younger children. These tumors are characterized by a cystic mass within the posterior fossa that has a nodular enhancing component. Hemangioblastomas of the spine can be cystic or solid.

Sellar and Suprasellar Tumors

Among sellar and suprasellar tumors, craniopharyngioma and chiasmatic/hypothalamic glioma are the most common. Also included in this category are hypothalamic hamartoma, pituitary adenoma, germ cell tumors, Langerhans cell histiocytosis, Rathke's cleft cysts, arachnoid cysts, and dermoid/epidermoid cysts.

Craniopharyngioma

Craniopharygioma is a benign (WHO grade 1) neoplasm arising in the suprasellar or intrasellar region; it is the most common non-neuroepithelial tumor in children [16]. These tumors arise from remnants of Rathke's pouch epithelium. Adamantinomatous craniopharyngioma is distributed bimodally: in children ages 5-15 and in adults ages 45-60. Papillary craniopharyngioma develops primarily in adults. Craniopharyngiomas constitute 50% of the suprasellar tumors seen in childhood. The clinical presentation includes headache, visual field defects, diplopia, and short stature, with occasional hydrocephalus and papilledema. These tumors are classically cystic in nature and filled with a cholesterol-rich fluid grossly resembling motor oil.

Craniopharyngiomas can compress, envelop, or infiltrate adjacent structures and produce a reactive gliosis, although they are histologically benign. In many cases, surgical extirpation is difficult; because of the high rate of recurrence, adjuvant radiotherapy is often necessary. On CT, 90% of craniopharyngiomas are cystic and calcified. On MRI, these tumors have variable signal characteristics depending on the contents of the cyst and the presence of calcium. On CT, the solid component of the tumor may be isodense or hypodense while on MRI it is isointense to hypointense on T1 and isointense to hyperintense on T2 (Fig. 9). The calcified component is of increased attenuation on CT and often T2 hypointense on MRI. The cystic component may be of high or low T1 intensity and T2 hyperintense. Following gadolinium administration, peripheral enhancement of the cyst as well as heterogeneous enhancement of the solid component generally occurs.

Chiasmatic/Hypothalamic Gliomas

Chiasmatic-hypothalamic tumors are often-low grade astrocytomas and pilocytic in appearance. Between 20 and 50% of patients with chiasmatic/hypothalamic tumors have neurofibromatosis type 1 (NF-1). NF-1 is the most common of the phakomatoses, affecting 1 in 3000 to 1 in 4000 individuals in the US, according to the NIH/NINDS. It is inherited as an autosomal dominant disorder localized to chromosome 17 and with variable penetrance. Among tumors of the CNS in NF-1, optic gliomas are the most common. These may involve any portion of the optic pathway including one or both optic nerves, the chiasm tracts, the lateral geniculate bodies, or the optic radiations. Other intracranial lesions that may be seen in NF-1 include vacuolization in the

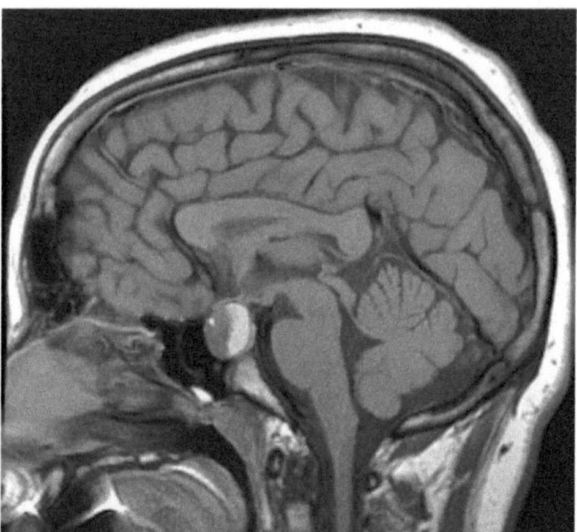

Fig. 9. Craniopharyngioma in a 15-year-old boy. Sagittal T1 image demonstrates a heterogeneous sellar mass with regions of hyperintensity and hypointensity extending into the suprasellar region, with mass effect on the optic chiasm which is displaced superiorly

myelin (i.e., NF spots), plexiform neurofibromas, and other astrocytomas. The chief clinical presentation of optic glioma is most often decreased visual acuity; other symptoms, including visual field defects, optic atrophy, hydrocephalus, or hypothalamic dysfunction and papilledema may be seen as well. These lesions are usually T1-hypointense and T2-hyperintense with typically homogeneous gadolinium enhancement; in large tumors, heterogeneous enhancement. MRI with fat suppression leads to optimal visualization of the optic pathways (Fig. 10).

Diencephalic syndrome is also commonly associated with hypothalamic/chiasmatic astrocytomas; in rare instances, it may be the underlying cause of failure to thrive in infancy. Clinical characteristics include severe emaciation in the setting of normal linear growth. The tumors associated with this unusual syndrome are often larger in size, occur in younger children, and are more aggressive than those associated with other presentations. Despite low-grade histologic findings, these tumors may seed throughout the CSF pathways. This syndrome serves as a model for studying growth hormone resistance and metabolic regulation of adiposity [29].

Hypothalamic Hamartoma

Hypothalamic hamartomas are masses of mature ganglionic tissue located between the pituitary stalk and mamillary bodies and involving the region of the tuber cinereum. They do not demonstrate invasion or growth. Often the patients are males who present with symptoms including precocious puberty, gelastic seizures, hyperactivity, and developmental delay. On CT, there is a suprasellar mass, isodense with gray matter, non-calcified, and rarely cystic. On MRI, a well-demarcated mass is present within or adjacent to the tuber cinereum or mamillary bodies. Hamartomas are T1-isointense and T2-isointense to slightly hyperintense to gray matter without enhancement. A subgroup of patients with hypothalamic hamartoma can also present with the clinical features of Pallister-Hall syndrome, an autosomal dominant disorder. The congenital anomalies associated with this syndrome include hypoplasia of the olfactory bulbs, absence of the pituitary gland, cardiac and renal anomalies, imperforate anus, craniofacial anomalies, syndactyly, and a short metacarpal. Mutations in the GLI3 zinc-finger transcription factor gene are also associated with Pallister-Hall syndrome [30].

Germ Cell Tumors

Germ cell tumors of the CNS that occur in children are commonly located in the suprasellar region and may be either germinomas or nongerminomatous germ cell tumors. Patients diagnosed with germ cell tumors may clinically present with central diabetes insipidus (DI), wasting, precocious puberty, or growth failure. On imaging, a mass involving the suprasellar region may be seen or there may be thickening of the infundibulum. On CT, these lesions are well-defined and slightly hyperdense. On MRI, they are T1-hypointense, T2-hypointense, and markedly enhancing. CSF seeding is not uncommon. On occasion, there is an associated pineal region germinoma, which may be metastatic or synchronous in character.

Patients with suprasellar germinomas often present with central DI. On MRI, the normally seen posterior pituitary bright spot is absent. The mechanism of central DI is thought to entail the interruption of vasopressin neurosecretory granule transport along the hypothalamic-neurohypophyseal pathway. Central DI and the absence of the posterior bright spot may present months or years before other clinical and imaging features of hypothalamic tumor are seen. In such cases, follow-up MRI with gadolinium is strongly recommended. In the

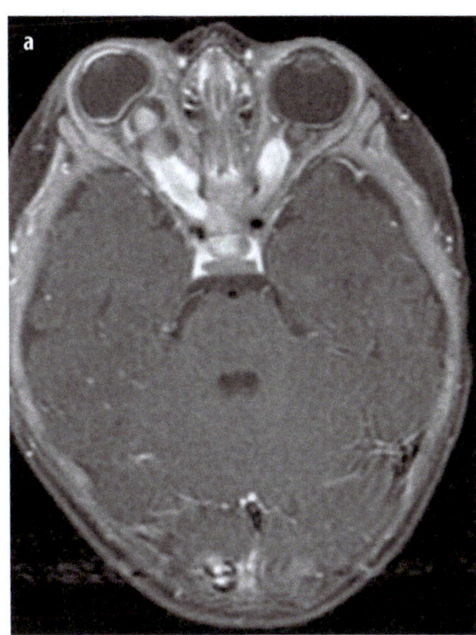

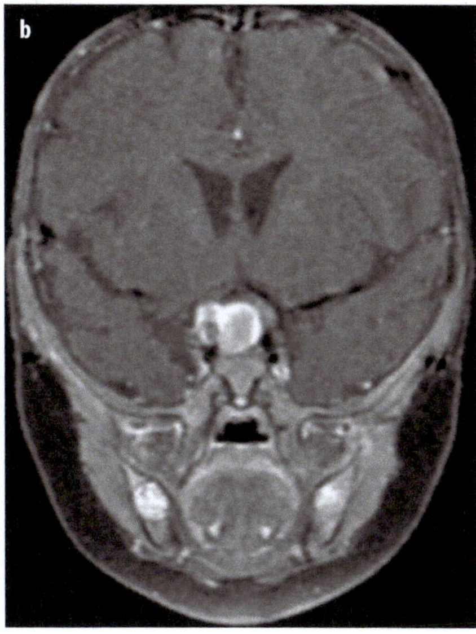

Fig. 10 a, b. Optic glioma in a 5-month-old. **a** Axial T1 image with gadolinium demonstrates the bilaterally enlarged, enhancing optic nerves. **b** Coronal T1 image with gadolinium demonstrates an enhancing mass in the optic chiasm

presence of a hypothalamic tumor, thickening of the pituitary stalk is sometimes seen. Langerhans histiocytosis, lymphocytic hypophysitis, and rare entities such as sarcoidosis and lymphoma may also give rise to pituitary stalk thickening.

Teratomas occur more often in the pineal region than in the suprasellar region. They are classified as mature or immature depending on whether the tissue components resemble mature adult tissues or immature embryonic tissues. On CT and MRI, the mass often contains fat, bone, or cartilage with heterogeneous density and intensity characteristics. These patients may present with precocious puberty.

Pituitary Adenomas

Pituitary adenomas are uncommon in childhood and represent <3% of all intracranial tumors. The clinical presentation depends on tumor size, hormonal activity, and extrasellar extent. Pituitary adenomas are divided into hormonally active and inactive types, with the majority being hormonally active and most commonly prolactin-secreting. These lesions tend to occur in adolescence; they are typically microadenomas (<1 cm), and are most often prolactinomas. Macroadenomas are >1 cm in diameter; in patients presenting with neuroendocrine symptoms, visual field deficits, and headache, they are often prolactinomas. Most macroadenomas diagnosed in adolescence are hemorrhagic and often occur in males [31].

On MRI, pituitary adenomas are T1-hypointense in most cases. Less frequently, adenomas are T1-isointense or hyperintense. On T2 images, adenomas are often hyperintense or isointense; macroadenomas are usually hyperintense. Macroadenomas may invade the cavernous sinuses, extend superiorly into the suprasellar cistern, and can compress the optic chiasm. Immediately following gadolinium administration, the lesion is hypointense compared to the normal gland.

Langerhans' Cell Histiocytosis

Systemic Langerhans' cell histiocytosis may involve the pituitary stalk and hypothalamus. These patients may present with DI; loss of the normal posterior pituitary bright spot is seen on MRI, which also may also demonstrate a solitary mass in the median eminence region of the pituitary stalk or thickening of the infundibulum. On CT, the mass is isodense; on MRI, the lesion is T1 isointense and T2 hyperintense. Following gadolinium administration, there is marked enhancement.

Conclusions

Of the pediatric malignancies resulting in death, primary brain tumors are second only to leukemia, and are the most frequently diagnosed type of solid tumor in children. Given the sobering rates of morbidity and mortality, the medical community is pressed to better understand the complex etiology of this often lethal disease and to develop more effective strategies for detecting, diagnosing, and treating brain tumors of childhood. With rapid advances in imaging technology, especially CT, MRI, and PET, physicians are increasingly able to identify pediatric brain tumors in their earliest stages and thus propose therapeutic options that improve patient outcomes and survival. However, understanding and mastering the numerous imaging features of more than two dozen subtypes of primary brain tumors affecting children remains a significant challenge.

References

1. Gurney J, Smith M, Bunin G (1999) In: Ries L, Smith M, Gurney J (eds) CNS and miscellaneous intracranial and intraspinal neoplasms. Cancer incidence and survival among children and adolescents: United States SEER Program 1975-1995 NIH Publication No 99-4649. Bethesda, MD: National Cancer Institute SEER Program, pp 51-63
2. Ries L, Melbert D, Krapcho M et al (eds) (2007) SEER Cancer Statistics Review, 1975-2004. National Cancer Institute. Bethesda, MD, http://seer.cancer.gov/csr/1975_2004/, based on November 2006 SEER data, posted to the SEER website
3. CBTRUS (2005) Statistical report: primary brain tumors in the United States, 1998-2002. Central Brain Tumor Registry of the United States, Hinsdale, Illinois
4. Poussaint TY, Rodriguez D (2006) Advanced neuroimaging of pediatric brain tumors: MR diffusion, MR perfusion, and MR spectroscopy. Neuroimaging Clin N Am 16:169-192, ix
5. Sorensen A, Reimer P (2000) Cerebral MR perfusion imaging. Thieme, New York
6. Barkovich A (2005) Pediatric neuroimaging. Lippincott Williams & Wilkins, Philadelphia
7. Kassner A, Roberts TP (2004) Beyond perfusion: cerebral vascular reactivity and assessment of microvascular permeability. Top Magn Reson Imaging 15:58-65
8. Barrett T, Brechbiel M, Bernardo M, Choyke PL (2007) MRI of tumor angiogenesis. J Magn Reson Imaging 26:235-249
9. Golay X, Hendrikse J, Lim TC (2004) Perfusion imaging using arterial spin labeling. Top Magn Reson Imaging 15:10-27
10. Gauvain KM, McKinstry RC, Mukherjee P et al (2001) Evaluating pediatric brain tumor cellularity with diffusion-tensor imaging. AJR Am J Roentgenol 177:449-454
11. Hamstra DA, Rehemtulla A, Ross BD (2007) Diffusion magnetic resonance imaging: a biomarker for treatment response in oncology. J Clin Oncol 25:4104-4109
12. Mabbott DJ, Noseworthy MD, Bouffet E et al (2006) Diffusion tensor imaging of white matter after cranial radiation in children for medulloblastoma: correlation with IQ. Neuro Oncol 8:244-252
13. Qiu D, Kwong DL, Chan GC et al (2007) Diffusion tensor magnetic resonance imaging finding of discrepant fractional anisotropy between the frontal and parietal lobes after whole-brain irradiation in childhood medulloblastoma survivors: reflection of regional white matter radiosensitivity? Int J Radiat Oncol Biol Phys 69:846-851
14. Jolesz FA (2005) Future perspectives for intraoperative MRI. Neurosurg Clin N Am 16:201-213
15. Pollack IF (1994) Brain tumors in children. N Engl J Med 331:1500-1507
16. Louis D, Ohgaki H, Wiestler O, Cavenee W (eds) (2007) WHO classification of tumours of the central nervous system. IARC, Lyon

17. Ball WS Jr, Holland SK (2001) Perfusion imaging in the pediatric patient. Magn Reson Imag Clin N Am 9:207-230
18. Rumboldt Z, Camacho DL, Lake D et al (2006) Apparent diffusion coefficients for differentiation of cerebellar tumors in children. AJNR Am J Neuroradiol 27:1362-1369
19. Law M, Yang S, Wang H et al (2003) Glioma grading: sensitivity, specificity, and predictive values of perfusion MR imaging and proton MR spectroscopic imaging compared with conventional MR imaging. AJNR Am J Neuroradiol 24:1989-1998
20. Goh S, Butler W, Thiele EA (2004) Subependymal giant cell tumors in tuberous sclerosis complex. Neurology 63:1457-1461
21. Parmar HA, Hawkins C, Ozelame R et al (2007) Fluid-attenuated inversion recovery ring sign as a marker of dysembryoplastic neuroepithelial tumors. J Comput Assist Tomogr 31:348-353
22. Wolff JE, Sajedi M, Brant R et al (2002) Choroid plexus tumours. Br J Cancer 87:1086-1091
23. Krieger MD, Panigrahy A, McComb JG et al (2005) Differentiation of choroid plexus tumors by advanced magnetic resonance spectroscopy. Neurosurg Focus 18:E4
24. Panigrahy A, Krieger MD, Gonzalez-Gomez I et al (2006) Quantitative short echo time 1H-MR spectroscopy of untreated pediatric brain tumors: preoperative diagnosis and characterization. AJNR Am J Neuroradiol 27:560-572
25. Aicardi J (2005) Aicardi syndrome. Brain Dev 27:164-171
26. Hargrave D, Bartels U, Bouffet E (2006) Diffuse brainstem glioma in children: critical review of clinical trials. Lancet Oncol 7:241-248
27. Laprie A, Pirzkall A, Haas-Kogan DA et al (2005) Longitudinal multivoxel MR spectroscopy study of pediatric diffuse brainstem gliomas treated with radiotherapy. Int J Radiat Oncol Biol Phys 62:20-31
28. Ternier J, Wray A, Puget S et al (2006) Tectal plate lesions in children. J Neurosurg 104:369-376
29. Fleischman A, Brue C, Poussaint TY et al (2005) Diencephalic syndrome: a cause of failure to thrive and a model of partial growth hormone resistance. Pediatrics 115:e742-e748
30. Johnston JJ, Olivos-Glander I, Killoran C et al (2005) Molecular and clinical analyses of Greig cephalopolysyndactyly and Pallister-Hall syndromes: robust phenotype prediction from the type and position of GLI3 mutations. Am J Hum Genet 76:609-622
31. Poussaint TY, Barnes PD, Anthony DA et al (1996) Hemorrhagic pituitary adenomas of adolescence. AJNR Am J Neuroradiol 17:1907-1912

Printed in March 2008

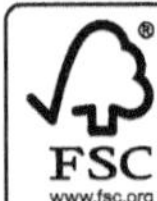

MIX
Papier aus verantwortungsvollen Quellen
Paper from responsible sources
FSC® C105338

If you have any concerns about our products, you can contact us on
ProductSafety@springernature.com

In case Publisher is established outside the EU, the EU authorized representative is:
Springer Nature Customer Service Center GmbH
Europaplatz 3, 69115 Heidelberg, Germany

Printed by Libri Plureos GmbH
in Hamburg, Germany